Nurses as Leaders

William "Billy" Rosa, MS, RN, LMT, AHN-BC, AGPCNP-BC, CCRN-CMC, Caritas Coach, is a nurse, author, and educator. He graduated with his bachelor of science in nursing, *magna cum laude*, from New York University (NYU) Rory Meyers College of Nursing, in 2009. While working as a critical care bedside clinician for four years at NYU Langone Medical Center (NYULMC), climbing to the top rung of the clinical ladder, he became committed to excellence in patient care delivery, advocacy for positive change within the profession, and the elevation of consciousness for nurses and nursing. After graduating as valedictorian of his master of nursing program at the Hunter–Bellevue School of Nursing at Hunter College in 2014, he moved into the role of nurse educator for critical care services at NYULMC.

He is a graduate of the Caritas Coach Education Program (CCEP) offered by the Watson Caring Science Institute (WCSI), the Integrative Nurse Coach Certificate Program (INCCP) offered by the International Nurse Coach Association, and the Clinical Scene Investigator (CSI) Academy of the American Association of Critical-Care Nurses (AACN). To date, these experiences have inspired over 65 publications in peer-reviewed and non-peer-reviewed journals, newspapers, magazines, and international platform blogs, such as *SpringBoard* and *The Huffington Post*.

Mr. Rosa has been recognized with the Association for Nursing Professional Development's national 2015 Excellence in Professional Development Change Agent/Team Member Award and the 2015 national AACN Circle of Excellence Award, and he was the winner of the 2012 National League for Nursing (NLN) Student Excellence Paper Competition. He was honored with the 2014 New York/New Jersey Rising Star GEM Award, the 2014 Dean's Prize for Outstanding Student Award from Hunter College, and the 2012 Rising Star Award from the NYU College of Nursing Alumni Association.

He has become passionate about cultivating a healthy environment for nurse leaders to thrive through his participation in the Nurse in Washington Internship and his organizational positions as U.S. board of advisors' member for the Nightingale Initiative for Global Health (NIGH), New York City chapter leader of the American Holistic Nurses Association (AHNA), and secretary for the New York City chapter of the Association for Nursing Professional Development.

As of this writing, Mr. Rosa is living and working in Kigali, Rwanda, as visiting faculty at the University of Rwanda and as an intensive care unit clinical educator at the Rwanda Military Hospital, Human Resources for Health Program in partnership with the NYU Rory Meyers College of Nursing. He contributes a weekly column on health and wellness to *The New Times*, Rwanda's leading English daily newspaper, and is currently working on his second book, *Dry Your Tears in Peace: Voices of a Rwandan Youth Village,* a project that chronicles the work of Agahozo-Shalom Youth Village in healing the most vulnerable young adults in Rwanda.

Nurses as Leaders
Evolutionary Visions of Leadership

William Rosa, MS, RN, LMT,
AHN-BC, AGPCNP-BC, CCRN-CMC, Caritas Coach

Editor

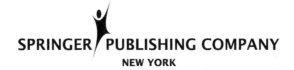

SPRINGER PUBLISHING COMPANY
NEW YORK

Springer Publishing Company, LLC
11 West 42nd Street
New York, NY 10036
www.springerpub.com

Acquisitions Editor: Margaret Zuccarini
Senior Production Editor: Kris Parrish
Composition: Exeter Premedia Services Private Ltd.

ISBN: 978-0-8261-3102-7
E-book ISBN: 978-0-8261-3103-4
Instructor's PowerPoints ISBN: 978-0-8261-3104-1

Instructor's materials are available to qualified adopters by contacting textbook@springerpub.com.

16 17 18 19 20 / 5 4 3 2 1

The author and the publisher of this Work have made every effort to use sources believed to be reliable to provide information that is accurate and compatible with the standards generally accepted at the time of publication. The author and publisher shall not be liable for any special, consequential, or exemplary damages resulting, in whole or in part, from the readers' use of, or reliance on, the information contained in this book. The publisher has no responsibility for the persistence or accuracy of URLs for external or third-party Internet websites referred to in this publication and does not guarantee that any content on such websites is, or will remain, accurate or appropriate.

Library of Congress Cataloging-in-Publication Data

Names: Rosa, William, 1982- , editor.
Title: Nurses as leaders : evolutionary visions of leadership / William Rosa, editor.
Description: New York, NY : Springer Publishing Company, LLC, [2016] | Includes bibliographical references and index.
Identifiers: LCCN 2016003519| ISBN 9780826131027 | ISBN 9780826131034 (e-book)
Subjects: | MESH: Nurse's Role | Leadership
Classification: LCC RT82 | NLM WY 105 | DDC 610.7306/9—dc23
LC record available at http://lccn.loc.gov/2016003519

Special discounts on bulk quantities of our books are available to corporations, professional associations, pharmaceutical companies, health care organizations, and other qualifying groups. If you are interested in a custom book, including chapters from more than one of our titles, we can provide that service as well.

For details, please contact:
Special Sales Department, Springer Publishing Company, LLC
11 West 42nd Street, 15th Floor, New York, NY 10036-8002
Phone: 877-687-7476 or 212-431-4370; Fax: 212-941-7842
E-mail: sales@springerpub.com

Printed in the United States of America by McNaughton & Gunn.

For Mom and Dad,
Beatrice and William Rosa Sr.,
for showing me love so that I might love,
for teaching me kindness so that I might be kind,
and for leading me with integrity so that I might lead.
I love you.

Contents

Contributors

Veda L. Andrus, EdD, MSN, RN, HN-BC, is vice president, Education and Program Development, for the BirchTree Center for Healthcare Transformation. She was founding president/CEO of Seeds and Bridges Center for Holistic Nursing Education (1983–2000), where she cocreated the certificate program in holistic nursing and other professional development continuing education programs. Dr. Andrus is past president and international director for the American Holistic Nurses Association (AHNA; 1991–1995) and a recipient of the 2004 Holistic Nurse of the Year award. She served as the delegation leader for the first holistic nursing delegation to China and Mongolia in 1994 through the Citizen Ambassador Program of People-to-People International. She serves on the board of directors for the American Holistic Nurses Credentialing Corporation (AHNCC) and editorial review board for the *Journal of Holistic Nursing*.

Jeanne Anselmo, BSN, RN, BCIAC-SF, HNB-BC, is a graduate of Cornell University–New York Hospital School of Nursing and a certified holistic nurse, educator, and consultant. In 1989, she was the first woman and the first nurse to be elected president of the Biofeedback Society of New York State, and she cofounded the Biofeedback Society of America's National Nurses Network. In 2001, she cofounded one of the first Contemplative Law Programs in the United States at City University of New York (CUNY) School of Law. For the past 25 years, she has studied with Nobel Peace Prize nominee and Vietnamese Zen Master Thich Nhat Hanh, who ordained her as a lay monastic in the Order of Interbeing in 1995 and as a lineage-holding Dharma Teacher in 2011.

Deva-Marie Beck, PhD, RN, is a nurse educator, multimedia journalist, keynote speaker, author, and Nightingale scholar, and serves in all these roles as international codirector of Nightingale Initiative for Global Health (NIGH) and as editor-in-chief of NIGH's "Global Online Portal" (www.NIGHVision.net). She mentors and collaborates with a volunteer team of nurses who serve as youth representatives at the United Nations in New York. In 2014, Dr. Beck was commissioned by the World Health Organization (WHO) to create a video, *At the Heart of It All: Nurses & Midwives for Universal Health Coverage,* which premiered at a WHO Global Forum for Chief Nursing & Midwifery Officers in Geneva, Switzerland. In 2008, she collaborated with WHO-affiliated nurses to produce the video *Health Professions' Role in Primary Health Care, Featuring Nurses and Midwives—Now More Than Ever for a Healthy World,* to celebrate WHO's 60th anniversary.

Michael R. Bleich, PhD, RN, FNAP, FAAN, is internationally recognized as a speaker on nursing trends and issues tied to leadership, health systems, and policy. Dr. Bleich has addressed major nursing, public, physician, and governance audiences. His awards include the 2011 Luther Christman Award by the American Assembly for Men in Nursing, the McArthur Award for work on the Institute of Medicine's report, *The Future of Nursing: Leading Change, Advancing Health,* the University of Minnesota's School of Nursing Humanitarian Award, and the Academy of Medical Surgical Nurses Anthony J. Jannetti award. He has been inducted as a Fellow of the American Academy of Nursing (FAAN; 2006) and the National Academies of Practice (2013). He is the current board president of Commission for Graduates of Foreign Nursing Schools (CGFNS) International. Dr. Bleich retired as the Maxine Clark and Bob Fox Dean and Professor at the Goldfarb School of Nursing at Barnes Jewish College, St. Louis, Missouri, in May 2016 to establish his own business, NursDynamics. His new venture is focused on faculty and leadership development, curricular innovations, and domestic and global workforce development.

W. Richard Cowling III, PhD, RN, APRN-BC, AHN-BC, FAAN, ANEF, is vice president of Academic Affairs for Chamberlain College of Nursing and editor of the *Journal of Holistic Nursing.* Dr. Cowling's most outstanding contributions to nursing have been in the area of unitary research and practice relevant to women's survivorship of childhood abuse and despair. His work is exemplified by the integration of theory, research, and practice from a unique unitary nursing perspective. His unitary appreciative inquiry praxis methodology has been used in a variety of projects to generate knowledge for the purposes of transformation and emancipation of participants in the support of healing. His most recent contribution to nursing science was a synthesis of his ideas into a conceptual model of unitary appreciative nursing.

Barbara Montgomery Dossey, PhD, RN, AHN-BC, FAAN, HWNC-BC, is internationally recognized as a pioneer in the holistic nursing and nurse coaching movements. She is codirector of the International Nurse Coach Association (INCA) and a core faculty of the Integrative Nurse Coach Certificate Program (INCCP) in North Miami, Florida. She is the international codirector and a board member of the Nightingale Initiative for Global Health (NIGH), Washington, DC, and Neepawa, Manitoba, Canada, and the director of Holistic Nursing Consultants (HNC), Santa Fe, New Mexico. Dr. Dossey is a Florence Nightingale scholar and has authored or coauthored 26 books.

Margaret A. Fitzgerald, DNP, FNP-BC, NP-C, FAANP, CSP, FAAN, DCC, is founder, president, and principal lecturer with Fitzgerald Health Education Associates, Inc. (FHEA). She maintains a clinical practice as a family nurse practitioner at the Greater Lawrence Family Health Center, Lawrence, Massachusetts. In 2006, Dr. Fitzgerald earned her DNP from Case Western Reserve University, Cleveland, Ohio, and in 2011 became certified by the American Board of Comprehensive Care as a Diplomate of Comprehensive Care. She was one of the first group of 20 nurse practitioner leaders to be inducted into the Fellows of the American Association (formerly Academy) of Nurse Practitioners in 2000. Dr. Fitzgerald is a Professional Member of the National Speakers Association and is the first nurse practitioner to earn the Certified Speaking Professional designation.

Terry Fulmer, PhD, RN, FAAN, is the president of the John A. Hartford Foundation in New York City, an organization dedicated to improving the care of older adults. Established in 1929, the foundation is world renowned for philanthropy devoted exclusively to the health of older adults. Dr. Fulmer is internationally recognized as a leading expert in geriatrics and is best known for her research on the topic of elder abuse and neglect, which has been funded by the National Institute on Aging and the National Institute for Nursing Research. She is a trustee for the Josiah Macy Jr. Foundation, the Clark Foundation, and the Bassett Healthcare System. She previously served as the chair of the National Advisory Committee for the Robert Wood Johnson Foundation Executive Nurse Fellows Program.

Laura Gasparis Vonfrolio, PhD, RN, has over 40 years' experience in critical care nursing and has held CCRN® and Certified Emergency Nurse (CEN) certifications for more than 13 years. She obtained an associate's degree from the College of Staten Island (CUNY), a BSN from Long Island University, Brookville, New York, an MA in nursing education from New York University, New York, New York, completed her doctoral courses in nursing at Adelphi University, Garden City, New York, and received her PhD in nursing education from LaSalle University, Philadelphia, Pennsylvania. She has held positions as a staff nurse, staff development instructor, and a tenured professor of nursing. Dr. Gasparis Vonfrolio has published more than 30 articles and authored 11 books. She was the publisher of *REVOLUTION—The Journal of Nurse Empowerment* from 1990 through 1998. She counts as her greatest accomplishment the Nurses March on Washington, in which more than 35,000 nurses participated and which served as the catalyst for nurse legislation improvements for safe nurse:patient ratios.

Joseph Giovannoni, DNP, PMHCNS-BC, APRN-Rx, Caritas Coach, is a doctor of nursing practice, advanced practice nurse with prescriptive authority, and sex therapist. He is founder and director of Joseph Giovannoni Inc., a clinic in Honolulu, Hawaii, where he provides holistic, compassionate, evidence-based, patient-centered mental health treatment. He has integrated Dr. Jean Watson's Theory of Human Caring into his forensic practice. Dr. Giovannoni conducts sex offense–specific evaluations; individual, couples, and family psychotherapy; cognitive behavioral group therapy; and psycho-pharmacological management for mental disorders. He has lectured internationally and conducts self-care workshops for Society's Safe-Keepers™ (law enforcement officers), forensic professionals, nurses, and health science professionals to lower stress, prevent burnout, and sustain a healthy quality of life.

Marlienne Goldin, MPA, BSN, RN, CNML, Caritas Coach, graduated from Bergen Community College, Paramus, New Jersey, in 1984 with an associate's degree in applied science and then served as the clinical coordinator at St. Joseph's Hospital and Medical Center in Paterson, New Jersey. While working in emergency medical services, she completed her BSN degree from St. Peter's College, Jersey City, New Jersey, in 1989. She discovered Caring Theory in 2002 when she traveled to Colorado and studied with Dr. Jean Watson. In 2008, she completed the Caritas Coach Education Program (CCEP) from the Watson Caring Science Institute. From 2008 to 2014, she served as associate faculty and registrar of the CCEP. Ms. Goldin has presented nationally and internationally on the application of Watson's caring theory.

Marcia Hills, PhD, RN, FAAN, is a professor at the School of Nursing, Faculty of Human and Social Development, University of Victoria, British Columbia, Canada. She was the founding director of the Centre for Community Health Promotion Research (2002–2009). She has been the principal investigator on several federally funded research projects aimed primarily at transforming health care systems, practices, and policies toward a primary health care and person-centered, caring approach. As a visiting scholar and a World Health Organization (WHO) Fellow, Dr. Hills worked and studied in Australia and England and at the National School of Public Health in Rio de Janeiro, Brazil. Dr. Hills has consulted extensively in the United States, the United Kingdom, New Zealand, Australia, Kenya, Brazil, and Canada.

Sara Horton-Deutsch, PhD, RN, PMHCNS, FAAN, ANEF, Caritas Coach, Heart-Math Trainer, graduated in 1986 with a BSN from the University of Evansville, Evansville, Indiana. She then moved to Chicago, Illinois, to take a position in inpatient adult and geropsychiatry at Rush Presbyterian St. Luke's Medical Center, where she simultaneously began work on her master's degree in psychiatric–mental health nursing at Rush University. After completing her doctorate and a one-year postdoctorate in psychoneuroimmunology there, she spent seven years on the faculty at Rush. In 2011 she was inducted as an Academy of Nursing Education Fellow (ANEF) by the National League for Nursing (NLN), and in 2014 as a Fellow of the American Academy of Nursing (FAAN). She has received many awards recognizing her excellence in creative work and leadership skill set. She is a graduate of the Watson Caring Science Institute Caritas Coach Education Program (CCEP).

Lynn Keegan, PhD, RN, AHN-BC, FAAN, is one of the founders of the holistic health focus in nursing and a leader in holistic nursing. She currently works as director of Holistic Nursing Consultants (HNC) in Port Angeles, Washington. Dr. Keegan was inducted in 1996 as a Fellow of the American Academy of Nursing (FAAN) and is board certified as an advanced holistic nurse by the American Holistic Nurses Association (AHNA). She is past president of the AHNA and has been on the board of many organizations and journals. In 1991, she received the Distinguished Alumnus Award from Cornell University–New York Hospital School of Nursing and later was named Holistic Nurse of the Year by the AHNA. She is a six-time recipient of the *American Journal of Nursing* Book of the Year Award. She is known for her focus on the development and advancement of holistic nursing and, in more recent years, on end-of-life care.

Mary Jo Kreitzer, PhD, RN, FAAN, is the founder and director of the Center for Spirituality & Healing at the University of Minnesota. She has more than 40 years of leadership and expertise in health care. In addition to her roles as nurse, teacher, health care administrator, and researcher, she is recognized as a pioneer and innovator in the field of integrative health and well-being. Dr. Kreitzer earned her doctoral degree in public health at the University of Minnesota, Minneapolis, Minnesota, her MA in nursing at University of Iowa, Iowa City, Iowa, and her BA in nursing at Augustana College, Sioux

Falls, South Dakota. Dr. Kreitzer regularly presents to practitioner and public audiences and to academic and health care conferences. She has authored more than 100 publications and is the coeditor of *Integrative Nursing,* published in 2014. Dr. Kreitzer also serves as coeditor-in-chief of *Global Advances in Health and Medicine*, an international journal focused on improving health and well-being worldwide.

Mary Rockwood Lane, PhD, RN, FAAN, is an associate professor at the University of Florida, a core faculty member of the Watson Caring Science Institute (WCSI), an artist/healer/painter, and a Caritas nurse. She experienced art, spirituality, and healing firsthand as she painted herself out of a severe depression. From what she learned through that experience, she became the cofounder and codirector of the UF Health Arts in Medicine program at the University of Florida, Gainesville, and founded the first hospital artist-in-residence program in the country. She has written many articles on art and healing and is a recognized leader in the field. She lectures and teaches workshops on art and healing worldwide and helps medical centers and artists set up art and healing programs.

Susan Luck, MA, RN, HNB-BC, CCN, HWNC-BC, is a holistic nurse educator and integrative nurse coach, medical anthropologist, clinical nutritionist, and a national speaker, writer, and consultant for organizations pioneering the emerging integrative health care paradigm. She is the clinical nutritionist for special immunology services at Mercy Hospital, Miami, Florida, and maintains a private practice in Miami as a wellness nurse coach and clinical nutritionist. She is codirector of International Nurse Coach Association (INCA) and core faculty for the Integrative Nurse Coach Certificate Program (INCCP). She was named Holistic Nurse of the Year by the American Holistic Nurses Association (AHNA) in 1987. Ms. Luck is on the editorial board of the *Alternative Therapies in Health and Medicine* journal and is a founding member of and consultant to the *Integrative Practitioner* newsletter. She is the founder and program director of EarthRose Institute (ERI), a nonprofit organization dedicated to women's and children's environmental health education.

Beverly Malone, PhD, RN, FAAN, was ranked among the 100 Most Influential People in Healthcare by *Modern Healthcare* magazine in 2010 and 2015. Her tenure at the National League for Nursing (NLN) has been marked by a retooling of the league's mission to reflect the core values of caring, diversity, integrity, and excellence. Throughout her career, she has mixed policy, education, administration, and clinical practice, working as a surgical staff nurse, clinical nurse specialist, director of nursing, and assistant administrator of nursing. During the 1980s, she was dean of the School of Nursing at North Carolina Agricultural and Technical State University. In 1996, she was elected to the first of two terms as president of the American Nurses Association (ANA). In 2000, she became Deputy Assistant Secretary for Health of the U.S. Department of Health and Human Services.

Phalakshi Manjrekar, MScN, RN, is the distinguished nursing director and board member at the P.D. Hinduja National Hospital & Medical Research Centre, Mumbai, India. She has served as a coresearcher on a team from the Missouri University of Science & Technology, Rolla, Missouri, the University of Cincinnati, Cincinnati, Ohio, and the

Sardar Patel University in Gujarat, India. She has conferred with global and regional nursing leaders in Canada, Great Britain, and other Commonwealth nations, as well as in Switzerland and India, and has attended World Health Organization (WHO) briefings in Geneva and at the WHO South East Asian Regional Office (SEARO) in New Delhi. She has served as Chairperson of Nurses' Welfare for the Maharashtra State Chapter of the national Trained Nurses Association of India (TNAI). Ms. Manjrekar presently serves on the executive committee of the Nightingale Initiative for Global Health (NIGH) world board of directors and oversees the development of the NIGH's worldwide presence in India.

Carla Mariano, EdD, RN, AHN-BC, FAAIM, was coordinator of the Advanced Practice Adult Holistic Nurse Practitioner Program in the Rory Meyers College of Nursing at New York University and developed the bachelor of science holistic nursing program at Pacific College of Oriental Medicine, New York, New York. She helped develop the scope and standards for practice as president of the American Holistic Nurses Association (AHNA) and spearheaded the initiative by the American Nurses Association (ANA) that gave holistic nursing official recognition as a distinct specialty. Dr. Mariano has been a member of the editorial review boards of *The Journal of Holistic Nursing* and *Advances in Nursing Science*. She chaired the Values and Competencies Task Force of the National Education Dialogue, the White House Commission on Integrative Health Care, and is the recipient of the AHNA Holistic Nurse of the Year Award and the distinguished Achievement in Nursing Education Award from Teachers College, Columbia University, New York, New York.

Diana J. Mason, PhD, RN, FAAN, is the Rudin Professor of Nursing and cofounder and codirector of the Center for Health, Media, and Policy (CHMP) at Hunter College, City University of New York (CUNY), and a professor at CUNY. She is past president of the American Academy of Nursing and serves as strategic adviser for the Campaign for Action, an initiative to implement the recommendations from the Institute of Medicine's *The Future of Nursing: Leading Change, Advancing Health* report. Dr. Mason served as copresident of the Hermann Biggs Society, a health policy salon in New York City (2012–2015) and was on the national advisory committee for *Kaiser Health News*. She was editor-in-chief of the *American Journal of Nursing* for more than a decade and has received numerous awards, including honorary doctorates from Long Island University and West Virginia University, a fellowship in the New York Academy of Medicine, and the Lillian Wald Service Award from the American Public Health Association.

Margaret L. McClure, EdD, RN, FAAN, is an adjunct professor at New York University (NYU). For more than 20 years, she was the chief nursing officer at the NYU Langone Medical Center, where she also served as the chief operating officer and hospital administrator. She is an active member of several boards, including Nurses Educational Funds and the Jonas Center for Nursing Excellence. She is past president of the American Academy of Nursing and the American Organization of Nurse Executives and has received numerous awards, including honorary doctorates from Seton Hall University and Moravian College. In 2007, she was named a Living Legend by the American Academy of Nursing. She retired from the United States Army Reserves with the rank of colonel.

Donna M. Nickitas, PhD, RN, NEA-BC, CNE, FNAP, FAAN, is the executive officer of the PhD in nursing program at the Graduate Center, City University of New York (CUNY), and a professor at the Hunter-Bellevue School of Nursing at Hunter College (CUNY). Prior to her appointment as executive officer, she was deputy executive officer of the doctor of nursing science program (2010–2013) and served as the graduate specialty coordinator for the first dual-degree program (master of science/master's in public administration) between Hunter College and Baruch College (2003–2011). She is the editor of *Nursing Economic$: Journal for Health Care Leaders* and manuscript reviewer for several peer-reviewed nursing journals. Dr. Nickitas is the cochair of the American Academy of Nursing, Raise the Voice Campaign Committee, and vice-chair of the nursing section for the New York Academy of Medicine. She earned a BSN from State University of New York (SUNY) Stony Brook University, Stony Brook, New York, an MSN from the New York University Rory Meyers College of Nursing, New York, New York, and a PhD in nursing from Adelphi University, Garden City, New York.

Daniel J. Pesut, PhD, RN, PMHCNS-BC, FAAN, is a professor in the Nursing Population Health and Systems Cooperative Unit of the School of Nursing at the University of Minnesota and director of the Katharine J. Densford International Center for Nursing Leadership. He holds the Katherine R. and C. Walton Lillehei Chair in Nursing Leadership. He was on active duty in the Army Nurse Corps from 1975 through 1978. He served on the faculty at the University of Michigan School of Nursing from 1978 through 1981 and completed his PhD in clinical nursing research there in 1984. He served as the director of nursing services at the William S. Hall Psychiatric Institute in Columbia, South Carolina (1984–1987), and at the University of Minnesota School of Nursing (2012–present). He is past president (2003–2005) of the Honor Society of Nursing, Sigma Theta Tau International (STTI). He is the recipient of the Army Commendation Award, and in 2005, the Daniel J. Pesut Spirit of Renewal Award was established through STTI, to honor his contributions and leadership legacy.

Janet Quinn, PhD, RN, FAAN, is an author, speaker, consultant, and retreat and workshop facilitator in several content areas, including integrative nursing and health care; caring and healing; and spirituality and healing. She is a pioneer in Therapeutic Touch practice and research and has taught worldwide. Among her numerous honors, Dr. Quinn is an elected member of the Hunter College Hall of Fame, an elected Fellow of the American Academy of Nursing (FAAN), and was named American Holistic Nurses Association (AHNA) Holistic Nurse of the Year in 1990 and Healer of the Year by Nurse Healers/Professional Associates in 1995. She is a trained spiritual director and spiritual coach in private practice, and founder/director of the Touching Body, Tending Soul™ program and cofounder/codirector of the InterSpiritual Mentor Training Program through the Caritas Institute.

William Rosa, MS, RN, LMT, AHN-BC, AGPCNP-BC, CCRN-CMC, Caritas Coach, is a nurse, writer, and educator. He graduated Magna Cum Laude with a BSN from the New York University (NYU) College of Nursing in 2009. While working as a critical care bedside clinician for four years at NYU Langone Medical Center, he became an advocate for positive change within the profession and the elevation of consciousness for nurses and nursing. He completed Caritas Coach Education Program (CCEP) of the Watson Caring Science Institute (WCSI) and the Integrative Nurse Coach Certificate Program (INCCP) of the International Nurse Coach Association (INCA). Mr. Rosa currently has over 65 publications for peer-reviewed and non-peer-reviewed journals, newspapers, magazines, and international platform blogs. He is a recipient of the Association for Nursing Professional Development's National 2015 Excellence in Professional Development Change Agent/Team Member Award and the 2015 American Association of Critical-Care Nurses (AACN) Circle of Excellence Award. He is currently working in Kigali, Rwanda, as visiting faculty at the University of Rwanda and as ICU clinical educator at the Rwanda Military Hospital, Human Resources for Health Program in partnership with the New York University Rory Meyers College of Nursing.

Bonney Gulino Schaub, MS, RN, PMHCNS-BC, NC-BC, is a psychiatric/mental health clinical nurse specialist and a transpersonal nurse coach. She is codirector of the Huntington Meditation and Imagery Center (HMIC) and director of HMIC's Transpersonal Nurse Coach (TNC) program. Ms. Schaub is cofounder of International Nurse Coach Association (INCA) and Integrative Nurse Coach Certificate Program (INCCP). She is a pioneer of the clinical use of meditation, imagery, transpersonal awareness, and energy practices as therapeutic tools that empower both the practitioner and patient. After working in medical–surgical nursing and inpatient psychiatry, she became a detox coordinator and psychotherapist in an alcohol and drug treatment program and subsequently formulated the Vulnerability Model of Recovery, a model of emotional and spiritual development that has been adapted by drug and alcohol treatment centers in the United States, Canada, and Italy.

Tilda Shalof, BScN, RN, CNCC(C), has been a nurse for 33 years and has worked in hospitals in the United States, Israel, and Canada. For the past 28 years, she has practiced in the medical–surgical ICU at Toronto General Hospital (TGH) and attained accreditation in critical care nursing from the Canadian Nurses' Association. Currently, she works in the immunodeficiency clinic at TGH, caring for people living with HIV. In the aftermath of the global severe acute respiratory syndrome (SARS) pandemic, she wrote *A Nurse's Story: Life, Death, and In-Between in an Intensive Care Unit* (2004), which became a national bestseller. As a speaker, nursing ambassador, and patient and nurse advocate, the common theme of all of her talks is how to be a mindful, engaged, creative, happy, healthy, and—above all—*brave*, nurse.

Marie M. Shanahan, MA, BSN, RN, HN-BC, is the founding president and CEO of The BirchTree Center for Healthcare Transformation, Florence, Massachusetts, which assists health care providers and organizations in creating caring cultures and vibrant work environments. The BirchTree Center also provides continuing education for nurses in holistic nursing and integrative health, leading to national board certification. She served on the board of directors of the American Holistic Nurses Association (AHNA; 2011–2013). Her nursing experience includes clinical, administrative, and educational roles, with research interests including self-care and restorative practices for nurses and nurse/patient satisfaction with therapeutic healing environments.

Leighsa Sharoff, EdD, RN, NPP, AHN-BC, is a board certified advanced holistic nurse, mental health nurse practitioner, nurse educator, and researcher. She is considered an advanced generalist in nursing, participating in the teaching–learning process in psychiatric nursing, maternal–child nursing, medical–surgical nursing, and a variety of other aspects within health care. In addition to being a mentor, Dr. Sharoff is an accomplished national and international author and presenter. In her view, the number of awards and accolades one receives does not equate to being a good nurse: It is how one looks at his or her own life that defines this. For Dr. Sharoff, her success lies in how her students think of her, how they remember her, and the awareness that she has touched many lives by participating in the teaching–learning process.

Marlaine C. Smith, PhD, RN, AHN-BC, FAAN, has had a 40-year career in academic nursing. She currently serves as dean and Helen K. Persson Eminent Scholar at the Christine E. Lynn College of Nursing at Florida Atlantic University (FAU), Boca Raton, Florida. Prior to joining FAU in 2006, she was on the faculty of the University of Colorado School of Nursing for 18 years, including 6 years as professor and associate dean for academic affairs and director of the Center for Integrative Caring Practice. She is certified as an advanced holistic nurse and her research has focused on the healing power of touch in various forms for patients with cancer. She is a recipient of the National League for Nursing (NLN) Martha E. Rogers Award and the Distinguished Alumna Award from New York University's Division of Nursing, and is a fellow in the American Academy of Nursing.

Isabelle Soulé, PhD, RN, earned her bachelor's degree in nursing at Walla Walla University, College Place, Washington, and her master's in family nursing and PhD at Oregon Health & Science University. Her professional work has been equally divided between neonatal intensive care unit (NICU) practice and academics, where she has specialized in immigrant and refugee health. Her nursing career has been informed by her interest in process work, deep democracy, neuro linguistic programming (NLP), indigenous cultures around the world, and being a practicing clay artist.

A. Lynne Wagner, EdD, MSN, RN, FACCE, CHMT, Caritas Coach, holds bachelor's and master's degrees in nursing and a doctorate of education in leadership. Recipient of several grants and awards in education and research, she currently works as a nurse educator-consultant, facilitating mentoring programs based on her Caring Mentoring Model. A former director of Watson Caring Science Institute's (WCSI's) Caritas Coach Education Program (CCEP), she currently serves as adjunct faculty at University of Colorado College of Nursing in the newly designed Watson Caring Science Center–CU CCEP program. A Caring Science scholar, Certified HeartMath Trainer, and published poet, her publications, presentations, and workshops address the development of caring practice from aesthetic personal and professional perspectives. A member of the American Nurses Association (ANA), Sigma Theta Tau International (STTI), and the International Association for Human Caring (IAHC), Dr. Wagner serves on the IAHC board of directors and is assistant editor for poetry for the *International Journal for Human Caring*. In 2013 she cofounded the Massachusetts Regional Caring Science Consortium.

Jean Watson, PhD, RN, AHN-BC, FAAN, is distinguished professor and dean emerita, University of Colorado Denver, College of Nursing Anschutz Medical Center campus, where for 16 years she held the Murchinson-Scoville Chair in Caring Science, the nation's first endowed chair in caring science. She is founder of the original Center for Human Caring in Colorado and is a fellow of the American Academy of Nursing, past president of the National League for Nursing (NLN), and founding member of the International Association of Human Caring (IAHC) and International Caritas Consortium (ICC). Dr. Watson is founder and director of the nonprofit Watson Caring Science Institute (WCSI).

Dr. Watson has earned undergraduate and graduate degrees in nursing and psychiatric–mental health nursing and holds a PhD in educational psychology and counseling. She is the recipient of many awards, including 11 honorary doctoral degrees. At the University of Colorado, she held the title of distinguished professor of nursing, the highest honor accorded its faculty for scholarly work. As author/coauthor of more than 20 books on caring (including *American Journal of Nursing* Book of the Year award winners), she seeks to bridge paradigms as well as point toward transformative models for the 21st century. In October 2013, Dr. Watson was inducted as a Living Legend by the American Academy of Nursing, its highest honor.

Foreword

When I was a little girl, I was sure that all the issues and problems would be resolved before I had a chance to make a difference. I had no idea that making a difference was a leadership role. I had myriad questions, ranging from "How would anyone ever know that I wanted to make a difference?" to "Would I ever be equipped with the knowledge, courage, and compassion to make that difference?"

Nurses as Leaders: Evolutionary Visions of Leadership would have been—and is—incredibly reassuring. For this book is full of reassurance from leaders who have made and continue to make a difference in the world of "health nursing," as Florence Nightingale would have called it. In these pages, you will find bridges connecting the leaders, shaped and molded by time and challenge, with those leaders delicately—and, sometimes, hesitantly—touching the newness of leadership. These bridges are awe inspiring. As you read, you will discover the opportunity to walk in the shoes of some of our well-known giants and, by simply continuing to read, you will find yourself in the shoes of those beginning or midway in their careers.

Amazingly, I still hear the anxiety emanating from both leadership sectors. From the well-developed leaders, I hear the echo of "Who will be my successor?" and from our formative leadership colleagues, "Will there be room for me in the arena often reserved for professional pioneers?" The chapters identify the trials of climbing the mountain to make contributions to the health of the nation and the global community. You will bump into teachable concepts like visioning, praxis, and resilience.

As the leadership dynamic unfolds, visioning tends to take center space. But visions cannot stand alone. So, in appreciation of praxis (moving the concept into action) as related to a vision, it is clear that a vision without action is a hallucination. The authors of the chapters present their testimonies of action and the challenges incurred along their life journey.

Interestingly, the precedent to a vision is the ability to dream, to see one's self in the role of *leader*. The writers invite us into their dreams and the evolution of their leadership. This book illustrates the links between the dream, vision, and action that so many of these leaders have practiced. With formidable resilience, it becomes clear that there really are multiple paths to leadership and to making the difference. Rather than a fork in the road with just two options, there frequently are many choices. Often, upcoming leaders lack clear planning or miss an opportunity due to life events and only later realize that the humility learned from those very events make one a better, more complete leader.

So, this is a book for little girls and little boys who lack the confidence that there will be issues and problems to resolve when they grow up. It is for the emerging voices that shout of a new time, a new day for health care; for the professional pioneers who can see their fingerprints on some of nursing's most notable innovations and discoveries of learning; and for the faculty who struggle with how to transfer the hunger for leadership and the humility to accept it to their students and, at times, to themselves. This book is a gift to mentors and mentees who continually build bridges of collaboration, partnership, and learning, and it challenges us to make a difference in the world of health and caring.

This book of leadership is for you.

Beverly Malone, PhD, RN, FAAN
CEO, National League for Nursing

Preface

> *. . . leadership [asks]:*
> **Do we have the courage to . . . show up . . . take risks, ask for help, own our mistakes,**
> **learn from failure, lean into joy, and . . . support the people around us in**
> **doing the same? . . .**
> *[It] requires leaders . . . willing to . . . show up as imperfect, real people.*
> *That's what truly, deeply inspires us.*
>
> —Brené Brown (2012)

In the 1870s, Florence Nightingale wrote that it would take 150 years to see the full embodiment of nursing as a profession—the kind of nursing she envisioned as its founder and first pioneering leader. She saw nursing as a calling and a must—a discipline without boundaries or limitations, built on a foundation of unrequited service to the public and globally relevant in research, education, journalism, clinical practice, policy, science, and environmental activism. As the year 2020 and the 150th anniversary of the aforementioned prediction approaches, nurses and nursing stand on the precipice of realizing this expansive professional aspiration. This book strives to usher in this Nightingalean ambition as its very aim and purpose.

The contributions compiled herein invoke the actualization of a mighty and innovative possibility, one that merges all corners of the discipline into a cohesive force for health and well-being; fully embraces the art and strategically engages the science of nursing; provides historical context and evolutionary foresight; and seeks to unveil and awaken the inherent leader dwelling within each nurse, regardless of position, title, credentials, or specialty. This book assumes that every nurse is a leader and provides guidance, opportunity, and the vision necessary to support making that leadership manifest in the world.

Nightingale proposed three sacred tenets of nursing foundational to the vitality of the profession and the health of the world at large: healing, leadership, and global action (Dossey, Selanders, Beck, & Attewell, 2005). As healers, we have defined scopes and standards for practice that are nursing's prerogative, specializing in the care of unique populations and translating humanistic and empirical paradigms into measurable outcomes. As global activists, we have advocated for the patients and families we serve across cultures, continents, and considerations and have positively impacted global health advancements through myriad contributions to research, education, and practice arenas. But as inspired and emboldened leaders, though the successes and accomplishments are many and the recognition from multidisciplinary partners substantial, we continue to fall just short of our highest collective potential: a unified, empowered, visionary, and globally informed profession, capable of redefining health care and creating a new understanding of health and well-being for ourselves and those we care for. We do not yet believe that we are the very ones we have been waiting for.

The World Health Organization (WHO; 2012) identifies us as the largest group of health care providers, with the number of nurses and midwives worldwide estimated to be well over 19 million. In the United States alone, nurses are represented by more than 200 state and national organizations (Matthews, 2012; Nurse.org, 2014–2015). We are positioned and mobilized for exceptional leadership opportunities—the "backbone of health care"—yet we remain divided over keystone issues and professional–cultural challenges. Internationally, disagreements persist over the entry-level degree requirement for a registered professional nurse and whether mandated nurse:patient ratios should be enforced. Interpersonally, horizontal violence still runs rampant in a multitude of settings, and nurses suffer from unacknowledged or disregarded symptoms of compassion fatigue, burnout, and moral distress. Conversations about the lived experience of each nurse—the challenges, frustrations, upsets, joys, and loves—often go unspoken; their candor and authenticity often unwelcome in an academic, quantitatively driven milieu. However, these are the conversations that hold the potential power of transformation. They require courage and fortitude and the audacity to be vulnerable, and they give voice to the unseen work of nurses and nursing. They are the stories and genuine expressions of humanity that have the potential to guide the profession from fragmentation toward wholeness.

This book forges an untraversed landscape of leadership in action—articulating the invaluable work and professional contributions of current-day nursing frontrunners, humanizing their experiences in a way that is accessible and tangible to the reader and creating a powerful worldview of possibilities for how nurses see who they are and what they are capable of achieving. These writings—composed by innovative and seasoned clinicians, nurse educators, deans, chief nursing officers (CNOs), executives, acclaimed authors, global advocates, policy experts, holistic guides, nurse coaches, editors-in-chief, organizational presidents, nongovernmental organization (NGO) founders, spiritual practitioners, and administrators—provide novice and beginner professionals the opportunity to arouse their own potential for nurse-driven leadership and explore realms beyond the finite outlines of traditional curricula. More experienced readers will have access to voices that support and nourish their need for professional development, wherever they are on their career path. Established leaders in nursing will be given ample and diverse opportunity to reflect on all aspects of their journey to date, as well as insightful considerations for their trajectory ahead.

The offerings of these authors and the tables they have earned seats at have disproven the notion of nursing as a historically subservient, "blinders on–bedside only" role and have elevated it to one of tremendous communal, societal, and global impact. This book introduces a first in nursing: subjective access to the inside details of this individual–collective journey and real-world education that flows from the richness of personal experience and professional wisdom. Each author has mastered an artful approach to writing, infusing the intimacy of personal storytelling with the science of scholarly expertise. This collection has the potential to create a mutually beneficial symbiosis for praxis between authorship and readership; a dialogue that serves as proof of theory in action as authors illustrate how their careers and life paths have exemplified their individual philosophies of nursing; an interplay that seamlessly merges the personal and professional. Never before has such a seemingly disparate group of authors been able to present their work side by side to create a unified front for nursing—a living testament of theory informing practice informing theory and so forth.

The authors write of their relationship with nursing and what drew them to the profession, the circumstances and experiences that sparked their interests and passions, their evolution within and contribution to the discipline, the morals and ethics that guide their practice, and their individual vision for a wholly embodied and fully expressed future of nursing. In essence, the contributors outline the part of the work, the area of their specialty, the heart of their purpose that has yet to be realized, so that up-and-coming nurse leaders may continue to expand upon it with confidence, direction, and intention. Through their artistic and scholarly approach, they outline the being, or current status, of the discipline while pointing us toward its very becoming. In this way, these writings move beyond a demonstration of leadership in action and become succession planning in action. Readers are handed both a guidebook and compass for personal–professional growth through the intimate narratives of nursing's most adventurous pioneers, boldest activists, and emerging voices.

The book is divided into two parts. Part I, "Laying the Groundwork," includes chapters from renowned leaders who discuss aspects of their professional contributions in detail and guide the reader to unleash his or her future potential through the lens of nursing. These chapters deeply connect the reader to one of the main intentions of the book: to assert and validate that nurses and a nursing sensibility are vital for the continued evolution of humanity and to ensure that dignity, humane caring, and compassionate, courageous leadership continue to pave the path for the profession and beyond.

Part II, "Building the Inroads," encapsulates the experiences, messages, work to date, and future directions of accomplished and inspiring nurses who are continuing the conversations started by those who have laid the groundwork or claiming a new domain with which readers can coidentify. These authors are adventurous scholars, doctoral students, and change agents who are continuing to shape the voice of the collective. Part II further provides alternate views of nursing as a discipline, promoting leadership capacity for the reader and encouraging individuality and authenticity in nursing praxis.

Each author's vision has been abbreviated and condensed to create their respective chapter title. Whether they view the full potential of nurses to be "translational and indispensable," "metaphorical and passionate," or "unitary and appreciative," the title of each chapter is an invocation for the future of the profession as it relates to the author's work. In fact, it is more than an invocation; it is an extension and reminder of the 150-year-old Nightingalean vision. Each author becomes an expert scholar and theorist in his or her own right, offering a lens through which to embrace, engage, and evolve nursing praxis. Reflection questions at the end of each chapter guide readers to contemplate presented concepts, merging the message of the authors with the individual perspectives of readership and grounding visionary possibilities in personal understanding and practice.

This book can be used as a primary text for undergraduate leadership and management courses; by graduate nursing administration students; as an adjunct book for nursing theory classes; and by those interested in deepening their understanding of global nursing, getting involved in policy and advocacy work, or fulfilling the potential of their role as advanced practice nurses. It is a tool for professional development specialists to guide the staff members they serve, a reference for managers to inspire their employee partners, and a resource for teachers to elevate the consciousness of students. It is a historical primer for those interested in how we got where we are and an action plan for those who want to be effective change agents. The novice can use it to encourage yet-to-be-known aspirations, and the expert will be humbled by its gentle return to nursing's most basic foundational values. The bedside clinician will find its bird's-eye perspective illuminating and the public health community worker can find inspiration to reintegrate the intimate specifics of human-to-human, one-on-one caregiving in an environment of cultural humility. More than any other single volume on the market, *Nurses as Leaders: Evolutionary Visions of Leadership* documents and celebrates the far-reaching, transcultural, and multidimensional impacts that nurse leaders have made and the guidance they continue to provide in health care and beyond. ***Qualified instructors may obtain access to ancillary instructor's PowerPoints by contacting textbook@springerpub.com.***

It is now up to you, the reader, to map out the journey and claim it as your own. After laying the foundations and building the inroads, the unwritten third part of this book will arise from what you choose to do with the insights provided. The next chapters will be lived out in how you translate this wisdom into everyday practice and the ways you choose to shepherd the profession as an evolutionary nurse leader. We will only realize our collective leadership potential when we, as a profession, become clear about what and how we are leading, and why our leadership matters.

This book is essential as we currently face the overt medicalization of the nursing profession and a disconnection from our unique and altruistic culture, with the resulting submergence of the ethic and ethos of nursing as both art and science. If nurses can no longer articulate what makes theirs a specialized profession, clearly express their thoughts, feelings, and emotions with confidence and consistency, or identify the challenges in the world they can address directly as the vanguards of human caring, then they will cease to be just that: nurses. At this moment in our professional development, our patients, colleagues, interdisciplinary partners, politicians, and the global society at large look to us for answers, guidance, and unwavering leadership. It is imperative that we remember who we are and who we were always meant to be as a collective. It is essential that we both claim and fulfill our individual roles as leaders for the betterment of ourselves and of those we serve.

It is time.

William Rosa

■ REFERENCES

Brown, B. (2012). Leadership series: Vulnerability and inspired leaders. *Impatient optimists: Bill & Melinda Gates Foundation.* Retrieved from http://www.impatientoptimists.org/Posts/2012/11/Leadership-Series-Vulnerability-and-Inspired-Leadership#.VwYmGccbqFI

Dossey, B. M., Selanders, L. C., Beck, D. M., & Attewell, A. (2005). *Florence Nightingale today: Healing, leadership, global action*. Silver Spring, MD: Nursesbooks.org.

Matthews, J. H. (2012). Role of professional organizations in advocating for the nursing profession. *Online Journal of Nursing, 17*(1), Manuscript 3.

Nurse.org. (2014–2015). Nursing organizations. Retrieved from http://nurse.org/orgs.shtml

World Health Organization. (2012). Enhancing nursing and midwifery capacity to contribute to the prevention, treatment and management of noncommunicable diseases. *Human Resources for Health Observer*, (12). Retrieved from http://www.who.int/hrh/resources/observer12.pdf

Acknowledgments

My friend and the author of the first chapter in this book, Jeanne Anselmo, wrote me a note some time ago that reads: "There is a great wealth of wisdom, compassion, innovation, vision, heart, diligence, insight, understanding, and love in our Nursing community that is not often given a venue to constellate and shine its light." I could not agree more.

I am deeply grateful for the countless nurses, change agents, leaders, mentors, teachers, students, and colleagues who have inspired me along my journey and whose impact on me has led to the realization of this book.

To the authors whose lived experiences grace these pages, there are no words to express my gratitude for you and your vulnerability, courage, and leadership. You are the vision! You are the living proof of what nursing can and might be. Thank you for trusting me with your stories. Thank you for taking a risk on a first-time book author. And thank you for your kindness and generosity as we partnered to ensure the integrity of this project.

Endless thanks to Springer Publishing Company for supporting me throughout this process.

Deep gratitude to my publisher, Margaret Zuccarini, for giving me this chance and believing in me from the start. Thank you for your caring presence and encouragement.

Amanda Carswell, Kris Parrish, and Jacob Seifert, thank you for your dedication to this project, for your quick responses, and for your patience as I navigated this learning curve.

Dr. Wendy Budin, without you, this book would not exist. Thank you for being you.

To my first nursing family at New York University Langone Medical Center, I am eternally grateful for all you have taught me over the years. I am thankful for your friendship and support. To the staff nurses I have worked with in the Critical Care Center, you are the most incredible and gifted group of people. Thank you for teaching me how to be a nurse and for inspiring me beyond words. To my nurse educator friends and colleagues, you have each taught me, in your own way, what it means to be of service through leadership. Loving gratitude to Roseann Pokoluk—thank you for your generous and unwavering support, your honesty, for always believing in me and for always giving me the chances I needed to grow and lead.

Thanks to all my teachers at the New York University Rory Meyers College of Nursing and the Hunter–Bellevue School of Nursing at Hunter College, especially

Dr. Grace Ogiehor-Enoma for being the very first teacher who made sure I knew that my ideas were "good enough" and that I needed to get clear about how I would lead.

To my caring science family, thank you for your magnificent and healing community. Special thanks and much love to Dr. Jean Watson, thank you for always being available to me, for always treating my words, thoughts, and dreams with kindness and openness, and for your constant support in all I do.

Many thanks to the International Nurse Coach Association (INCA) for creating new possibilities of leadership for nurses. A note of gratitude to Barbara Dossey, for your unending support in this project; and to Susan Luck, thank you for being a part of this, even in the face of challenging circumstances—your dedication to this book has meant the world to me.

Thank you to the national and international organizations that have supported me in my growth as a leader and writer, particularly the American Association of Critical-Care Nurses (AACN), the Association for Nurses in Professional Development (ANPD), the American Holistic Nurses Association (AHNA), the American Nurses Association (ANA), the National League for Nursing (NLN), and the Nightingale Initiative for Global Health (NIGH).

To my personal and creative inspirations, you have not only changed my views on the world of leadership but have touched my heart with your audacity, boldness, and truth. Brené Brown, thank you for daring greatly and teaching me the power of vulnerability as a person, professional, friend, family member, and leader; Elizabeth Gilbert, thank you for your words that have helped me to rediscover and celebrate my creativity and returned me to myself in my most challenging times; and Jacqueline Novogratz, thank you for your advocacy work in procuring human equality and dignity on a global scale and for inspiring me to live a life of immersion each and every day.

For my dear friends who have opened my heart and filled my life with joy. You know who you are. I love you.

In memory of my grandparents, Canio and Jennie Bartolini and William Rosa I, immigrant laborers who worked hard with minimal reward so that one day their grandchildren might be educated, find happiness, and write books.

My family, thank you for loving me, celebrating me, and for allowing me the privilege of loving you.

My brother, Kief, I am so happy you are in my life. Thank you for being a part of all of it.

Mom and Dad, words will fall short, regardless of what I try and say. Thank you for always being there.

My beautiful, loving, kind, and unbelievably caring husband, Michael, thank you for your unquestionable support throughout this project and in all I do. You are whole, perfect, and complete, and I love you just the way you are.

Nurse as Leader: A Journey of Privilege

William Rosa

The nurse belongs to the collective of nursing; we are all responsible for creating a community of compassionate, moral empathy that lifts the veil of silence and promotes healthy, respectful, clear and truthful articulation of our inner lives. . . . Nurses do not practice in silos. We all attend to the needs of humanity, and we all deserve to process this intimate, multi-faceted gift in environments of support [and] understanding (Rosa (2014a, p. 20). As nursing evolves . . . and procures [its] legacy, there is a sacred opportunity to merge the theoretical underpinnings of the profession with . . . [the] clinical realities. . . . It is in returning to the basics of our discipline that our dutiful complexities within the healthcare system will be understood, valued, and promoted (Rosa (2014b, p. 76).

■ LEADERSHIP AS PRIVILEGE

The essence of leadership, although considered one of the domains most discussed and written about in professional sectors the world over, often remains elusive in its application to practice. Leaders who innovate and implement an evolutionary vision of "how things could be" often personify concepts that we may tend to believe exist only in theory. But, somehow, they have figured it out—they have grasped that fine and delicate space of praxis, the congruence of theory in action.

Think of the most notable leaders in recent history and consider the words that come to mind in their wake: Mohandas K. Gandhi—truthful and nonviolent; Nelson Mandela—focused and determined; Martin Luther King Jr.—courageous and unwavering; Mother Teresa—compassionate and loving; Winston Churchill—confident and resolute. Now, the words listed to describe these individuals may differ from the ones you would use and may even seem to limit the depth of their persona and myriad contributions to humanity somewhat, but encapsulated in these words may very well be the vision they have left behind for all who follow. For example, Gandhi believed that through nonviolence, what is known as *ahimsa*, the truth of equality would be revealed and sociopolitical integrity would prevail in India. Mother Teresa showed the world that through demonstrable compassion and extending love toward those closest to each of us, we can change the world one person at a time. To these historical figures, leadership was a platform upon which they lived and practiced the precepts of social justice and human rights. For them, leadership was more than a power differential used to arouse notoriety. Leadership, for the Kings, Churchills, and Mandelas, will forever be a privilege—a life practice of wielding those ideals considered most sacred to the preservation and dignified existence of humanity.

It causes one to wonder, what are the words—the ideals, principles, and visions for a healthier world—that I will leave behind in my wake? What ethics do and can I employ, as a nurse, to positively impact another human being and, therefore, the world around me? What is the platform I hold and the privilege of leadership I possess in my daily practice, regardless of the setting? And, how do I begin to translate the concepts and ideas I have about leadership into practice, where who I am as a leader is received, felt, and understood for my good and the good of those I serve?

The literature is overwhelmed by scholarly contributions that attempt to define, delineate, and project the role of the nurse leader across specialties (Elwell & Elikofer, 2015; Plonien, 2015; Hart et al., 2014); differentiate between the types of leadership considered most effective (e.g., authentic, ethical, aesthetic; Mannix, Wilkes, & Daly, 2015; Spence Laschinger, Borgogni, Consiglio, & Read, 2015; Makaroff, Storch, Pauly, & Newton, 2014); promote a lens, program, or training through which leadership education can or should be imparted (Stikes, Arterberry, & Logsdon, 2015; Day et al., 2014); and question or inquire about leadership practices and discuss varied perceptions of leadership in nursing (Cutcliffe & Cleary, 2015).

None of these more traditional approaches to the ongoing dialogue on leadership are addressed in this book. This is not a training course and it is not an educational perspective. It is an offering. From this offering springs forth considerations and reflections, tools and options, interpretations and understandings, invitations and opportunities, and diverse paths and innovative aspirations. In this book, you hold the journeys of nurse change agents who have dealt with personal setbacks and tribulations, professional doubts and disappointments, and learned, through willingness and flexibility and self-honoring, how to elevate nursing to its place as a professional body of influence and major global leader in health care delivery and development. In fact, in this book you hold the ethos of what it means to be a nurse leader—the very essence of those who have laid the groundwork and those who continue to build the inroads of the discipline. In this book, you hold their stories, and in these stories, you hold the heart of nursing.

The misnomers may be more common than we would like to think: Bedside nurses who lack positions of authority or do not possess a lofty credential may continue to believe they are not leaders. The long-term impact they have on patients' lives, and therefore the families, communities, and societies those patients are a part of, frequently goes unrealized. The bedside clinician's abilities to coordinate the interdisciplinary care provided at any given time, to direct the flow and output of major health care facilities, and to create environments of healing and preserve the dignity of another amid their suffering and health challenges, all the while maintaining and implementing exemplary clinical skills and knowledge, is nurse leader work. Nurse authors who contribute articles, letters, and poetry to publications may think they are not leading—but what thought patterns and professional trends are you exploring or challenging or expanding upon? Who will think differently after reading your words? That is nurse leader work. At times, teachers and instructors may be unable to fully comprehend the sphere of their influence beyond the time limitations of the term or the students who sit in front of them at any given moment, but this is the workforce of the next generation being trained to evolve and expand the minds and hearts who will advance nursing toward what it was always meant to be, and that is nurse leader work.

Nurse leader work is about who we are being and who we are aspiring to become. Nurse leader work is relational; it occurs at the interface of our individual ethics and how we show up to collaborate with others in partnership and service. Nurse leader work makes itself known through our words, behaviors, and actions, and reflects to others what is most important to us as people and as professionals. Leadership is an inherent aspect of being a nurse and so nurse leader work is always being done, consciously or unconsciously, knowingly or unknowingly. When we adopt the title "nurse," we implicitly come to shoulder the responsibilities, ethical obligations, and privileges that comprise leadership. And the question is: What will we do with it?

■ AN EMERGING CONCEPT OF LEADERSHIP AS STARTING POINT

In order to more consciously engage the innate aspects of leadership within the nursing role and to have a premise with which to mature throughout the process of this book journey, a starting point lens is offered through which to think of leadership and how it is practiced. The *Holistic Leadership Model* (HLM) is "a participative leadership model in which people, regardless of formal titles, engage in a constructive process as equal partners to influence an affirming, sustainable, and humanistic outcome" (Andrus & Shanahan, 2016, p. 591). Holism is a cornerstone of the nursing profession, as suggested and discussed by Nightingale. *Holistic nursing* may be defined as "all nursing practice that has healing the whole person as its goal and honors relationship-centered care and the interconnectedness of self, others, nature, and spirituality" (Dossey, 2016, p. 3). One does not have to "become" a "holistic nurse" in order to utilize or apply this model to practice. In fact, given the definition in the preceding text, holistic nursing is a philosophy that can be embodied by multi-specialty clinicians, educators, administrators, policy advocates, teachers, or any role informed by the moral and ethical principles of nursing's scope and standards. It is a way of being; a currency with which we practice the art and science of nursing. It can be used by bedside nurses in the emergency department and intensive care unit as easily as it can in outpatient psychiatry or advanced private practice, by the chief nursing officer and director of nursing research, as well as the unit manager and professional development specialist. It is a way of understanding and approaching one's relationship with self and other, upon which other theories, skills, competencies, and personal ideals can be layered. The HLM is an inclusive worldview that invites all nurses, regardless of beliefs, preferences, or judgments, to partake in its emerging and ever-evolving concept of the nurse as leader.

This particular model is considered a synthesis of other participative leadership models, incorporating the idealized influence, inspiration and vision, intellectual stimulation, and individual consideration known as the core characteristics of *transformational leadership* (Burns, 1978); the principles of self-awareness, collaboration, and connection that Frisina (2011) discusses as central to *influential leadership*; and the emphasis of *servant leadership* on the primary desire to serve and be of service, the main focus of which is the growth and well-being of others (Greenleaf, 2002).

In order to make the HLM more relatable to nursing-specific considerations, several nursing professional practice models are used to help operationalize its theoretical perspectives and frameworks.

The BirchTree Center Model™ (Andrus & Shanahan, 2016; Shanahan, 2014; see Chapter 17 for more information on the BirchTree Center Model™ and Figure 17.1 for an illustration of its components)

- Serves as an integrative, interdisciplinary, progressive practice model of personal and professional transformation
- Promotes capacity building for individuals to develop a caring-healing ethic in transforming both personal practice and organizational culture
- Incorporates self-care, self-reflection, self-renewal, and self-awareness as essential to leadership competency
- Reorients shared values, behaviors, and actions of health care institutions toward healing and caring
- Links a cultural anchor of compassion to a standard of excellence for performance-based outcomes

The Quality Caring Model© (Duffy, 2009, 2015)

- Integrates the processes of caring with quality health care outcomes to promote nursing excellence
- Incudes structures involved in health care delivery: care providers, patients/family, and the health care organization/system
- Supports relationship-centered care informed by caring values, attitudes, and behaviors
- Focuses on improved interpersonal and clinical outcomes for the care provider and patient/family and economic, safety, and quality outcomes for the organization/system

The Caring in Nursing Administration Model (Nyburg, 1998)

- Promotes leadership actions that stem from an ethical core of the caring sciences
- Supports evidence-based caring research frameworks
- Requires nurse administrators to partake in and role model self-care and to extend that caring to create healing environments in organizations
- Identifies nurse administrators as leaders who have the potential to link the humanistic value of caring and the economic realities of health care to transform practice settings

The HLM includes all ways of knowing in the form of qualitative and quantitative research, narrative research inquiry, and appreciative inquiry (Andrus & Shanahan, 2016). In summary, the model:

- Recognizes that leaders working from this perspective will take on innovative roles in the transformation of health care
- Assumes that everyone is a leader, regardless of position or title
- Acknowledges that every nurse is a partner in the transformation of any given system

Additionally, the HLM identifies seven core characteristics of a holistic nurse leader that can be viewed along with brief explanations in Table I.1.

The HLM is just one perspective with which to more deeply engage the narratives of leadership and personal growth discussed in this text. It is a lens through which to remain open and available to the ideas and lived experiences of accomplished nurse leaders who share the vision of all nurses as cocreators in the future of the profession. It also serves as a canvas upon which to create and explore new ways of thinking about your own individual leadership capacities and potentials. It acts as a mirror while observing demonstrated leadership in the world, helping you to question if what you are seeing is representative of the highest good in nursing; aiding you to determine what you can do

TABLE I.1   **Core Characteristics of a Holistic Leader With Brief Descriptions**

Core Characteristics of a Holistic Leader	Brief Description
1. Visionary	"Open to learning from other points of view through evolving the art of full presence, deep listening, and a nonjudgmental attitude . . . understands the deeper spiritual needs of people by caring for souls of individuals as well as the soul of the organization . . . see[s] the big picture and utiliz[es] out-of-the-box thinking" (p. 598)
2. Inspirational presence	"Inspires people to be their best selves through inclusion, respect, caring, and acknowledgment . . . foster[s] collaboration, teamwork, and shared information . . . embodies a sense of personal integrity that radiates to others as respect, kindness, and genuine, authentic caring" (pp. 598–599)
3. Role model	"Set[s] standards of excellence in clinical nursing . . . serve[s] as a positive example for other nurses to follow and emulate . . . There are four core principles that serve as pillars for role modeling: maintaining integrity, upholding ethical standards, demonstrating bold and courageous actions, and being visible-approachable-accessible" (p. 599)
4. Mentor	"View[s] mentorship as a mutually beneficial shared, rather than hierarchical, process where both people, as partners, learn and grow from one another's insights and wisdom . . . allowing for acceptance, cooperation, appreciation, and inclusivity—a circle of influence" (p. 600)

(continued)

TABLE I.1   **Core Characteristics of a Holistic Leader With Brief Descriptions (*continued*)**

Core Characteristics of a Holistic Leader	Brief Description
5. Champion for clinical excellence	"[Links] the *caring case* of bedside care with the *business case* of healthcare transformation . . . promot[es] education and learning at every level . . . hold[s] nurses accountable for clinical excellence . . . intentional about . . . implementing progressive, innovative strategies . . . [and the] cultivation of true collaboration . . . elevate[s] the professionalism of nurses by encouraging . . . ongoing professional development and clinical competence" (pp. 600–601)
6. Courageous advocate	"Support[s] and enrich[es] all dimensions of . . . nursing practice, from bedside to boardroom . . . creat[es] a work environment and culture that fosters caring for nurses . . . [cultivates] [a]n innovative culture and workplace environment that enhances the patient experience and . . . satisfaction . . . build[s] . . . partnerships with community organizations . . . include[s] environmental health as a nurse competency" (pp. 601–603)
7. Cultural transformational agent	"Works to actualize a plan to transform the culture of an organization to become a caring, healing environment . . . supports nurse well-being, nurse-patient engagement, and a collaborative partnership among healthcare providers . . . create[s] avenues and opportunities for *nurse empowerment* . . . develops an infrastructure for an innovative, collaborative practice environment by providing *structural empowerment*" (p. 603)

As defined by Andrus and Shanahan (2016).

as a change agent—empowered with a vast array of leadership tools and perspectives—to better it. As the term *holistic* implies, we are integral to each other's growth and experience of nurse leadership and interconnected in the healing of the collective, helping the profession move from the current-day status of professional fragmentation experienced at institutional, national, and international levels to a unified, singular, and powerful whole through shared and mutually beneficial leadership.

■ EVOLUTIONARY LEADERSHIP ASSUMPTIONS

Several diverse and varying approaches are offered throughout this volume as possible paths to potentiating and realizing one's inner and outer nurse leader. Contributing authors have found inspiration and direction through committing to higher education and participating in interdisciplinary collaborations, through adversity and hardships, and through opportunities for self-growth they never could have imagined. In preparing oneself for this writer–reader dialogue, there are several assumptions that may assist you in getting the most out of this experience. These assumptions in no way intend to create global statements or definitions on what leadership is and they do not account for all cross-cultural considerations or limitations some leaders may currently experience. They are simply suggestions that have been extrapolated from the themes expressed by the

TABLE I.2 **Evolutionary Leadership Assumptions**

- Evolutionary leadership embraces vulnerability.
- Evolutionary leadership calls for a state of openness and self-awareness.
- Evolutionary leadership requires self-renewal and self-reflection.
- Evolutionary leadership implies a willingness to mature in ways of being, doing, thinking, seeing, and knowing.
- Evolutionary leadership acknowledges the difference between striving and perfectionism.
- Evolutionary leadership is "both/and" and not "either/or."
- Evolutionary leadership respects all voices in the room.
- Evolutionary leaders rehumanize work environments to promote ethical engagement and meaningful partnerships.
- Evolutionary leaders work to unveil and promote the truth.
- Evolutionary leaders allow for the transformation of self and systems.

authors herein. The list is in no particular order of importance or relevance and is by no means exhaustive of idealistic leadership qualities. Rather, it is intended to support the reader in releasing self-imposed limitations that may abbreviate or negate the learning possibilities while reading and reflecting upon the wisdom of the following chapters. See Table I.2 for a list of these Evolutionary Leadership Assumptions (ELAs) followed by further explanation in the following text.

EVOLUTIONARY LEADERSHIP EMBRACES VULNERABILITY

Brown (2012) defines vulnerability as "uncertainty, risk, and emotional exposure" and acknowledges it as "the birthplace of love, belonging, joy, courage, empathy, and creativity . . . the source of hope . . ., accountability, and authenticity . . . [and the way to gain] greater clarity in our purpose . . . and more meaningful . . . lives" (p. 34). Brown (2012) writes that to "dare greatly" is to meet the fear of vulnerability head-on and to muster the strength to be our fully expressed selves in environments that do not give any guarantees. Ultimately, she goes on to say, "*Vulnerability sounds like truth and feels like courage*" (p. 37).

If a nurse is going to own and demonstrate behaviors representative of leadership, such as questioning the tasks presented, forming individual opinions, taking risks, relationship-building, showing excitement about work, creating adventure, providing something to believe in, and inspiring others (Taffinder, 2006), then learning to navigate and embrace vulnerability is essential. Having the courage to embrace and relate to one's own vulnerability and that of another contributes to developing a compassionate practice and the ethical formation of nursing care (Thorup, Rundqvist, Roberts, & Delmar, 2012; Curtis, 2014). In fact, it has been noted that in environments where nurses' vulnerability is acknowledged and their whole person is honored and celebrated, beyond the limitations of their technical skills and abilities, human flourishing for both nurses and those they care for is possible (Sumner, 2013). (See Chapter 27 for more information on the importance of deepening our understanding of vulnerability.)

EVOLUTIONARY LEADERSHIP CALLS FOR A STATE OF OPENNESS AND SELF-AWARENESS

As a leader, as one whose actions will impact those around him or her either through influence or direct action, it is vital to maintain an attitude of openness. Openness requires suspending preconceived judgments and being willing to see things from another's point of view. It can also be thought of as "coming from nothing" or surrendering the automatic labels and meanings we tend to place on anything and everything that hinder our abilities to grow and consider life from a different perspective (DiMaggio, 2011a). "The *nothing* that's available for us to experience is not nothing as a negation of self . . . [but the ability] to create, design, and live with a freedom that's not available when we create from *something* . . . a clearing that frees [us] from [our] own self-imposed restrictions" (DiMaggio, 2011a, p. 18).

We can also think of the application of openness as the concept of the *beginner's mind* in Zen practice (Suzuki, 1983), or *unknowing*, releasing previously held beliefs as a way of experiencing a phenomenon in nursing practice (Munhall, 1993). Coming from nothing, employing a beginner's mind, and applying unknowing are all forms of openness that allow for a clean slate in the teaching–learning process and create space for new possibilities to emerge that are inaccessible when coming from something, employing an expert's lens, and honoring previously held knowing as fact.

Maturing in self-awareness and taking action to improve upon observed growth opportunities increases the nurse's capacity to provide caring and healing to self and others (Thornton & Mariano, 2016). As it pertains to the learning process and the work milieu, self-awareness can alert us when we are attaching to outdated beliefs and patterns that prevent us from being open and available to the concepts presented. Self-awareness may assist you in identifying and acknowledging those areas where you are resistant to growth and evolution, and may also engender the willingness necessary to surrender those self-imposed limitations that no longer serve you. (See Chapter 9 for more on how openness and self-awareness facilitate healing in nursing.)

EVOLUTIONARY LEADERSHIP REQUIRES SELF-RENEWAL AND SELF-REFLECTION

Nurse leaders "reflect on action to become aware of values, feelings, perceptions, and judgments that may affect actions, and they also reflect on their experiences to obtain insight for future practice" (Mariano, 2016, p. 66). These reflections are just one component of the self-renewal work needed to meet the anticipated demands of effective leadership. This ELA is deeply related to increasing self-awareness and helping one to remain open to what is available in the moment, as mentioned above, but maintains further implications in the development and application of leadership-based ethics. While the questions offered at the end of each chapter provide one avenue for ongoing and progressive introspection, self-renewal and self-reflection work can also take the form of journaling, storytelling, meditation, creative expression, and other mindfulness practices. These outlets allow the nurse leader to process the events and people around him or her, reframe experiences from a different perspective, reconnect and recommit to inner purpose and intention, and come to know the self at a deeper level. Quite simply: "Reflection is a means of renewal" (Pesut, 2005, p.1). Responsibility for self-renewal is necessary for the individual mental, emotional, and spiritual well-being of nurses who are committed to the delivery of humane, quality care (Pesut, 2012). Reflective practice, while shown to improve individual performance outcomes, can also elevate organizational consciousness when applied at a systems level (Sherwood & Horton-Deutsch, 2012, 2015).

EVOLUTIONARY LEADERSHIP IMPLIES A WILLINGNESS TO MATURE IN WAYS OF BEING, DOING, THINKING, SEEING, AND KNOWING

Willingness suggests one who is flexible and adaptive, tolerant and mindful, in touch with one's inner wisdom, and appreciative and stable in one's sense of self (Schaub & Schaub, 1997). All ways of being, doing, thinking, seeing, and knowing are invited to expand and mature throughout this book journey. It is not a task you are asked to complete. Rather, it is an offering that implores you to acknowledge and personalize that which is beneficial to your journey as a nurse leader from the wealth of the authors' lived experiences. As you read and reflect upon the histories of these nurse leaders, continue to ask yourself important questions such as, Who am I being? Does that way of being support me in realizing my highest potential as a nurse leader? Would doing things in a new way contribute toward the betterment of myself or another? How can I think about my leadership from a different vantage point? Would it benefit me to release what I know in order to relearn and reconsider? Leadership becomes stagnant without a willingness to unravel previously held, long-standing beliefs and emerge into a way of being-doing-thinking-seeing-knowing you may never have considered before. (See Chapters 13 and 30 for more on new ways of engaging the world.)

EVOLUTIONARY LEADERSHIP ACKNOWLEDGES THE DIFFERENCE BETWEEN STRIVING AND PERFECTIONISM

Brown (2010) states that the quest for perfectionism is very different from healthy striving and a desire to be one's best:

> Perfectionism is *not* about healthy achievement and growth. Perfectionism is the belief that if we live perfect, . . . we can minimize or avoid the pain of blame, judgment, and shame. . . . *Perfectionism is* not *self-improvement*. . . . Healthy striving is self-focused—*How can I improve?* Perfectionism is other-focused—*What will they think?* (pp. 94–95)

Healthy striving keeps our contributions as unique individuals and our journeys of self-growth, self-realization, and self-expression rooted in personal integrity. The process of striving helps us to understand that leadership is not about perfection and that the idea of perfect outcomes of any kind is a drain on our energy and interpersonal resources. In fact, the nurse leader who can acknowledge mistakes, ask for help, take risks, and share creative ideas without fear of others' judgments or opinions is living authentically (Brown, 2012). Striving is an inherent aspect of the human experience (Watson, 2012), the quest to become more evolved and grounded in who we are, the unyielding motivation to improve upon ourselves mentally, emotionally, and spiritually, and the desire to reconnect with our inner and highest wisdom. Striving calls for the authentic integration of the personal and professional: in other words, fostering the integrity of a unified self. Inversely, the path of perfectionism further compartmentalizes how we see ourselves, our lives, and our contributions. It is in our commitment to healthy striving and releasing the need for perfectionism that we find the freedom to embrace our individualism as nurse leaders (See Chapters 28 and 29 for more on merging the personal and professional for a healthy and unified self.)

EVOLUTIONARY LEADERSHIP IS "BOTH/AND" AND NOT "EITHER/OR"

There is no need for inner fragmentation: for a mental–emotional separation of our personal–professional life, as previously noted, or for the self-limitations that keep us from experiencing a reality of inclusivity. Nurse leaders do not have to choose between leadership methodologies: between being holistic or not, incorporating nurse theories or not, believing in caring as the essence of nursing or not. Leadership is an adventure into "both/and." As an intelligent and accountable nurse leader, you have the opportunity to select the concepts, ideas, and inquiries that will support you in becoming an effective force or positive change, as you are, with what you have to contribute at this point in time. Pressuring ourselves to choose between "either/or" diminishes the integrity of our innate human complexities and creates barriers to our wholeness. Living an undivided life and reading the pages that follow from a perspective of "both/and" can help one in learning how to shape an integral experience, derive meaning and value in community, teach and learn for transformation, and understand how to influence valuable and peaceful social change (Palmer, 2004). (See Chapter 4 for more on integral leadership and wholeness.)

EVOLUTIONARY LEADERSHIP RESPECTS ALL VOICES IN THE ROOM

Provision 1 of the American Nurses Association's (ANA, 2015) *Code of Ethics for Nurses With Interpretive Statements* is clear that "the nurse practices with compassion and respect for the inherent dignity, worth, and unique attributes of every person" (p. 1). Attention to this provision ensures that human dignity is preserved in all interactions and that people feel heard and acknowledged. As you read, you may see statements or opinions you disagree with or doubt. Feel free to reflect upon any resistance you encounter, but do your best to respect each chapter as an expression of an author's lived experience and as what the author knows to be true. Consider the context from which the insight was offered, glean what you can, and remain open to what it can teach you.

Provision 5 of the ANA (2015) *Code of Ethics* states that "the nurse owes the same duties to self as to others, including the responsibility to promote health and safety, preserve wholeness of character and integrity, maintain competence, and continue personal and professional growth" (p. 19). This means that self-respect is integral to this journey of learning and expansion. Strive to cultivate self-respect as you challenge yourself, explore new perspectives, and engage in self-development. (See Chapter 21 for more on the power of caring collaboration and leading from beside.)

EVOLUTIONARY LEADERS REHUMANIZE WORK ENVIRONMENTS TO PROMOTE ETHICAL ENGAGEMENT AND MEANINGFUL PARTNERSHIPS

Leaders and those they partner with thrive in environments where creativity is valued, vulnerabilities are embraced, and people are respected for who they are and what they bring to the table. Brown (2012) points out in the "Daring Greatly Leadership Manifesto":

> When learning and working are dehumanized—when you no longer see us and encourage our daring, or when you only see what we produce or how we perform—we disengage and turn away from the very things the world needs from us: our talent, our ideas, and our passion. (p. 212)

It is no secret that many health care environments have become dehumanized by succumbing to bureaucratic dictates (Watson, 2005, 2008) that focus on employee output, patient outcomes, insurance reimbursement, regulatory standards, and the adage, "Do more with less." Nursing has witnessed the submergence of its humanistic core values—its own dehumanization of value and purpose (Watson, 2012).

This fact is not something to resist or resent but something to acknowledge in one's evolving nurse leader journey. The business of health care is a reality that must be considered and included in nurse leadership dialogue at this time. All nurses need to be educated to understand and respect the places and spaces where business and nursing merge. The altruistic ethics of nursing are vital for the preservation of dignity wherever it is threatened,

> but empathy is only our starting point. It must be combined with focus and conviction, the toughness to know what needs to get done and the courage to follow through. . . . We will only succeed if we fuse a very hardheaded analysis with an equally soft heart. (Novogratz, 2009, p. 284)

In rehumanizing our learning experience, in coming to value both the experiential wisdom of others and our own individual uniqueness, we create new possibilities for our understanding of both nursing and leadership. (See Chapters 16, 19, and 23 for more on rehumanizing health care on a global scale.)

EVOLUTIONARY LEADERS WORK TO UNVEIL AND PROMOTE THE TRUTH

When nurses are taught how to complete a thorough pain assessment, they are reminded about the subjective truth of the patient: "Pain is whatever the patient says it is." It is with the same nonjudgmental and available approach that the nurse leader seeks out the subjective truth of the populations and communities they serve. Ethical commitments to beneficence and social justice guide our leadership on a truth-seeking journey to ensure the equitable access to and delivery of services. It is this mission to engage, acknowledge, and understand the truth of another that allows the nurse leader to be sure he or she is acting from a place of moral and ethical integrity. Quality, dignified health care is a human right and it is the nurse leader's role to honor and procure this truth. (See Chapters 5 and 11 for more on the role of nurse leaders in promoting truth through beneficence and social justice.)

EVOLUTIONARY LEADERS ALLOW FOR THE TRANSFORMATION OF SELF AND SYSTEMS

Transformation may be simply defined herein as allowing for the positive and reflective growth of self so that we are never the same. It is a bold action—a commitment to learning new ways of interacting with the surrounding world, exploring previously untapped parts of ourselves, and teaching-learning-role modeling with consideration to "what is" while believing in "what could be."

> Transformation has the power to upset the status quo, to unseat us from business as usual—it gives us a platform for being all we can . . . to live consistent with what we know is possible. . . . Transformation carries with it . . . a knowing that we have a choice about who we are. (Dimaggio, 2011b, p. 49)

Transformation of self and systems go hand-in-hand. As individuals transform how they engage with health care, the infrastructures they create and sustain will come to reflect their heightened ethics and values. Individual transformation on a mass scale advances systems toward the ideals of a caring society (See Chapters 17 and 26 for more on the transformation of self and systems.)

■ ONWARD

While reading the words and life lessons of the leaders presented here, allow your understandings of nursing and health and well-being and leadership to shift, expand, and mature into something beyond your current understanding. Release the need to control the experience and give yourself permission to remain vulnerable, open, and self-aware in the process; maintain your willingness to redefine how and who you are; observe your need for perfection and recommit to healthy striving; be inclusive and undivided in your journey; respect all voices and perspectives for what they offer; rehumanize the learning experience through an honoring of creativity, expression, and passion; and seek to unveil and promote your own truth. Transformation of self in this context allows one to embrace the current status of health care and the nursing profession with hope for positive and mutually beneficial change, guided and supported by an individually constructed, evolutionary vision of leadership.

The HLM and ELAs provide a framework and foundation from which to explore your personal understandings, expressions, and commitments to yourself as a nurse leader. Now is the time to put the theory into action to create new possibilities for yourself and those you are leading and will lead. I leave you to continue your journey with the inspired and powerful words of global citizen entrepreneur, author, change agent, and leader, Jacqueline Novogratz (2009):

> Every one of us . . . has something important to give. . . . *Build a vision for the people and recognize that no single source of leadership will make it happen.* . . . We have only one world . . . and the future really is ours to create, in a world we dare to imagine together. (pp. 281, 283–284)

■ REFERENCES

American Nurses Association (ANA). (2015). *Code of ethics for nurses with interpretive statements*, Washington, DC: Author.

Andrus, V. L., & Shanahan, M. (2016). Holistic leadership. In B. M. Dossey & L. Keegan (Eds.), *Holistic nursing: A handbook for practice* (7th ed., pp. 591–607). Burlington, MA: Jones & Bartlett.

Brown, B. (2010). *The gifts of imperfections: Letting go of who we think we should be and embracing who we are.* Center City, MN: Hazelden.

Brown, B. (2012). *Daring greatly: How the courage to be vulnerable transforms the way we live, love, parent, and lead.* New York, NY: Gotham.

Burns, J. M. (1978). *Leadership.* New York, NY: Harper & Row.

Curtis, K. (2014). Learning the requirements for compassionate practice: Student vulnerability and courage. *Nursing Ethics, 21*(2), 210–223.

Cutcliffe, J., & Cleary, M. (2015). Nursing leadership, missing questions, and the elephant(s) in the room: Problematizing the discourse on nursing leadership. *Issues in Mental Health Nursing, 36,* 817–825.

Day, D. D., Hand, M. W., Jones, A. R., Kay Harrington, N., Best, R., & LeFebvre, K. B. (2014). The oncology nursing society leadership competency project: Developing a road map to professional excellence. *Clinical Journal of Oncology Nursing, 18*(4), 432–436.

DiMaggio, J. (2011a). Something about nothing. In J. DiMaggio & N. Zapolski, *Conversations that matter: Insights & distinctions: Landmark essays* (Vol. 1., pp. 13–18). San Francisco, CA: Landmark Worldwide.

DiMaggio, J. (2011b). Big shoes to fill—there's no going back. In J. DiMaggio & N. Zapolski, *Conversations that matter: Insights & distinctions: Landmark essays* (Vol. 1., pp. 45–49). San Francisco, CA: Landmark Worldwide.

Dossey, B. M. (2016). Nursing: Holistic, integral, and integrative—local to global. In B. M. Dossey & L. Keegan (Eds.), *Holistic nursing: A handbook for practice* (7th ed., pp. 3–52). Burlington, MA: Jones & Bartlett.

Duffy, J. (2009). *Quality caring in nursing: Applying theory to clinical practice, education, and leadership.* New York, NY: Springer Publishing Company.

Duffy, J. (2015). Joanne Duffy's Quality-Caring Model©. In M. C. Smith & M. E. Parker (Eds.), *Nursing theories and nursing practice* (4th ed., pp. 393–410). Philadelphia, PA: F.A. Davis.

Elwell, S. M., & Elikofer, A. N. (2015). Defining leadership in a changing time. *Journal of Trauma Nursing, 22*(6), 312–214.

Frisina, M. (2011). *Influential leadership: Change your behavior, change your organization, change health care.* Chicago, IL: American Hospital Association.

Greenleaf, R. K. (2002). *Servant leadership: A journey into the nature of legitimate power and greatness* (25th anniversary ed.). Mahwah, NJ: Paulist Press.

Hart, P. L., Spiva, L., Baio, P., Huff, B., Whitfield, D., Law, T., . . . Mendoza, I. G. (2014). Medical-surgical nurses' perceived self-confidence and leadership abilities as first responders in acute patient deterioration events. *Journal of Clinical Nursing, 23*(19/20), 2769–2778.

Makaroff, K. S., Storch, J., Pauly, B., & Newton, L. (2014). Searching for ethical leadership in nursing. *Nursing Ethics, 21*(6), 642–658.

Mannix, J., Wilkes, L., & Daly, J. (2015). Grace under fire: Aesthetic leadership in clinical nursing. *Journal of Clinical Nursing, 24*(17/18), 2649–2658.

Mariano, C. (2016). Holistic nursing: Scope and standards of practice. In B. M. Dossey & L. Keegan (Eds.), *Holistic nursing: A handbook for practice* (7th ed., pp. 53–76). Burlington, MA: Jones & Bartlett.

Munhall, P. (1993). "Unknowing": Toward another pattern of knowing in nursing. *Nursing Outlook, 41*(3), 125–128.

Novogratz, J. (2009). *The blue sweater: Bridging the gap between rich and poor in an interconnected world.* New York, NY: Rodale.

Nyburg, J. (1998). *A caring approach in nursing administration.* Boulder, CO: University Press of Colorado.

Palmer, P. (2004). *A hidden wholeness: The journey toward an undivided life: Welcoming the soul and weaving community in a wounded world.* San Francisco, CA: Jossey-Bass.

Pesut, D. (2005). Foreword to The scholarship of reflective practice (resource paper). Retrieved from https://www.nursingsociety.org/docs/default-source/position-papers/resource_refl ective.pdf?sfvrsn=4

Pesut, D. (2012). Self-renewal. In H. R. Feldman, R. Alexander, M. J. Greenberg, M. Jaffee-Ruiz, A. McBride, M. McClure, & T. D. Smith (Eds.), *Nursing leadership: A concise encyclopedia* (pp. 337–338). New York, NY: Springer.

Plonien, C. (2015). Perioperative leadership: Using personality indicators to enhance nurse leader communication. *AORN Journal, 102*(1), 74–80.

Rosa, W. (2014a). Caring science and compassion fatigue: Reflective inventory for the individual processes of self-healing. *Beginnings, 34*(4), 18–20.

Rosa, W. (2014b). Nursing is separate from medicine: Advanced practice nursing and a transpersonal plan of care. *International Journal for Human Caring, 18*(2), 76–82.

Schaub, B., & Schaub, R. (1997). *Healing addictions: The vulnerability model of recovery.* Albany, NY: Delmar Publishers.

Shanahan, M. (2014). The BirchTree Center Model: Transforming healthcare with heart! *Beginnings, 34*(3), 6–9, 30.

Sherwood, G., & Horton-Deutsch, S (Eds.). (2012). *Reflective practice: Transforming education and improving outcomes.* Indianapolis, IN: Sigma Theta Tau International.

Sherwood, G., & Horton-Deutsch, S (Eds.). (2015). *Reflective organizations: On the frontlines of QSEN and reflective practice implementation.* Indianapolis, IN: Sigma Theta Tau International.

Spence Laschinger, H. K., Borgogni, L., Consiglio, C., & Read, E. (2015). The effects of authentic leadership, six areas of worklife, and occupational coping self-efficacy on new graduate nurses' burnout and mental health: A cross-sectional study. *International Journal of Nursing Studies, 52*(6), 1080–1089.

Stikes, R., Arterberry, K., & Logsdon, M. C. (2015). A nurse leadership project to improve health literacy on a maternal-infant unit. *Journal of Obstetric, Gynecologic, & Neonatal Nursing, 44*(5), 665–676.

Sumner, J. (2013). Human flourishing and the vulnerable nurse. *International Journal for Human Caring, 17*(4), 20–27.

Suzuki, S. (1983). *Zen mind, beginner's mind.* New York, NY: Weatherhill.

Taffinder, P. (2006). *The leadership crash course: How to create personal leadership value* (2nd ed.). Philadelphia, PA: Kogan Page.

Thornton, L., & Mariano, C. (2016). Evolving from therapeutic to holistic communication. In B. M. Dossey & L. Keegan (Eds.), *Holistic nursing: A handbook for practice* (7th ed., pp. 465–478). Burlington, MA: Jones & Bartlett.

Thorup, C. B., Rundqvist, E., Roberts, C., & Delmar, C. (2012). Care as a matter of courage: Vulnerability, suffering and ethical formation in nursing care. *Scandinavian Journal of Caring Sciences, 26*(3), 427–435.

Watson, J. (2005). *Caring science as sacred science.* Philadelphia, PA: F.A. Davis

Watson, J. (2008). *Nursing: The philosophy and science of caring* (Rev. ed.). Boulder, CO: University Press of Colorado.

Watson, J. (2012). *Human caring science* (2nd ed.). Sudbury, MA: Jones & Bartlett.

PART I

Laying the Groundwork

Mindful and Intentional: Embodying Interbeing Awareness in Grassroots Leadership

Jeanne Anselmo

We touch dimensions of the sacred each day in nursing. Understanding how spirit and our sense of interconnectedness, meaning, and purpose impact our health and life continuously offers us new opportunities for growth, renewal, deepening, and learning. Whether we are new nurses or experienced practitioners, the journey continues to unfold.
    —Anselmo and O'Brien (2013, p. 226)

■ WHY NURSING?

I would like to begin by offering a meditation practice, the first of three kitchen-table wisdoms found in this chapter. If you like, you can do this practice along with me as you read this. Thich Nhat Hanh, also known as Thay, taught me this practice in the early 1990s in the kitchen of a prewar building on the Upper West Side of Manhattan. It was late afternoon and Thay was seated at a small table covered with a blue-and-white checkered oilcloth as a few of us drank small cups of tea. We had all been sitting quietly together when Thay slowly raised his right hand in the air above his head and began to glide it vertically downward in front of him and shared something like, "All the ancestors of the spiritual and blood families who have gone before us." Pausing at an imaginary midpoint for just an instant, he then continued his hand's gentle movement downward, "And all those descendants yet to be born." He then moved his hand to the far left and moved it across his body to the right on an invisible horizontal axis, "And all people and all species alive in the world in this moment." He then raised his hand once again above his head and began drawing a circle in the air around the invisible horizontal and vertical axes as if his hand were a great brush, offering, "I let go of the idea that I am this body and my life span is limited" (Nhat Hanh, 2007, p. 48).

The practice Thich Nhat Hanh shared with us that afternoon touched a deep truth, a truth that I knew from my own inner experience. That is, each of our lives has arisen from an interconnected web of ancestors, nature, and life, and the gifts we offer the world have also arisen from both what we have inherited and what we have cultivated. As nurses and as leaders, we each have a great inheritance of love, wisdom, compassion, skillfulness, and awareness that comes from nursing, our families, and our spiritual and land ancestors. Knowing our multirooted map anchors us in a great mystery that supports and guides our lives and practice of nursing in ways beyond our own efforts and awareness.

I am aware that this year marks my 40th anniversary as a nurse. For these past decades, nursing is and has been a path of personal and professional self-development and spiritual discovery, an awakening to self, compassion, life's mystery, and our interconnectedness (what I now call *Interbeing*). In many ways, I take no credit for what has unfolded along this path. I say this not with any self-deprecation, for I acknowledge the deep intention, study, and effort I have invested in my life and this nursing path and have done so with real heart and commitment. But shared in the meditation in the preceding text, along with my own efforts and presence, are the gifts and challenges of those who have gone before, those who will come after, and all beings, whether animal, plant, mineral, or human, alive in the here and now. For each of us, all these dimensions come together, composing a life, composing a path, offering a life message, a life teaching. Every nurse has the capacity to embody her or his gifts and offer them to life, to those we serve: our patients, families, and communities. In this way, every nurse is a leader, offering a life teaching through her or his embodied study and practice of nursing, paraphrasing what Thich Nhat Hanh shares, and Gandhi before him: "Our life is our message." So in this spirit, I offer a few pivotal awareness moments still alive in my heart that embody this nurse's life message and path of nursing. I offer these in the hope that you can touch the wisdom and wonder in yourself.

I would never have imagined that as a first-year new nursing student, listening to Dean Eleanor Lambertsen's orientation welcome to us as the incoming class of 1975 at Cornell New York Hospital School of Nursing, I would experience a moment of awakening. And yet I did. Her talk focused on what lay ahead for us as we embarked on our path to becoming a nurse. As I listened, something opened in me as clarity, a larger sense of self, of life, and a deeper and greater experience of nursing. In that moment, I experienced nursing as a great vehicle to support human beings embody being truly alive, fully human, and humane. I became aware that for this vision to unfold, nursing's gifts would have to be deeply embedded and embodied within humanity in all forms, beyond what was known as nursing in 1973. It also became clear that many of my previous life experiences had led me to this moment of listening to this orientation. This made becoming a nurse a real calling that had been evolving all my life, even from before I was born. Both sides of my family were immigrants to this country, carrying with them deep spiritual Catholic roots, Irish on my mother's side and Sicilian on my father's, so healing, community, service, connection to nature, and spirituality were just natural elements of my life growing up. Though both of my parents' lives included what many immigrants experienced—poverty, illness, early death of loved ones, and discrimination—they also carried personal true spiritual aspiration, love, connection to family, community, nature, and strong faith.

My mother's deeply devotional prayer life opened doors for me to St. Theresa of Avila, St. Therese (The Little Flower), St. Francis of Assisi, and Thomas Merton; my father's spiritual life brought me many devotional blessings, play, and the positive vision of Dr. Norman Vincent Peale. Mom's family were farmers, intuitive dreamers, and horse whisperers in Ireland, and district nurses and handy women in northern England, and they all knew herbal and natural remedies to care for illnesses. My father and his brothers learned natural remedies working in their uncle's pharmacy in the Hell's Kitchen section of Manhattan during the early 20th century. For both sides of my family, healing was local and natural, providing health care for the poor, whether through the village handy women, like my mother's Aunt Alice, or English district nurses, like her cousin Rose, or pharmacists, like my great-uncle Peter of Anselmo's Pharmacy. In poor mill and mining villages, handy women "took the place of doctors (who were few) and prepared poultices, salts, herbs, and offered nursing care" (M.D. Anselmo, personal communication, 1989). Great-uncle Peter was known to treat whoever needed care, regardless of their ability to pay. His inspiration led to a number of his nephews (my uncles) following in his footsteps, becoming pharmacists themselves and studying at St. John's University School of Pharmacy. In the 1990s and 2000s, I had a family full-circle continuation experience when the faculty of St. John's School of Pharmacy, the same school my father's brothers attended, invited me to teach the current pharmacy students about holistic nonpharmacological approaches to healing.

Entering nursing school, I was not truly aware of how much my family members' gifts and efforts had guided me toward not only becoming a nurse, but also becoming a holistic nurse focused on natural approaches to healing, especially for the disadvantaged. As a student, I also was unaware of the true impact Cornell's faculty would have, as they introduced me to Dr. Martha Rogers's little-known Science of Unitary Human Beings, which offered a new revolutionary quantum-based theory in nursing. Many of Cornell's faculty members were students of both Dr. Rogers and Dr. Delores (Dee) Krieger at New York University's (NYU's) graduate nursing program. In the fall of 1973, we students would soon be struggling to comprehend Rogers's new paradigm and reflect on Dee Krieger and Dora Kunz's therapeutic touch, a practice of *Renaissance Nursing* (Krieger, 1981).

Cornell's Dean Lambertsen had a commitment to cultivating nursing leadership for a new revolutionary era of wellness health care, so its nursing program focused on the profession as a path of lifelong study, evolution, and continuous learning. Cornell developed a progressive, yet controversial, curriculum offering more nursing science classroom hours and fewer hospital-based clinical hours, the backbone of most other programs at the time. This radical departure from standard nursing education supported our capacities for developing innovative practice but became a source of criticism in some circles for both Cornell's program and its graduates. Dean Lambertsen was a woman of great vision and determination.

> She pioneered the concept of "team nursing," revolutionizing the organization and delivery of nursing and health care by placing registered professional nurses in the primary interdisciplinary leadership role. . . .
>
> Her influence made it possible for generations of clinical nurse specialists and nurse practitioners to practice their art and science independently. (American Nurses Association [ANA], 2012)

During the 1970 senior convocation, then newly appointed Dean Lambertsen spoke of "nurses capable of developing innovative patterns of patient care while others practiced within the framework of the existing structure" (Fondiller, 2007, p. 185). Truly, the program at Cornell gave me a foundation for adapting to changes in health care and developing new and innovative approaches, not only within nursing but also within holistic nursing, applied psychophysiology, and biofeedback, and later within social justice and public interest lawyering.

The spirit and vision of celebrated alumna, community health innovator, and women's rights activist Lillian Wald was also a very active dimension of our education at Cornell, as all students served as community health nurses at Wald's Visiting Nurse Services of New York (VNSNY), founded in 1891. Wald's commitment to social reform and improving the quality of life for the poor and disadvantaged was reflected at VNSNY and at Henry Street Settlement founded in 1893. Wald told her nurses: "Nursing is love in action, and there is no finer manifestation of it than the care of the poor and disabled in their own homes" (Lundy & Bender, 2016, p. 90). Wald's vision of nursing as "love in action" not only guided my own practice working in the community and underserved areas, but also surfaced decades later in a new form when I was invited to teach young social justice law students. I shared that I saw them as healers, building beloved communities, and they responded with echoes of Lillian Wald, asking me to teach them "law based in love."

All these elements of the past, present, and possible future were woven into that first awakening that I experienced during orientation in 1973. It was a reorienting of my heart, a fresh understanding and perspective of nursing as a spiritual path of practice, which continues within me today. From that moment on, my inner compass became activated within my nursing study and practice. This did not mean that I did not experience disappointments, challenges, and frustrations that were a part of nursing, especially during the 1970s, when nursing was far from being positively valued (not only by some men, but also by some progressive women of the day). But from then on, my path as a nurse was connected to an inner awareness that has continued to unfold and guide me beyond what may be visible and clear. This inner guidance has offered a path I could never have imagined. The links and connections that have led me along this path may seem in some ways obvious now, but were not obvious or clear to me then.

■ EARLY IMPRESSIONS

As a student nurse, I had the opportunity to learn a great lesson as I cared for a first-time young mother during my labor and delivery clinical rotation. "Sarah" was having a difficult labor and though I had yet to learn therapeutic touch, I discovered, as I was breathing with her and massaging her back, that a deeper connection unfolded between the two of us, so much so that my hands seemed to know exactly where to go. Everything became *flow*. I realized that Sarah and I had touched a true communion in the nurse–patient relationship, but that this was not able to be supported by the staff nurses on the floor, though they were doing their best. At the end of my shift, my instructor had me leave even though Sarah pleaded that I be allowed to stay. We both had been touched by the deep connection we shared and I saw the beauty and healing potential of cultivating a nurse–patient relationship akin to what doulas or midwives offer for all clients/patients; for some time thereafter, I strongly considered becoming a nurse midwife.

Years later, I established a community-based holistic nursing private practice in my hometown, in which I midwifed the deathing of a small number of clients who had cancer or AIDS. Doing so, I was able to travel with them and their families through their healing journey of illness and end-of-life experience (Hostutler, Kennedy, Mason, & Schorr, 2000). This healing relationship with my clients became a key dimension of my private practice and required a deeper self-awareness and more profound level of personal and professional self-care, which included personal retreats. These seeds for midwifing within my professional practice may have been sown in me through my great-aunt Alice, the handy woman delivering babies on Puddlers Row in North England, and through caring for Sarah as a student.

Upon graduation, I chose to work at Memorial Sloan Kettering Cancer Center (MSKCC), as it would take me "into the fire" of my own growing edge, allowing me the opportunity to be with life-challenging illness, face fears, and be with death and dying. In 1975, working at MSKCC was considered high risk, as the incidence of cancer among MSKCC staff was far greater than at any other institution, so there was a belief, at that time, that cancer was contagious. This risk did not factor into my decision; my inner guidance did. Working at MSKCC opened me to deep teachings of the heart and offered many opportunities for cultivating equanimity (nondiscrimination or inclusiveness).

A very meaningful experience of equanimity unfolded as I was assigned both an elderly Holocaust survivor and a young male from Argentina, who was the child of a former Nazi soldier. Both had cancer and both became teachers of my heart as I served, supported, and cared for them. Though they did not know each other, together they opened my heart to a deeper calling and understanding of nursing: the gifts of compassion, going beyond all concepts of discrimination, views of right and wrong, touching our shared humanity, and cultivating true openhearted inclusiveness within ourselves. Once begun, this inclusive opening, expanding process of the heart has continued to guide my study and practice of moving beyond discrimination and the boundaries of nonduality.

■ PROFESSIONAL EVOLUTION/CONTRIBUTION

I continued to work with people living with cancer and AIDS for the next 25 years and learned through lived experience that

> Nurses have access to clients in their most vulnerable . . . moments—the birth of a child, the moment of death, and the . . . joys, and fears of life. Many times we are the spiritual support that holds the hand, witnesses the first . . . or the last breath, and offers solace and understanding. (Anselmo & O'Brien, 2013, p. 239)

Through this work, I found that the same levels of love and attention were required for both illness and wellness care, including the wellness self-care needed to sustain oneself as a nurse. In fact, I realized it was essential to integrate wellness for all into every form of health care, especially during end-of-life practice. Walking in the last moments and breaths of life with my patients opened me to experience a greater connection to all that is, the birthless/deathless consciousness that continues, whether we are in bodily form or not.

After leaving MSKCC in 1976, I was hired as a nurse biofeedback and stress management therapist at an executive health clinic in Manhattan. The position offered the autonomy of the nursing private practice Lambertsen envisioned, while offering the wellness-based, nonpharmacological holistic interventions of biofeedback and relaxation embedded with the health care teaching and counseling that Krieger and Rogers espoused. Most biofeedback practitioners of the time were not nurses, so my inclusion of health care teaching, counseling, and hands-on healing, combined with my comfort level with experimental protocols after working at MSKCC, offered unique nursing dimensions and contributions to biofeedback professional practice.

In the 1970s, it was not widely accepted that the psychophysiology of mind and body (let alone mind, body, and spirit) were interconnected and influenced each other. Therefore, I was fiercely challenged as I taught at biofeedback workshops to researchers, neurologists, psychiatrists, and psychologists, who seemed appalled that a young nurse was attempting to teach them something that flew in the face of all they had studied and believed as scientific fact. Rather than trying to convince them that mind and emotions influenced physiological responses, I offered them the opportunity to experience biofeedback themselves and let their own experience provide their answer. The unbiased technology registered a psychophysiological response reflecting their cognitive or emotional states and, most times, opened them to the possibility of a new understanding of themselves and psychophysiology: body, mind, and emotion connectedness.

I have continued to offer this practice as an experiment for nurses developing body-mind-spirit self-awareness (Anselmo, 2016). Biofeedback was also a method for tracking psychophysiological responses to therapeutic touch by NYU graduate nurse researchers. In 1979, I was invited to join Janet Macrae, Marie Therese Connell Meehan, and Patricia Heidt as core faculty of NYU's postgraduate, yearlong Integrative Nursing Certificate Program, which hosted many of the nursing pioneers found in Dee Krieger's 1981 book *Renaissance Nursing*.

Graduates from that program continued to embrace a nursing pioneering spirit and practice over the ensuing decades and became innovative leaders themselves. I felt humbled and grateful to have the opportunity to study, share practice, and teach with these nursing visionaries, whether students or faculty. Among this rich tapestry of nursing heart paths, Marie Therese Connell offered us her definition of nursing at the time: "Nursing is tending the flow of Life." *Tending the flow of life* spoke deeply to a larger communion and commitment that nursing has with life. Her words echoed Nightingale's deep resonance with nature, our communion with this planet, and all our relations. Being with the flow of life, practicing healing and therapeutic touch, working with patients, and reflecting on myself led me to naturally change my diet and lifestyle, explore spiritual practices and study healing, energy practices, and oneness/interconnectedness with Native Americans, Chi Kung masters, and Armenian healers. All these teachers embodied this communion and connection with life, sharing nondual wisdom, what some call "Big Sky Mind" or "All That Is."

As I went deeper into studying healing, my work evolved and I began to be called to work in community health projects in underserved communities, consult in larger organizations and corporations, and serve in leadership positions. While working in these projects, the vital importance of community, especially addressing larger systems challenges, became even more evident. A vision of beloved community, in which every member is also a leader/healer, arose within me and I then viewed and experienced each community as a spiritual community, whether they did so themselves or not. Bringing this spiritual dimension into the community's and my own mutual awareness elevated our work together and offered new collective potentials beyond what seemed available or possible at the time.

In 1989, I was elected the first nurse and first woman president of the Biofeedback Society of New York State. It marked a turning point in the organization's history, for even though biofeedback was founded on interdisciplinary principles, practice, understanding, collaboration, and insight (all of which had been very inspirational and resonant with my own values and vision), neither its board members nor the actual workings of the organization, like many at that time, reflected such an enlightened view. One of my goals as president was to actualize the true interdisciplinary potential professional biofeedback held. So, over the next few years, and not without great challenges and resistance, the organization became more inclusive, reflecting the professionals, healers, and educators who made up this unique and diverse community, as well as beginning a multiyear expansion from a state to a regional organization. This vision continues to be lived today.

In late 1989, Susan Luck (see Chapter 24) and I met at her East Village apartment where, at her kitchen table, we began to weave together the first threads of Holistic Nursing Associates for teaching and mentoring nurses interested in healing and transforming themselves and their practice. Susan knew Bonney Schaub (see Chapter 27), a nurse psychosynthesis practitioner, who we invited to join this new initiative. Together, the three of us wove together our knowledge, experience, and practice offering a continuing education certificate program called Caring for Ourselves, Caring for Others: The Holistic Nursing Process. Our goals were to support nurses to reconnect with their roots, values, and inspirations that first brought them to nursing, learn holistic self-care, develop professional holistic nursing patient care practices, and pioneer new paths for both living and implementing these practices, all within an unfolding, safe, and supportive nursing community. For 10 years, nurses found their way to us in the West Village and began their own journey of personal and professional transformation. What arose within these participants was truly inspiring for us all and, at times, offered stunning transformations, as some were impelled to leave jobs and personal relationships no longer serving them and began to journey into their own personal and professional unknown, while others found renewal for reentering their work, relationships, and roles, imbuing them with new vision, compassion, and practice skills.

In the mid-1990s, a small grassroots movement in the Northeast arose to address a nationwide challenge to the profession of nursing. Begun as a reorganization of health care, it included downsizing and reengineering of hospitals, massive nursing layoffs, and a campaign to replace licensed RNs with less-costly hospital-trained technicians. Local nurses were understandably caught by the fear generated by this crisis, and at one local nursing conference, I was asked to offer stress management to help address this challenge. I realized that what was being called for was more than stress management, which could possibly mask what was happening. This was nursing's health challenge/life-threatening illness, as we faced our own uncertain future, both individually and collectively.

At the time, it was unclear if nursing, as a profession, would survive, so walking into this unknown, unclear, and uncertain future, I saw this challenge as an invitation for personal and collective reflection, whether this was truly the end of our profession or not. Along with stress reduction, I invited reflection on the following: How would we want our collective/profession to spend these precious days together during this great challenge? What healing would we want to offer ourselves and each other, and model for the world? As I contemplated these questions myself, a cognition arose that we needed a way to apply our collective gifts and insights as well as embrace and be with the pain, fear, loss, and challenge unfolding.

To explore these questions, a "kitchen cabinet" of friends and colleagues gathered in Soho around Barbara Glickstein's kitchen table, including Barbara, Diana Mason (see Endnote), Barbara Joyce (then New York State Nurses Association's [NYSNA's] president), and myself. Together we crafted a grassroots nursing movement, which continued for the next five years. Holding nursing town meetings, we offered inspiration, time for sharing, meditation, and reflection, while updating nurses with reliable information from NYSNA regarding the crisis and encouraged the creation of healing circles so nurses had continuing local support. These simple approaches helped build community, reduce fear of the unknown, and reduce the chaos generated by the continuous unexpected layoffs and a dearth of communication from administration to staff nurses and managers.

As the crisis continued to mount, we realized that we needed to expand our efforts by reaching out regionally to as many nursing organizations as possible. Gathering a diverse group of nurse leaders who represented local and national nursing organizations, we planned a regional nursing summit. Our monthly planning meetings, truly, were the living summit process we aspired to for our community as we shared our hearts, cultivated our intention to heal our personal and collective fears, and grieved the loss of our colleagues and the failing health care system in which we had attempted to sustain quality patient care. As we dialogued, we realized that we needed to present possibilities for the future, so we invited innovators from across the country, including our friends and colleagues at the University of Minnesota, Mary Jo Kreitzer (see Chapter 8), Sue Towey, Joanne Disch, and Barbara Dossey of Holistic Nursing Consultants (see Chapter 4), to share their visionary initiatives. These initiatives offered inspiration and an alternative to solely being angry, numb, in denial, or paralyzed by fear. Guided by Native American council circle wisdom, our intention was to gather, share our collective wisdom, learn from each other, and heal together so we could return to our lives and "dance with the chaos." Nurses were invited to enter the summit heart-to-heart, nurse-to-nurse, leaving roles, positions, titles, and credentials at the door. To support and grow grassroots nursing leadership, we attempted to turn expectations upside down by mentoring staff nurses and students to be facilitators at the summit rather than turning to the innumerable, highly skilled leaders attending. These grassroots nurses, who did not see themselves as leaders, facilitated sharing circles, which included national/international nurse leaders, thereby offering real-life leadership experience and building their self-confidence.

Our first regional summit was held at Omega in 1997, followed by another in 1998, mirroring the same yearlong presummit process, but this time its focus was diversity and community. To emphasize our deep and true commitment to explore our society's most challenging and important issues, we opened the second summit with a joint welcome by nurses of color and those not of color introducing a video of Lani Guinier speaking about race as society's "canary in a coalmine" and the importance of grassroots/bottom-up change (Guinier, 1998). Many nurses attending were moved to tears by our collective's willingness and openness to look into issues of race and racism from the very inception of our gathering. Both summits were committed to healing the wounds in ourselves, our profession, and relationships with and between each other, as a foundation for taking on the systemic challenges unfolding. They offered inspiration, community, connection, and innovation in a time of real crisis. Our collective efforts culminated in a presentation by members of the summit community at the 100th Anniversary London Conference of the International Council of Nurses in 1999. In many respects, the vision and contributions of this book are a continuation of this movement, for many contributors found in this book were a vital part of these summits.

In 2000, Rachel Gluckstein—a friend, colleague, and gifted nurse yoga and shiatsu teacher/practitioner working in community health and private practice—and I both received calls from Fred Rooney, founding director of the Community Legal Resource Network (CLRN) at the City University of New York (CUNY) School of Law. Fred wanted to provide law graduates yoga and meditation techniques to assuage the mounting drug self-medication and alcohol abuse and in order to relieve the painful realities and stresses found in social justice law practice. CUNY was one of the most diverse law schools in the country, drawing to its program nontraditional law students from underserved communities from across the country and around the world. These graduates then planned to return to their home communities to offer previously unavailable local access to justice. They were a legal interpolation of Wald's vision of community nursing serving the poor and, like my own alma mater, Cornell, CUNY was based on a progressive educational vision. Its founders wove principles of humanistic psychology into its core structure for teaching "Law in the Service of Human Needs" (as their maxim states).

At first, I was greatly conflicted about the possibility of teaching outside my commitment to community health and my own private practice clients. Then, Rachel offered the first yoga class on September 10, 2001, the day before September 11. All my doubts fell away on 9/11, as my inner compass helped to reorient me once again and I recognized that we were being *called* to this law school, no matter how foreign or unlikely it appeared at the time. Almost as confirmation, on September 13, when the law school reopened, I was invited by Dean Kris Glen to address the entire law school community and share how meditation could help us heal during this time of uncertainty, as well as assist law students with their studies. My planned one-hour visit for a meditation class turned into five hours as I was introduced to faculty, staff, and students throughout the school.

There was no roadmap for this contemplative law venture; it had not been done before. These students were living a deep calling, intention, and commitment, as they were coming from and going to what Thich Nhat Hanh called the "blue flame," the hottest part of society's candle, living and working in some of the most disenfranchised, marginalized, forgotten, violent, and abandoned communities found in our culture and the world. I could see myself as a young nursing student in them, as they too were deeply committed to relieving suffering of those in need, especially the poor.

I began to investigate more about the history of the law school and through my inquiries, discovered that every dean since the law school's inception meditated. To support my initial efforts, I began breathing with "not knowing" and called on those who came before us, including the previous deans, Dr. Martin Luther King Jr., the humanistic psychologists who inspired the progressive curriculum, Thich Nhat Hanh, Merton, Nightingale, Wald, and the Native American ancestors who had originally lived on this small plot of land in Flushing, Queens, inviting from them all of their guidance and support. I found myself hugging exhausted and beleaguered students as I made my way down law school hallways and, like my teachers Thich Nhat Hanh and Dora Kunz, I wanted to offer them an engaged mindfulness practice based in compassion and self-care that was applicable to the challenges they were facing. I shared how to apply the energy of mindfulness to their everyday life and work and included what I had learned myself about resilience, self-compassion, and self-care from my studies and practice as a holistic nurse in underserved communities.

As in the past, I found myself once again in a situation with few resources and little support, but shared that we could be fueled by inner resources—loving-kindness, forgiveness, compassion practices, and a growing energy of mindful awareness within our community. Based on more than two decades' experience of transforming health care through the inclusion of new healing paradigms, I explored, discovered, and included new worldviews of legal practice, offering healing alternatives for contemplative law students to forge their own pioneering path in social justice and public interest law. I invited pioneering attorneys who wielded innovative law initiatives to our contemplative, communitarian, and nonadversarial gatherings—the ushering in of a new healing legal paradigm. Sustaining social justice through love, when traditionally it had been fueled only by anger and outrage, is a real *koan* (unanswerable paradoxical story or question that can open us to a greater insight/awakening, beyond reason) for our society. By including therapeutic presence exercises (Anselmo, Bryant, & Goode, 2006) and heart-centered compassion practices to offset the heavy intellectual demands of law, my intention was that these students be guided not only by their heads but also by their hearts, their connection to purpose, and their spiritual awareness to become inspirational leaders themselves, ready to continuously transform themselves, their law practice, and society. These contemplative law students were being fostered by both law and nursing as they entered social justice. As such, they were spiritual offspring of both healing and justice, hopefully holding the best of what both our professions had to offer.

I found that my experimentation with personal and professional contemplative practice within the law offered a universal understanding that transcended any professional differences and emphasized our connectedness and the shared human experience of encountering suffering in ourselves and in the world, and underscored the vital importance of self-care in the face of human challenges. In 2015, our community, including faculty members Victor Goode, Maria Arias, Liz Newman, and myself, celebrated our 15th anniversary. Now hundreds of our students and graduates, along with once-skeptical colleagues, are practicing, writing, and teaching contemplative practice in law and social justice (Anselmo & Goode, 2016; Anselmo, Bryant & Goode, 2006).

■ MORAL/ETHICAL FOUNDATION

After the tragic death of a peace activist friend in the late 1980s, I found myself in deep shock, beyond the reach of any of the spiritual traditions I had studied or practiced. Unexpectedly, I learned of Vietnamese Buddhist monk and Zen master, Thich Nhat Hanh, who was coming to the United States to offer healing to the American soldiers who had killed his own people. This was truly remarkable to me, as I was trying to heal from the tragic death of one friend, while Thay had lost hundreds of friends and family and thousands in his country and yet was coming to support those who called him an enemy.

In 1966, he founded the Order of Interbeing, a lay and monastic order practicing nonviolent precepts to guide their mindful, peaceful, and engaged actions and helping those in the midst of the war. For his work and stand for peace for all people, Thich Nhat Hanh was both exiled from his own country as well as nominated for the Nobel Peace Prize by Dr. Martin Luther King Jr. (King, 1967) and was called "my brother" by Thomas Merton (Merton, 1966, p. 18). Connecting with Thich Nhat Hanh—who, like Dr. King, Florence Nightingale, and Lillian Wald before him, has given his whole life to his deepest purpose, intention, and aspiration—and practicing in his Plum Village community of committed, engaged mindfulness practitioners, applying engaged mindfulness practice to my own life reflects my own true commitment to live authentically with integrity and intention. This living practice has enriched, opened, and deepened my spiritual path as a holistic nurse and as a human being. Many people ask me why I am vegan, do not drink alcohol, and make the life choices I make. Studying and practicing holistic nursing and healing since 1975, as shared previously, I found a natural coherence unfolding within me, moving me to change life habits incrementally, over time, without effort. The healing I was practicing was also healing me, working synergistically as a mutual simultaneous interaction, guiding me to live more in accord with my experience of nature's wisdom and my deepest aspiration to be compassionate to all beings and the Earth. So, eating less meat until I became a vegan and eliminating caffeine and alcohol were all just natural progressions over the first two decades of my holistic nursing practice.

Then, in 1991, I met Thay and heard his mindfulness trainings, both the 5 (Sitzman & Watson, 2014) and the 14 (Order of Interbeing, 2012). As I studied and practiced these trainings in my life and work, they elevated my own natural precepts to a new level. The 14 mindfulness trainings were written as Interbeing insights and global ethics in response to deeply held, underlying, unhealed personal and collective misunderstandings and disharmonies that lead to war, and, therefore, are a universal teaching for our times. Through living these trainings, Thay's early students developed a resilient and healing path through some of Vietnam's most difficult moments. Each training is an invitation to live more consciously, to *be* peace, and develop awareness of the ways we contribute to violence and suffering in ourselves, others, and the world. Reflecting a universal humanism, beyond the confines of religions, they focus on growing our understanding, compassion, and openness, beyond ideas of right or wrong, to become insightful practice partners. They do not require that we agree with each training to practice with them, as they remind us of the deep interconnectedness that is alive in every dimension of life and help us become conscious of the impact and implications of our choices, actions, words, and understandings or misunderstandings.

Along with these trainings, I have found the work of Laura van Dernoot Lipsky's (2009) Trauma Stewardship and David Berceli's (2008) Trauma Releasing Exercises (TRE) to be invaluable. These two resources have been a wonderful accompaniment to my mindfulness practice, helping me grow my capacity to be with what is, while becoming more attuned to my body's natural capacity to shake off tension and steward trauma, supporting my best efforts to embody inclusiveness, consciousness, healing, and compassion, especially during times of real personal and community challenge. I found these to be especially helpful resources for rebalancing after a car accident in 2010 and helping my local meditation community recover from the impact of Hurricane Sandy in 2012. At Blue Cliff monastery retreats, I integrated TRE, Trauma Stewardship, and Neff's (2011) Self-Compassion practice, with mindfulness and loving-kindness practice (Anselmo, 2016) during a retreat for healing professionals and one for Iraq and Afghanistan veterans, their families, and caregivers, with very positive responses.

From my own personal and community mindfulness practice experience, what has become even more clear is that integrating mindfulness practice *with* personal and collective values/precepts/guideposts *within* a committed contemplative community offers real potential for personal and community well-being and resilience, especially during the inevitable times of natural disaster or societal crisis (Anselmo, 2016). I have realized that throughout my life and career, there have been ever-widening circles of Interbeing awareness (all things change/are impermanent); we are not separate selves but inter-are with all beings in the cosmos; all is a continuation of all who have gone before and all yet to come and we are *life* without boundaries, like energy, neither created nor destroyed; and self-compassion (compassion for self, all beings, the Earth) naturally unfolds within me and guides me to deepen my commitment to Zen and holistic nursing practice.

I was ordained as a lay monastic in the Order of Interbeing by Thich Nhat Hanh in 1995 and received lamp transmission from him as a teacher/dharma holder in 2011 on the 45th anniversary of the founding of the Order. Traveling to Hanoi with Thay and the Plum Village international delegation during his last visit to Vietnam for the 2008 UNESCO Vesak Celebration and Conference, I held a Nightingale moment at a former Communist compound. Later that same week, I presented on "Mindfulness and Social Justice," weaving together the inspirational threads and teachers of my life: Nightingale, Wald, Thich Nhat Hanh, and Dr. King. During the presentation, I evoked Dr. King's definition of *justice*: "Justice is love correcting everything that stands against love."

■ VISION

Over the last decade, Barbara Joyce, Jane Seley, Linda Saal (another Cornell graduate), Rosemary Sullivan, and I have worked within the former Cornell-New York Hospital (now New York-Presbyterian, NYP) to reintegrate the holistic wellness teachings and quantum nursing theory originally taught at Cornell and NYU 40 years ago. During these last few years, Jane Seley and the Cross Campus Nursing Practice Council have developed, received approval for, and integrated the NYP hospital policy on integrative health care modalities (IHM). Staff nurses who have gone through the NYP holistic nursing education program are now able to offer bedside holistic nursing practices and easily chart IHM. In the 1970s, Dee Krieger predicted that this integration would take 20 years, and it has proved, at least in New York, to be more challenging than she imagined, taking twice as long. At NYP, we offer not only holistic/integrative practice and the reintroduction of the Rogerian theory, but also the work of nurse theorists Jean Watson (see Chapter 16), Margaret Newman, Rosemary Parse, Elizabeth Barrett, and Barbara Dossey, as well as Nightingale and Wald. In this work, my intention has been, once again, to seed new inspiration and practice for this new generation at NYP, so they themselves can further this unfolding continuation begun more than 100 years ago.

If I were to invite any consideration for what vital work we, as nurse leaders, have yet to complete, I would invite that we mindfully embody true *public health* for our global family to support well-being and justice for all, including the Earth herself. This would require a reorientation of our hearts beginning with a mindfulness-based personal and collective examination of ourselves and our society. If done with compassion and insight, such a reflection may open us to a new consciousness to understand the impact that we and our society have on each other, our global family, and our planet. Many, including Thay, see this awareness of our shared humanity, our Interbeing with all species and the Earth, as the next human evolution, becoming "homo conscious" (Nhat Hanh, 2010).

This radical departure from our current societal experience of well-being is not dependent on any personal or societal wealth, possessions, or consumption, but on the well-being of all as a capacity of our interconnectedness. How to begin? Start where we are. Walking mindfully down a hall, administering medication mindfully (Anselmo, 2016), or eating mindfully, we begin to embody this new possibility for ourselves, our families, our colleagues, our society, and our world. These practices may seem very ordinary, but offer a powerful way to embed mindful nurse leadership in everyday living.

If we choose to cultivate present moment awareness throughout our life, from my experience to date, embodying this Interbeing consciousness will naturally open us to ever-widening circles of awareness and compassion. Doing so, animated by this wise energy, we are gently guided toward living peacefully, healingly, and resiliently, even in times of great uncertainty. Nurturing this capacity, we ground ourselves in the present moment, so not to get as caught in fears of "what ifs?" It is natural that we may at times lose heart or inspiration, or become fearful or discouraged. In such times, two things are essential: first, stopping not only our activity but also our thinking, and taking a breath to embrace and calm our fears and be in deeper awareness; and second, practicing within a committed community, where we can lovingly remind ourselves and each other that as we cultivate cosmic homo consciousness, this collective evolutionary human consciousness is *cultivating us,* offering renewal and recognition that this endeavor is not ours alone.

Nurse healers know not to be attached to outcome and instead to trust the healing process. Applying the trust inherent in the healing process to our global environmental/social justice crisis is a very difficult and challenging practice in itself, yet, if we take this on and walk together in this great not-knowing, once again nurses, as society's trusted profession of healing and compassion, will offer a path through whatever unfolds. As I look back at the vision of nursing I had as a new student nurse during orientation, I see it again with new eyes and recognize that it continues to invite me/us to grow beyond conventional borders of practice for nursing to be a great vehicle in supporting human beings to embody being truly alive, fully human, and humane. Nursing's gifts need to be deeply embedded and embodied within humanity in all forms, beyond what is known as "nursing" in this present moment.

Ending this chapter, may we each, in our own way, awaken to our personal and collective heart's healing and embody our true Interbeing humanity for ourselves, all beings, and our Earth.

■ REFLECTIONS

1. *Reflecting on my journey, what has led me to nursing as my life path? What influences, connections, and ancestors have inspired my path?*
2. *What early experiences formed me as a nurse? How have they informed my practice as a leader and as a human being?*
3. *How is nursing a spiritual path for me in my life? What do I see as the message my life as a nurse offers? In what ways have I experienced this message embedded in myself and my work?*
4. *How have my values, understanding, and vision as a nurse expanded my sphere of professional practice? What role do I see contemplative practice/centering/mindfulness playing in my life and nursing practice?*
5. *What roles do nurses, spiritual practice, and spiritual community play in cultivating collective resilience, healing, compassion, and justice? In what ways, besides writing, do I transmit or embody these dimensions of nurse practice and leadership?*

■ REFERENCES

American Nurses Association. (2012). *Eleanor C. Lambertsen, EdD, RN, D.Sc (Hon.), 2012 Inductee, ANA Hall of Fame.* Retrieved from http://www.nursingworld.org/EleanorCLambertsen

Anselmo, J. (2016). Relaxation. In B. M. Dossey & L. Keegan (Eds.), *Holistic nursing: A handbook for practice* (7th ed., pp. 239–267). Burlington, MA: Jones & Bartlett Learning.

Anselmo, J., Bryant, S. J., & Goode, V. (2006). *Connection to purpose, law in the service of human needs: Social justice and contemplative practice.* Presentation in Cultivating Balance in Legal Education Section at Association of American Law Schools (AALS), Washington, DC.

Anselmo, J., & Goode, V. (2016). Contemplative practice for social justice lawyering: From the cushion to the very heart of the struggle. In M. Silver (Ed.), *Transforming justice: Lawyers and the practice of law.* Durham, NC: Carolina Academic Press.

Anselmo, J., & O'Brien, P. (2013). Holistic nursing and complementary modalities. In P. O'Brien, W. Kennedy, & K. Ballard (Eds.), *Psychiatric mental health nursing: An introduction to theory and practice* (2nd ed., pp. 225–243). Burlington, MA: Jones & Bartlett Learning.

Berceli, D. (2008). *The revolutionary trauma release process.* Vancouver, CA: Namaste Publishing.

Fondiller, S. (2007). *Go, and do thou likewise: A history of Cornell University-New York Hospital School of Nursing.* New York, NY: Cornell-New York Hospital.

Guinier, L. (1998). *Lift every voice: Turning a civil rights setback into a new vision of social justice.* New York, NY: Simon & Schuster.

Hostutler, J., Kennedy, M. S., Mason, D., & Schorr, T. (2000). Profiles: Then and now: Nurses and models of practice. *American Journal of Nursing, 100*(2), 82–83.

King, M. L., Jr. (1967). *Letter nominating Thich Nhat Hanh for Nobel Peace Prize.* Retrieved from http://www.thekingcenter.org/archive/document/letter-mlk-nobel-institute

Krieger, D. (1981). *Foundations of holistic health nursing: The renaissance nurse.* New York, NY: Lippincott, Williams & Wilkins.

Lundy, K. S., & Bender, K. (2016). History of community and public health nursing. In K. S. Lundy & S. Jones, *Community health nursing: Caring for the public's health* (3rd ed., pp. 90–93). Burlington, MA: Jones & Bartlett Learning.

Merton, T. (1966). Nhat Hanh is my brother. In T. Merton (Ed.), *Collected essays* (Vol. 8). Louisville, KY: Merton Center Reading Room.

Neff, K. (2011). *Self-compassion: The proven power of being kind to yourself.* New York, NY: HarperCollins.

Nhat Hanh, T. (2007). *Chanting from the heart: Buddhist ceremonies and daily practice.* Berkeley, CA: Parallax Press.

Nhat Hanh, T. (2010). *Reconciliation: Healing the inner child.* Berkeley, CA: Parallax Press.

Order of Interbeing. (2012). *Fourteen mindfulness trainings, Thich Nhat Hanh biography, history of the order.* Retrieved from http://www.orderofinterbeing.org

Sitzman, K., & Watson, J. (2014). *Caring science, mindful practice: Implementing Watson's human caring theory.* New York, NY: Springer.

van Dernoot Lipsky, L. (2009). *Trauma stewardship: An everyday guide to caring for self while caring for others.* San Francisco, CA: Berrett Koehler.

CHAPTER TWO

Translational and Indispensable: Using the Gift of Foresight to Reenvision Nursing

Michael R. Bleich

As a discipline nursing has been cautious, steady, and ever caring, traits that are desirable but insufficient in a time of unprecedented chaos and complexity. . . . The pool of talent . . . is formidable. In fact, we see "translational workers" emerging— people who see a bigger picture, think through the options for and impact of care delivery changes, embrace solutions that include policy development, utilize research for promulgating evidence-based clinical practices, and value research with an eye toward organizational systems and administrative best practices. . . . The value worker of the future may likely be the person who moves fluidly between academic and service settings, demonstrating expertise in both.
—Hewlett and Bleich (2004, pp. 273–274)

■ WHY NURSING?

My early career experiences shaped my sense of the variety of roles nurses could play, the possible accomplishments of nurses over a career, and the human resource potential of nurses. From designing hospital-based care systems in two acute care hospitals to creating forums for advancing nursing roles through educational achievements and making complex ideas applicable to nurses and the health team, it was obvious to me that nurses would attend to a range of human responses.

The human response to health and illness meant nurses would promote health, intervene in the presence of disease, and champion disease abatement efforts while coordinating care to enrich human functioning. I call this the gift of foresight: sensing the future of nursing and leading efforts toward a preferred future for the discipline. Through it, the opportunity to serve on the Institute of Medicine (IOM) committee that would write the report *The Future of Nursing: Leading Change, Advancing Health* would emerge. Interacting with the public, nurses, health providers, and health system leaders in governance roles; the opportunity to champion the discipline, both in the United States and abroad; and the chance to address diversity and inclusion of the workforce through systems design and structural barrier removal continues to resonate through my work. Given experiences in both service and academics, I envisioned myself as a translational worker, someone to bridge both aspects of the discipline.

Without question, I did not grow up wanting to become a nurse. Being a music teacher was my destiny. But piano lessons led me to a job in a county-operated psychiatric facility, as the administrator's daughter took piano lessons before my half-hour turn at the keyboard. Always early, the hospital administrator talked with me and put it out there that on my 18th birthday state law would permit me to work in a mental health facility. So it came to be. Living in rural Wisconsin and needing to pay my own college expenses, my birthday marked my entrée into health care. While donning a white *Ben Casey*–style side-button top, white pants, and shoes, I was called to duty.

Many stories can be tied to this first position as an orderly. A licensed practical nurse (LPN) taught me to administer medicines and perform treatments for which I had no clinical knowledge (her duty hours ended when feeding patients dinner concluded, leaving me alone on a 36-bed ward until the third shift arrived). No telephone communication existed between the buildings. Rather, communication between buildings was possible through the use of an archaic intercom system. By pulling a lever, clicking sounds to another building *might* work and could be heard if the lone RN on the other side was close to the nurses' station. Patients were expected to help provide care to other residents, a situation not uncommon in custodial settings. The 4–2 work schedule allowed you to plan your work schedule for years in advance. Four days on, two days off, with one full weekend off, each seven weeks apart. With a stable patient census, this plan was highly efficient, yet offered no work–life balance. It was never questioned in the several years I worked under those circumstances.

In spite of the obvious challenges, the work held allure for me. Another classmate from the high school I attended was hired and started a day later than I did, coinciding with his 18th birthday. During my first year attending a teacher's college, Steve convinced me to leave the college I was at and commute with him to attend the LPN program in Madison, Wisconsin. Steve and I commuted for the year and leaned on each other, quickly coming to grips with being outliers in a female-dominated profession. Although many professors were kind and encouraging, there were those who made being male tense and difficult. Youth served us well, not knowing whether we were experiencing inequitable education or clinical opportunities from these few faculty.

At the onset of my career and education, nursing was about helping others, performing tasks, and communicating observations, especially through charting. In my mind, it really was not more complicated than that. And I learned that fewer questions about masculinity would be asked if I quickly stated that my interest was in mental health, or later, orthopedics, where having men help with lifting justified being present on the unit.

■ EARLY IMPRESSIONS

My first role as an LPN was in a state facility, caring for men who were profoundly developmentally disabled. As I reflect, this was another setting where being a male was not questioned. Professional staffing was sparse and unionized nursing assistants (NAs) provided care based on their NA career ladder ranging from NA1 to NA5, with the top (NA4 and NA5) being supervisory over a cottage, where residents lived, or a cluster of cottages. NAs did not report to either an LPN or an RN, so one learned quickly that *relationships* and *collaboration* meant everything if a nurse was to survive or thrive through a shift. Fortunately, the NA4 who was my link to the core NA workforce was older, wiser, and collaborative. She provided me with important insights on the various medical conditions that impacted the residents, the most prevalent being seizure disorders, where at any given time, three to five residents could be experiencing a seizure. I recall that individuals who were developmentally disabled were afflicted with many rare clinical disorders well beyond what would be covered in traditional nursing education.

With this first nursing position came a stark realization that many parents had abandoned their children, essentially making them wards of the state. This instilled in me a sense of being responsible for the *quality of life* and *functional existence* of these residents, who ranged in age from early childhood through senescence. Safety and security were a paramount nursing focus, but so was bringing small bits of joy into the workplace. Caring for a minimum of 90 residents demanded a high level of organization and time management in medication administration, treatment provision, charting, and emergency management. Communicable disease outbreaks were not uncommon. Shigellosis, a bacterial infection impacting the digestive system, meant that the cottage was placed on isolation and extreme procedures were implemented, including administering antibiotic regimens for all residents.

In this first year as a nurse came the jolting knowledge of *patient advocacy*. One full-time physician covered 1,200 residents, performing perfunctory history and physical examinations, addressing medical emergencies, and prescribing medications that today would stun the public. An African American teen on my assigned cottage was unusual in that his intellect and verbal communication skills were of a much higher level than the other residents who were nonverbal. This made him eligible to participate in a sheltered workshop day program. The female physician had expressed to the NA4 her fear of his size and race and so placed him on a drug to diminish his sex drive, the side effect of which was breast development.

The young man came to me and expressed—in today's terms—that he was bullied by others on the bus ride to and while at the workshop because of his breasts. Following a communication protocol, I queried the physician by leaving a note as to whether an alternative drug could be used and mentioned that the resident was able to discern the side effect of breast enlargement.

Two days later, while pulling into the parking lot, the evening supervisor, an RN, informed me I was in trouble. Stunningly, it was because of the note. The physician demanded a reprimand for questioning her order. On entering the building, I was queried, "What were you thinking? Do you not respect physicians' orders? Do you realize the physical harm this resident could do?" My answers were direct:

> The resident realized he was shaped differently than other boys. His behavior on the cottage, before the drug was prescribed, was always docile and he was easygoing. I was asking if there was an alternative to the prescribed drug, not suggesting one nor saying that the order was not justified.

Lesson learned: Patient advocacy involves risk-taking and remembering that not all health providers are patient advocates. Back then, physicians wielded power beyond my youthful and naïve imagination. Most disappointing, I learned that the director of nursing was said to have stated, "He will never amount to anything if he does not adhere to physicians' orders."

Standing up for this resident was frightening and anxiety provoking in that I could have lost my job. The tact of the evening supervisor who believed that I did the right thing led to calming the situation, but there was no change in the resident's prescription. The RN supervisor became my first role model. The role of the nurse as an advocate remains central to my practice today and was a driver to return to school.

In the nursing shortage of the 1970s, many employers were eager to hire nurses. I started my second job as an LPN at the conclusion of an interview with the human resource director, who rode with me on the elevator and, upon arrival at the third floor, introduced me to the evening charge nurse. That was the extent of orientation and I worked a partial shift that very evening. Orthopedics was considered an ideal setting for men, as the heavy hip spica casts and need for lifting assistance were plentiful. Nurse after nurse and patient after patient would tell me how good I was good at lifting and how I was needed on that unit. No mention was made of any other abilities I may have possessed. In this acute care setting, LPNs were active caregivers in a team-based care model, meaning that we performed specific nursing tasks for a group of patients and, if assigned as a team leader, provided supervision to NAs.

Survival on orthopedics required team efforts so the staff worked in tandem. In this team care model, the RN was poised at the nursing station to take phone calls and round with physicians, make assignments, perform the task of checking off orders with the ward secretary, and answer questions from visitors or family. RN engagement in care delivery was limited to critical situations; offering nonemergency assistance to the team was not a charge nurse responsibility. Again, I observed hierarchy and role delineation that made me question wanting to become an RN, although I was in a diploma school at the time.

Over the years, some have asked why I chose a diploma program. The choice of this type of nursing program was made for three reasons: The diploma program I attended had a history of admitting and *graduating* men (one regional college had a policy where you could be admitted, but they would not offer a degree to a male), and there were still other nursing programs that would not admit male students. Practicing nurses said that diploma programs reflected excellence and real-world knowledge. Finally, once accepted into the program, a clinical placement was assured. This was unlike state school baccalaureate students who, after two years of study, went into a lottery to determine if they would have a clinical placement (if not, these students would be required to change majors, a risk many were unwilling to take).

These early positions provided me with few role models, an uncertain perspective on the discipline as anything more than serving physicians, and feeling used by females in positions of hierarchy. At the same time, I enjoyed my peers and the work of patient care. To remove myself from the role of full-time lifting, the only other viable option available was to become a float nurse. It proved to be a wise decision.

The success that went along with becoming a float nurse was as much psychological as anything. Every unit to which I was assigned was happy to accept the resource. Floating demanded less engagement in unit politics, and I could differentiate how various units performed. Although rare, access to other men who were successful as nurses made me feel less an outlier as I witnessed their integral function in the emergency department, surgical intensive care, and surgery. Mostly, my skills were sharpened by learning new procedures and techniques. But the primary lessons as a float nurse were found in the close working relationships with the evening supervisors, three very strong and patient-centered nurses (Dianne Younk, Sr. Gabriel, and Margaret Krummel). They helped me link and understand patient needs as universal, across clinical unit boundaries. For instance, treating surgical pain may be different from orthopedic pain, but it is still pain that has to be managed, and I had a role in that. These broad perspectives led me to appreciate *patient-centered care*.

■ PROFESSIONAL EVOLUTION/CONTRIBUTION

After becoming an RN, emergency nursing was next in line. Working in an inner-city hospital, many victims of violence and trauma presented. Intense teamwork, strong clinical reliance on professional peers, and high volumes of patients made the work seem important—and we did save lives. It was also a time where issues in the public's health ended up at our doorstep. Air pollution led to asthma attacks. Obesity and smoking led to heart attacks. Heavy equipment and chemical-based industries led to workplace injuries, often musculoskeletal in nature. Sexual freedom led to sexually transmitted diseases, which were treated and referred. From this role, and without having a formal name for it, I grasped how social determinants impacted emergency and acute care services, a perception that was strongly reinforced several years later while pursuing a graduate degree in public health nursing and patient care administration.

After cutting my teeth in emergency nursing, I was called to the nursing office to meet with the director of nursing—a very different experience than with the first nursing director. She knew of my work and my work ethic and offered me a role in staff development to assist in the development of a new medical center. The clinical pace and challenges of emergency nursing were appealing but the opportunity to teach resonated. In staff development, my earliest desires to be an educator could be fulfilled. In terms of working with the development of the new medical center, it sounded exciting yet I had no context for what it would mean and how it would change my career trajectory.

At this juncture in my career, serendipity led me to an interest in hospital design and how it was linked to nursing practice and patient outcomes. In the late 1960s and early 1970s, Canadian architect and hospital administrator, Gordon Friesen, made waves in the design of hospitals, not unlike Nightingale's impact in hospital reform (Bellwether League, Inc., n.d.; http://www.bellwetherleague.org/bellwethers-2009/hall-of-fame/2009-honoree-Friesen-Gordon.html). The new medical center I was to be part of creating was modeled after the Friesen concept. Learning about this concept and representing nursing on architectural planning groups was extremely stimulating. Two site visits to hospitals built using Friesen's innovations opened my mind to how care could be delivered in a decentralized model, where each patient room was designed to be the nursing station.

Friesen had a great affinity for nurses and nursing from a health systems perspective. He believed in the use of technology to enable care, so pagers were employed to facilitate communication, a major breakthrough for its time. Nurses' stations were eliminated and work redesigned so that charting, medications, and treatment supplies were housed at the point of care in Nurservers, air pressure–balanced cabinets to keep clean supplies clean, and soiled linens and equipment portioned off to reduce contamination. Replacing semiprivate and wardrooms, all rooms were private, allowing for improved patient–nurse communication and accommodating the presence of family. These were but some of the concepts that made Friesen hospitals unique from the traditional ward structures that emanated from Victorian principles of work design and orderliness. All of the activities linked with the construction of this hospital catapulted my beliefs about nurses as value-added care providers, granting me granular insights into the centrality of the discipline from an interdisciplinary perspective. Whether materials distribution, food service, life safety systems, or communications equipment, all had to be designed to intersect with point-of-care service from the first patient on.

Many of the Friesen concepts have been reintroduced in recent years with the Transforming Care at the Bedside (TCAB) initiative, speaking to the foresight and clear end-point vision that Friesen had for work design and optimal patient experience (Rutherford, Lee, & Greiner, 2004).

Throughout these experiences, as I reflect, there were individuals who strongly believed in me and offered encouragement. Two names come to mind, of many: Sr. Catherine Albers and Catherine Kirk offered encouragement and prayer, which impacted my self-confidence and motivation to be and do the best I could.

When coupled with the emerging practice of primary nursing, also prevalent in the late 1970s and 1980s, I found myself on a team creating a care delivery model that fully aligned with my personal thoughts and beliefs about what nursing could be.

The experiences throughout my 20s and 30s profoundly impact me today. The following are some of the leadership lessons learned during this time frame:

- Social determinants and public and environmental health issues shape the nature and type of acute care services that are delivered.
- Nursing is relationship centered and the work environment can be designed through structures and processes that increase the opportunity for positive clinical outcomes directly influenced by nurses.
- Systems thinking is an essential leadership skill. Systems are embedded in other systems. A hospital is a set of commingling disciplines sharing space, which if not designed with intent, often results in chaos, parallel play, or medical error. If job role and the care delivery system are designed with intention, then seamless and collaborative patient and family care emerges that feels organic to health care workers. Alternatively, processes that develop unilaterally without systems awareness often exist with historical roots. Symptoms of poor work design can be found in the statement, "That is the way things are done here," an overdependence on coordinators to navigate poor systems, and patient care being a neglected by-product, where nurses nurse the processes rather than the patient.
- Too few leaders are willing to take on complex systems design because it disrupts job roles and power structures and involves risk, conflict, and negotiation skills.
- Teaching is a leadership and management skill. Teaching can be synonymous with communication but it implies more. When leaders teach, they are in relationship with their stakeholders in a manner that models caring through a developmental commitment.

In more recent decades, the influence of strong leaders has led me to value being mentored and being a mentor, especially in organizational science and scholarly development. With an acute care nursing background, teaching in a degree completion program for RNs and developing a consulting practice linked to the Joint Commission on Accreditation of Healthcare Organizations (JCAHO) gave me substantive exposure to health care organizations within the United States and abroad. Each of these experiences, in addition to doctoral studies in human resource and organizational development, strengthened the way I embodied how an organization's mission, vision, and values drive the nature of the work to be accomplished; all of which are insufficient without aligning structures and processes to support human resource optimization. Comfort in acute care and other clinical settings complemented my interest in educational roles.

After being so close to patient care providers and organizational leaders, and engaging with them to solve complex organizational problems, the need to publish and develop a scholarly portfolio was a practical solution to give something back to the field, where too little was in the literature. To this end, Dr. Sue Ellen Pinkerton and her team at St. Michael Hospital in Milwaukee, Wisconsin, were impactful in modeling that doctoral education provided unique ways of thinking, new tools to use in decision making, and expanded contributions to the profession. Nursing process, nursing documentation, quality improvement, standards development, access to care, and other organizational topics led to an editorial appointment on the board of the *Journal of Nursing Care Quality*.

Mentors Drs. Karen Miller, Jan Bellack, Shirley Chater, Maryann Fralic, and Jona Raasch, all leaders with substantive organizational, policy, governance, and leadership competence, nudged me to look at expanded leadership opportunities. The University of Kansas School of Nursing was my entrée into academic medicine, academe, and expanded interprofessional teaching in organizational leadership and health policy and management. The School of Nursing and the School of Allied Health had separate practice incorporation as part of their respective missions. Serving as an associate dean with responsibilities for the practice mission, exposure to governance structures, and bridging faculty practice with student learning to serve the public helped students learn the organizational side of patient care. Note the confluence, once again, of practice, teaching, role development, and policy aimed at systemic change.

One of many highlights of this experience was the privilege of leading a community-based clinic, exposing students to diverse, underrepresented, and un- or underinsured residents. Faculty and students in organizational leadership, advanced practice nursing and advanced therapies, health care informatics, and basic nursing and medical students cut their teeth on designing patient-centered processes for each program that expanded the growth of the clinic.

Part of an academic's career is pursuing an area of scholarship. The portfolio of publications I had contributed to the field at that time consisted of field-based necessities, but was insufficient to claim as part of an academic profile. As an academic, two areas surfaced that fueled my interests and built on my past: systems leadership and workforce development, including supply and demand.

Clinicians, especially at the advanced level, are dependent upon the structure of organizations and how work is designed. Quality science had advanced to the point where each improvement project required its own processes. When implementation plans failed, it was often because the improvement strategy stood as a separate set of practices from existing processes. Stand-alone protocols, those disconnected from organizational processes, accelerated *work-arounds*, a term synonymous with a set of actions outside acceptable routines. Work-arounds provided evidence of a protocol's lack of fit within existing processes. Teaching about and modeling the design of systems was an important contribution to quality and implementation science, preparing a workforce to enable systems leadership. Work-arounds add complexity to routine practices, which could include bypassing safeguards that ensure the quality and safety linked to patient care.

Concomitantly, the National Research Corporation that sponsored the Picker Institute afforded me the opportunity to serve as an expert panel member to focus on access to care. The work of Harvey Picker, an important manufacturer of radiologic equipment for use in health care, was advanced largely due to the illness of his wife. Dr. Picker was the first to promote patient-centered care from the perspective of organizational systems and processes. Picker bridged technology with patient experience and developed instruments to measure the effectiveness of the patient's perspective in the design of care processes. In addition to the focus on access to care, Picker's research (Gerteis, Edgman-Levita, Daley, & Delbanco, 1993) named several patient care principles, such as respect for the patient's values and expressed needs, care coordination and integration, high-quality communication used to educate the patient and family, physical comfort, emotional support, family and friend engagement, and seamless care transitions, all of which align with today's commitment to care through the Affordable Care Act.

Analyzing the needs of the workforce from a perspective of supply and demand also seemed important, having worked for years on the demand side (service) before moving to the supply side (academia). Nursing curricula development is not a nimble process. Creating enrollment targets and hiring faculty to fulfill the needs of those targets is a longitudinal initiative. The national Colleagues in Caring: Regional Collaboratives for Nursing Work Force Development program, my first interaction with the Robert Wood Johnson Foundation (RWJF), which funded national workgroups on workforce supply and demand, seriously examined workforce issues. Here, with colleagues in the greater Kansas City bistate region, we developed a role- and function-based data collection instrument. Rather than capturing subjective data about the anticipated numbers of nurses needed, the instrument measured projected knowledge and skill sets needed to ensure that nurses would be prepared *with requisite competencies* to align with the employment opportunities, which today I refer to as "staging the workforce."

What this essentially means is that academic institutions must align their graduates for the job opportunities available. Too many nurses available without work can become demoralized and/or deskilled. Too few nurses available, for a prolonged period of time, creates critical gaps in patient care. The workforce model that I explored with Dr. Peggy Hewlett called for bridging supply with demand, competency attainment based on a continuum of workforce settings where nurses were employed, and staging a workforce to ensure a relatively steady state of employable nurses. These data fostered a stronger bridge between academic and service partners.

RWJF was instrumental in my leadership development, and I became the first man to be accepted into their Executive Nurse Fellows program. Later they would fund the Wisdom at Work project, which examined the issues of the impending loss of senior nurses with years of experience. This contribution led many to examine the impact of lost knowledge and develop workforce plans to shore up programs to recognize the importance of mid-career hires and to use technology to capture the wisdom of experienced nurses. The work of David Delong (2004), a national expert in the impact of workforce turnover, knowledge capture, and talent management, profoundly informed the Wisdom at Work project.

This leadership development afforded me experience in academic–service partnerships that spanned a career, and the interest in workforce pipeline led to the privilege of leading two nursing schools at Oregon Health and Science University and at the Goldfarb School of Nursing at Barnes-Jewish College. Both schools are embedded in a service milieu with ties to major academic health sciences programs. Both have achieved renown for innovations in education and research, with strong alliances to practice, including Magnet hospitals. Both were environments where opportunity presented itself to implement the findings of the IOM's (2011) report entitled *The Future of Nursing: Leading Change, Advancing Health.*

In what was a career-changing opportunity, I received the call to interview to serve on the committee for the RWJF Initiative at the IOM. It was both humbling and daunting. The interview clarified the diversity of the committee and that five nurses would serve on the group. By regulatory design, the committee would be interprofessional and the study would meet the rigorous criteria established for all IOM reports. The chair would be Dr. Donna Shalala, past secretary of the U.S. Department of Health and Human Services and known to me from my days in Wisconsin, where she was chancellor at the University of Wisconsin–Madison. My role would be to represent nursing education from a futures perspective. And for the first time, the IOM would partner with the RWJF with the aim that the foundation would support implementation funding.

Serving on such a committee is an experience that I wish could be shared with others. From the onset, where the charter is reviewed, to when committee members formally introduce their biases such that all are aware of the perspectives represented, to the rigor of accepting only the highest quality of research from which to write the narrative and recommendations, yields a process that affords great confidence in how science serves our nation.

Dr. Shalala masterfully framed that the report was to reflect the public's current and future expectations of the nursing discipline, not a report about nursing for the benefit of nurses. With agility, she engaged each committee member and the formidable and far-reaching expertise each possessed. With policy awareness, she maintained astounding insights into how the Affordable Care Act was progressing to ensure that our report was contextually relevant. Dr. Shalala also modeled something that we, as nurses, may often be too timid to confront: to immediately seek out the brightest and best talents when confronting complex and difficult situations. Go to the top players in any given field to expedite knowledge generation that may already exist—a lesson that I have grown into.

Along with Dr. Linda Burnes-Bolton as cochair, and Dr. Susan Hassmiller, the senior adviser for nursing at the RWJF, resources were plentiful as the depth and breadth of nursing's contribution to health care unfolded. National hearings on acute care and technology, community-based care and public health, and nursing education were conducted. Each hearing was rich with evidence from experts, public testimony, and opportunities to clarify and expand on issues. Commissioned papers were summoned. Research was conducted when needed by health systems scientists.

Throughout the nearly two-year process, several aspects struck me as crucially important. The first is that when you are trained as a professional and gain a particular framing lens (in this case, nursing), it becomes increasingly difficult to see the discipline through the lens of those you serve (the patient) and other disciplines. The time to listen through the patient's eyes revealed more than just their trust of the discipline. It showed how critical nurses are in every venue where nurses practice and through every stage of the life span. Since the IOM's (2011) final report, *The Future of Nursing: Leading Change, Advancing Health*, was released, I have shared this message with thousands of nurses whom I have encountered and addressed.

Second, health care is complex, but not less complex than nursing's own history and role within the health system. Consequently, messaging to all stakeholders is essential. Complexity must be expressed through messaging that is accessible. That the report had four key messages and eight concise recommendations was by design. The title of the report was carefully constructed. The tone and inclusivity of the writing was thoughtfully executed to be accessible to the public, policy makers, other health disciplines, and to nurses. Transforming complex messages into language that has functional utility is anything but simplistic; it is artful and requires great skill to achieve.

Third, emotion trumps the facts. Repeatedly, individuals and groups would attend hearings, wanting to be heard. They had stories, good and bad, sad and hope filled. When their emotions were released, only then could their minds handle the data that was being accumulated and synthesized. Skillful negotiations, being comfortable with conflict, and using evidence is a powerful combination when creating a blueprint for social change.

There are many ways that *The Future of Nursing* report has influenced and is changing the nature of the discipline. State action coalitions continue to create agendas around the report's findings. Many professional nursing organizations have used the IOM report as a stimulus for their specialty work. Nursing journal editors have spread the messages and recommendations to multiple stakeholders. Policy makers have responded to the call to expand the role of advanced practice registered nurses (APRNs). Nurses have returned to school to complete their BSN degrees in record numbers, as health care institutions and states realize that nursing is a high-stakes profession. New research has been generated to support policy development aimed at fulfilling public expectations, documenting the public's readiness for nursing to expand its scope of practice. Nursing curricula have been revised and reshaped to accommodate seamless education through to the doctoral level of preparation.

Knowing how this report has catapulted nursing into expanded arenas and has educated the public as to the nature of the discipline is beyond anything I could have imagined during the intense efforts it took to create this scholarly work. Beyond extensive efforts to bring the messages to countless audiences, there are several postreport developments that resonate with the contributions I am trying to make:

- I have accepted a volunteer role with the Governance Institute, a formidable organization that deals with board development for major health care institutions and systems across the United States. Initially, too few boards were aware of the report. Once they were, their attention turned to nursing education, particularly surrounding APRN roles. APRN roles (nurse practitioners, clinical nurse specialists, midwives—who may or may not be nurses—and nurse anesthetists) are poorly grasped and confused with the physician assistant and primary care physician roles. The effort to educate and advise boards on these roles, and to press for the inclusion of nurses on boards and board committees, remains important to me.

- The global context of nursing is expanding my way of being. The fortunate relationship I have chairing the board of the Commission on Graduates of Foreign Nursing Schools (CGFNS) International has connected me to the issues of global nursing and other health discipline migration, no longer just in the United States but in a variety of global locations. How professional credentials are evaluated, authenticated, and verified, along with certification and assessment examinations, is a field of expertise that addresses new issues surrounding supply and demand and changes in educational requirements. The focus of this work is to protect the public through the preparation of practitioners who can deliver safe, quality care.

- Research has become increasingly important and my advocacy efforts have expanded. The role of the National Institutes of Health, especially the National Institute for Nursing Research, is important to expand clinical research through a nursing model. Few other health disciplines attend to symptom management, end of life, and other forms of science that bridge the human response to disease. But advocacy for organizational research, including care delivery evaluation and impact across an expanding health care continuum, and informing state and national policy agendas has never had more meaning to me. Having examined the relevance of the latter forms of research through the IOM (2011) study, we have too few scientists informing health systems and policy. If nursing is to influence the systems of care, including economics, then we must advance nursing research to these broader perspectives. These are the messages and initiatives I support through current involvement with the Friends of the National Institute for Nursing Research (FNINR). The message here is that a personal passion has a home, somewhere, with like-minded advocates.

- Last, but not least, I have taken time to deeply commit to the diversity and inclusion agenda to enrich the discipline. Serving on the national Bipartisan Policy Center's Health Professional Workforce Initiative Expert Advisory Panel, it was stunning to realize the advancement of every health profession with regard to diversity with the exception of nursing (Keckley, Coughlin, Gupta, Korenda, & Stanley, 2011). While writing the report, too few studies on diversity and inclusion were available. What was known is that national demographics are shifting, and without men entering the profession and cultural and ethnic expansion into the discipline, workforce shortages will be extremely exacerbated. The reduction or elimination in service and academic structures of an existent and willing workforce to accept modified ways of teaching and being a nurse will seriously challenge those who remain in health care.

■ MORAL/ETHICAL FOUNDATION

I started this chapter by saying that nursing had never entered my mind as a profession. Let me now add that I grew up with a stern father who believed in traditional discipline and hard work and a mother and maternal grandmother who were extraordinarily kind. My siblings and I were taught to "do unto others as you would have done unto you." We were expected to demonstrate respect to those who were older, in how we addressed them, and even how to walk on the outside of the sidewalk so they would be protected from the street. It was very important to my parents that all people be treated with dignity. In reflection, these childhood values and expectations are ideal nursing traits.

There were but five or so Catholic families in the small village where I grew up, mine among them. Most of the residents of Rio, Wisconsin were staunch Lutherans, first and second generation from Norway. Church and public school was commingled, without separation of church and state, and the teaching faculty were primarily local. This is to say that I felt like an outsider even though my entire grade and high-school years were spent in Rio.

When I was 10, my maternal grandmother became very ill (she was in her late 50s at the time). In an era where there were still "hospital zones" where noise was to be limited, children were not allowed into hospitals. Realizing how grave my grandmother's health was, we were taken to the hospital to see her for what would be the last time. We stood out on the sidewalk looking up at my grandmother's hospital room and a white-capped and uniformed nurse eased my grandmother to the window. I can still see my grandmother's faint smile and gentle wave of her hand as my two brothers and I waved back. This went on for several minutes. It is the last remembrance I have of my grandmother before she passed away.

This story is a reflection of the kindness of the nurse and the respect she had for my grandmother's grandchildren. It represented an era in time where patient-centered care was not a strong value. Rituals, protocols, and a lack of evidence-based practice, instilled with European norms, reigned. Social justice, valuing relationships, and doing the right thing as a way of adapting to different realities were what morally made sense to me.

The most tragic—yet values-clarifying—experience of my career came about after accepting my second position as a chief nursing officer at a hospital in the heartland. On my first day at work, the last of a series of patients died from cardioplegic solution contamination. The moral–ethical dilemma related to the pressure placed on a pharmacist provider to follow a mandate enforced by authority figures, forcing the pharmacist to create a solution from a protocol that was later deemed as "manufacturing a drug," which was not allowed in a hospital setting and subject to Food and Drug Administration regulations. The subsequent deaths of patients served as strong reminders that each health professional has a moral duty and obligation to serve in the best interests of the patient. Beyond the tragedy of patients' lives lost, after regulatory reprimand, the pharmacist committed suicide. Although extreme, this scenario reminds us that there is moral–ethical distress in the high-stakes business of health care, where values and beliefs are tested routinely. Today leaders are, hopefully, more likely to recognize and respond to the moral and ethical stress and distress that a crisis can create but also the toll of caregiver compassion fatigue over time.

As the opportunity to be in service and academic leadership positions has filled my career, and opportunities to influence social policy as described earlier continue to present, I have tried to find the balance in providing structures that offer a sense of direction and orderliness, but have done so with an eye on the end point vision. The Picker work on patient-centered care and the Friesen work on design reflect the creation of spaces to provide structures that address doing the greatest good for the greatest number, yet find a balance in personalizing care. As a dean and college president, I try to find the balance in ascribing to academic and professional standards needed to model expert and vigilant nursing care to the public, while encouraging faculty innovation and adaptation to address the learning and personal needs of students; and ensuring policies, procedures, and practices as adjunctive support to aid faculty and staff who benefit from structure, while also honoring academic freedom to stimulate creativity. Academic environments are best served when students find respect, balance, creative outlets, and rich and diverse perspectives to stimulate holistic growth. In this kind of environment, moral and ethical development can evolve and flourish.

■ VISION

In a world that is complex in many ways (socioeconomically disparate, ethnically and culturally expansive, religiously ideological, violent, technologically sophisticated, environmentally challenged, and more), nursing has never been more needed. Nurses are, at the end of the day, when all knowledge of disease and the treatments that accompany the eradication of disease are exhausted, the instruments of healing. Comfort, hope, encouragement, and gentleness may be all that is left when each of us experiences the final pages of our life.

The scope of nursing practice should not be constrained in any manner. Holistic care that aligns with human responses to life challenges are fitting dimensions of nursing practice. That the science of our discipline can enrich the alleviation of pain, manage self-care deficits, or elevate the patient's acceptance of self and family provides nondisease-based treatment options. Nurses can expand their practice to include diagnosing and treating disease as a natural part of a nursing portfolio, but view care through the lens of a nurse, not of a physician. For this reason, I envision a stronger presence of nursing in all parts of the community: churches and schools (where individuals and families gather and where health and well-being are introduced), hospitals and ambulatory care settings (where humanistic care is critical when disease is being diagnosed and treated), primary and specialty clinics (where a nurse is an adjunct and a team member to physicians), palliative and hospice care (where pain management and psychosocial and spiritual presence is offered), correctional facilities (where we have come to house too many with mental health disorders), and public health and transitional care and other settings.

The vision here is that we nurses will remain present in the social situations where people live and reside, in the spirit of Nightingale and Lillian Wald. We will remain educated to have exposure across the life span and to experience the onset and ending of life. We will be advocates for those whose voices cannot be heard, representing their strengths and dignity, not as a discipline that dwells on incapacitation.

Education will vitalize the discipline. A strong foundation remains important, where in addition to all aspects of disease and illness care, nurses will prevail in developing more than how to "do" nursing (tasks and procedures), but become role models of how to "be" a nurse (as a healer and advocate). Diverse and inclusive teams will bring enriched knowledge and sensitivity to care settings, and there will be space for all who have the traits to engage in nursing.

Our science will be used in new and expanded ways. Physicians will come to realize that nursing science is a necessary complement to medical science; all disease and treatment options create human responses, which must be understood to be acceptable. Bench science will enrich physiologic knowledge; translational science will provide the context and use for what is discovered at the bench level. Individualized care will be strengthened through personalized medicine. The ethical dimensions of personalized medicine will require examination and understanding from both a use and a risk perspective.

Nurses in advanced practice roles will complement physician-delivered care in a balanced manner. Turf wars (mostly driven by concern for loss of reimbursement) will diminish as newer generations of physicians and other health professionals realize that *all* citizens need health and illness care. The mindset of only providing care to those with fiscal access will be recalibrated as nurses speak to this imbalance. The public and legislators will come to realize that a healthy citizenry is linked to an educated and able workforce. It is in the best interest of businesses to work with nurses and other health team members to invest in wellness.

Finally, health systems will be designed to be seamless and continuous rather than needlessly complex and disjointed. Nurses will play a strong role in the design of these systems through education, training, and presence in settings where care is needed. Nurses will play a role in ensuring that patients and families are also at the table where care design takes place. Our role in care design at the institutional level will not be trumped at the policy level as we bridge institutional policies and practices with state and national policies and practices. Our contribution will be to bring coalitions together to afford needed change in the health system.

This may sound too idealistic to classify as a vision. Perhaps. But I know of nurses who are champions in each and every one of these areas today: nurses who are systems leaders and who have the public's interests at heart to ensure that a workforce is present that is cognitively, technically, and morally/ethically able to communicate and function independently and in teams. Nurses with foresight need to act as translational workers, a necessary part of the hub of social change.

■ REFLECTIONS

1. *Who have I experienced in my career that meets the definition of a translational worker, someone who can transcend service and academics? How does this professional play an important role when interacting with others?*

2. *In thinking about the IOM report,* The Future of Nursing: Leading Change, Advancing Health, *what has this blueprint for the public's health done to elevate nursing from my vantage point? Have the findings and recommendations from this report changed my practice or career trajectory?*

3. *When someone says that he or she is a "systems thinker," how does this differ from someone who says he or she thinks systematically?*
4. *How does the physical and process design of a health care facility influence clinical care delivery and patient outcomes? Think of an example that would enhance care and one where care was impeded.*
5. *What are the work-arounds I have observed in my clinical, educational, or research setting? How do the work-arounds affect safety and outcomes? Which protocols are not in congruence with the existing processes? How can I go about fixing it to improve quality, safety, and outcomes?*

■ REFERENCES

Bellwether League, Inc. (n.d.). *Gordon A. Friesen.* Retrieved from http://www.bellwetherleague.org/bellwethers-2009/hall-of-fame/2009-honoree-Friesen-Gordon.html

Delong, D. W. (2004). *Lost knowledge: Confronting the threat of an aging workforce.* New York, NY: Oxford University Press.

Gerteis, M., Edgman-Levita, S., Daley, D., & Delbanco, T. O. (1993). *Through the patient's eyes: Understanding and promoting patient-centered care.* San Francisco, CA: Jossey-Bass.

Hewlett, P. O., & Bleich, M. R. (2004). The reemergence of academic-service partnerships: Responses to the nursing shortage, work environment issues, and beyond. *Journal of Professional Nursing, 20*(5), 273–274.

Institute of Medicine (IOM). (2011). *The future of nursing: Leading change, advancing health.* Washington, DC: National Academies Press.

Keckley, P. H., Coughlin, S., Gupta, S., Korenda, L., & Stanley, E. (2011). *The complexities of national health care workforce planning.* Washington, DC: Deloitte Development, LLC.

Rutherford, P., Lee, B., & Greiner, A. (2004). *Transforming care at the bedside* (IHI Innovation Series white paper). Boston, MA: Institute for Healthcare Improvement.

CHAPTER THREE

Unitary and Appreciative: Nourishing and Supporting the Human Spirit

W. Richard Cowling III

With unitary appreciative nursing, we are often shocked by the grasping of wholeness in human life. We come to understand and appreciate that disease, symptoms, and specializations are a place for presenting of the whole . . . an awareness that has been stolen from us by the dominance of the biomedical worldview.

—Cowling and Swartout (2011, p. 64)

■ WHY NURSING?

In 1964, as a young boy of 15, I felt very much a loner in high school for a variety of reasons. I grew up in a family of four brothers and sisters and a stream of foster children: infants and toddlers for the most part. I was not a very social child and spent lots of my time helping care for these small children from the time I was 10 years old. My sister, a nursing assistant at a local hospital, suggested that I become a candy striper—not perceived as a cool thing to do by my teenage peers of the day. Although I went through the training program at the local Red Cross during the summer of 1964, I was reluctant to pursue this endeavor, mostly out of fear of being seen as less than masculine by my peers. However, during the Christmas break that year, my nursing assistant sister suggested I come to the hospital with her on the evening shift. Purely out of boredom, I agreed.

That night was a turning point in my life. I was assigned to help out on a medical–surgical unit in a male ward at Lewis Gale Hospital in Roanoke, Virginia. Two wonderful things happened that first night. I was welcomed with open arms by the charge nurse and the nursing staff, including the nursing assistants. They took me into their fold and wanted to teach me what I needed to know and do to help them and, ultimately, the patients. In addition, I felt needed—deeply needed by the staff and the patients. This was such a profound experience for me that I wanted to come back the following night and every night—literally, every night—thereafter.

A series of events followed that led to my choice of nursing as a career. I developed a very close and deep connection to the patients on the unit. One patient in particular made an indelible impression on my life. This middle-aged man was hospitalized on several occasions over a period of a year or so with vague neurological symptoms. I became very connected to his wife and she relied on me for support for him and to share her anxieties about his condition. When he passed away years later she reached out to me. This was one of many deep connections I felt with patients and their families.

One of the enduring feelings of that period of time in my young life was the sense of belonging based on two aspects of my work. One was providing basic, intimate care for patients and observing the power of small acts that provided comfort, such as bathing, bed making, and back rubs, and responding to calls for assistance. The second was the strong relationships that I developed both with patients and their families, as well as with the nursing staff and physicians. The nurses and nursing assistants were willing to provide guidance and appreciated any help I could provide.

I loved this work so much that I almost immediately began skipping my last two periods of classes in high school so I could be on the unit. It was difficult for my parents to understand how I could skip school to go to the hospital to work. I was at the hospital every evening, including weekends. At one point I was called into a meeting with the director of nursing who offered me a job as a nursing assistant. When I asked her what I would be doing, she said essentially the same thing, only I would get paid for it and I would be required to take one day off a week. She was also willing to have me work around my school schedule.

I also developed a positive relationship with the nursing students who were attending the hospital's diploma in nursing program. The hospital was preparing to merge with another local hospital to form the Community Hospital of Roanoke Valley and merge the respective diploma programs. One of the nursing students asked me one day what I was planning to do after graduating from high school. I told her that I was going to be either an accountant or a teacher. My grades were actually very poor in high school due to the amount of time I was spending at the hospital. She asked me why I was not interested in becoming a nurse and I was entirely shocked because I did not know that men could pursue a nursing career. I had certainly never seen one in my experience. I learned from talking to her and others that there were men in nursing. However, I would become only the second man in Virginia to become a nursing student in a diploma program.

Becoming a nurse excited me because I admired what I saw nurses do during those many hours I spent at the hospital. I saw them be the source of comfort and advocacy for the well-being of patients. I experienced the care they gave patients and families that was as reliant on understanding the human condition as much as it was on understanding the medical condition and diagnosis. What I noticed was that nurses were there for their patients in a way that was different from any of the other health care providers and it seemed to me, even at that very young age, that nurses were the most likely to make the greatest difference in the recovery process. Before I knew what nursing was, I cherished what nurses did and was amazed that it might be possible for me to become a nurse. The vision I had of nursing was shaped by those experiences and it drove the intention I had of becoming the kind of nurse I had known at that time. I believe it is still an enduring and accurate image of nursing in my consciousness.

■ EARLY IMPRESSIONS

Further impressions of nursing were shaped by my experiences as a nursing student and later as a beginning nurse in practice. What was most striking about my educational experience in a diploma school was the substantial amount of knowledge and skill development necessary for practice. My first two semesters of study were devoted to general science courses, a rather progressive approach at that time for a diploma school when most students were immediately immersed in practical learning. The depth and breadth of knowledge was beyond my expectations, but clearly formed the basis of how we practiced and learned new skills. In reflecting upon my early experiences with nurses as an aide, I realize that I had no concept of the knowledge that was necessary to provide the exquisite care I observed and experienced. In 1966, my first year in nursing school, I read *Educational Preparation for Nurse Practitioners and Assistants to Nurses: A Position Paper* published by the American Nurses Association (ANA; 1965). I still own this document today. It impressed upon me the importance of being prepared at the baccalaureate level to effectively respond to the needs of patients and their families and to be equipped for the future of health care and my contributions as a nurse. I decided that I must enroll in a BSN program immediately upon graduation from my diploma program. So in 1969 I entered the BSN program at the University of Virginia.

While a student in my diploma program, I developed an interest in the activities of the student nurses association and got highly involved in this organization at the school, district, and state levels. In 1968, after serving as school president, I was elected as the president of the Student Nurses Association of Virginia. This involved me in meetings and conferences with the state nursing association leadership group I was a member of their board of directors and was asked to represent nursing students on a board of nursing panel to advise legislators on the revision of the Virginia Nurse Practice Act from 1969 to 1970.

In the beginning years of my career in nursing, I worked as a floating nurse in a variety of units in a large community hospital in Roanoke, Virginia while I was pursuing my BSN. What I noticed from the onset was the ongoing need to focus on the person underneath the disease or diagnosis. It seemed that the primary demand of the health care system was for a primary focus on the medical condition, often at the expense of the factors associated with the psychosocial well-being of the person or family. I think these observations and experiences were what led to my interest in psychosocial nursing and later evolved into a strong passion for holistic nursing grounded in the Science of Unitary Human Beings (SUHB). Most nurses deeply cared about the whole person but operated in environments where the major frame of reference on caring was medical in nature. What was compelling to me was that most nurses found a way to accomplish the overwhelming medical tasks they were delegated while simultaneously looking out for all the nonmedical aspects of the human experience that contributed to the conditions their patients were experiencing. These same observations continued to inform my career choices over several years that included roles as a director of in-service education, a director of nursing in a long-term care facility, and a staff nurse in a veterans hospital.

What I most desired to change was the creeping de-emphasis in acute care on the human condition at the expense of the need to perform medical tasks. In particular, little attention was given to the psychosocial aspects of care from either a person- or family-centered perspective. Over time, I saw a growing trend in nurses being less involved in direct patient care and having growing responsibilities associated with documentation of nursing care, much of which was medical in focus. Additionally, many nurses were not prepared to manage the psychosocial aspects of the complexity of disease and recovery processes with the challenges in their own personal lives. Many nurses with whom I worked in these early settings of my career provided extraordinary integrated care and my belief in the power of nurses and nursing care to make a positive difference in the lives of patients and their families remained very strong. There was compelling evidence of this in many documented cases of nursing care provided that resulted in improved outcomes despite overwhelming odds against successful recovery.

These experiences and the emerging sense of concern were driving forces in my decision to pursue a master of science degree in psychiatric mental health nursing. At one point, because of my particular experiences in long-term care, I sought a program that would allow me to combine psychiatric mental health and gerontological nursing specialties into a single program. Unable to find such a program, I accepted admission into a program with a major in psychiatric mental health nursing at Virginia Commonwealth University. The philosophical and conceptual framework of that program was existentialism and I had four extraordinary professor mentors in that program who contributed greatly to my thinking and attitude about the science and art of advanced practice nursing: Patricia Wiley, Barbara Munjas, Gloria Francis, and Jack Duncan. Each contributed, in some unique way, to my thinking and attitude about the value of relationships and care for one another while being considerate about the quality and discipline of one's professional work. The experiences I had with the faculty, students, and clients in that learning environment, steeped in the philosophical values of existentialism, confirmed my focus on and commitment to more humanistic nursing care.

Just as I moved directly from my diploma education to BSN education, I graduated from my MSN program in May of 1979 and started my PhD program at New York University in July of that year. What sparked my interest in doctoral education evolved from a graduate-level course in nursing theory as part of my MSN program; I began to appreciate the role of theory in guiding the science and practice of nursing and, although, I considered many programs, I chose to apply solely to New York University for a PhD in theory development in nursing science. The summer of 1979 was a turning point for me, both professionally and personally, as I sat through a four-day-a-week four-week course, "The Science of Unitary Man," taught by Dr. Martha E. Rogers. My exposure to Martha, as a person and a scholar, was pivotal in my development, subsequently affirmed and encouraged with the guidance and support of John Phillips throughout my dissertation studies. I was deeply attracted to the SUHB because it provided a lens and frame of reference for understanding and appreciating the wholeness of human beings, which I always intuitively comprehended was the basis for extraordinary nursing care. The most effective nursing care I had seen, and which I created in my own career, was based on knowing people as whole and using that knowledge to guide practice, often transcending the limits of a purely diagnostic approach to care.

■ PROFESSIONAL EVOLUTION/CONTRIBUTION

The accomplishments that I am most proud of stem from the body of work associated with the development of nursing knowledge grounded in the SUHB (Rogers, 1992) and the impact it had on the lives of students and participants in my practice and research. The body of work is best categorized as:

- Developing pattern appreciation as a method for unitary nursing research and practice (Cowling, 1997)
- Articulating a unitary-transformative view of nursing science that transcends methodological dichotomies (Cowling, 1999)
- Conceptualizing healing as appreciating wholeness (Cowling, 2000)
- Articulating a unitary participatory vision of nursing knowledge (Cowling, 2007)
- Developing and refining unitary appreciative inquiry (UAI; Cowling, 2001, 2004a; Cowling & Repede, 2010)
- Applying UAI to a praxis of healing for women in despair and surviving abuse as children (Cowling, 2004b, 2005, 2006, 2008)
- Synthesizing the unitary foundations for a nursing healing praxis focused on wholeness and life patterning (Cowling & Repede, 2009; Cowling & Swartout, 2011)
- Collaborating on the creation of the Nurse Manifest website and addressing the medicalization of human experience forthrightly (http://nursemanifest. com/a-nursing-manifesto-a-call-to-conscience-and-action/; Cowling, Shattell, & Todd, 2006; Kagan, Smith, Cowling, & Chinn, 2010; Cowling, Chinn, & Hagedorn, n.d.)
- Describing connections of consciousness, caring, and wholeness in nursing praxis across paradigms (Cowling, Smith, & Watson, 2008)

I think I would characterize my life's work thus far as participating in the creation of a context for the development of nursing knowledge grounded in the SUHB (Rogers, 1992). My particular contributions within a family of dedicated scholars of unitary nursing science have stemmed from the stream of ideas outlined in the preceding text. The intense intellectual attraction I found in unitary science was accompanied by a profound sense of knowing from the heart, resonating with my experiences as a nurse and with people in general, and creating a reality for nursing that was intensely meaningful and enthusiastically innovative. I hope that my work will promote human flourishing through nursing that is attuned to the wholeness and life patterning of people. Fragmentation of human experience persists in health care, and I believe that what I have offered is one alternative to that approach to healing and well-being. This is embodied in unitary appreciative nursing, which is an outgrowth of UAI and not yet fully articulated and elaborated as a conceptual system. The enterprise of writing about and publishing these ideas has been rewarding in both creative and challenging ways. There is an incredibly expansive knowledge development in nursing and it is a struggle to push the boundaries and really make a compelling case for an alternative view of nursing as both a science and an art.

The most satisfying aspect of my work has been in the research, practice, and educational applications of unitary appreciative nursing. I think the desire to bring the SUHB to life through applications is probably the most prevailing force in my professional life. Although UAI, formerly called unitary pattern appreciation, began as a research method, it also evolved into a practice method. Because UAI mutually informs the dual purposes of knowing, within both research and practice, it is really a praxis method. My current work is focused on developing a conceptual model of Unitary Appreciative Nursing (UAN).

I am most proud of the accomplishments of sharing UAI with students and colleague scholars who have found it useful and meaningful in their work. Examples of this include working with doctoral students who have conducted research using the method in relation to healing environments; supporting women survivors of child abuse, midlife transitions in women, veteran women traumatized by sexual abuse, men living with depression, posttraumatic experiences of boys, spinal cord injuries, alcoholism, and chemotherapy for breast cancer; empowerment of elderly people; and the impact of social work education on students. Although each of these studies was unique, what they shared in common was that UAI offered the participants an opportunity to deepen and broaden their understanding of the experience that was the focus of the study. When the wholeness and life patterning of these experiences were explored, new insights and opportunities for healing emerged. UAI is designed as a form of participatory inquiry where knowledge is generated, practice is informed, and research questions are addressed. It is also intended to be emancipatory and transformative in its application, such that human lives are bettered and new potentialities are revealed when applied in practice and research studies.

I am also proud of the work I have done using UAI in my own research related to despair and adult survivorship of childhood abuse (Cowling & Swartout, 2011). The first application of UAI was directed at understanding the life patterning of despair. As a clinical specialist in psychiatric mental health nursing, I was intrigued by the predominance of depression in the vast majority of clients. Depression is primarily treated as a medical diagnosis and is addressed symptomatically with good results using medications and various forms of psychotherapeutic interventions. Yet, repeatedly, I heard clients describe how medications deadened or ameliorated the sensation of depression but never really got at the nature of it. In some cases clients said that they would rather feel something than nothing at all as a result of being medicated. Many revealed that improvement in symptoms, although valued, did not necessarily improve their sense of well-being or the quality of their lives. Rather than focus the research on depression with its diagnostic connotations, I chose despair as the focal phenomenon. The advertisement of the research study led with "Despair: Your Story?" The response was overwhelming from the first day of the study. Seeking stories of despair inevitably opened up possibilities for understanding depression as well.

With one exception, women were the ones who responded to this call for participants, and many reported childhood abuse as a source of their despair. This study led to a program of research aimed at the life patterning of women in despair related to childhood abuse. These studies were both *appreciative*—acknowledging the wholeness of life patterning associated with despair—and *participatory*—empowering women to be actively engaged in pursing the understanding of their despair as coresearchers. These studies led to the development of empowerment and self-healing efforts by the women, including some groups formed for mutual support to improve their lives.

As a leader of academics for a large nursing college, I have found a strong relationship between appreciating wholeness and life patterning in individuals and appreciating the wholeness and patterning within organizations. I appreciate the pattern of the organization I work in, which manifests itself in the values and strategies that infuse the culture of care for colleagues and students alike. One example of this is the way in which we approach the success of our students. We appreciate them fully for what they bring, both academically and beyond, knowing their success can be fostered by mobilizing resources that facilitate their transformation into extraordinary nurses. We share stories of who we are, both personally and professionally, in our daily work lives so that we appreciate and acknowledge the uniqueness of each person and create a culture of care.

The evolution of my view of nursing has not changed significantly from those early days of realizing the centrality of nursing's role in bettering the lives of human beings through recognizing and appreciating the "person underneath the disease or diagnosis." I continue to believe that nurses are in a unique position to support people during those times that are most challenging and when opportunities to improve health are evident. Nursing makes a difference through its emphasis on wholeness and is at its best when the life patterning of people is the focus of care rather than the disease. My view of nursing remains best expressed in the language that I helped craft for the Nurse Manifest Project (http://nursemanifest.com/a-nursing-manifesto-a-call-to-conscience-and-action; Cowling et al., n.d.; Kagan et al., 2010); see Chapter 14 for more on the Nurse Manifest Project.).

- It is our firm conviction that there is a body of knowledge that is specific, if not unique, to nursing's concerns and interests. We think that this knowledge is grounded in the appreciation of wholeness, concern for human well-being, and ways in which we accommodate healing through the art and science of nursing. We value theoretical and practical plurality with the centrality of nursing knowledge at the forefront of practice and knowledge development.
- We advocate for a critical formulation of the educational enterprise of nursing that places a greater emphasis on personal and professional sovereignty and that nurtures the development of action generated from reflection, contemplation, and recognition of values. We believe that it is time to attend to inherent wholeness and natural healing tendencies that are often educated out of nurses as students.
- Nursing practice is guided by conscience, competence, connection with individuals and communities, and a belief in the essential worth of all beings. We own our power to transform.

■ MORAL/ETHICAL FOUNDATION

Beyond the formal sense of moral and ethical foundations, I believe that there are moral and ethical perspectives that flow from each of the streams of knowledge that I have sought to develop in my work. I share these not as an alternative to standard moral and ethical principles associated with the discipline of nursing but as a complement to those enduring beliefs. The perspectives that I share are driven by the core ideal that nursing is a service to humankind.

I have previously conveyed (Cowling & Swartout, 2011) that I agree with the ethical perspective of Schaef (1992) of "how important it is to 'name' our experience and reality" and to question what she saw "as violence done in the name of science and healing in the helping professions" (p. 10). She further inquires,

> If psychologists and people in the helping professions are open to asking themselves the question, "Is the unspoken worldview that underlies the assumptions from which I practice my profession perhaps, unwittingly, contributing to the very problems I am committed to solve?" (p. 10)

Schaef argues forcefully for every person in the helping professions to struggle with this question and to clearly articulate assumptions.

There are guiding core ethical principles, which I espouse that are grounded in unitary appreciative nursing (UAN) and its assumptions (Cowling & Swartout, 2011). In naming them, I suggest corollary ethical imperatives.

1. *Inherent wholeness.* Wholeness is a given and not a state to be achieved and, therefore, reaching to know the wholeness of another honors the fullness of his or her being and existence. Even though it may seem impossible to know the wholeness of another, the act of reaching for that wholeness signifies the desire to go beyond seeing a person as the disease, symptoms, or diagnosis. Yet, knowing one's wholeness requires a willingness to embrace all the aspects of the being, including disease, symptoms, and diagnosis. It is an ethical imperative in UAN to avoid the tendency to fragment human experience.

2. *Patterning appreciation.* Appreciation is the act of reaching for and knowing wholeness and represents a willingness to embrace the infinite possibilities of healing as it unfolds continuously. To appreciate is to consider all the aspects of human experience, regardless of how these experiences might be socially relegated, such as healthy or unhealthy and evil or good. To appreciate wholeness is to promote healing and infinite possibilities. Appreciation is an ethical imperative of UAN that creates the personal and professional comportment one must acquire to be open to all the potentialities and possibilities of the human experience associated with wholeness.

3. *Human life patterning.* From a UAN perspective, human life patterning is the focus of nursing. Human life patterning is reflected in all phenomena associated with human experience: physical/physiological, mental/emotional, spiritual/ mystical/metaphysical, and social/cultural. However, human life patterning cannot be reduced to any singular phenomenon or set of phenomena. Life patterning represents the wholeness of human beings and therefore requires use of a synoptic lens by nurses. An ethical imperative of UAN is to resist the propensity of reductionism when seeking to appreciate and understand human experience, health, and well-being.

4. *Validity of the individual experience.* All experiences are considered valid in UAN. "Individual experiences and perceptions are recognized and affirmed as being central to understanding and appreciating life patterning" (Cowling & Swartout, 2011, p. 58). An egalitarian relationship between nurses and the

people they serve is intentionally created "to honor the voice of the other as a credible source of information" (p. 58). An ethical imperative that emerges is to foster the time and space for the fullest sharing of the unique expressions of each person's life patterning.

5. *Healing as emancipation.* The goal of UAN is to promote conditions allowing for the deepest expression of freedom that support healing. This involves the highest degree of collaboration with and participation by the people being served by UAN It is acknowledged that there are socially contrived constraints placed upon the human experience and, thus, one of the primary purposes of UAN is to help people develop ways of alleviating or mediating these constraints. An ethical imperative of UAN as emancipatory healing is to promote those conditions that are most congruent with personal freedom and self-directed health.

■ VISION

Nurses have made incredible contributions to the health and well-being of humankind. Nursing as a discipline has a unique mission that is even more relevant today because of its focus and accountability to society, which has now been and continues to be legislated. Furthermore, nursing is a body of knowledge that is constantly being refined, and it contributes to improving health and well-being. In accord with Martha Rogers, I envision a world of infinite potentials (1993). She described a new reality based on a synthesis of emerging knowledge and creative ideas. Rogers believed that

> Experiencing expanding horizons can help us gain a vastly greater understanding of people and their evolutionary potential. The nature of it is going to vary as we move into a future with more new ideas that will transform what we know now. (p. 3)

Her view of nursing science was an optimistic one in which people could employ their capacity to knowingly participate in change to their greatest advantage. I believe that one vital capacity of humankind is to participate appreciatively in ways that will be transformative and emancipatory.

Nursing will evolve and continuously capture its richest potential as nursing grows with the needs of human beings. The enduring nature of nursing resides in its connection and relationship to people who are experiencing challenges to well-being and health and who want to improve these. Health systems continue to be dominated by an acute care model in spite of the decades of calls for a primary care focus. The predictions of a pending nursing shortage and, more recently, of a less severe shortage, are based on limited ways of thinking about what nursing means or may mean to society. A shift is required to go beyond the discourse of the quantity of nurses needed to the quality and forms of nursing that can be pivotal in improving the health of all. Nursing will discover new territories of service that are likely to grow and emerge as an alternative to health care institutions that currently exist and expand existing ones. As always, nursing will thrive as it promotes human flourishing. It is clear that people are seeking alternatives to current systems of care. It is clear that digital information is a common resource of information for those seeking to promote healing and improve health. There will be no boundaries for nursing as it inhabits communities, the digital world, and space and responds to calls for care in many forms.

There is a great deal of emphasis on a fully embodied nursing profession, particularly with the national call for nurses to practice to the fullest extent of their preparation (Institute of Medicine, 2011). Although this is a worthy call and should be a guiding principle in designing an enriched nursing profession, a nursing future shaped on ongoing embodiment personified by creative responsiveness to the flourishing of humankind is most important. Rather than advocate for a single road for nursing, I would resist the temptation to tell a single story or define the perfect road to embodying nursing fully. One path would be incomplete. The bold future of nursing I subscribe to requires many paths that support nourishing and inspiring the human spirit, appreciating the wholeness of human life, promoting healing through freedom and self-determination, and seeking novel ways of caring that expand the infinite potentials of human beings.

A common way of assessing one's professional contributions is to focus on what has been unrealized in a life of work. This has great value in that it gives one a context of where one would like to go next. However, I resist this temptation to fully base an assessment of my work from this perspective, because it seems counterintuitive to the notion of appreciation and might limit the many possibilities of what would come next. The power of writing this chapter for me is that it required me to go back and look at my work and to appreciate what I had done and also to see it with new eyes and richer understandings, and consider novel ways of expanding and enriching this work. As I write this section, I am personally inspired to take my thinking in unique directions, considering its relevance to my current endeavors in nursing education and beyond.

I think most nurses know what they need to know if they follow their passions. What I did not know early in my nursing experience was that what was most important was not *why I wanted to be a nurse* but *what it felt like to be a nurse*. Being a nurse as a man in the early 1960s was illogical in many ways. It went against conventions of what men were "supposed to be" doing with their lives at that time. I endured some experiences from peers and male patients that bordered on ridicule and seem unheard of today. Little taunts provoked a sense of doubt and shame that diminished the real joy I felt in doing what nurses do. This was also woven into my dawning realization that I was gay, although I did not have a word for those feelings. On the other hand, I experienced resentment from nurse peers for the opportunities that were unfairly given to me based on my gender. It felt right to be a nurse and it has always felt right to be a nurse.

What I would say to anyone about his or her profession, nursing or otherwise, that I did not know then, is pay attention to your heart, because it is likely telling you what your head needs to know. And when you appreciate this inherent wholeness of all the aspects of who you are, your spirit thrives.

■ REFLECTIONS

1. *As I think about my own journey in nursing, where I am right now on this journey, what is the dominant force that drives me to do nursing? What does it feel like when I believe I am practicing nursing to my fullest potential? Can I describe anything common in the author's and my shared journeys in nursing?*

2. *In what ways have I been unknowingly reductionistic in my attempts to appreciate and understand human beings, health, and well-being? How can I integrate a lens of wholeness into my practice?*

3. *If I accept the idea that humans and groups are inherently whole, and the goal is not to help people become more whole but to appreciate the power of their innate wholeness, what kinds of power would that bring to their lives?*

4. *What is my vision for the future of nursing and how can I participate knowingly in that future, as Rogers (1993) has described?*

5. *With regard to healing as emancipation, which conditions, congruent with freedom and self-directed health, should be promoted and strengthened in my life?*

■ REFERENCES

American Nurses Association. (1965). *Educational preparation for nurse practitioners and assistants to nurses: A position paper.* New York, NY: Author.

Cowling, W.R., III. (1997). Pattern appreciation: The unitary science/practice of reaching for essence. In M. Madrid (Ed.), *Patterns of Rogerian knowing* (pp. 129–142). New York, NY: National League for Nursing.

Cowling, W. R., III. (1999). A unitary-transformative nursing science: Potentials for transcending dichotomies. *Nursing Science Quarterly, 12*(2), 132–135.

Cowling, W. R., III. (2000). Healing as appreciating wholeness. *Advances in Nursing Science, 22*(3), 16–32.

Cowling, W. R., III. (2001). Unitary appreciative inquiry. *Advances in Nursing Science, 23*(4), 32–48.

Cowling, W. R., III. (2004a). Pattern, participation, praxis, and power in unitary appreciative inquiry. *Advances in Nursing Science, 27*(3), 202–214.

Cowling, W. R., III. (2004b). Despair: A unitary appreciative inquiry. *Advances in Nursing Science, 27*(4), 287–300.

Cowling, W. R., III. (2005). Despairing women and healing outcomes: A unitary appreciative nursing perspective. *Advances in Nursing Science, 28*(2), 94–106.

Cowling, W. R., III. (2006). A unitary healing praxis model for women in despair. *Nursing Science Quarterly, 19*(2), 123–132.

Cowling, W. R., III. (2007). A unitary participatory vision of nursing knowledge. *Advances in Nursing Science, 30*(1), 61–70.

Cowling, W. R., III. (2008). An essay on women, despair, and healing: A personal narrative. *Advances in Nursing Science, 31*(3), 249–258.

Cowling, W. R., III, Chinn, P., & Hagedorn, S. (n.d.). *A nursing manifesto: A call to conscience and action.* Retrieved from https://nursemanifest.com/a-nursing-manifesto-a-call-to-conscience-and-action/

Cowling, W. R., III., & Repede, E. (2009). Consciousness and knowing: The patterning of the whole. In R. C. Locsin & M. J. Purnell (Eds.), *A contemporary process of nursing: The (Un)bearable weight of knowing persons* (pp. 73–98). New York, NY: Springer.

Cowling, W. R., III., & Repede, E. (2010). Unitary appreciative inquiry: Evolution and refinement. *Advances in Nursing Science, 33*(1), 64–77. doi:10.1097/ans.0b013e3181ce6bdd

Cowling, W. R., III., Shattell, M., & Todd, M. (2006). Hall's essay on an authentic meaning of medicalization: An extended discourse. *Advances in Nursing Science, 29*(4), 291–304.

Cowling, W. R., III., Smith, M., & Watson, J. (2008). The power of wholeness, consciousness, and caring: A dialogue on nursing science, art, and healing. *Advances in Nursing Science, 31*(1), E41–E51.

Cowling, W. R., III, & Swartout, K. M. (2011). Wholeness and life patterning: Unitary foundations for a healing praxis. *Advances in Nursing Science, 34*(7), 51–66. doi:10.1097/ANS.0b013e3182094497

Institute of Medicine. (2011). *The future of nursing: Leading change, advancing health*. Washington, DC: National Academies Press.

Kagan, P., Smith, M., Cowling, W. R., III., & Chinn, P. (2010). A nursing manifesto: An emancipatory call for knowledge development, conscience, and praxis. *Nursing Philosophy, 11*(1), 67–84.

Rogers, M. E. (1992). Nursing science and the space age. *Nursing Science Quarterly, 7*(1), 27–34.

Rogers, M. E. (1993). Comments from Dr. Rogers on the birth of the journal. *Visions: The Journal of Rogerian Nursing Science, 1*(1), 3–4.

Schaef, A. W. (1992). *Beyond therapy, beyond science: A new model for healing the whole person*. San Francisco, CA: Harper Press.

CHAPTER FOUR

Integral and Whole: Embracing the Journey of Healing, Local to Global

Barbara Montgomery Dossey

Healing is a lifelong journey into understanding the wholeness of human existence. Healing occurs when we help clients, families, others, and ourselves embrace what is feared most. It occurs when we seek harmony and balance. Healing is learning how to open what has been closed so that we can expand our inner potentials. It is the fullest expression of oneself that is demonstrated by the light and shadow and the male and female principles that reside within each of us. It is accessing what we have forgotten about connections, unity, and interdependence.

—Dossey (2016, p. 23)

■ WHY NURSING?

I was born in Little Rock, Arkansas, followed 13 minutes later by my fraternal twin brother; our dear sister was born three and a half years later. I was blessed to be part of a close family from whom I learned about unconditional love. My immediate family and my grandparents were all blessed with good health.

Education was valued in my family and my parents were both college graduates. I always knew I wanted to go to college. I gave no thought to a professional career until my junior year in high school. My cousin, 15 years older, was a nursing supervisor and a very wise woman. Her stories about nursing and the hospital were always fascinating to me. Soon after this, my cousin's two younger sisters became nurses, so I then had three cousins who were nurses. During one visit to these relatives, my uncle was the first to suggest the value of a nursing career. I was impressed when he told me that I could always find work as a nurse anywhere in the world. I had already spent a summer traveling from London to Helsinki, Finland, where I lived with a family for five weeks and I knew

I wanted to do more traveling. Several weeks after this visit my junior counselor asked me what I wanted to study in college; my reply was nursing. Thus began the journey.

In the fall of 1961, I was off to Baylor University, Waco, Texas, with no idea of what the nursing profession was or how it would change my life. The first two years of science courses and labs were challenging. In the fall of 1963, my nursing class began our clinical rotations at Baylor University Medical Center in Dallas, Texas. This was the beginning of national discussions on the entry into professional nursing practice at the baccalaureate level that was to begin in 1965, the year of my graduation.

Our nursing school was not accredited, and my classmates and I did not understand the implications of this national mandate or the importance of graduating from an accredited school of nursing. However, we soon realized the importance of the credential when our school applied for national accreditation with increased emphasis on course objectives, curriculum, and clinical practicum outcomes. National nurse examiners came to our classes and our clinical rotations and all nursing students were interviewed.

Two events in my senior year were to have an impact on the rest of my career. The first was that, as students, we were being encouraged to join the American Nurses Association (ANA). I did join and have been a member now for 50 years. I remember the thrill of belonging to my first professional nursing organization. The second event occurred during my senior leadership course, where we were encouraged to attend a national nursing theory conference where three esteemed nurse theorists—Ernestine Wiedenbach, Lydia Hall, and Virginia Henderson—discussed the importance of theory development and their personal conceptualizations of nursing. Their words about the nursing profession as an art and a science and its unique contributions to society were profound. From the beginning of my career, I always tried to apply theory to my practice.

This was a progressive and innovative time at Baylor University Medical Center with the development of many new cardiothoracic surgery procedures and protocols that were also happening in all the specialties. Following cardiothoracic operations and other procedures, patients required 24-hour monitoring and the recovery room was open continuously. Nursing students were allowed to do basic nursing care to assist these nurses and I began working weekends to gain more skills. Soon several medical and surgical floor rooms were converted to small intensive care units, followed later on by elaborately designed intensive care units. I let the intensive care unit supervisor know that I wanted to work on her unit after graduation. In the summer of 1965, I became an intensive care unit nurse and discovered both my passion and the formidable challenges within the complexity of what later was named critical care. I had no idea what was to open for me in those early years of my career.

■ EARLY IMPRESSIONS

I entered critical care nursing at a time when the thoughts, emotions, and beliefs of patients and their families were valued and considered. As technology increased, so did impersonal interactions and a focus on the curing of symptoms. When a patient got well, it was attributed to the physicians, machines, and potent medications. The meaning of illness and its place and purpose in a person's life became anachronistic.

My colleagues and I began to write critical care protocols and I remember placing the words "body, mind, and spirit" in my contributions. In 1974, I joined the American

Association of Critical-Care Nurses (AACN) and also attended my first National Teaching Institute (NTI). It was thrilling to be with critical care nurses from all over the country. I became certified in critical care in 1977 and that helped me understand the significance of the national certification process.

Early in my career, I became aware of the power of a person's belief systems. My first supervisor taught me the importance of what it meant to serve another in the midst of the fast-paced, technological critical care environment. She emphasized the nurse's presence and the quality of being present with a person without doing anything. She told me to listen with my heart and to feel as much as possible what a patient believed to be true. As I listened to the rich tapestry of patients' life stories, I realized that the meaning they gave their lives and the healing rituals they were incorporating, for the most part, directed how they would heal, with little influence of the medical technology or treatments used.

The first example of this was when patients were given placebos and their pain was relieved. Although many physicians and nurses laughed at how easy it was to fool a patient, I began to see a pattern of a placebo working and most often knew who would respond and who would not. If the physician or nurse engaged with an authentic presence with the patient, then the placebo would relieve the pain.

Another example pertained to a patient, a Gypsy king, who was being treated with intravenous medications secondary to a myocardial infarction. Two days after being in the critical care unit, he told me that his personal medicine woman had given him a copper bracelet the evening before and he was feeling well. He announced to me that he would be leaving in several hours. About this time, his physician came in and told the Gypsy king that if he left he would have to find another physician and that he would probably die. My supervisor's response was that he was welcome to come back if needed. I saw this Gypsy king a year later very alive and well.

In 1967, my interests and passions were ignited with a series of events that have shaped my professional and personal life endeavors. I became interested in the emerging field of holistic health and became aware of setting new personal health goals, meditating, learning self-regulations strategies, and eating healthier. I was also fencing competitively and engaging in a disciplined training program that included stretching, strength training, and running. I began to study and attend workshops on ideas related to holism and the body-mind-spirit connection, as well as read other disciplines such as systems theory, quantum physics, integral, Eastern, and Western philosophy and mysticism, and much more. I also read nurse theorists and other discipline theorists who informed my knowing, doing, and being in caring, healing, and holism. I joined the Texas Air National Guard (first lieutenant 1968–1970; captain 1970–1972) as a nurse in the medical department. I traveled to Europe in the summers where we set up our field hospital to prepare our unit for emergency readiness, as this was during the Vietnam era.

In 1967, I was blessed to have Larry Dossey walk into the critical care unit where I worked and where he completed his critical care rotation during his last month in medical school. Thank you, Universe! Yes, it was love at first sight! He was, and still is, a lovely, handsome man and the love of my life! It was beyond exciting to meet Larry as our interests were so compatible. As they say, the rest is history. We met in our 20s and we have grown together, challenging and supporting each other with creative ideas and new possibilities that were then outside of mainstream health care. It just seems to be richer now that we are in our 70s and we continue thinking about new potentials and ideas. Larry also has an identical twin brother; thus since both of us were twins, we had fascinating and remarkable conversations related to a special kind of knowing about our twin before an event happened or a simultaneous event occurring while our twin was at a distance miles away. This became part of our exploring expanding states of consciousness that continues to this day.

In 1981 and 1982, we both found our voices and discovered a passion for writing. Each of us published our first books, which have been followed by many more books, articles, and contributions at regional, national, and international conferences and other venues.

After Larry returned from serving in Vietnam and completed his second year in the military in 1970, followed by a two-year residency, he began his practice of internal medicine. As we cared for critically ill patients and their families, some of our greatest teachers, we were able to reflect on how to blend the art of caring and healing modalities with the science of technology and traditional ones. We held salons in his large office meeting room with 30 to 40 interprofessionals who were also interested in consciousness studies, holistic health, and healing modalities.

In 1965, I had a health challenge that began my deep education about personal health responsibility and self-regulation. I was in Mexico on a vacation and ate some contaminated food that resulted in a 24-hour course of a 102° fever, diarrhea, and vomiting. Two days later after returning home my right eye became swollen shut. I was diagnosed with dendritic keratitis, an infection of the cornea caused by the herpes simplex virus. At this time, antiviral medications were still experimental; I was placed on topical ointment and it cleared up after six weeks. However, whenever I was under any type of stress over the next 10-year period my eye would flare-up, and with each one, I developed more scar formation on my cornea and eventually had no vision in my right eye.

By the end of 1975, I had gone a full year without a flare-up, which was then the criterion for a corneal transplant. Six weeks after my corneal transplant, I had two bouts of acute rejection that were managed by the injection of a steroid into my cornea. An eyelid stretcher was placed around my right eye to keep it open while receiving the injection. Although my eye had been anesthetized so I would not feel pain, my anxiety in seeing the needle coming toward my eye and the helplessness I felt has never left me. I can still remember holding my breath, bracing, and tensing my shoulders and jaws. How I wish I had known more about distraction, relaxation, and rhythmic breathing practices. This event made me aware of the need to be more present with my patients before I poked, suctioned, and performed all the procedures and treatments on them that were part of caring for a critically ill patient. It also let me know that I never really or truly know a person's story and I must listen deeply.

According to the statistics, I ran the risk of a 20% to 30% rejection rate for my corneal transplant for the rest of my life. My eye is currently in a healed state and I have a perfectly clear cornea. But when I am tired, stressed, or overworked, my right eye aches, tears, and hurts, and my vision becomes cloudy. But instead of worrying about a rejection of my corneal transplant, I know that I must take a break, let go of some of the deadlines, and engage in self-care. I have learned to incorporate technology, mind, and spirit. I always travel with an antiviral medication in case I get a flare-up and cannot manage it with my relaxation, imagery, and self-care. I know my eye well. When it begins to bother me I get a subtle sensation like a single hair that sweeps above, under, and in the center of my right eye. This is the first step in inner self-awareness—listening to my body and acknowledging the sensation. I say to myself, "Okay, I feel you. Thank you!" This has been a great gift, as it has helped me recognize what it is to live with a chronic condition. It also has helped me explore the wonderful journey of health responsibility, self-care, and the use of healing rituals to understand more about human consciousness and self-regulation, and to incorporate it into my life and work.

Larry was also having severe migraine headaches and was in search of something else rather than medicine. We both began to take courses related to body-mind-spirit therapies (biofeedback, relaxation, imagery, music, therapeutic touch, meditation, and other reflective practices) and began to incorporate them into our daily lives. As we strengthened our capacities with self-regulation and self-care modalities, our personal lives and our professional philosophies and clinical practices also changed. We took seriously teaching and incorporating these modalities into the traditional health care setting that today is called integrative health care.

Within his internal medicine practice, Larry began a large biofeedback practice with four biofeedback therapists. When any of them needed time off, I began to work there. It became very clear that we used the same type of equipment in the critical care unit but did not engage patients to use their consciousness for healing as was done in the biofeedback lab. This observation began my steady integration of relaxation, music, and imagery in my critical care practice. We had many colleagues who did not understand the relevance of consciousness and healing as an adjunct to traditional medicine. However, there was no way we could engage in our professional practices without integrating these modalities. From these experiences, our philosophies were a "both/and," not "either/or." We began to find and continue to have many professional and interdisciplinary health care colleagues with whom to discuss concepts, protocols, and approaches for practice, education, research, and health care policy.

■ PROFESSIONAL EVOLUTION/CONTRIBUTION

Around 1975, I began to ask myself, "What might I do to engage in and create innovative changes in nursing and health care?" Practicing as a critical care and cardiovascular nurse, I was intensely aware that the emphasis was on the latest technology. A patient may have open-heart surgery or thrombolytic therapy to limit or stop an evolving heart attack and save his or her life. These technological interventions take only minutes to hours, but it may require years to bring about a fundamental shift in one's consciousness to reshape the thoughts, emotions, and behaviors that contributed to the heart disease in the first place. I am referring to how patients choose to live their lives, to create healthy lifestyle patterns including one's spirituality, meaning, and purpose, life balance and satisfaction, loving relationships, and health promotion activities such as exercise, stress management, and nutrition. This area of wellness and well-being continues to be my focus after 50 years in nursing.

I could see ways to weave and integrate holistic concepts into clinical practice and was already doing this, although many colleagues thought it took too much time and there were no scientific data to support its use in critical care. I began my master's program in 1975 so that I could learn more about this expanded role. I identified many opportunities to incorporate these concepts and modalities into nursing education in traditional core courses and technology. Practicing nurses could join nursing faculty to come together and determine the best way for the integration to take place in their particular institution, hospital, or academic setting. The biggest challenge was in how to use an integrative approach when the health care system was driven by a disease-based model, which functioned as a disease management industry. In order to meet the needs of patients and their families, we needed to follow models of caring and healing. The challenge was to bring our intuition, compassion, and presence into all corners of health care, even when technology nudged them out, and to recognize that patient care also required "being with" rather than always "doing to."

From 1965 to 1972, I worked full-time in critical care. From 1972 until 1982, I worked part-time in critical care and also began teaching critical care in a university setting. I joined with a critical care and cardiovascular nursing colleague and soul mate, Cathie Guzzetta, to advance holistic ideas in our teaching protocols and critical care courses, as well as write textbooks and articles with other contributors. We published *Critical Care Nursing: Body-Mind-Spirit* (Kenner, Guzzetta, & Dossey, 1981), released by several different publishers with different titles until 1997. In 1984, Cathie and I published *Cardiovascular Nursing: Bodymind Tapestry* (Guzzetta & Dossey, 1984), which also had several editions. Both books had holistic nursing and integrative modalities woven throughout.

In 1981, I became a founding member of the American Holistic Nurses Association (AHNA; 2016). The AHNA and ANA (2013) define *holistic nursing* as a philosophical foundation that can be practiced at any time and anywhere—local to global. It embraces all nursing that has the enhancement of healing the whole person, from birth to death, as its goal. It is a perspective that addresses the body, mind, and spirit of not just the patient but of the nurse as well. This philosophy or way of being supports the holistic nurse in her or his personal life, as well as in clinical and private practice, education, research, and community service. It can be practiced in any hospital, clinical, community, or global setting.

I have made many contributions to holistic nursing and the AHNA, with my first committee chair position working with colleagues to draft the first *AHNA Scope and Standards of Practice* in 1985, revised several times over the next five years and first published in 1990 (AHNA, 1990). The AHNA and ANA *Holistic Nursing: Scope and Standards of Practice* is now a joint publication (AHNA/ANA, 2013). In 2006, the ANA recognized holistic nursing as a specialty as a result of the work of many holistic nurse colleagues and myself since 1981.

Holistic nurse colleague and soul mate, Lynn Keegan, and I began our Bodymind Systems business teaching workshops and published our *Self-Care: A Program to Improve your Life* (Keegan & Dossey, 1987). We have both been very active in the AHNA (see Chapter 7 for more informationon the AHNA and our collaboration). Next, we coauthored *Holistic Nursing: A Handbook for Practice* (Dossey, Keegan, Guzzetta, & Kolkmeier, 1988), which is now in its seventh edition. Our new editors are Cynthia Barrere, Mary Helming, Deborah Shields, and Karen Avino, and the textbook has many online support resources.

In 1995, with Noreen Frisch, we chaired the AHNA Core Task Force that reviewed 10 years of literature on holistic nursing and related fields. From that review, an Inventory of Professional Activities and Knowledge of a Holistic Nurse (IPAKHN) questionnaire was published and the AHNA membership responded. From the data analysis, we were able to establish the essential holistic nursing core content and core concepts and 24 of the most frequently used interventions in holistic nursing practice. Because of this work I was appointed the first editor of the *AHNA Core Curriculum for Holistic Nursing* (Dossey, 1997). This work became a blueprint for the basic, and later the advanced, holistic nursing certification (American Holistic Nurses Credentialing Corporation, n.d.).

In 1997, the AHNA entered into a contract with the National League for Nursing for the writing of the certification examination. This work has now been expanded into the *AHNA Core Curriculum for Holistic Nursing* (2014), with editors Cynthia Barrere, Mary Helming, Deborah Shields, and Karen Avino.

My passion for nursing theory led me to pursue my doctoral degree in 2000 at the Union Institute & University in Cincinnati, Ohio. During my doctoral studies, I began the development of my Theory of Integral Nursing (TIN). However, I completed the theory after finishing my doctoral studies, as I needed to finish my doctorate and the theory development needed much more time.

The TIN is a grand theory that guides the art and science of integral nursing practice, education, research, and health care policy. It incorporates physical, mental, emotional, spiritual, cultural, and environmental dimensions and includes an expansive worldview. It invites nurses to think widely and deeply about personal health, client/patient/family health, as well as that of the local community and the global village. This theory recognizes the philosophical foundation and legacy of Florence Nightingale (1820–1910; Dossey, 2010; Dossey, Selanders, Beck, & Attewell, 2005), healing and healing research, the metaparadigm of nursing (nurse, person[s], health, and environment [society]), the six patterns of knowing (personal, empirics, aesthetics, ethics, not knowing, sociopolitical), integral theory, and nonnursing theories. It builds on the existing integral, integrative, and holistic multidimensional theoretical nursing foundation and has been informed by other nurse theorists. It incorporates concepts from various philosophies and fields that include holistic holism, multidimensionality, integral and chaos theories, spiral dynamics, complex systems, and many other paradigms.

I am excited to say that TIN is being used in practice, education, research, health care policy, and global nursing. Darlene Hess used the TIN as a template to design an RN-to-BSN curriculum based at Northern New Mexico College in Espanola, New Mexico. Darlene's endeavors were recognized when she received the 2015 Excellence in Holistic Nursing Education Award at the AHNA's 35th Annual Conference.

Like most of my colleagues in nursing, I gained only a meager and essentially trivialized picture of Florence Nightingale (1820–1919) during my professional education. In 1992, my breath was taken away when I obtained a 42-second voice recording of Nightingale's voice from the Thomas Alva Edison Museum in East Orange, New Jersey, that had been recorded by Edison's assistant in London on July 30, 1890. Nightingale speaks the following words: "When I am no longer even a memory, just a name, I hope my voice perpetuates the great work of my life. God bless my dear old comrades of Balaclava and bring them safe to shore" (Florence Nightingale's voice, 1890).

From 1992 to 1998, with many trips to London to read Nightingale's original letters at the British Library, the Florence Nightingale Museum, the Wellcome Trust, and the Greater London Record Office, I explored her life deeply and was awed by what I found. In 1995, I traveled to Istanbul, Turkey, and visited the Barracks Hospital where she worked during the Crimean War (1854–1856).

Like a fiery comet, Florence Nightingale streaked across the skies of 19th-century England and transformed the world with her passage (Dossey, 2010). She was a towering genius of both intellect and spirit, and her legacy resonates today as forcefully as during her lifetime. Her legacy was far more magnificent than I had imagined, and she, as an individual personality, was more complex than I could have dreamed. The farther my research took me, the larger Nightingale loomed—not just in nursing but in other fields as well, such as public health, statistics, hospital design, philosophy, and spirituality. By any measure, she is one of the most influential figures in the Victorian age, with her long life that spanned 90 years and 3 months. Indeed, it is difficult to find her equal on the entire canvas of the 19th-century Western world.

I felt a compelling inner tug to write an illustrated biography through my nursing lens that was published as *Florence Nightingale: Mystic, Visionary, Healer* (Dossey, 2000; 2010 Commemorative edition). To date, I am her only nurse biographer. The work that I am most proud of within the biography is bringing Nightingale forward as a 19th-century mystic using Evelyn Underhill's five phases of mystical spiritual development, making the case for her illness being due to chronic brucellosis, exploring her personality type using the Myers-Brigg Type Indicator* (MBTI), and finding an article that Mohandas K. Gandhi wrote on Nightingale in 1915.

In 1995, while in London during my research, I attended the Florence Nightingale Service at Westminster Abbey that was filled with nurses from around the world. When I returned home I began inquiring about why we had no such service in the United States at the Washington National Cathedral that is under the direction of the Episcopal Church of the United States. Months earlier, I had met Louise Selanders, a nurse and Florence Nightingale scholar, who was an Episcopalian and knew the church protocols. I contacted The Reverend Canon Ted Karpf, my dear Episcopal priest friend, who at the time was with the National Episcopal AIDS Coalition (NEAC). I shared how Louise and I would like to work with him and create a Nightingale Service at the Washington National Cathedral and to have her name placed on the church calendar. He listened to our strategies and also told us that Nightingale had already been denied on the calendar; however, we were not to be deterred.

We began our scholarship to secure the approval for reliability of the case and reasonableness of reconsideration of Nightingale's place on the calendar. I wrote three of five articles, Louise wrote two, and we acquired two additional contributed articles. Each of the seven articles also had a reflection. Just before the document was sent forward, I was introduced via e-mail to Deva-Marie Beck, who had written a poem titled "The Flame of Florence Nightingale's Legacy." The poem, seven articles, seven reflections, and the Resolution Proposal requesting the reconsideration of Nightingale's commemoration and for her name to be placed on the church calendar list of *Lesser Feasts and Fasts* in the *Book of Common Prayer* were compiled and sent to the Episcopal Church Standing Liturgical Commission before the 72nd General Episcopal Church Convention in Philadelphia in June 1997. It would take another three years before the outcome was revealed. The official vote to accept Nightingale to the church calendar occurred at the General Convention in Denver, Colorado, in July 2000, and she was entered into the church calendar on August 12, 2000.

The AHNA published these articles in a special issue of the *Journal of Holistic Nursing* in 1998 ("Florence Nightingale and her legacy," 1998), reprinted them in the special issue of the *Journal of Holistic Nursing* in her centennial year ("Florence Nightingale and her legacy," 2010, March), and in another special issue some months later ("Florence nightingale and her legacy . . . Part II," 2010, December). The inaugural Florence Nightingale Commemorative Service was held on August 12, 2001, at the Washington National Cathedral, Washington, DC.

Louise, Deva, and I finally met in person at the Florence Nightingale Museum in London during the 1999 International Council of Nurses convention. Following our meeting, we continued to further our conversations, as we knew there was more to be done to carry Nightingale's legacy forward. In 2004, we established the Nightingale Initiative for Global Health (NIGH, 2016) and the "Nightingale Declaration for A Healthy World" (Nightingale Declaration, 2016), which was the first ever Nightingale global nursing Internet signature campaign (see Chapter 18 for more information on NIGH, the Nightingale Declaration, and our collaboration.).

In 2005, we coauthored *Florence Nightingale Today: Healing, Leadership, Global Action* (Dossey, Selanders, Beck & Attewell, 2005). Together with NIGH and Sigma Theta Tau International (STTI), and our sponsors' financial support, we planned the Florence Nightingale Centennial Service on April 25, 2010, at the Washington National Cathedral, which is archived (Florence Nightingale Service, 2010). The NIGH is now in global conversations with the Florence Nightingale Museum and others in the planning of the 2020 Florence Nightingale bicentennial celebration (1820–2020).

In 2010, I began to bring all of my career passions together to focus on the role of nurses in health and wellness coaching. I became a codirector of the International Nurse Coach Association (INCA) with Susan Luck (see Chapter 24) and Bonney Gulino Schaub (see Chapter 27). Our coauthored book, *Nurse Coaching: Integrative Approaches for Health and Wellbeing* (Dossey, Luck, & Schaub, 2015), is the first nurse coaching textbook to be published. Currently, Susan and I continue as codirectors of INCA and are the core faculty of the Integrative Nurse Coach Certificate Program (INCCP).

Susan, Bonney, and I developed the Theory of Integrative Nurse Coaching (TINC), which is a middle-range theory as well as a philosophy, framework, and methodology. Healing, the metaparadigm, and patterns of knowing in nursing (personal, empirics, aesthetics, ethics, not knowing, sociopolitical) are integrated in the TINC. The TINC has five components as follows: (a) Nurse Coach Self-Development, (b) Integral Perspectives and Change, (c) Integrative Lifestyle Health and Wellbeing, (d) Awareness and Choice, and (e) Listening with HEART© (Healing, Energy, Awareness, Resiliency, Transformation).

To further the role of nurse coaching, Susan and I developed the Integrative Nurse Coach Leadership Model© (INCLM). The INCLM components are the same as those of the TINC. The INCLM expands nursing's visibility in creating a culture of health and well-being. Nurses are challenged to be leaders and the driving force both in health care reform and in the health and wellness coaching movement. Integrative nurse coaches are uniquely positioned to coach and engage individuals in the process of behavior change in hospitals, clinics, and communities, and to advance steps toward healthier people living on a healthy planet—local to global.

Parallel to this process, we worked with three other nurse coach colleagues, Darlene Hess, Mary Elaine Southard, and Linda Bark, and drafted a document that was vetted through nurse coach experts and a thorough peer review process to fully describe the professional nurse coach role. The ANA and 19 other organizations officially recognized our endeavors. This work was later published as *The Art and Science of Nurse Coaching: The Provider's Guide to Scope and Competencies* (Hess et al., 2013).

These endeavors led to conversations with the American Holistic Nurse Credentialing Corporation (AHNCC) regarding the paradigm shift toward health and wellness inherent in the Affordable Care Act (ACA) and the importance of developing the nurse coach role. Given that holistic nurses specialize in the practice of health and wellness, it was mutually determined that AHNCC was the appropriate venue for a national certification program for professional nurse coaches. After lengthy discussions, the six authors entered into an agreement with AHNCC, whereby AHNCC would sponsor our work (Hess et al., 2013) in exchange for the rights to establish a national certification process for nurse coaches that began in January 2013 (AHNCC, n.d.).

■ MORAL/ETHICAL FOUNDATION

To me, a holistic ethic is the moral fiber of nursing. The basic underlying concept is unity and integral wholeness of all people and of all nature. From the beginning of my career, I have been aware of a professional nursing code of ethics, which I have integrated with my personal ethical code. This has influenced the way I work with clients/patients in their care, with other interprofessional colleagues, and how I think about my role in society. I find that ANA's (2015) revised *Code of Ethics with Interpretative Statements* can assist nurses and the nursing profession to translate ethics into daily practice and life.

My early childhood upbringing and my nursing foundation have always guided me to reach a decision about the choice of the right thing to do and to enact chosen behavior/s and action/s. Since this includes an expansive consideration from "me" to "us" to "all of us," it has often been very challenging. To strengthen my moral capacity, I strive to access the deep place of my "soul's purpose" and stay in touch with what I have been called to do in this lifetime. This is the ethical character that I believe is inherent in nursing. To deepen this capacity of ethical connectedness, I find that creating time to enter into a sacred space or a nonordinary state of consciousness is essential. Thus my awareness is to tell the truth to myself without judging, to touch my sense of inner worth, and recognize what and who really matters. This is also the opportunity to explore the "shadow" and to be with what is not working and where I feel vulnerable. This requires that I move to a reflective place and allow clarity of thought, actions, and next steps to emerge.

For me, a constant metaphor and image of clarity for more than 40 years comes from the first time Larry took me backpacking to Warbonnet Lake in the Sawtooth Mountains in Idaho, which is at an altitude of 10,000 feet. I often go to this place in my mind and step into the sounds, sensations, and feelings, and imagine sitting by this pristine jewel of blue-green clear, cold, deep water where I can see to a depth of 20 feet. Using the metaphor of water and going deep below the water surface requires that I shift my consciousness from the busy, day-to-day activities and the superficial awareness and enter into this image and experience—to see new images, patterns, processes, and possibilities that feel authentic and true for the greater good of a project or endeavor.

To bring this moral awareness to my work requires that I am sourcing my wisdom from the deepest possible place so that my words and behaviors can flow from this authentic space. This creates a feeling of abundance that empowers me in my collective mission of health and healing of humanity. If I operate from a place of scarcity my best will not come forward. This space also allows me to form different levels of partnerships and be very supportive of the many creative ideas of others; there is no one way to accomplish the vast work needed in the healing of health care and society. The words I use to describe this inner space may seem trite, but there is a profound feeling and inner experience that occurs. My goal is to live life from this space as much as I can.

For me, nursing has always been an ethics of caring and compassion, and striving to maximize the good (autonomy, comfort, dignity, quality of life) and minimize the bad (pain, suffering). It is listening with intention and from a heart space to the client's stories/narratives, history, experiences, and perceptions. It is to ask curious questions such as, "What do you need right now?" and, "What do you want me to know most about you?" This conveys, "I see you," "I hear you," "I am walking with you," and, "I am learning and understanding how you relate to the world and others." From an integral perspective, these questions reflect the subjective "I" that explores the many dimensions of being in the world, while assisting the client to reflect and respond in her or his own time to what is manifesting and emergent in the moment. It is also the "we" of the shared intersubjective presence and the interactions between the nurse and client. We, as nurses, do our best when we are fully engaged with clients, which implies a capacity to connect to and be with another in an intersubjective, mutual, and authentic manner, while honoring complexity and ambiguity. When I view clients, others, and society from unity and integral wholeness, the fundamental values of a client-centered, integrative, integral, and holistic relationship are experienced. The profound privilege of being called to a profession of service is sacred. In the everyday of nursing practice, nurses come to know people in the most intimate ways, particularly when a person is very ill and her or his bodily functions are beyond control. This has been called the *ethic of intimates* and is consistent with nursing's history of orienting our moral compass toward issues of everyday practice (Wright & Brajtman, 2011). Every nurse knows this intimacy as a past experience or a present lived experience that resides in the deep understanding of another and in the nursing role. Thus this embedded consciousness and intimacy live within the soul of each nurse and are part of "being with" another.

A holistic and integral moral/ethical foundation must include respect. *Respect* is the act of feeling esteem for or honoring another; it is an act that demands we have a sense of authenticity, integrity, self-knowledge, and appreciation of the uniqueness of another as well as of ourselves (Rushton, in press). It is rooted in our internal beliefs about how we value another human being. Respect is central and foundational to the ethical framework that guides our professional roles, relationships, and responsibilities. It helps us recognize the dimensions of multiculturalism, understandings of culture, and the rich understanding of self and others that must be included in practice, education, research, and health care policy.

I believe that nurses' moral and ethical foundation includes Earth ethics (Burkhardt, 2016). *Earth ethics* is a code of behavior that incorporates the understanding that the Earth community has core value in and of itself and includes ethical treatment of the nonhuman world and the Earth as a whole. This influences the way that we individually and collectively interact with the environment and all beings of the Earth. A major focus of all my collaborative endeavors in holistic nursing (Dossey & Keegan, 2016), nursing coaching (Dossey, Luck, & Schaub, 2015), and the NIGH (Dossey et al., 2005; Dossey, 2000; Nightingale Declaration, 2016) have included Earth ethics as essential for healthy people living on a healthy planet. Our "Nightingale Declaration for A Healthy World" (Nightingale Declaration, 2016) is a way to increase the awareness of nurses and the global public about the priority of human health and an Earth ethic. To truly understand Earth ethics requires a shift in consciousness and in our beliefs, attitudes, and worldviews about the interdependence of all of life. An Earth ethic declares that we are all "one mind" and that our individual minds are part of a greater consciousness (Dossey, 2013), and this matters in how we see our role with all humanity and a healthy world—local to global These ideas are inherent in my vision of nursing.

■ VISION

I have a vision of nursing as integral, integrative, and holistic that weaves together our Florence Nightingale legacy, our science, and our art. My hope is for nurses to be kinder to each other and respect each other, and for all nurses to stand in their power and see themselves as change agents for health and healing. This is foundational to increasing our understanding of being a nurse and a citizen activist at our deepest and highest expression of self, nature, and culture. We must focus on both the individual and the collective, the inner and outer, and human and nonhuman concerns. This challenges us to strengthen and to engage ourselves fully at the individual, shared, and collective levels to heal Earth and its people. The time has come to increase our message of wellness and integrative health combined with traditional technology when appropriate.

We nurses must continue to expand our consciousness and our role and awareness as global citizens. We are challenged to act locally and always think globally as we strive to achieve a healthy world by 2020—the bicentennial of Nightingale's birth—and beyond. Nurses must see themselves as health coaches and health diplomats who are advocates for integral, integrative, and holistic health. This applies to any environment, whether we work in a hospital, a clinic, a home, a community setting, school of nursing, or an underdeveloped rural village.

We are 21st-century Nightingales who can transform health care and carry forth her caring–healing vision of social action and sacred activism to create a healthy world (Beck, Dossey, & Rushton, 2011). Nurses can be the driving force to bring scholarly caring and healing to the forefront. We must stay steady to further the language of healing interactions and strategies for practice, education, research, and health care policy. We can also bring concerned citizens to unite their voices, capacities, wisdom, and works of service to create a healthy world. Nurses must shine their commitment to compassion, caring, and wholeness on the common quest of healing, health, and well-being for all humanity and planet Earth.

Dr. Monica Sharma (2004, 2007) believes that our current and future work needs to be a *full-spectrum initiative*. She describes this as an emerging paradigm, recognizing that the source of all sustained strategies and action includes sourcing personal awareness and wisdom that results in transformation. It addresses immediate systems and root causes of a problem or condition using appropriate assessments and technologies.

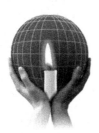

"We, the nurses and concerned citizens of the global community, hereby dedicate ourselves to achieve a healthy world by 2020.

We declare our willingness to unite in a program of action, to share information and solutions and to improve health conditions for all humanity—locally, nationally and globally.

We further resolve to adopt personal practices and to implement public policies in our communities and nations—making this goal achievable and inevitable by the year 2020, beginning today in our own lives, in the life of our nations and in the world at large."

www.NIGHvision.net/Nightingale-Declaration.html

FIGURE 4.1   Nightingale Declaration for A Healthy World.

We are anchored in one of the most dramatic social shifts in health care history. We are part of all nurses and midwives in the global village working with other concerned citizens to create a healthy world amid complex societies with many entangled systems. We must seek all opportunities to unite in the countless forums available to us, including the Internet, in order to create a healthy world. I invite you to read and sign the Nightingale Declaration (Figure 4.1) at www.NIGHvision.net/nightingale-declaration.html

■ REFLECTIONS

1. *In what ways am I consciously aware of the daily opportunities to increase my health and well-being?*
2. *What can I do to increase my conscious awareness of fully participating in life?*
3. *What do I experience when I acknowledge that I am sourcing from my personal wisdom?*
4. *How am I guided by a nursing theory in my professional endeavors?*
5. *What is my vision for a healthy world?*

■ REFERENCES

American Holistic Nurses Association. (1990). *Holistic nursing: Scope and standards of practice*. Raleigh, NC: Author.

American Holistic Nurses Association. (2016). Mission statement. Retrieved from http://www.ahna .org/About-Us/Mission-Statement

American Holistic Nurses Association and American Nurses Association. (2013). *Holistic nursing: Scope and standards of practice* (2nd ed.). Silver Spring, MD: Author.

American Holistic Nurses Credentialing Corporation. (n.d.). Retrived from http://www.ahncc.org/ certification/nursecoachnchwnc.html

American Nurses Association. (2015). *Code of ethics for nurses with interpretive statements*. Silver Spring, MD: Nursesbooks.org.

Barrere, C. C., Helming, M. A. B., Shields, D. A., & Avino, K. M. (2014). *AHNA core curriculum for holistic nursing practice* (2nd ed.). Burlington, MA: Jones & Bartlett Learning.

Beck, D. M., Dossey, B. M., & Rushton, C. H. (2011). Integral nursing and the Nightingale Initiative for Global Health (NIGH): Florence Nightingale's legacy for the 21st century—Local to global. *Journal of Integral Theory and Practice, 6*(4), 71–92.

Burkhardt, M. A. (2016). Holistic ethics. In B. M. Dossey & L. Keegan (Eds.), *Holistic nursing: A handbook for practice* (7th ed., pp. 121–134). Burlington, MA: Jones & Bartlett Learning.

Dossey, B. M. (1997). *AHNA core curriculum for holistic nursing practice.* Gaithersburg, MD: Aspen Publishers.

Dossey, B. M. (2000). *Florence Nightingale: Mystic, visionary, healer* (Commemorative ed.). Springhouse, PA: Springhouse.

Dossey, B. M. (2010). *Florence Nightingale: Mystic, visionary, healer* (Commemorative ed.). Philadelphia, PA: F. A. Davis.

Dossey, B. M. (2016). Nursing: Integral, integrative, and holistic—Local to global. In B. M. Dossey & L. Keegan (Eds.), *Holistic nursing: A handbook for practice* (7th ed., pp. 3–49). Burlington, MA: Jones & Bartlett Learning.

Dossey, B. M., & Keegan, L. (2016). *Holistic nursing: A handbook for practice* (7th ed.). Burlington, MA: Jones & Bartlett Learning.

Dossey, B. M., Keegan, L., Guzzetta, C. E., & Kolkmeier, L. G. (1988). *Holistic nursing: A handbook for practice.* Rockville, MD: Aspen Publishers.

Dossey, B. M., Luck, S., & Schaub, B. G. (2015). *Nurse coaching for health and wellbeing.* North Miami, FL: International Nurse Coach Association.

Dossey, B. M., Selanders, L. C., Beck, D. M., & Attewell, A. (2005). *Florence Nightingale today: Healing, leadership, global action.* Silver Spring, MD: Nursesbooks.org.

Dossey, L. (2013). *One mind: How our individual mind is part of a greater consciousness and why it matters.* Carlsbad, CA: Hay House.

Florence Nightingale and her legacy for holistic nursing. (1998). *Journal of Holistic Nursing* [Special issue], *16*(2), 1–124.

Florence Nightingale and her legacy for global nursing. (2010, March). *Journal of Holistic Nursing* [Special issue], *28*(1), 1–108.

Florence Nightingale and her legacy for global nursing: Part II. (2010, December). *Journal of Holistic Nursing* [Special issue], *28*(4), 221–339.

Florence Nightingale service. (2010). Retrieved from http://www.cathedral.org/exec/cathedral/mediaPlayer?MediaID=MED-4LD39-PT000P&EventID=CAL-4CS30-C8000B

Florence Nightingale's voice. (1890, July 30). London. Retrieved from https://www.youtube.com/watch?v=ax3B4gRQNU4

Guzzetta, C., & Dossey, B. M. (1984). *Cardiovascular nursing: Bodymind tapestry.* St. Louis, MO: Mosby.

Hess, D. R., Dossey, B. M., Southard, M. E., Luck, S., Schaub, B. G., & Bark, L. (2013). *The art and science of nurse coaching: A provider's guide to scope and competencies.* Silver Spring, MD: Nursesbooks.org.

Keegan, L., & Dossey, B. M. (1987). *Self-care: A program to improve your life.* Temple, TX: Bodymind Systems.

Kenner, C. V., Guzzetta, C. E., & Dossey, B. M. (1981). *Critical care nursing: Body-mind-spirit.* Boston, MA: Little, Brown, & Co.

Nightingale Declaration for a Healthy World. (2016). Retrieved from www.nighvision.net/nightingale-declaration.html

Nightingale Initiative for Global Health. (2016). Retrieved from http://www.nighvision.net

Rushton, C. H. (in press). *Moral resilience: An antidote to moral distress.* New York, NY: Oxford University Press.

Sharma, M. (2004). Conscious leadership at the crossroads of change. *Shift, 12*, 17–21.

Sharma, M. (2007). World wisdom in action: Personal to planetary transformation. *Kosmos Fall/ Winter,* pp. 31–35.

Wright, D., & Brajtman, S. (2011). Relational and embodied knowing: Nursing ethics within the interprofessional team. *Nursing Ethics, 18*, 20–30. doi:10.1177/0969733010386165

Powerful and Beneficent: Seizing Opportunity in Practice and Equality in Health Care

Margaret A. Fitzgerald

Nurses must keep in mind that only the powerful are a threat, and every time there is pushback to what we do as nurses, that means we are so powerful that we are seen as a threat. As exhausting as this can be, we have to recognize this opposition is a very good thing, because people without power are not a threat and they don't get pushback. Only the powerful are a threat.

—Fitzgerald (2015a)

■ WHY NURSING?

I had an aunt who I was very close to—she was my mother's older sister and a public health nurse in the city of Boston where I grew up. When I was quite young, probably only six or seven years old, she would take me out on rounds with her as she went around to see patients with infectious diseases and decide whether the family needed to be quarantined. My aunt also provided treatment for these patients. These early experiences greatly influenced me. I could see the power of public health, especially when I heard my aunt's reports of delivering some of the first vaccines against polio and other communicable, often fatal illnesses that were present in Boston.

My choosing to become a nurse reflects a melding of two driving interests: my love of science and my desire to work with people. I seriously thought about going into a laboratory-based science like medical technology, but I realized I would not have any clinical contact with patients in that field. Conversely, I also thought about becoming a social worker, but I realized that as a social worker I would have a lot of human contact but very little science. At age 16, I somehow managed to figure this out and decided to become an RN.

I was young when I graduated high school and went directly into an associate's degree program. So I have been an RN since I was 19 years old, which means I have been in nursing for 45 years! There are not many people 45 years into a career who still love what they do, but I am one of them.

I would love to say that at age 19 I had a great vision about nursing—I actually did not. But back in the early 1970s, I was very much drawn to critical care. At that time, critical care was likely the most science-based, high-tech part of health care. By comparison to what we do now, it was not particularly technologically advanced but I was very much attracted to taking care of patients with extraordinarily complex health problems and working very closely, shoulder to shoulder, with other health care providers to ensure that patients achieved optimal outcomes.

What I thought a nurse was when I started out is very much the way I still think about it: A nurse is an advocate for people and for families and is one of the most public faces of health care. This idea of advocacy has been in the forefront of my mind throughout all these years. And now what I do as a family nurse practitioner (FNP) is advocate for best health practices for entire families. So this concept of nurse as advocate has been at the core of what I have done since the very beginning. Now, however, I am able to accomplish more than I could when I first started out, in part because of being a nurse practitioner (NP). And that actually is one reason why I sought the NP role: to have a much higher-level skill set that would allow me to advocate for and benefit a family in more ways.

■ EARLY IMPRESSIONS

Some of my earliest experiences as an RN were in a community hospital intensive care unit (ICU), where I could see that nurses were truly practicing at the RN level—very much to the full extent of their license and experience. That might not sound like a revolutionary idea now, because what we are all talking about in health care these days is just that: practicing to the very fullest scope of our license, experience, and knowledge base. But back then, it was a revolutionary idea because several influences on nursing practice at that time would encourage RNs to limit their practice expertise.

For example, this was a time in nursing practice when an RN could not document that a patient was bleeding from a surgical wound but rather would be directed to say that red fluid was noted on the wound. The origin of this now laughable limitation on nursing assessment is that RNs were not thought to be capable of making such a sophisticated observation. Despite this, I found in my early days of critical care that those external limits on nursing practice had been moved aside. Our mindset was:

> We are RNs. We have a very, very high skill and knowledge level and, to do best by these critically ill patients we must practice to the very edge of that knowledge—to the full extent of what is allowable by our license.

And that is what kept me in critical care for 16 years.

I wanted to move nursing practice along by directly impacting the health care system and role modeling new ways of working with fellow nurses, patients, and interprofessional colleagues. After a very successful career in critical care where I was a staff nurse, staff resource educator, and nurse manager, I was ready for graduate school. Rather than stay in critical care, however, I decided to become an FNP. I had thrived both professionally and personally in critical care and had enjoyed great recognition for the work that I did; in fact, many people thought I was deviating from a very successful career path when I decided to leave. However, one of the driving forces in my decision to move on was that I viewed the NP role, which was only 20 years into its existence at the time, as one where I would be able to advocate for and work with my patients and in the community to keep people out of the ICU. During my 16 years of working in critical care, I could walk through the unit many days and just see one person after another with what I knew were easily preventable diseases, had the patient had access to primary health care services. It was these recurrent observations that led me to leave and begin practicing in the community. I knew I could do something about it.

I have to say that the transition was an extraordinarily uncomfortable one because I went from being the expert critical care nurse to being the novice NP. Sixteen years into being an RN, I was not all that thrilled to be wearing a pair of novice shoes—they were awfully uncomfortable! At times, during my first year as an NP, I recall thinking to myself, "My brain just hurts." For the first time in a long time, I had to think about and often rethink every single thing I was doing. It was all brand new. But within about a year those novice shoes started to feel much more comfortable and I became gradually more expert in how I was practicing, and I have enjoyed a tremendously successful career since then.

In critical care I had, if you will, done it all—clinically speaking—and I had done a very good deal on the administrative side as well. The next step in my critical care career likely would have been to go to a larger hospital and assume a higher level administrative role, perhaps a director of critical care services for nursing. I was quite good at administration and had enjoyed tremendous success. For example, I had turned around a failing ICU that was in chaos when I stepped in as the leader and helped organize a regional critical care consortium that exists to this day and has served as a national model. Although continuing on in administration was really the next logical step in my career, I found that, despite contributing toward a tremendous number of very rewarding accomplishments, with every rung I climbed on that ladder, the more distanced from patient care I was becoming, and I wanted to get back to taking care of patients. My choosing to move away from critical care was more of a personal evolution of where I wanted to go next rather than being a response to anything inherently wrong with nursing practice at that time. There were actually several different directions I was considering when I decided to go to graduate school. These included law school, where many RNs in the mid-1980s were deciding to go, or getting a master's degree in health care administration and staying on the aforementioned trajectory. There was also a clinical nurse specialist role in critical care but that role again was more taking care of cohorts of patients and not individuals. And then there was the NP role, which drew me to it with the inherent implications of clinical expertise and sense of possibility.

■ PROFESSIONAL EVOLUTION/CONTRIBUTION

My view of nursing has matured over time parallel to the evolution of the profession, getting back to the concept that all nurses, whether they be at the RN or the advanced practice registered nurse (APRN) level, need to be educated and cognizant of their immense knowledge base and be able to apply it to clinical practice so that they are the best possible advocates for their patients. I believe my greatest contribution has been hammering that message home to a vast array of nursing groups over and over again.

Going back to my critical care days, we worked very much in geographic isolation from one another through the 1970s and early to mid-1980s, even in hospitals that were sometimes only 5 to 10 miles away from each other. The term you would use now is practicing in our own *silos*. We did not talk about silos back then, but as we practiced in our own little critical care worlds, separate from one another, a group of us came together and decided we really needed to regionalize nursing practice. Our group decided that we were all going to teach the exact same clinical topics, particularly for all new critical care nurses. To do that, we needed to have the nurses we worked with travel as much as 20, 30, or 40 miles in order to meet with a group of like-minded colleagues to bring the highest level of nursing practice possible to the bedside. I was one of the cofounders of this regionalized approach to critical care education in the Merrimac Valley, which is in northeast Massachusetts. And we did get together: We had people from 5-bed and 25-bed ICUs, shoulder to shoulder, learning with and from one another. That was our first iteration of an evolution in nursing education.

A secondary intention of that regionalized approach to education was bringing physicians in to learn alongside the NPs. Thirty years ago this was a big deal! By bringing our physician colleagues to learn and teach in partnership with us, we all were better able to appreciate the unique contributions of our roles and acknowledge that none of us could successfully work independently from one another. On the contrary, we realized we were incredibly dependent upon one another's skill sets and knowledge bases and we had to work collaboratively, not just cooperatively, with one another. That program continues to this day. I am very proud of that accomplishment.

I was also of the first generation of nurse managers (head nurses, as we were called then) of a critical care unit. I was actually the first in the hospital where I practiced to institute a self-governing model where we kept most of our decision making within the unit. With this model, we could take care of things on our own and, ultimately, make the best decisions for our patients and staff.

I was the first NP in the community health center where I still practice today (the Greater Lawrence Family Health Center in Lawrence, Massachusetts) to hold a leadership role. I was brought on to fulfill a dual role as both a clinician and to lead the opening and establishment of the health center's first satellite clinic. My task then was to define those roles, that of clinician and leader, within the satellite and to determine what would work best in that particular neighborhood to meet patients' needs.

After setting up the clinic, I became a full-time faculty member in an NP program at Simmons College in Boston, Massachusetts, and I was the first person to start up an FNP program in the city of Boston, also at Simmons College. When I began the FNP program around 1990, there were no FNPs to be found in Boston. There were many adult, pediatric, and women's health NP programs, but they were very much focused on specific patient cohorts and not the overall concept of caring for families. I started the FNP program to introduce that missing component of family-centered care through a nursing lens into the city of Boston, which was considered visionary at the time.

I was also the first NP faculty at Simmons College to teach pharmacology. It is very rewarding to be able to take my very strong science background, along with my interest in pharmacology, and apply that in the classroom with a group of students, rather than have a pharmacist or a person who does not write the prescription teach the pharmacology course.

Among my accomplishments, the one that I am most proud of is creating Fitzgerald Health Education Associates, Inc. (2015). At the time I started it, I did not realize I was starting a company. I was trying to fill a void. This was around 1988, when I was teaching part-time and precepting and my student asked me to provide a review course to help her and her classmates get ready for the NP boards.

At that time, I had done some teaching at the associate, baccalaureate, and master's levels, and I had done a tremendous amount of continuing education teaching. So I was not new to teaching. I had only been an NP a couple of years myself but I was practicing what I call "full-contact primary care": caring for an ethnically diverse patient population, some of whom had tremendously complex physical health and psychosocial needs. Although I was early in my career, I thought I could help these students get ready for the NP boards.

The question that comes up is this: Why were there no courses around to help these NP students prepare for their boards? This gets into the idea of *exploiting opportunity*. I think many people see "exploit" as a bad word, for example, one person exploits another person. But I would like nurses, regardless of their level of education, to rethink the negative connotation of "exploit" and start looking at it from a viewpoint of exploiting opportunity. The opportunity that presented itself in 1988 was that the state nurses' association, which had offered a review course in the Northeast every year for many years, was moving in the fall. As they moved their offices, they decided they simply did not have the resources to orchestrate the review course simultaneously. Back then there were only two other NP review courses being offered: one held annually in Washington, DC, and the other in San Diego, California. The business model for the companies holding courses in DC and San Diego was along the lines of, "You come to us and we'll help you get ready for boards." As it was, there was no other course available in the Northeast in 1988 other than the one I taught.

We began with six students around my dining-room table that year. I conducted a second course in the fall again around that same table. In fact, at that time, the NP boards were only offered once a year, so students really only needed a review course in the fall. Word about my certification review course got around very quickly in eastern Massachusetts. In January of the next year, 10 months before the NPs boards were being offered, I was getting phone calls from people saying, "You're going to do that NP review course again, aren't you?" and I said, "I guess I am." During the first two years, I literally ran the course out of my dining room, accepting registrations and putting the checks in a shoebox on top of my desk.

Due to family and professional responsibilities, I did not begin offering the program nationally until 1993. This was during the Clinton administration and NP programs were growing because there was talk of national and overall health care reform with an expanded role for APRNs. As the number of NPs in the early 1990s increased, the NP exam became available twice a year rather than once and the demand for the course became higher. My husband started working with me in the company and we very quickly moved away from the competitor model of "You come to us" and embraced an open and available "We will come to you." We traveled and provided certification preparation support in varied and geographically diverse parts of the United States. That is how we have survived and emerged as the industry leader in NP board review. As technology has advanced, we are now able to offer multiple ways of delivering NP review via in-person seminars, online trainings, and MP3 recordings.

What I learned was simple: There was the lack of an NP course and a clear, unacceptable vacancy in the market. I offered a product to fill the void. I looked at the opportunity. The company continues to grow on new and evolving waves of opportunity. We continue to look for the voids and vacancies and not at what our competition is doing. We have multiple distinct product lines aside from NP review, including continuing education, university courseware, and consultation. Our company has grown to include 20 faculty consultants who, aside from my work, develop and teach courses. None of this came about without examining the emerging and current market, carefully evaluating the market needs and trends, and exploiting the available opportunity.

I earned my DNP after two decades of NP practice and 36 years after entering the nursing profession. I am often asked why I chose to return to school. The entire time I had a master's degree, I felt that I was doing doctoral-level work, and I had this intense desire to finally be degree congruent—to hold a degree that matched what I do clinically, what I do in my writing, and what I do in my consulting. The DNP was a way of doing this. Having completed my DNP studies, I finally feel as if my education and professional responsibilities are much more closely matched. I completed my studies at age 55, so nobody can ever tell me they are too old to do it.

In addition, because of the DNP studies I am far more skilled at evaluating clinical evidence and research. I feel like a chamber in my brain that I did not know I had was opened during my doctoral studies at Case Western Reserve University, where I had amazing faculty, mentors, and classmates. Furthermore, the DNP has opened up countless prospects for me as a speaker, consultant, author, and clinician. I am blessed with ample professional opportunities! At the same time, many previously unavailable venues for professional development have come my way after gaining the DNP, particularly when a group is looking for a doctorally prepared, actively practicing NP to participate in a given project. My zeal for being a lifelong learner is even keener now. I believe most of my DNP colleagues feel the same.

I am credentialed as a DCC, having successfully completed the requirements of the American Board of Comprehensive Care examination. This credential wields two main benefits. First, I was eligible. I viewed it as an opportunity to be tested on the broad content of primary and emergency care it covers. I view myself as a role model, particularly for NPs new to practice. I wanted to demonstrate that after 25 years I have breadth and depth of practice and hold myself to the high standards that I ask new graduate NPs to strive toward. I performed very well in all areas of this examination and I was very happy and proud of my performance.

Second, I wanted the experience of taking a high-stakes exam. I teach a review course for those taking a high-stakes examination and so I wanted that opportunity myself. After more than 25 years as an NP the DCC credential a way to demonstrate a high level of practice.

I believe this certification is the wave of the future and will be a sought-after one as more NPs are prepared with the DNP degree. There is a DNP page on Facebook to which I am a frequent contributor and where I counsel people on preparing for this examination. Although I do not reveal the exam content, I mentor and plant the seed for those considering whether or not to test. I do believe this certification will one day be eligible for nursing licensure purposes.

One of the things for which I am well recognized, and for which I was awarded the National Organization of Nurse Practitioner Faculties' Lifetime Achievement Award and the Sharp Cutting Edge Award from the American College of Nurse Practitioners, is my work in educating NPs to the highest knowledge and skill level they can possibly possess so that they are able to practice to the full extent of their license (Fitzgerald, 2015b). I have done this through clinical education, authorship, and mentorship, and through helping people pass their NP boards and demonstrating to them that, yes, this in fact is the knowledge and skill base that NPs possess and apply. I have role modeled and demonstrated that approach to advanced practice nursing through my ongoing clinical work at a federally qualified health center for nearly 30 years. Envisioning the broad-spectrum embodiment of the NP role to the full extent of the knowledge base, the full extent of the skill base, and the full extent of the licensure is really what has driven everything else I have done.

■ MORAL/ETHICAL FOUNDATION

For me, the ethical fiber that is most important to nursing is the concept of equality: equal care to all populations with no stratification of its delivery. This, unfortunately, does not exist across health care today. If you speak English, you are likely going to get easier access and better care than a person who does not. If you have financial means, you will likely get better care than somebody who does not have the same socioeconomic status. That is unacceptable.

The stratification of care that we have in the United States due to issues of poverty and racial, ethnic, and sexual orientation discrimination prevents many people from accessing high-quality care. We as nurses, including NPs, are at the absolute front line and must carry with us, in the very core of who we are, the ethical concept of *beneficence*, which is the idea that everybody benefits in the same manner from the health care system and that there is no stratification due to income, ethnicity, sexual orientation, gender, or any other factor. We must be constantly vigilant to those barriers that are thrown in front of us.

I have chosen to practice my entire career in the poorest urban neighborhood in a six-state region, and one of the reasons I have stayed in that practice is because the quality of care that we collectively render is on par with anything that the wealthiest person can get, and I pride myself on that. It is exceptional care without discrimination, and it is not I alone who provide this care, but rather my 120 clinical colleagues who care for patients along with me. A message I have tried to impart to NPs throughout my career is to align themselves with organizations that have an impeccable moral code and that treat people in an equitable manner, regardless of personal characteristics.

I also want nurses to realize that practicing in an underserved community is not just an option when you cannot find a job anyplace else; rather, it is a choice one can make to move along the profession, and health care in general, and to maximize the overall health of this great nation.

I do a good deal of role modeling with other health care providers where I practice. In particular, I have developed a concept called *micro-mentoring*, which involves integrating short, highly focused mentoring efforts with people who are rising through the ranks in health care. I also carry these concepts of beneficence, equality, and practicing to the full extent of knowledge base and skill set into my clinical presentations when I speak at various meetings. My message is this: Exploit your entire knowledge base and practice to the full edge of your license and your skill set, but at the same time, treat all patients with dignity and respect, regardless of their background or how they got to the place where they are right now with their health. Treat everybody as if you were caring for a member of your own family or a loved one. There are no shortcuts.

By role modeling and speaking about these concepts to individuals, I believe I have helped move the profession along in many ways. And, with the Affordable Care Act, these concepts must truly be embedded at the core of nursing practice. Many people have joined the rolls of the health care insured who have never had access before. At this time, we need to be even more cognizant of treating everybody with the same degree of respect, bringing our best and most knowledgeable selves to the table, and striving to be those persons who will advocate for every single patient and family.

■ VISION

Now is nursing's time to shine. For many years, we have not been at the table in care. Increasingly, at all levels of nursing, we are at countless tables and are part of the major decision making taking place in health care. This steady rise in nursing power has, in many locations, upset the status quo and, therefore, we might see some pushback. We cannot backslide in asserting our nursing power in the face of this opposition. Instead, we must dig in our heels and affirm that this is our time; we are at the table and we are here to stay.

Sometimes it can become exhausting to hear others constantly say, "Oh, the nurses shouldn't be doing this, the nurses shouldn't be doing that, the APRNs are trying to take over health care." My keynote speech quote that introduced this chapter (Fitzgerald, 2015a) bears repeating again and again to all nurses who are leaders in the evolution of modern healthcare:

> Nurses must keep in mind that only the powerful are a threat, and every time there is pushback to what we do as nurses, it means we are so powerful that we are seen as a threat. As exhausting as this can be, we have to recognize this opposition as a very good thing, because people without power are not a threat and they don't get pushback. Only the powerful are a threat.

I pose a challenge to nurses, particularly those in early career: Think of yourself as the CEO of your own nursing career. What opportunities can you exploit? How can you best direct where your nursing career goes? How can you be that powerful threat?

In regard to advanced practice nursing, I believe within the upcoming years the DNP will be required for certification. Setting the DNP as the entry into advanced practice nursing not only helps recognize the rigor of the current master's-level education in nursing but also provides a way for the APRN student to study areas not currently included, or which are presented less formally, in the current programs. Such areas include, but are not limited to, education in evidence-based practice, quality improvement, and systems leadership. The DNP also offers an alternative to research-focused doctoral programs.

DNP-prepared nurses can facilitate the implementation of the science developed by nurse scientists prepared in PhD and other research-focused doctorates.

Another important factor is the need for APRNs to achieve educational parity with other professions that have established the practice doctorate as the degree requirement for entry into practice including law, dentistry, social work, pharmacy, medicine, and physical therapy. This parity is critically important to NP advancement in the area of health care policy and leadership. The NP profession has survived and thrived since the transition from the certificate course to the master's degree as the requirement for entry into practice. I believe the transition to the DNP will yield similar results.

Over the years, the requirements for the profession of nursing have evolved in response to the needs of the health care environment. To transform its delivery it is critically important for nurses and other clinicians to design, evaluate, and continuously improve the context within which care is rendered. Nurses prepared at the doctoral level, with a blend of clinical, organizational, economic, and leadership skills, are the ones most likely to be able to critique nursing and other scientific findings and design programs of care delivery that are locally acceptable, economically feasible, and significantly impact health care outcomes. This will help advance the NP profession beyond its current considerable reach.

The part of my work that has not yet been fully realized for me and my fellow DCCs is to grow the number of people who hold this designation. The DCC is an extremely high level of certification for NPs who hold a doctoral degree. We need to make the DCC more visible and to better communicate to the health care community its meaning, the accomplishment in the testing of our clinical expertise, and the exceptional level of knowledge and skills we have demonstrated.

What I would like nurses to know that I did not know earlier is what a fantastic career this can be if you keep your eyes open and you exploit every opportunity that is presented to you. I have had at least six very distinctly different careers in my 45 years as an RN. Each one of them has carried its own challenges, but each one of them has also gleaned tremendous reward. All RNs and APRNs should be looking ahead to what they can do in the future with this great career. Always be taking a look at what you are going to do next while you continue to work very hard at maximizing what you can get out of your current experience; this will keep your career both novel and interesting. In this way, you will help move forward both the great profession of nursing and the multiple dimensions of modern health care itself.

■ REFLECTIONS

1. *As a nurse, have I gained as much knowledge as I possibly can to bring to my practice?*
2. *Am I fully utilizing all the knowledge I have gained to practice to the full extent of my role and license?*
3. *Am I actively looking for the next opportunity in my profession?*
4. *Am I consistently acting as a role model of compassionate, high-quality nursing care for others?*
5. *Am I practicing in a manner such that, occasionally, I am viewed as a threat to the status quo?*

■ REFERENCES

Fitzgerald, M. A. (2015a). *Keynote presentation.* 50th Anniversary of the NP role celebration, American Association of Nurse Practitioners™ 2015 National Conference, Philadelphia, PA.

Fitzgerald, M. A. (2015b). *Nurse practitioner certification and practice preparation* (4th ed.). Philadelphia, PA: F.A. Davis.

Fitzgerald Health Education Associates, Inc. (2015). *The leader in NP certification and continuing education.* Retrieved from https://fhea.com

CHAPTER SIX

Influential and Determined: Assuring Integrity in the Care of Older Adults and Beyond [1]

Terry Fulmer

My career has been a series of remarkable opportunities—each has unfolded in ways I could never have imagined. It is all about watching for the right opportunities and taking the leap!
        —Terry Fulmer (personal communication, November 12, 2015)[1]

■ WHY NURSING?

It is a great honor to be invited to participate in this exciting book that shares stories of key change agents in nursing, a profession that has so many remarkable leaders! My passion lies in the care of geriatric patients and all of my leadership experience has been informed by what I have learned in delivering that care. When invited to participate, I let our editor know that I had recently published the story of my nursing career journey and, with his permission, would share it again in this book.

So, why nursing? Both the incredible progress and the goals we have yet to attain in geriatric health care provide me with an answer to that question. Simply: I wanted to make a difference in this field and I felt called to do it as a nurse.

The past 50 years have been a time of dramatic change and exceptional progress in the care of older adults. Back then, if geriatric patients were incontinent, we inserted a Foley catheter. If they stopped eating, a nasogastric tube was placed for feeding. If they were confused, we gave a medication and put on a restraint device. We have come a long way, as chronicled by many pioneers who have written about the history of gerontological nursing (Ebersole, 1999; Ebersole & Toughy, 2006; Fulmer & Mezey, 1998; Mezey,

---

[1] This chapter has been adapted from Fulmer, T. (2015). Geriatric nursing 2.0. *Journal of the American Geriatrics Society, 63*(7), 1453–1458.

Amella, & Fulmer, 1995). In particular, the book *Geriatric Nursing: Growth of a Specialty* by Pricilla Ebersole and Theris Toughy (Ebersole & Toughy, 2006) is the most comprehensive history we have of the field to date, spanning from the 1800s to the present. These authors painstakingly document the early elements of geriatric nursing, especially from the 1940s until the present, with an outstanding narrative of our early iconic leaders, including Irene Burnside, Barbara Davis, Thelma Wells, Edna Stilwell, and Doris Schwartz. They also trace geriatric nursing from the early "poor houses" that were essentially the places where the indigent—and particularly the elderly indigent—received care and went to die, up to the nursing home reform movement, and finally to the remarkable improvements in geriatric education and care led by the Hartford Institute for Geriatric Nursing (HIGN) at New York University (NYU) and the Hartford Centers for Gerontological Nursing Excellence we have today. Within the profession, I have been referred to as a "second-generation" (2.0) geriatric nurse pioneer, and I welcome the opportunity to reflect here on the growth and development of gerontological nursing and the transformational changes I have witnessed over the course of my own career.

When I graduated from Skidmore College in 1975 and began my search for a staff nurse position in Boston (where my soon-to-be husband would begin graduate school), the nation was in the throes of a terrible recession with double-digit inflation, accelerating gasoline prices, and Watergate. Medicare and Medicaid celebrated a 10th anniversary. There were few jobs available and I was very fortunate to accept a position on a general medical unit at the Beth Israel Hospital (BIH). I accepted this position without any foreknowledge of the extraordinary talent I would encounter and the dynamic nursing model at the BIH, or any appreciation of the aging demographics and imminent momentum in geriatrics and gerontology.

■ EARLY IMPRESSIONS

Mitchell T. Rabkin, then president and chief executive officer (CEO) of the organization, was committed to "primary nursing" (Clifford, 1980) as a model that instilled and required accountability, responsibility, and authority of nurses over the care and nursing practice of their patients. Joyce Clifford was the chief nursing officer and already a national figure for her advancement of this primary nursing model as a way to engender leadership and responsibility in all nurses as they cared for their patients. I thrived under Dr. Clifford's leadership and her extraordinary commitment to primary nursing. This nursing model is based on continuity of care and nurse answerability to the patient on a 24-hour basis. Clifford knew the demands and requirements of the model and, thus, required a baccalaureate degree for all new nursing hires—long before the Robert Wood Johnson Foundation (RWJF) Initiative on the Future of Nursing at the Institute of Medicine (IOM, 2011) report was published.

As I began my practice, it was immediately apparent that the majority of the patients on my unit were very old and frail, and that most of the physicians and nurses found caring for these older adults unexciting and certainly not as prestigious as the intensive care units. The book *House of God* (Shem, 1978, 2003) had been published in 1978 under the pseudonym Samuel Shem by Steven Bergman, an intern at the BIH. The theme of the book not only centered on some of the difficulties and working conditions of interns at that time, but also was filled with disparaging remarks related to the geriatric patients. The term "GOMER"—which stands for "Get Out of My Emergency Room"—reflected the annoyance that staff felt in caring for geriatric patients, who were thought of as either futile in terms of medical care outcomes or unworthy of that same care. It was in that context that I discovered the power of geriatric nursing.

As a new nurse, I learned that when I paged an intern or resident and asked what to do if, for example, my geriatric patient had a pressure ulcer, the answer was, "Do whatever you usually do" or something along the lines of "That's your job, not mine." These interns and residents were exceptionally smart, but nervous themselves—afraid to make mistakes or admit a lack of know-how. They were clearly telling me that my questions, as far as I could gather, were in the domain of nursing and that I should know or figure it out. It was actually quite refreshing to be in the middle of a Harvard teaching hospital and have full scope of practice for what I later termed "SPICES: Skin problems, Problems with eating and feeding, Incontinence, Confusion, Evidence of falls, and Sleep disorders" (Fulmer, 2007; Wallace & Fulmer, 1998, 1999). I was free to examine whatever small amount of literature was available and create solutions for these syndromes that have now become such a part of the lexicon of both geriatric nursing and geriatric medicine. I got the message, took it, and ran with it, never looking back, and happily began my geriatric nursing career.

For me personally, a lasting influence on my career was the return from the National Institutes of Health (NIH) of Jack Rowe to be the chief resident of internal medicine at the BIH in 1975. Rowe would go on to be the first director of the Division on Aging in Harvard Medical School and chief of the Gerontology Division of the BIH from 1977 to 1988. His legendary ascendance in geriatric medicine began then, and I had the full benefit of his success. Another vector of major impact for me was the publication of Robert N. Butler's book *Why Survive? Being Old in America,* which won the Pulitzer Prize for general nonfiction in 1976 and laid out what has been referred to as "the dismissive and contemptuous attitude toward the elderly and their diseases by many of his teachers and medical schools" (Wikipedia, 2014). He coined the term *ageism* and directed a spotlight exactly onto the propositions being laid out in Shem's book (Butler, 1975). Butler railed against the term GOMER and other acts of cruelty, injustice, and ageism. His message really resonated for me.

As freshmen at Skidmore, my classmates and I were asked what our plans were for our doctoral education, and although many of us laughed, that question immediately arose again for me in the context of the BIH. By 1976, I had enrolled in a graduate course on gerontological nursing with Marion Spencer at Boston University. The following fall, I enrolled full-time at Boston College in a medical–surgical graduate nursing program with the support of a full scholarship from the Department of Health and Human Services. Since Boston College did not have a geriatric specialty track, I focused all my required papers and projects on geriatric nursing topics. In this way, I believed that I was independently completing a minor in geriatric nursing. (As a young adult, the scholarship support far outweighed the necessity to enroll in a very specific geriatric nursing master's program!) The professors of Boston College were very supportive of my plan and at the completion of my master's in 1977, I accepted a faculty position in rehabilitative nursing at Salem State College, where I immersed myself further in geriatric nursing. I continued working part-time at the BIH and began my participation at geriatrics seminars and clinical rounds with its Gerontology Division.

Let me again emphasize the leadership of Mitchell T. Rabkin and Joyce Clifford, who created a medical center environment that completely supported advancing geriatrics and interdisciplinary team care. I was recruited the next year back to Boston College for a faculty position and, for the next several years, I advanced the geriatric curricula at the now "Connell School of Nursing." The Harvard Division on Aging was established in 1980 and I began attending those weekly seminars and conferences. In 1983, the year I completed my doctoral degree, I was invited, as a Boston College faculty member, to work with the Division on Aging on a Health Resources Services Administration Geriatric Education Center (GEC) grant application. We were funded and I served 50% in that Center from 1983 to 1987. My relationship with that outstanding division on aging faculty was forever cemented. Jack Rowe, Richard Besdine, Ken Minaker, Fox Wetle, Jerry Avorn, Paul Cleary, Allen Jette, Larry Branch, Sue Levkoff, Barbara Berkman, Lew Lipsitz, Neil Resnick, Peggy Edson, Kate Morency, Mark Beers, and Liebe Kravitz (I know I have left some key people out) were all there; each has been extremely influential in geriatrics and gerontology and on my career.

The aforementioned coincidences, circumstances, and opportunities came together with my realization that I could have a major impact on the practice and academic leadership of geriatric nursing while doing what I loved, which was taking care of geriatric patients, teaching, and developing research that would improve their care. The nursing care was extremely compelling and the complexity a real challenge. My patients did not ask to live to be 80 or 90 years old, but the array of life-saving technologies and pharmaceuticals made them almost prisoners of the health care system (U.S. Congress, 1987). The "save them and scorn them" mentality of Dr. Shem's book, juxtaposed with the "Why survive?" narrative of Dr. Butler, made it the best time to accelerate geriatric nursing and I wanted to be a part of it. Medicare and Medicaid changed the health care landscape for older adults and their families. How much care was enough? Under what conditions? We are still grappling with these issues today and the recent IOM (2014) report *Dying in America: Improving Quality and Honoring Individual Preferences Near the End of Life* sheds new light on a decades-old set of conundrums.

■ PROFESSIONAL EVOLUTION/CONTRIBUTION

Medicare and Medicaid were passed as Social Security Amendments on July 30, 1965, as President Lyndon Baines Johnson proclaimed universal access to health care (then thought of as "hospital care") as a key component of the "Great Society" (Berkowitz, 2008). Many presidents before him had tried to advance legislation for health funding and access, but he did it and it changed care delivery and cost of care indelibly. This also had a great impact on those of us in the clinical setting—especially in academic medical centers—who were learning how to become expert clinicians, and on many expert researchers. The late 1960s and early 1970s were a time of major transformation and progress for gerontological and geriatric nursing. With the passage of Medicare (Frank, 2000), there was an increased attention to working with older populations. Availability of funding for research and education led to a rise in research studies and new knowledge related to aging and geriatric care.

The further context was the women's movement, the reimagining of women's work from that of homemaker, nurse, teacher, and secretary to the then less traditional, male-dominated roles of law, medicine, and business. I was one of those women who made the conscious decision to choose nursing, and did it in direct opposition to my parents' recommendations. The "Why nursing and why not medicine?" was a bitter question to swallow. I did not yet have the ready vocabulary of today for the differences, except to explain that "medicine served to treat disease, and nursing treated human responses to disease" (American Nurses Association [ANA], 1980, 2015; Silva, 1983).

Significant milestones for nursing were emerging, such as the creation and publication of the *Standards for Geriatric Nursing Practice* (ANA, 1970) and the certification process for recognizing expertise in the field. In the mid-1970s, I was among the first 74 nurses to be certified as a gerontological nurse and, in 1976, ANA certification for the geriatric nurse practitioner (GNP) specialty was initiated. As certified gerontological nurses, we focused on promoting healthy aging and wellness, not just concentrating on the illness care of older adults. One of the changes that exemplified this shift was renaming the ANA *Geriatric* Nursing Division the *Gerontological* Nursing Division in order to reflect an emphasis on health promotion as distinct from disease management. Until that time, nurses who were attracted to and experts in the care of older adults had no such mechanism to be critically evaluated for expertise and knowledge. With certification and ANA standards came the recognition of a specialty long discussed but less well understood or measured. There was a great need for advanced practice gerontological nurses, as many physicians were still indifferent, if not averse, to caring for the elderly. For me, the gerontological nursing specialty certification gave me a credential I needed to be recognized by my interdisciplinary peers. The momentum that had started in the 1970s continued to accelerate into the 1980s. In 1981, the first International Conference on Gerontological Nursing was held and ANA's Division of Gerontological Nursing published a statement on the scope of practice.

The Teaching Nursing Home Initiative, funded by the RWJF from 1982 to 1987, was created to improve the quality of nursing home care and the clinical training of nurses by linking nursing schools with nursing homes. Codirected by Drs. Mathy Mezey and John Lynaugh of the University of Pennsylvania School of Nursing, it was the first of its kind. This collaboration between nursing homes and 11 different nursing programs was specifically intended to upgrade the clinical care in nursing homes by placing advanced practice nurse faculty in the homes, create an environment supportive of education, and promote clinical research. This important initiative brought awareness to the need for innovative solutions for geriatric education and care (Fulmer & Mezey, 1994; Mezey, 1989; Schneider, Ory, & Aung, 1987). It was found to improve care in the nursing homes and, at the same time, improve the geriatric curriculum in schools of nursing (Shaughnessy, Kramer, Hittle, & Steiner, 1995). It served as the inaugural program to understand the ways in which the more than 6,000 nurse practitioners and RNs in practice today, 80% of whom work in nursing homes, can improve the quality of care for older adults. The program was based on a medical model where residents get their training in teaching hospitals and schools of medicine and assume responsibility for quality of care. The limitations of the program had to do with poor financial resources in nursing homes and the continued problem of attracting nurses to long-term care. Although the RWJF did not continue this program, it set the course for improving the standards and quality of care by nurses in nursing homes. It should be noted that the Teaching Nursing Home Initiative was later adapted by the National Institute on Aging's (NIA's) program for medical schools for the teaching of geriatric medicine (Schneider, Ory, & Aung, 1987). This important initiative brought awareness to the need for innovative solutions for geriatric education and care (Fulmer & Mezey, 1994; Mezey, 1989; Schneider, Ory, & Aung, 1987).

A few schools began inaugural master's programs in geriatric nursing in the late 1960s. In 1966, Duke University, led by Virginia Stone, who had incredible foresight and vision for the specialty, opened the first master's program to prepare clinical nurse specialists in gerontological nursing. Case Western Reserve University and Boston University (Ebersole & Toughy, 2006) followed suit, but there was, by no means, an abundance of programs or a clear understanding of what the curricula should look like (Ebersole & Toughy, 2006). Further, there was no stampede by nursing students to the programs. Geriatric nursing was not yet seen as a bona fide specialty; instead, geriatric nursing was equated with nursing homes, and the practice of nursing in nursing homes was considered substandard—it meant you were not good enough to get a job in acute care. The 1980s had experienced a proliferation of graduate programs in other areas of nursing (Fulmer & Matzo, 1995). In 1982, the first endowed chair in gerontological nursing was established at the Frances Payne Bolton School of Nursing at Case Western Reserve University. In 1988, a new milestone was achieved with the first PhD program in gerontological nursing established at Case Western Reserve University.

Gerontological nursing, however, was lagging behind other specialties. In 1987, only 37 academic programs prepared GNPs, 27 awarding advanced degrees and the balance providing certificates of advanced study (Fulmer & Mezey, 1994, 1998). At best, these programs were graduating fewer than 300 GNPs annually. Mezey referenced evidence, as late as 1995, which showed that elder care in hospitals and long-term care facilities continued to be substandard and far from the ideal (Fulmer & Matzo, 1995; Mezey, 1995).

In 1990, the Association for Gerontology in Higher Education (AGHE) published a status report on nursing and gerontology (Johnson & Richard Connelly, 1990). In that report, they laid out the issues and shortcomings of geriatric curricula and, in 1995, they again documented the extraordinary shortcomings of nursing curricula and need for change (Fulmer & Matzo, 1995). Long-term care, home health care, and other clinical options such as adult day care have only recently been embraced as important elements of primary care. Today, there are more than 80 graduate-level specialty programs with a very specific set of competencies and extremely rigorous criteria for certification in the specialty, as well as demanding requirements for recertification (The John A. Hartford Foundation [JAHF], 2010, 2012). This is only a start, given that there are more than 4,500 nursing schools in the country. All accredited programs must have curricula that address the entire life span, but my hope is that in the future, all schools will have qualified faculty and a formal curriculum dedicated to the care of older adults.

It is important to note here the role of the GEC initiative, a part of the Health Service Act Title VII, which was inaugurated in 1983 by the U.S. Department of Health and Human Services. The GECs have done an outstanding job of providing "care for older adults" education to nurses in all settings, including faculty. The original four GECs included SUNY at Buffalo, Michigan University, the University of Southern California, and Harvard

University at the Division on Aging, where I served as the associate director under Richard Besdine. The initial four grantees, known in 1985 as the "four-fathers," were soon joined by an additional 16 grantees known as the "Sweet 16." The Association of Geriatric Education Centers was formed in 1989, with more than 30 GEC members, and became an important new partner organization allowing the coordinated voice of the centers to be heard in lobbying activities that have been important in continuing the GEC initiative to date. The GEC was an enormous step forward for interdisciplinary geriatric education across an array of disciplines and levels of practice from assistive personnel to doctorally prepared faculty. It represented, in no small measure, new territory for many of us advancing the GECs, and we can look back with pride and accomplishment on the many successes and ongoing efforts of these GECs for nurses and all interdisciplinary team members.

Obviously, government funding and foundation support for geriatric nursing science has been essential for the growth of new knowledge in our field. The NIH has played a pivotal and powerful role in the advancement of geriatric nursing science, especially the National Center for Nursing Research, founded in 1985 and then elevated to the National Institute for Nursing Research (NINR) in 1993, along with the NIA and the National Institute for Mental Health. Early examples of funded research include the seminal work of Strumpf and Evans in the elimination of restraint use in older adults funded by the NIA (R01-AG08324; Evans & Strumpf, 1989; Evans et al., 1997; Strumpf & Evans, 1988), that of May Wykle with Jaclene Zauszniewski (R01-NR04428) on "Teaching Resourcefulness to Chronically Ill Older Adults," and Ann Whall's "Factors Associated With Aggressive Behavior Among Nursing Home Residents With Dementia" (IRPG RO1-NRO4568). Since that time, the NIH has funded dozens of nurse investigators who are transforming our understanding of the still relatively young field of gerontological care and science.

With the accelerated focus on science, gerontological nursing leaders were also alerted to the need for a stronger body of literature on the care needs of older adults, and new journals were needed to disseminate the science. The *Journal of Gerontological Nursing,* founded in 1974 by the Slack Corporation with Edna Stillwell as editor, was the first of its kind to specifically define gerontological nursing as a content area; currently, Donna Fick, professor of nursing at the Penn State University, is the editor. *Geriatric Nursing* was established in 1980 by Elsevier with Cynthia Kelly as the founding editor; it is currently edited by Barbara Resnick, professor of nursing at the University of Maryland. More recently, in 2008, Slack added *Research in Gerontological Nursing* to its portfolio; Dr. Christine Kovach from the University of Wisconsin/Milwaukee now serves as editor. These journals have dramatically improved the quality and distribution of the science of gerontological nursing and have evolved into world-class journals.

In 1977, my first article, "On Vitamins, Calories, and Help for the Elderly," was published in the *American Journal of Nursing* (Fulmer, 1977) and was a result of my master's thesis entitled *Dentition and Nutrition in the Elderly.* My interest in the topic came directly from my clinical practice in the hospital where older adults would lose weight, their dentures would no longer fit, and they could no longer chew food. The downward spiral of poor nutrition during hospitalization was a major concern for me. Many years later, as the founding dean of the College of Nursing at the College of Dentistry at NYU, I was able to proudly point out my long-standing commitment to oral health in older adults.

Obviously, journals such as the *Journal of the American Geriatrics Society, The Journals of Gerontology, Gerontologist*, and a multitude of others are also available for disseminating our research. Specifically dedicated gerontological nursing journals, however, have greatly accelerated the transmission of our science. Finally, I would be remiss if I did not point out the obvious impact of the American Geriatrics Society (AGS) and the Gerontological Society of America (GSA) and their extraordinary influence on geriatric nursing progress. The abstracts and papers presented at these national meetings have had an enormous effect on the mainstreaming of our science into interdisciplinary research and practice teams. As the first nurse board member for the AGS and first nurse president of the GSA, I can attest to the way those organizations and their meetings and collaborations have changed my approach to elder abuse research and scholarship.

Our success and progress in geriatric nursing are directly related to those who provided crucial financial support to our enterprise. I am certain, and there is general agreement, that the story of contemporary gerontological nursing education has been defined by the JAHF of New York City, a foundation that has been a tireless champion of geriatric nursing since the early 1990s when few other foundations had this focus. The JAHF, under the exceptional leadership of Corinne Rieder, executive director and treasurer, and Norman Volk, chairman of the board, was an early leader in the transformation of geriatric medicine through funding geriatric medicine centers of excellence and fellowships in major academic medical centers. By the late 1980s, its three areas of grant making had narrowed to two: increasing the supply of academic geriatricians through the centers of excellence and improving delivery of health care services to older adults. From 1980 to 1995, the JAHF had made awards of more than $58 million to its aging and health program to train physicians to care for the elderly. Then, starting in 1992, the JAHF introduced its Hospital Outcomes Program for the Elderly (HOPE) initiative to "alleviate the negative effects of hospitalization and emergency care on older patients." The original HOPE geriatrician-as-principal investigator (PI) grants had embedded within them three major nursing projects that formed the basis for many of the nursing programs we have today. These were the Geriatric Resource Nurse Model I developed in the context of the Yale-New Haven project; the Delirium Nurse Specialist Model, led by Marquis Foreman, within the University of Chicago HOPE project; and the ACE (Acute Care of the Elderly) Unit Model led by Denise Kresevic at the Case Western Reserve/University Hospital's project in Cleveland, Ohio (Foreman, 1984, 1993; Fulmer, 1991a, 1991b; Inouye et al., 1993; Kresevic & Naylor, 1995; Landefeld, Palmer, Kresevic, Fortinsky, & Kowal, 1995).

Each of these embedded nursing projects was carefully scrutinized by the program officer, Donna Regenstrief, who had already begun to explore with the board the potential of funding a nursing initiative. The resultant two-year pilot project, awarded to me as PI at the Columbia University School of Nursing with Mathy Mezey at NYU and Cheryl Vince at Education Development Corporation as the co-PIs, was the Nurses Improving Care to the Hospitalized Elderly (NICHE) program. NICHE featured specific nursing interventions that could be tailored to geriatrics in the acute care practice setting. The NICHE "toolkit" allowed nurses to measure elements of the impact of their care. NICHE gave the JAHF the opportunity to see firsthand a successful nurse-led program grant and support to go on to make a more robust investment in nursing leadership with further funding of that program at NYU, as well as funding the Geriatric Interdisciplinary Team

Training (GITT) program in 1995. I served as director for the GITT Resource Center, which was housed at NYU.

Finally, the pinnacle for me was the JAHF's support for the HIGN in 1996, also at NYU and led by codirectors Mathy Mezey and myself. The HIGN, through its websites, publications, and presentations, disseminates cutting-edge materials to promote best practices in geriatric care, including the Try This® assessment series, Nursing Counts, and policy white papers. This kind of extraordinary support for geriatric nursing was unimaginable when I was graduating from college, and my depth of gratitude for the opportunity to work with the wonderful Mathy Mezey on so many crucial initiatives can never be fully expressed. She is more than a pioneer. She is a legend.

A project of the HIGN and the Foundation of the ANA, which had significant influence on improving care for older adults, was the Nurse Competence in Aging project and, subsequently, the Resourcefully Enhancing Aging in Specialty Nursing (REASN) project. This project, funded in 2002 for five years, addressed the need to ensure competence in geriatric nursing among nursing specialty organizations. It provided grants to specialty organizations and developed a critical mass of well-prepared nurses from other nursing specialties who had a desire to improve their knowledge and skill in geriatric nursing. Each of these grants was transformative to the field of geriatric nursing and spawned dramatic change in the way both American nursing and American medicine thought about geriatric nursing.

The JAHF's largest commitment to geriatric nursing came through its Building Academic Geriatric Nursing Capacity (BAGNC) initiative, endorsed by the JAHF trustees in March 2000. The main mission of the BAGNC initiative was

> to create well-prepared, productive academic geriatric nurses who are able to conduct research that underpins care, teach the next generation of nurses so that they are enthusiastic and knowledgeable in the care of elders, and lead change in schools of nursing and health care systems (JAHF, 2010).

BAGNC supported pre- and postdoctoral training in geriatric nursing and awarded funding to schools of nursing which were known for their exceptional geriatric nursing faculty, geriatric nursing science, and commitment to the preparation of the next generation of geriatric nurse scholars. Because of the partnership with Claire Fagin, dean emerita of the University of Pennsylvania School of Nursing, and Corinne Rieder as the brilliant architects of the program, five schools were supported initially for a five-year period, and in 2006, they were each renewed for an additional five years. These schools were the University of Arkansas for Medical Sciences, University of Iowa, University of Oregon Health Sciences Center, University of California at San Francisco, and University of Pennsylvania. In 2008, four new centers (University of Minnesota, Pennsylvania State University, University of Utah, and Arizona State University) were funded. The JAHF was clear that its funding would not extend beyond an initial 10-year span, after which the centers were expected to be self-sustaining. As part of that process, the centers and training support program were transitioned in 2013 from their original home at the American Academy of Nursing (AAN) to the GSA under the leadership of J. Taylor Harden (McBride, Watman, Escobedo, & Beilenson, 2011). A membership organization of former Archbold Scholars and Fagin Fellows (geriatric nurse leaders), as well as newly participating schools, now help form the National Hartford Centers of Gerontological

Nursing Excellence (NHCGNE)—the latest evolution in advancement among geriatric nursing leadership organizations. Now with more than 30 schools participating, the NHCGNE is an important new way to bring leaders together for progress.

Support for one additional exceptionally important nursing program was initiated in 2008. The JAHF awarded the AAN and the Universities of Arkansas, Iowa, and Pennsylvania a four-year collaborative project to enhance the cognitive and mental health of older Americans by increasing the knowledge and skills of nurses. Also known as the Geropsychiatric Nursing Collaborative (GPNC), this work included development of competency enhancement statements and educational materials (made available via the Portal of Geriatric Online Education) on the care of elders suffering from depression, dementia, and other mental health disorders to guide preprofessional, graduate, and continuing education of nurses who work with older adults (Beck, Buckwalter, & Evans, 2009; Beck, Buckwalter, Dudzik, & Evans, 2011). The work begun by this project is now being furthered by the next generation—members of the Hartford geriatric nurse leaders.

■ MORAL/ETHICAL FOUNDATION

The moral and ethical foundation of my work is based on several questions that I reflect upon daily. Why is it that we develop mechanisms to keep people living longer and then fail to provide expert care? How is it possible that there is elder abuse that goes undetected because we only look for abuse in children and younger women? How can I, as a nurse, influence my profession and the public in a way that enhances the care of older adults? I hope that this chapter provides insight into the progress we have made and the journey in front of us in caring for older adults.

■ VISION

With great pride and humility, I know that the HIGN at NYU has become the definitive beacon for advancing progress in geriatric nursing, and it continues today under the leadership of Tara Cortes. Further, the NICHE program, also at NYU and led until recently by Dr. Elizabeth Capezuti (now at Hunter College), is currently present in more than 500 hospitals nationally and internationally. I would argue that the success of NYU's HIGN opened the gates to the funding of the additional centers of geriatric nursing excellence. It is an understatement to say that the commitment of the JAHF has been transformative. I certainly want also to recognize the ongoing funding by the Department of Health and Human Services Division of Nursing, the NIA, the NINR, the U.S. Department of Veterans Affairs, the Brookdale Foundation, the Gordon and Betty Moore Foundation, the Reynolds Foundation, and the RWJF among those entities that have also made significant contributions toward the advancement and progress of geriatric nursing.

Clearly, great strides have been made in the field of gerontological nursing to date, and its future warrants exponential effort and advances to stay abreast of the needs of our aging society. Longevity, caregiving needs, self-management strategies for chronic disease, telehealth, virtual monitoring, bioanalytics, and designer medicines are on the horizon for older adults, and the need for highly educated, patient-centered nursing will only accelerate. A key mandate is that we build on what is already known in order to generate tomorrow's evidence for care models, clinical strategies, and excellence in team care. The teams of tomorrow have not yet been invented, and the goal will be to prepare a workforce that can anticipate and move quickly to assimilate new paradigms. Nursing has benefited from the programs and people discussed here and the shape of things to come will require even more inventive strategies, public–private partnerships, and a true reckoning of how the voice of older people will guide us. I have loved the opportunity to help shape the change and look forward to the next wave of innovators (the 3.0s!), my daughter Holly among them!

I want nurses who have read this chapter to gain an appreciation for all that must be done to improve the quality of care for older adults, and I hope this chapter will inspire people to gain expertise in geriatric nursing. All of us have had friends or relatives who experienced care that was unacceptable. I firmly believe that it is the profession of nursing, and *only* the profession of nursing, that has the intellectual and numeric power to create the change we need for the future.

■ REFLECTIONS

1. *In thinking about my career, can I articulate my passion, and is it a passion that will last me a lifetime?*
2. *Everyone needs mentors. Can I identify at least one or two mentors who will help me along my journey as I address my passion?*
3. *All careers have significant setbacks. There will obviously be disappointments along the way. Do I consider myself resilient, and how have I demonstrated resilience in the face of adversity?*
4. *Everyone needs to consider their legacy and create the next generation of nurse scholars who will carry on their work. Am I actively engaged in creating the next generation who can address my work?*
5. *In order to make true progress, there has to be an element of fun in all that one does. How do I keep joy in my work?*

■ REFERENCES

American Nurses Association. (1970). Standards for geriatric nursing practice. *American Journal of Nursing, 70*(9), 1894–1897.

American Nurses Association. (1980). *Nursing, a social policy statement.* Kansas City, MO: Author.

American Nurses Association. (2015). *Code of ethics for nurses with interpretive statements.* Silver Spring, MD: Nursesbooks.org

Beck, C., Buckwalter, K. C., & Evans, L. K. (2009). *Geropsychiatric Nursing Collaborative.* Retrieved from http://www.aannet.org/geropsychiatric-nursing-collaborative

Beck, C., Buckwalter, K. C., Dudzik, P. M., & Evans, L. K. (2011). Filling the void in geriatric mental health: The Geropsychiatric Nursing Collaborative as a model for change. *Nursing Outlook, 59*(4), 236–241.

Berkowitz, E. (2008). Medicare and Medicaid: The past as prologue. *Health Care Financing Review, 29*(3), 81.

Butler, R. (1975). *Why survive? Being old in America.* New York, NY: Harper Torchbooks.

Clifford, J. C. (1980). Primary nursing: A contemporary model for delivery of health care. *American Journal of Hospital Pharmacy, 37,* 1089–1091.

Ebersole, P. (1999). The dynamic duo: Mathy Mezey, EdD, RN, FAAN, FGSA and Terry Fulmer, RN, PhD, FAAN, FGSA. *Geriatric Nursing, 20*(2), 106–107.

Ebersole, P., & Toughy, T. A. (2006). *Geriatric nursing: Growth of a specialty.* New York, NY: Springer Publishing Company .

Evans, L. K., & Strumpf, N. E. (1989). Tying down the elderly: A review of the literature on physical restraint. *Journal of the American Geriatrics Society, 37*(1), 65.

Evans, L. K., Strumpf, N. E., Allen-Taylor, S. L., Capezuti, E., Maislin, G., & Jacobsen, B. (1997). A clinical trial to reduce restraints in nursing homes. *Journal of the American Geriatrics Society, 45*(6), 675.

Foreman, M. D. (1984). Acute confusional states in the elderly: An algorithm. *Dimensions of Critical Care Nursing, 3,* 207–215.

Foreman, M. D. (1993). Acute confusion in the elderly. *Annual Review of Nursing Research, 11*(3), 30–98.

Frank, R. G. (2000). The creation of Medicare and Medicaid: The emergence of insurance and markets for mental health services. *Psychiatric Services, 51*(4), 465–468.

Fulmer, T. (1977). On vitamins, calories, and help for the elderly. *American Journal of Nursing, 77*(10), 1614.

Fulmer, T. (1991a). The geriatric nurse specialist role: A new model. *Nursing Management, 22*(3), 91–93.

Fulmer, T. (1991b). Grow your own experts in hospital elder care. *Geriatric Nursing, 12*(2), 64–66.

Fulmer, T. (2007). How to try this: Fulmer SPICES. *American Journal of Nursing, 107*(10), 40–48; quiz 48–49.

Fulmer, T. (2015). Geriatric nursing 2.0. *Journal of the American Geriatrics Society, 63*(7), 1453–1458.

Fulmer, T., & Matzo, M. (Eds.). (1995). *Strengthening geriatric nursing education.* New York, NY: Springer.

Fulmer, T., & Mezey, M. (1994). Nurses improving care to the hospitalized elderly. *Geriatric Nursing, 15*(3), 126.

Fulmer, T., & Mezey, M. (1998). Contemporary geriatric nursing. In W. R. Hazzard, J. P. Blass, W. H. Ettinger, J. B. Halter, & J. G. Ouslander (Eds.), *Principles of geriatric medicine and gerontology* (4th ed., pp. 355–363). New York, NY: McGraw-Hill.

Inouye, S. K., Wagner, D. R., Acampora, D., Horwitz, R. I., Cooney, L. M. J., & Tinetii, M. E. (1993). A controlled trial of a nursing-centered intervention in hospitalized elderly medical patients: The Yale Geriatric Care Program. *Journal of the American Geriatric Society, 41*(12), 1353–1360.

Institute of Medicine. (2011). *The future of nursing: Leading change, advancing health.* Washington, DC: National Academies Press.

Institute of Medicine. (2014). *Dying in America: Improving quality and honoring individual preferences near the end of life.* Washington, DC: National Academies Press.

John A. Hartford Foundation. (2010). 2010 annual report. Retrieved from http://www.jhartfound .org/ar2010/index.html

John A. Hartford Foundation. (2010). *Adult-gerontology primary care nurse practitioner competencies.* New York, NY: Author.

John A. Hartford Foundation. (2012). *Adult-gerontology acute care nurse practitioner competencies.* New York, NY: Author.

Johnson, M. A., & Richard Connelly, J. (1990). *Nursing and gerontology: Status report.* Washington, DC: Association for Gerontology and Higher Education.

Kresevic, D., & Naylor, M. (1995). Preventing pressure ulcers through use of protocols in a mentored nursing model. *Geriatric Nursing, 16*(5), 225–229.

Landefeld, C. S., Palmer, R. M., Kresevic, D. M., Fortinsky, R. H., & Kowal, J. (1995). A randomized trial of care in a hospital medical unit especially designed to improve the functional outcomes of acutely ill older patients. *New England Journal of Medicine, 332*(20), 1338–1344.

McBride, A. B., Watman, R., Escobedo, M., & Beilenson, J. (2011). Clustering excellence to exert transformative change: The Hartford Geriatric Nursing Initiative (HGNI). *Nursing Outlook, 59*(4), 189–195. doi:10.1016/j.outlook.2011.04.008

Mezey, M. (1989). *The teaching nursing home program: Outcomes of care.* Philadelphia, PA: W.B. Saunders.

Mezey, M. (1995). *Strengthening geriatric nursing education.* New York, NY: Springer Publishing Company.

Mezey, M., Amella, E., & Fulmer, T. (1995). Gerontological nursing: Successes of the past, visions for the future. *Journal of the New York State Nurses Association, 26*(1), 25–27.

Schneider, E. L., Ory, M., & Aung, M. L. (1987). Teaching nursing homes revisited: Survey of affiliations between American medical schools and long-term-care facilities. *Journal of the American Medical Association, 257*(20), 2771.

Shaughnessy, P. W., Kramer, A. M., Hittle, D. F., & Steiner, J. F. (1995). Quality of care in teaching nursing homes: Findings and implications. *Health Care Finance Review, 16*(4), 55–83.

Shem, S. (1978). *House of God.* London, UK: Corgi.

Shem, S. (2003). *House of God.* New York, NY: Delta Trade Paperbacks.

Silva, M. C. (1983). The American Nurses' Association's position statement on nursing and social policy: Philosophical and ethical dimensions. *Journal of Advanced Nursing, 8*(2), 147–151. doi:10.1111/j.1365-2648.1983.tb00305.x

Strumpf, N. E., & Evans, L. K. (1988). Physical restraint of the hospitalized elderly: Perceptions of patients and nurses. *Nursing Research, 37*(3), 132.

U.S. Congress, Office of Technology Assessment. (1987). *Life-sustaining technologies and the elderly* (OTA-BA-306). Washington, DC: U.S. Government Printing Office.

Wallace, M., & Fulmer, T. (1998). Try this: Best practices in nursing care to older adults. Fulmer SPICES: An overall assessment tool of older adults (reprinted with permission). The John A. Hartford Foundation Institute for Geriatric Nursing, Vol. 1, No. 1, August 1998. *Journal of Gerontological Nursing, 24*(12), 3.

Wallace, M., & Fulmer, T. (1999). Fulmer SPICES: An overall assessment tool of older adults. *Viewpoint, 21*(2), 6.

Wikipedia. (2014). *Robert Neil Butler.* Retrieved from http://en.wikipedia.org/w/index.php?title=Robert_Neil_Butler&oldid=631383460

CHAPTER SEVEN

Present and Humbled: Leading the Conversations That Matter Most

Lynn Keegan

Remember to imagine and vision. When you dream, dream big!
For all things are possible.
My hope is that each of us can live from a place of personal peace.
That each of us will develop a sense of spirituality and treat one another as
they wish to be treated,
And I wish for others to come to believe, as I do,
That our primary purpose on planet earth
Is to grow and develop our soul.

—Keegan (2013, pp. 144–145)

■ WHY NURSING?

My first nursing experience was in the 1950s at age 14, caring for my mother after surgery. By default, I also cared for the whole ward of postoperative patients at John Sealy, the then charity hospital in Galveston, Texas. Since those days, it has become a large, renowned teaching hospital, a branch of the University of Texas system.

For two days and nights, I shuttled between the patients in the poorly staffed, old-fashioned open ward, tending to helpless, very ill women through insufferable pain and vomiting episodes, doing my best to help, especially while the busy night nurse dispensed her medications and treatments. All she had time for was an impossible list of tasks. She did not have a single moment to pause . . . sit beside a woman in discomfort . . . hold her hand . . . moisten her parched lips . . . pass a cooling cloth across her brow . . . speak a loving word. Many of these women either sobbed softly by themselves or asked me to help. It was in the midst of that emotionally and physically intense experience I decided to become a nurse. In the eyes of that 14-year-old, there was a critical need for more people to help the patients; they needed focused, whole-person, caring attention during those critical postsurgical hours.

During the balance of my high-school years, I supported my family in any way possible: cooking, cleaning, and tending the younger children, as my mother had become too ill to do so. These were tiresome and difficult teenage years. To kindle a sense of hope and intention, I carefully plotted and planned, dreaming about how to begin a better life for myself elsewhere.

I had absolutely no money and, at best, mediocre grades, since after school, home responsibilities left me no time for homework or study. However, I joined the Future Nurses Club and was able to volunteer once a month on Saturday mornings as a candy striper at the local hospital in order to learn as much as I could about nursing. At school, I talked with the resident nurse about how to get myself to college and the path she followed to becoming a nurse. In the late 1950s and early 1960s, she only knew about local diploma schools, but she helped and encouraged me to start searching for a program that provided a college degree for nursing.

All I knew was that I wanted to be the best nurse possible. I had an inherent need to help reduce the suffering of the many, many women I had witnessed at John Sealy Hospital. With the help of the county librarian, I explored how to accomplish that goal. After library reference searches and writing for catalogues from all over the country, I decided that Cornell or Columbia, both in New York City, seemed to be the two best schools at the time and I prayed one of them would accept me. Both were five-year programs requiring two years of college prior to acceptance. My mission during the final years of high school was to develop an action plan of great personal significance: how to get out of poverty in a small town, go elsewhere—anywhere—to make something worthwhile of my life and be able to serve others.

To begin, I made my way to the cheapest college in the United States (Western State College of Colorado in Gunnison). I was drawn there by the pictures in their paper catalog, and it was what I needed—affordable and away from home. Once there, I studied diligently to complete the initial college requirements for admission to nursing school: biology, zoology, chemistry, and the slate of required liberal arts, including French, English literature, psychology, and sociology. Indeed, these are very different than the requirements today. Two years later, I was accepted and finally made it to Cornell University–New York Hospital, School of Nursing (CU-NYHSN) to embark upon the final three academic and clinical years of the five-year baccalaureate curriculum.

■ EARLY IMPRESSIONS

After completing the first year at Cornell, I was eligible to take the New York State board exam to become a licensed practical nurse (LPN). Weekend and summer LPN assignments, coupled with *more* student loans and small scholarships, got me through to graduation. After 5 bone-crunching, challenging student years and two years of part-time, summer, and school-year LPN clinical care, I finally felt experienced. I was a graduate nurse ready to "change the world!" My first job was a half-year stint as the emergency department evening charge nurse in a community hospital back in Texas. Here I witnessed many serious traumas and illnesses and discovered how quickly life can end. I often wondered if any of these people were *ready* to die. Certainly, I came to recognize that life is fleeting. But in those days, in my 20s, I did not stay focused there, and instead rushed forward into the busy, developing profession and the fast pace of acute care practice.

My next job was as a bedside nurse at St. Luke's Hospital in New York City. The challenge I discovered here: There were more things I wanted to improve than I could possibly accomplish as a bedside nurse. I thought I had the knowledge and skills, but the hierarchy declared that I needed more credentials to have any relevant say in instituting changes or enhancing care quality. Needless to say, my eyes were further opened to how the units could be better organized and how the care team might facilitate a more effective rapport. I wanted to know how a nurse might alter her schedule to create pauses—to interweave the *art* of nursing with the *science* and to enliven more spirit-directed care during the nurse–patient exchange. Even though I disagreed that additional credentials should be the requisite stature necessary to contribute input into greater management and operational decision making, I acquiesced and created a new life plan to obtain an MSN degree. After working for a year, I chose Loma Linda University in California to continue my education with a master's degree. I was ready to leave the East Coast and wanted to explore a new part of the country.

At Loma Linda University, I was introduced to the Seventh-Day Adventist spiritual approach to health care. Nurses awakened patients by singing hymns in the hallways and prayed with patients before they went for surgery. What a joyful experience! It embodied the spiritual element that secular Cornell had not even mentioned. The two years at Loma Linda further opened my spiritual calling to serve as a guide for others and challenged me, academically, in new ways of working with the sick.

Graduating with an MSN from Loma Linda at age 26, I was ready to charge into an advanced nursing practice and I hoped to further serve the ill and suffering. My first position with a graduate degree was as a nurse manager at the now University of California Medical Hospital at San Diego. In the late 1960s and early 1970s, it was the County Hospital. Also, during this time, the first intensive care units (ICUs) opened as partitioned spaces of four to six beds in the middle of step-down units that housed acutely ill patients. I relished the management/practice position until my husband's military assignment caused us to move.

Prior to the 1960s, most students attended a hospital-based, three-year diploma school and completed all of their education and clinical work in one hospital. They were identified by their unique cap and lapel pin that was specific to each school. During the 1960s, both associate degree and many new baccalaureate programs began. Many, like Temple University in Philadelphia, morphed from diploma to university while others emerged in primary university settings. It was from 1965 forward that nursing leadership debated having the BSN as the recognized professional nursing degree. Anyone with less than baccalaureate education would be an associate nurse. Needless to say, that concept never took root. However, it was this push to the BSN that finally propelled nursing to emerge out of its perceived technical status to become accepted as a profession.

I was blessed to be a part of this time in nursing history. At Philadelphia's Temple University, I was one of four core faculty who took one year to develop curriculum, negotiate clinical rotation venues, and prepare labs and classrooms for Temple's new baccalaureate program. After successfully implementing the program, we relocated to Charleston, where I procured another academic appointment at the Medical University of South Carolina. Baccalaureate education was setting deep roots and I loved all of it, especially seeing students grow and flourish. Having moved out of the era of a solo hospital diploma setting, these students were exposed to a much larger breadth and depth of education, including arts and science, inpatient and community settings, as well as physical, mental, and spiritual components of both illness and health. They emerged from this type of education able to see a broader picture of both needs and possibilities.

From South Carolina and academia to Maine and jumping back into clinical practice, I had our first child, who brought new meaning to work–life balance. With a baby in tow and schedules changed, the ability to do what I wanted had been modified; another's needs had to supersede my goals.

■ PROFESSIONAL EVOLUTION/CONTRIBUTION

Relocating back to Texas for the next 22 years, I applied for a position at Texas Women's University to coordinate an off-campus MSN program in the community. Once in the job, I was informed that one of the criteria to retain the position was the pursuit of a doctoral degree. What? I now had a full-time academic teaching job, a three-year-old, and a new baby. It seemed impossible; get my doctorate at the same time? Not at all interested in my personal situation, the dean was adamant and I succumbed. I decided I could divide and spend my teaching and program administration income between tuition and a full-time babysitter.

In the summer of 1980, fortune smiled on me. The University of Texas at Austin (UTA), an hour's drive down Interstate 35, accepted my student application and, within months, I now had a third full-time job as a nursing doctoral student. I quickly learned that the formula to success was not to tell the doctoral faculty and classmates about my other two jobs: motherhood and the master's program I led up the road. Thus, for three years I kept my two identities separate, that of a dedicated doctoral student in one city and that of lead faculty and mother in another.

It was during this academic immersion in 1981 that the American Holistic Nurses Association (AHNA) announced its first annual meeting. Leaving the children with the babysitter and studies dangling, I spontaneously took the plunge, boarded a plane, and disembarked into unknown territory. It was a heaven-sent opportunity and the holistic content looked tantalizing and different.

And what a surprise it was. Checking in at the conference site at the University of Wisconsin in rural La Crosse was a unique experience, but it was late, I was tired from travel, and so went straight to bed in one of the dormitory residences. Now, that in itself was quite an experience. All the professional meetings I had attended during the past 15 years had been in convention centers in cities, so being in a dorm room again was very different. Early the next morning, I followed others who made their way cross-campus. I slugged forward in desperate need of morning coffee. Along the way, in the grassy hillocks beside paved sidewalks, was a group of individuals in flowing white garb doing odd hand/arm/leg/foot movements. They appeared to be floating as we approached the school cafeteria building. "What," I asked, "are these people doing?" The group I had linked with looked at me oddly and said, "Well, tai chi, of course." "Okay, well, that's certainly something uniquely new to me," I thought to myself.

The next surprise greeted me in the food line. First, there were only herbal teas—no coffee. (Oh, how I wanted coffee!) I "needed" coffee but there was none, and I simply had to adjust. Then no bacon and eggs or pancakes and syrup; only plain, homemade yogurt, berries, and nuts, along with miso soup and other assorted unusual health foods. True, I had become accustomed to a vegetarian regime in grad school, but that was years before and this was even more unusual. I later discovered that the menu had been set by Norm Shealy, the then president of the American Holistic Medical Association (AHMA), our cosponsor of the conference. Shealy was a serious holistic health advocate. As it so happened, all the meals followed the same formula: vegetarian, low fat, low sugar, and good for you.

Next came the plenary sessions and breakout workshops. I had become so immersed in secular, linear, academic curriculums and practice that I actually felt my mind expanding while engaged in the host of nontraditional, alternative, and transformational didactic and practice session content. We learned about guided imagery, touch therapies, spiritual dimensions, alternative nutrition, and environmental factors in health, along with many other new focus areas. Attention to introspection, self-development, and personal insights, along with innovative patient/client application models, were novel and exciting. Remember now, this was 1981, what many consider the birth year of holistic nursing.

Another refreshing component of this meeting was the emphasis on interpersonal relationships. These were not the networking, job-shopping type of relationships so often encountered in traditional association meetings. Here, the participants seemed to relish getting to the essence of one another. One's goals, purpose, and application of self and self-care to work, family, and colleagues were valued and important.

A mere five-day immersion at a unique conference during the inception of a new national nursing organization changed me. The draw of this emerging worldview, along with professional intentions to teach health and wellness and guide others toward an experience of wholeness, was compelling. I was hooked. From that moment onward, I dedicated myself to living both a personal and professional life according to holistic nursing principles.

Back at UTA, I changed my focus of study to holistic nursing. I even met with Billie Brown, then the UTA dean, and told her about the AHNA, its mission, and goals. She applauded the idea and encouraged me as I explained my redirected pursuit.

I quickly learned that, in essence, holistic nursing is self-living awareness and working with others within a framework of body-mind-spirit consciousness. From a holistic perspective, a person—oneself or one's client—is seen or perceived based on the knowledge that the whole is greater than and different than the sum of its parts. The objective is to bring oneself or another back to a state of health as it relates to feelings of harmony and unity. Illness, in contrast, is perceived as dissonance and separation from the whole. In the holistic model, the overall focus is on creating health and healing, whereas the traditional medical model has been focused on curing. Over the past few decades, it has been wonderful to watch, as well as to be involved in, the change, as many in mainstream medicine and nursing have adapted their practice to a more holistic model.

When working with others or oneself from a body-mind-spirit framework, the person is considered a part of an ever-changing environment, which includes both internal and external elements. The *internal environment* relates to the subjective nature of people's own observations and perceptions, as well how they think, process, cope, and perceive outside events from their own mental and spiritual development. The *external environment* relates to components of the physical milieu, such as temperature, sound, visual stimuli, comfort or discomfort of settings, and people. Within this context, we are all interconnected. This concept moves us to understand that all sentient beings share the same planet and, thus, share the same physical environment. It also recognizes that, regardless of the barriers of politics, religion, or culture, people can share in a universal reciprocity of love and responsibility. We exist in dual simultaneity, alone in our internal environment and sharing the space and experience of the external environment (Dossey & Keegan, 2016; Keegan, 2001, 1994).

It is so fulfilling to know that for more than 30 years I have been an active part of the seeding and growing of the AHNA and been present to watch it bloom and flourish. The AHNA has grown to become a nonprofit membership association for nurses and other holistic health care professionals, with more than 5,700 members and 125 local network chapters across the United States and abroad. Accredited by the American Nurses Credentialing Center (ANCC), the AHNA approves over 150 educational activities every year through the quarterly *Journal of Holistic Nursing*, monthly *Beginnings*, the annual AHNA conference, the *Foundations of Holistic Nursing Course*, and other continuing nurse education (CNE) activities. See Table 7.1 for a description of the AHNA (2016) goals, guiding principles, and purpose.

Once holistic nursing was identified and defined, my path was chosen. I became a part of this emerging focus, both living the philosophical tenets and teaching the specialty, while at the same time working with colleagues to further develop the science. After tailoring as much independent coursework as possible in a holistic direction, in 1983 I completed my doctoral dissertation on an aspect of wellness lifestyle behaviors and their impact on recent illness. I discovered that subjects who maintained more vigorous wellness lifestyle behaviors had fewer recent illnesses than those subjects who did not practice such behaviors.

TABLE 7.1 **Goals, Guiding Principles, and Purpose of the American Holistic Nurses Association (AHNA)**

The AHNA goals are	• To provide continuing education in holistic nursing
	• To help to improve the health care workplace by promoting the incorporation of the concepts of holistic nursing
	• To educate professionals and the public about holistic nursing and integrative health care
	• To serve as a resource to members
	• To promote research and scholarship in the field of holistic nursing
The guiding principles include	The *mission*: The mission of AHNA is to advance holistic nursing through community building, advocacy, research, and education.
	The *vision*: Our vision is a world in which nursing nurtures wholeness and inspires peace and healing.
	The *purpose* as described next

(continued)

TABLE 7.1   **Goals, Guiding Principles, and Purpose of the American Holistic Nurses Association (AHNA)** (*continued*)

The *purpose* is	• AHNA promotes the education of nurses, other health care professionals, and the public in all aspects of holistic caring and healing. The efforts of AHNA resulted in the recognition of holistic nursing as an "official nursing specialty" by the American Nurses Association.
	• AHNA advances the profession of holistic nursing by providing continuing education in holistic nursing, helping to improve the health care workplace through the incorporation of the concepts of holistic nursing, educating professionals and the public about holistic nursing and integrative health care, and promoting research and scholarship in the field of holistic nursing.
	• AHNA has taken positions on the practice of complementary and alternative medicine (CAM), holistic nursing ethics, and research and scholarship within the field of holistic nursing. In addition, AHNA monitors and responds to government policy initiatives around the United States. Most recently, AHNA issued a response to the Food and Drug Administration (FDA) in its draft document: *Guidance for Industry on Complementary and Alternative Medicine Products and Their Regulation* by the Food and Drug Administration.
	• As a resource to its members, AHNA provides a supportive community, informative publications, continuing education, local networking opportunities, liability insurance, and a focus on self-care and wellness, among others.

Adapted from www.ahna.org

Following the intensity of three nonstop years, I drew back from academia to take a much-needed break and spend more time with family. In 1984, I opened The Wellness Center. As the first independent nurse-run practice in our small, medically dominated, traditional town, it was a novelty. During this same period of time, I became the president of the AHNA, and spent more volunteer work time building and strengthening the national organization.

In 1986, my colleague and friend, Barbara Dossey, and I began a long-term journey of coauthoring books and partnering a wellness-based business, BodyMind Systems. Our four-time American Journal of Nursing Book of the Year award-winning textbook, *Holistic Nursing: A Handbook for Practice,* was first published in 1988. Since that time, we have added six more editions and, working alongside a growing editorial team of nurse educators, have completed the seventh edition (2016). Over the course of our 30-year partnership, we have developed and carried the message of holistic nursing wherever we could, all over the world (see Chapter 4, written by Barbara Dossey, for more information about our coauthoring and collaboration).

■ MORAL/ETHICAL FOUNDATION

Moving into the new millennium, I left both academic work and the state of Texas and moved with our family to a remote, aesthetic location on the edge of the sea in the

Pacific Northwest. It was a move designed as a new beginning. We bought a house on a mountainside looking out to the sea. I put aside my books and plunged into a home garden, hiking the rural fresh paths and coastal fishing villages and towns. The local flora and fauna and landscape of Washington State's wild Olympic Peninsula became the fresh focus.

By this time in my career, I had worked to develop holistic content and books and taken and taught courses about complementary and alternative therapies (CAM), today also known as *caring–healing modalities* (Watson, 2012), taught in university programs, and traveled worldwide to present these ideas to others. I had studied, taught, experienced, and written about caring–healing modalities as aspects of holistic nursing for application in health and wellness improvement. With 19 published books to date and numerous scholarly articles and chapters in books, my professional mission was one of being a part of a dedicated team to develop a holistic nursing focus. It was time to take a break.

This time was not without some continued replay of past life experiences. As a child and into adulthood, attention was focused on the needs of my mother, my children, and then, later on, came the intense needs of my grandmother during the last decade of her life. She split time between living with us and in a local nursing home in Texas for the last 10 years of her life, until she died at age 97. Shortly after our arrival in Washington, my husband's uncle required a decade of end-of-life care when he came to us, until his death at 93. Ultimately, the lived experience and many inpatient clinical episodes taught me that each of these loved ones needed better, more compassionate end-of-life care when they finally ended up in hospitals or nursing homes. Thus, after almost a year in the garden, on the trails, and doing firsthand care of dying relatives, I was fully prepared when the commencement of a next phase opened me to more formal methods of helping evolve end-of-life practices.

I knew there had to be a better way to help people through their final transition. Back in the 1970s, I was thrilled to hear Dr. Cicely Sanders when she came from her practice in London, England, to the University of Pennsylvania to introduce the hospice concept to the United States. I so enthusiastically embraced her ideas that later, during my doctoral program, I had actually initiated dissertation work in this area before I discovered the AHNA and holistic nursing, which subsequently changed my focus of study.

In 2008, after an annual meeting of the AHNA, a longtime friend and colleague, Carole Ann Drick, suggested that we write another book together. I had previously read and written a formal endorsement of her first book about an end-of-life perspective (Drick, 2008) and we had previously coauthored the AHNA history book (Aime, Keegan, & Drick, 2008). We worked well together and, as it turned out, were both passionate about changing the settings and consciousness in end-of-life care. So this was to be another new beginning.

We delved into the field to learn as much as we could and talked to as many people as possible to help consolidate and conceptualize our beliefs about how life endings could become so much better. It seemed that my childhood passion for helping the suffering had never ended; it had only taken a small hiatus. Thus, with a new coauthor and a new location, I began writing again. Springer Publishing in New York, in conjunction with Watson Caring Science Institute in Boulder, Colorado, contracted us to deliver a book. We spent two years in the research, development, and publication of *End of Life: Nursing Solutions for Death with Dignity* (Keegan & Drick, 2011a). It explores society's experience with death and dying and details a novel approach, describing why new locations and caregiving ethics for actively dying patients are needed. We use multiple anecdotes to describe what happens to many patients during their last days in multiple current clinical settings. Ample theory and text are provided to demonstrate methods of substantial improvement. The book went on to receive two of the prestigious *American Journal of Nursing* Book of the Year Awards in hospice and palliative care and gerontology nursing in 2011. The book is used in nursing classrooms and continuing education to prepare students with innovative end-of-life theory and practical caregiving skills.

What we discovered later is that we needed a similar book written for the lay public. This led us to create another volume, *The Golden Room: A Practical Guide for Death with Dignity* (Keegan & Drick, 2013a). This work serves to introduce the next level in the evolution of palliative and hospice care. It requires a shift in consciousness and attitude toward death so that dying is accepted as a sacred process deserving of compassion, dignity, and beautiful surroundings. The Golden Room is a dedicated place for those within a week or two of dying (Keegan & Drick, 2011b, 2013a). Later, we produced a pocket guide booklet, *Quality of Life at End of Life* (see Keegan & Drick, 2013b), to give to participants at seminars and presentations.

Currently, end-of-life costs are very expensive; the bulk of one's health care dollars are spent in the last six months of life. In contrast, the development of such restful places like Golden Rooms, an extension of the hospice concept, would cost only a fraction of the amount of high technology care, which is currently spent in the last few days and months of life. Our mission is to reverse the all-too-common trend of expensive technology overuse during futile care at end of life and replace it with a dignified and holistic approach (Keegan & Drick, 2012) and a humane, pleasant environment that aids loved ones in contributing toward the patient's peaceful transition.

> Indeed, contributing toward the consciousness shift in how individuals view and society approaches end of life is an ethical platform that speaks not only to how we die, but also to how we live. The moral and ethical considerations involved call us to delve inward, evaluate the decisions we make, and refocus our energies on fostering nursing practice, education, and research that prioritizes caring and humane expressions of healing beyond the inadequate and restrictive medical model confines of curing. Furthering this crucial dialogue is a demonstration of holistic perspectives regarding the interconnectedness of Self and Other, an offering of peace and well-being for those enduring unnecessary suffering at end of life, and a way of creating harmony between patients' internal and external environments, which often remain dissonant and overlooked in their final moments. The conversations surrounding end-of-life care and dying with dignity help to deepen one's ethical awareness of humanity's most sacred transition, weaving threads of compassion and reverence throughout the tapestries of living and learning. These are the conversations that matter most. (W. Rosa, personal communication, November 21, 2015)

■ VISION

In 2013, I wrote about some of my dreams for children born in the future. Reexpressed and reworded here, these include the following:

- I wish that children be born into a world of planetary peace.
- I hope today's wars, replete with weapons and identifying one another as the enemy, will be a thing of the past. I hope the only wars they hear about are in the history books.
- I wish that new generations come into a "green" world; one that is self-sustaining, using natural resources. I hope they learn early in life to recycle everything—that nothing is wasted; everything is reused and recycled.
- I hope that some of their behaviors will revert to the past, when daily life was more natural. In the winter they keep the heat low and wear warm clothes and sweaters, that in the summer they adapt to warm temperatures and wear natural fibers designed to keep them cool, that they lower the thermostats in the winter and raise them in the summer and save on abundant overuse of resources that we see today.
- I hope they live in houses and work in buildings with windmills and solar panels and other new technological devices to better utilize resources.
- I hope living spaces and communities are better designed for more environmentally friendly living, less reliance on automobiles, and improved public transportation.
- I hope there are more individual and community gardens so that people have fresher food to eat, and better appreciate where it comes from and the labor involved in bringing food from seed to the table.

(Keegan, 2013, pp. 144–145)

For this book, I expand my desired vision to all peoples, and that is to mirror the intent so aptly voiced in John Lennon's 1971 song, "Imagine." In this best-selling single of his solo career, the lyrics encourage the listener to imagine a world at peace without the barriers of borders or the divisiveness of religions and nationalities and to consider the possibility that the focus of humanity should be living a life unattached to material possessions. Today, more than 40 years later, think of how much better we could all be if we still collectively pushed for this vision.

Since the publication of our end-of-life books, my career-specific vision is to guide others to grow in their knowledge about end-of-life philosophies and practices and to help both laypeople and health care professionals to understand that by working together, we can bring more compassionate care to those undergoing the transition. This important work occurs by beginning the conversation about death. Nurses can help those at the end of life to consciously face their fears and process their concerns about their journey. Death comes unbidden to all of us. For many, it is one of the most difficult things to think or talk about. For the most part, this is because our society has moved us away from the place of sacredness and importance that death once held. Today, death is a subject that is just not part of contemporary conversation. The more we know about death and dying, the more comfortable we become. Knowing does not take the sting of loss and sadness away. But knowing does help us to prepare so everyone can move through death and dying with a higher degree of comfort and understanding.

It is my belief that nurses must lead the movement to establish the conversations everyone needs to have about death and dying. These conversations are rapidly being established by well-meaning laypeople and organizations, but this domain should be captured by nurses. Nurses are the ones who understand not only the pathophysiology but also the mind, spirit, and psychology of the whole person, as well as leadership theory. Groups such as Death Cafes, Dinner Over Death, and others are rapidly forming with lay volunteer leaders. Organizations such as Visiting Angels, a national syndicated home health agency, staffed mostly by unskilled or certified nursing assistants, are advertising and offering end-of-life home care. Their business and others like them are booming. My question is: Where is the professional nurse in this equation? Nurses need to be at the forefront guiding, teaching, and honing these end-of-life workers. Let us not surrender this sacred, significant work to others. Let us claim and focus our nursing skills with our most vulnerable, vastly increasing aging population. Discussions and conversations about public health and end-of-life care should be at the heart of this area.

Most people who die are old and sick. Certainly, there are those taken in their youth or others in midlife who depart unexpectedly in accidents and injuries or even an early onset of fatal disease. The vast majority of us, however, die at the end of our physical life cycle when the body can no longer remain in balance because of illness or old age. The fact is that eventually all of us, 100% of us, will die. That is the heart of what we must come to grips with and prepare for. To better prepare, each of us needs to begin to consider:

- Where do you want to be at end of life?
- How do you hope your life will end?
- Who do you want with you at end of life?
- Are you ready to go?
- What can you do to better plan for your death now?
- What do you want to happen after you pass on?
  (Keegan & Drick, 2013a, pp. 11–12)

These can be challenging questions to ask, and you may tend to rapidly read over them or think, "I'll look at these later." This is the telltale sign of being scared and denying. If this is the case, the question to ask is, "If I don't face this now, then when?"

The greatest human freedom is to live and die according to one's own desires and beliefs. The most common desire among those with a terminal illness is to die with some measure of dignity. From advanced directives to physician-assisted dying, death with dignity is a goal for all of humanity. Each of us needs to learn all that we can about this so as to be able to make our own end-of-life care decisions. Essentially, death with dignity means concluding this physical life with composure, peace, and compassion in the way that has meaning to you.

We all are learners and we all are teachers. What we learn we can pass along to others to assist them in their journey. My vision is that each of us can begin to educate nurses, physicians, caregivers, and the lay public about the concept of Golden Rooms. Learn more about this concept from our website http://www.GoldenRoomAdvocates.org. As with anything, the more a topic is talked about and shared, the more power and awareness it generates. As we share Golden Room ideas and end-of-life information, there can be a giant groundswell that stimulates a change in the health care profession and how we view death and dying. Already, selected hospitals are considering incorporating Golden Rooms in their new architectural designs and care philosophies. Once one or two units are complete, we anticipate that others will quickly adapt the designs into their towns and cities. It all starts with small steps. Ask and keep asking, and eventually people will become curious and begin to search out information. Each small step forward becomes one giant leap for quality of life at the end of life.

As we continue to walk our talk, it is good to reflect on the wisdom of Mother Teresa, who declared that we should begin our caring practice close to home. In one of her hundreds of quotes, she says: "You aren't asked to be kind to everyone, only to those close around you. Love is practical and do-able, and always starts with the people nearest to you."

If we can follow these words in our personal lives, then it becomes easier to extrapolate them to our extended family—our health care teammates. Let us be kind to one another so as to facilitate care for the others in our own environment. It is not necessary to change the world, although many leaders may want to. If each of us can offer our finest selves to what we do, then we can serve as an example of leadership to others. Each of us can light the allegorical candle to illuminate the path for those around us and for those who shall follow. As I conclude, I am both present and humbled to have had the opportunity to consider and relate personal thoughts and experiences, which I hope will help stimulate the conversations that matter most.

■ REFLECTIONS

1. *How do I describe my understanding of holistic nursing?*
2. *Am I attuned to body-mind-spirit orientation when I work with patients and during self-care?*
3. *In which areas of caregiving could I apply holistic principles during nursing interventions?*
4. *When and how will I begin to discuss end-of-life issues? How do I begin to change my relationship with and understanding of end of life, acknowledging it as a natural part of life's process?*
5. *What is the vision I have for how I would like to prepare myself and my patients for the end of life? If I do not have a vision, what is a first step I can take toward creating one? What can I do to make the process more comfortable and more meaningful?*

■ REFERENCES

Aime, D., Keegan, L., Drick, C. A. (2008). *American holistic nurses association: Implementing visions of health and healing.* Topeka, KN: AHNA publication.

American Holistic Nurses Association. (2016). *Goals and purpose of the American Holistic Nurses Association.* Retrieved from http://www.ahna.org

Dossey, B., & Keegan, L. (Eds.). (2016). *Holistic nursing: A handbook for practice* (7th ed.). Burlington, MA: Jones & Bartlett.

Drick, C. A. (2008). *Mother stories: Through our mothers' death and dying.* North Charleston, SC: Create Space.

Keegan, L. (1994). *The nurse as healer.* Albany, NY: Delmar.

Keegan, L. (2001). *Healing with alternative and complementary therapies.* Albany, NY: Delmar.

Keegan, L. (2013). Lynn Gates Keegan: Leader, author and woman of vision. In K. H. Shames (Ed.), *Amazing mentors* (pp. 131–145). Scottsdale, AZ: Inkwell Productions.

Keegan, L., & Drick, C. A. (2011a). *End of life: Nursing solutions for death with dignity.* New York, NY: Springer Publishing Co.

Keegan, L., & Drick, C. A. (2011b). A new place for death with dignity: The golden room. *Journal of Holistic Nursing, 29*(4), 287–291.

Keegan, L., & Drick, C. A. (2012). Death with dignity: a holistic approach. *Beginnings, 32*(3), 4–6.

Keegan, L., & Drick, C. A. (2013a). *The golden room: A practical guide for death with dignity.* North Charleston, SC: Create Space.

Keegan, L., & Drick, C. A. (2013b). Quality of life through the end of life. *Beginnings, 33*(1), 14–7.

Watson, J. (2012). *Human caring science* (2nd ed.). Burlington, MA: Jones & Bartlett.

CHAPTER EIGHT

Integrative and Evolving: Advocating a Whole Person and Whole Systems Perspective

Mary Jo Kreitzer

For decades, the hierarchical command and control style of leadership was embraced as the most effective way to tackle problems and lead change. . . . What is now clear is that the nature of our work settings and the problems we face require a fundamentally different approach.

—Kreitzer (2014a, p. 47)

■ WHY NURSING?

When I reflect on my career path, I have deep gratitude that I chose nursing as the foundation of my work. Although I began with a sense that nursing would afford me interesting and diverse career options, I did not anticipate the joy that the profession would bring me or the incredible opportunities that I would have to serve.

My mother, Dr. Nancy Freeman, was a nurse and an educator. She worked part-time when I was young, then went back to school for her master's and, ultimately, doctoral degrees when I was in middle school, and had a long career as a nurse educator. Her clinical passion was in psychiatric/mental health nursing and she had a deep interest in death and dying. Although I was well aware of how much she loved nursing and her work and I thought that nursing looked interesting, I still was not sure when I started college whether I would choose it as a profession. I was drawn to being in health care and at first considered social work or medicine. I think that part of my initial reluctance was related to feeling very adventuresome and independent, and I was not at all certain that I wanted to follow in my mother's career path. Ironically, once I decided to pursue nursing, I can remember saying that I surely would not get a master's degree or a doctoral degree or become a teacher. Of course, I did all three of these things!

It is hard to know for certain, but I sense that one of the things that drew me to nursing was an experience I had as a young child. When I was about four years old, I was hospitalized for a relatively minor medical procedure. From what I recall my mother telling me, I must have had an adverse reaction to anesthesia and the surgery had to be canceled and then rescheduled. Although I do not have distinct memories around this experience, I do not recall being frightened or feeling vulnerable and I do recall feeling comfortable with the nurses and well cared for. I sense that this experience influenced me initially to become a pediatric nurse.

Early in my career, I was drawn to work in settings where I could be very independent. My first graduate degree was a master's in the nursing of children, during which I also completed a pediatric nurse practitioner program. I completed this degree in 1974—which was quite early in the nurse practitioner movement (see Chapter 5 for more information on nurse practitioner history and evolution). Drs. Henry Silver and Loretta Ford began the first nurse practitioner program at the University of Colorado in 1965. I remember feeling as though I was part of a new generation of nurses pioneering a very bold and innovative role. The challenges and constraints that nurse practitioners experienced in these early years likely sensitized me to the importance of policy issues. I also learned early on another very important lesson: the importance of listening to patients and the discovery that they often had a much better sense of what they needed than I did. It was humbling to figure out that I did not have the answers, that healing was a very complex endeavor, and that there was a world of healing practices out there that I had never been exposed to in nursing school.

As I look back on my career, I am struck by my deep interest in both being in the trenches and part of making change within the "system" of health care and also the equally strong pull that I felt toward academia. The attraction of academia was the rigor of research and the importance of generating new knowledge and the desire to prepare the next generation of nurses. Early in my career, I went back and forth several times between academia and service. Much to the chagrin of some of my colleagues, the year I was first tenured in a university, I left to take a position as a nurse leader at the University of Minnesota Hospital and Clinic. Job security was of much less interest than the chance to be part of a dynamic team of nurse leaders boldly leading change in a large health care system.

■ EARLY IMPRESSIONS

I have a great love of nursing history, and early in my career, I was frustrated by what I saw as a lack of bold leadership and innovation in contemporary nursing. I earnestly pored over the biographies of leaders such as Florence Nightingale, Lillian Wald, Lavinia Dock, and Isabel Hampton Robb. In addition to being the founder of modern nursing in the Western world, Florence Nightingale was renowned for her work in sanitary reform and statistics. It was only after her death that her extensive work on religion and mysticism was published (see Chapters 4 and 18 for more on Nightingale's legacy). Lavinia Dock was the foreign editor of the *American Journal of Nursing*, a staunch advocate for legislation to regulate nursing practice, and worked with Lillian Wald at Henry Street Settlement and with Isabel Hampton Robb at the Johns Hopkins School of Nursing.

Throughout her life, she was a suffragette and political activist. These early nursing leaders fought ferocious battles to gain control of nursing practice to better serve patients, whether in the hospital wards, settlement houses, or homes. I was impressed by their extensive worldwide networks in eras when communication was limited to letters and overseas travel was very slow. I was also struck by their immense visions and capacity to lead systems change beyond nursing. They had seats at the table and seemed unwilling to accept the status quo. They also held in common a keen understanding of politics and the need to be politically engaged.

Another seminal paper I read early in my career that significantly shaped my thinking was "The Proletarianization of Nursing in the United States, 1932–1946," by David Wagner (1980), which was published in the *International Journal of Health Services*. The paper chronicles the migration of nursing from the autonomy of private homes to the institutionalization of nursing in hospitals and nursing homes. It was an era when hospitals required cheap labor and offered job security, yet many nurses resisted the change by criticism, sabotage, and walking away from jobs. By the end of World War II, according to Wagner, the majority of nurses were employed by institutions and an era began, marked by regimentation, rigid division of labor, and intense supervision characteristic of modern hospitals. I have thought often and hard about the implications of this shift relative to control over nursing practice.

The nursing world that I faced in 1973 when I graduated from a baccalaureate nursing program had evolved from the depiction characterized by Wagner, yet there were elements that were alive and independently expressed. My class, for example, received traditional white nursing caps and many of us had photos taken in them, yet we never wore them in clinical practice. A few years before my graduation in 1969, Marie Manthey implemented *primary nursing*, a system of nursing care delivery that emphasized continuity of care and RN accountability for a group of patients throughout their stay in a hospital (see Chapter 6 for more information on primary nursing). Although it was adopted in many settings, *functional* or *team nursing* was even more prevalent. Over the next 10 years, advanced practice roles continued to emerge, directors of nursing roles with narrow scopes of responsibility evolved into directors and vice presidents of patient care services, and there was a technology explosion in the hospital environment. Interestingly, the hierarchy of roles, shift mentality, and bureaucracy changed very little during this time.

In choosing a focus for my doctoral education in 1983, I opted to pursue a PhD in public health with a focus in health services research, policy, and administration. It made sense, given my deep interest in knowledge development, leadership, systems change, and policy. My supporting program was in strategic innovation.

From 1987 until 1997, I was the director of nursing practice and research at the University of Minnesota Hospital and Clinic. These years were formative for me in many respects. I deepened my understanding of clinical practice and the art and science of nursing. I also honed my leadership skills and had many opportunities to lead complex systems change. It was also a time during which I broadened my expertise by taking on responsibilities beyond nursing, as in the latter years of this decade when I also became the administrator of quality for the health system and spiritual care services. It was the confluence of these roles that provided the insight and inspiration for creating the Center for Spirituality & Healing in 1995, a center that has embodied my vision for systems change and transformation over the past 20 years.

■ PROFESSIONAL EVOLUTION/CONTRIBUTION

I am often asked why I created the Center for Spirituality & Healing (www.csh.umn .edu). The most honest answer I can offer is that I wanted to do a better job of caring for patients. My sense was that people were yearning for care that was more holistic—attentive to the whole person: body, mind, and spirit. We were caring for an increasingly diverse patient population, many of whom highly valued cultural healing traditions. I was also aware of the growing interest in what was then called alternative or complementary medicine. Patients were asking about therapies such as healing touch, massage, imagery, and aromatherapy, and research was beginning to emerge, demonstrating that some of these approaches were both safe and effective. Our focus in the first year and a half of the center was informal education and support of a nursing network that was beginning to offer some of these therapies as a routine part of care. From the onset, it was apparent that demand was high, as was interest from a broad range of health professionals in both nursing and beyond.

In the fall of 1996, when the center was a little over a year old, I approached the senior vice president of the Academic Health Center, Dr. Frank Cerra, and the dean of nursing, Dr. Sandra Edwardson, with the idea of offering a couple of academic courses. I had created a spreadsheet with a listing of what some other universities were doing and was prepared to talk about what I perceived to be important trends on the horizon. Dr. Cerra, a surgeon, responded in an interesting way. He noted that what I was proposing was bigger than a couple of courses; it would ultimately transform health care. I left the meeting with the charge of coleading a task force that would focus on the bigger question of what the role of the University of Minnesota should be in this realm of complementary, cross-cultural, and spiritual care.

The task force was composed of approximately 50 people representing a number of different disciplines and included faculty with teaching and research expertise, clinicians, and people with expertise in complementary and alternative medicine (CAM). Our sense was that we needed to create a big tent with lots of diversity to craft the vision. While we were having lots of discussions and reviewing information on trends and research data, we made a very critical decision. Instead of just talking among ourselves, we would listen to the community. Looking back, this was a very big step. Universities and organizations then often assumed that they knew what was best and made decisions on behalf of those they were serving—and they often still do. We invited into the conversation patients, community leaders, representatives of health systems, hospitals and cultural groups, and legislators. In addition to asking them about needs, trends, and opportunities, we asked them specifically what competencies they wanted health professionals to have and what role they wanted the university to assume in the growing field of CAM. What emerged from the task force was a report that laid out a bold vision and strategies for the center. As the university hospital was sold to a community hospital system, a decision was made to keep the center within the university, and it became a freestanding academic unit with a blueprint for change, strong support from the university and community, and a scope that included education, research, and clinical care. With this transition, a new chapter for the center unfolded.

As of this writing, the center offers more than 55 academic courses, most of them for graduate credit, though many are open to undergraduate students as well. Although students in nursing and other areas of health science are drawn to the courses, students come from all sectors of the university, including music, architecture and design, food science and nutrition, business, and law—literally every college and school. Examples of graduate-level courses offered include:

- Integrative therapies: Aromatherapy; Acupressure; Botanical Medicine; Reiki; Energy Healing; Functional Nutrition; Ethnopharmacology; Introduction to Integrative Therapies and Healing Practices
- Arts and Healing: Healing Imagery; Creative Arts in Health Care; Movement and Music for Wellbeing; Music and Healing
- Nature-Based Therapeutics: Journey Into Nature; Animals in Healthcare; Therapeutic Landscapes; Therapeutic Horticulture; Horse as Teacher
- Culturally Based Healing: Ayurveda Medicine: The Science of Self-Healing; Traditional Tibetan Medicine; Yoga, Ethics and Spirituality; Traditional Chinese Medicine; Foundations of Shamanism; Cultural Awareness, Knowledge and Health; Latinos: Culture and Health; Amazonian Plant Spirit Medicine; Indigenous Hawaiian Healing
- Mindfulness: Meditation; Advanced Meditation; Mindfulness-Based Stress Reduction; Emotional Healing and Happiness; Hatha Yoga
- Health Coaching: Health Coaching Fundamentals I and II; Health Coaching Practicum; The Business of Health Coaching; Lifestyle Medicine
- Self-Care: Art of Healing/Self as Healer; Wellbeing; Self-care and Resilience
- Spirituality: Peacemaking and Spirituality; Forgiveness and Healing; Spirituality and Resilience; Spiritual Aspects of Palliative Care
- Leadership: Mindfulness in the Workplace; Whole Systems Healing

Students may earn a graduate minor or graduate certificate in integrative therapies and healing practices, and/or a certificate or a master's degree in health coaching.

At the undergraduate level, there is a high demand for courses such as:

- Creating a Meaningful Life
- Living on Purpose: An Exploration of Self, Purpose, and Community
- Food Choices: Healing the Earth, Healing Ourselves
- Ecosystems of Wellbeing

Many undergraduate and graduate students in nursing enroll in the center's courses, often as electives, though the Introduction to Integrative Therapies and Healing Practices course is required in most DNP specialties.

The center cohosts with the School of Nursing a DNP in Integrative Health and Healing (http://www.nursing.umn.edu/DNP/specialties/integrative-health-and-healing/index.htm), the first established in the United States. I cofounded that specialty area and continue to colead it. We draw students from throughout the United States and prepare them for leadership roles across clinical settings and patient populations. Our graduates are leading integrative health programs in the Veterans Administration (VA) Medical Center, community-based and university hospitals, mental health centers, community organizations, and corporations.

The research portfolio of the center reflects the diversity of the faculty interests and areas of expertise. Center faculty conduct clinical and basic science research, as well as health services research, utilizing a wide range of qualitative, quantitative, and mixed-method approaches. Most research is conducted by teams of interdisciplinary faculty, and the center has extensive research partnerships with many university departments as well as community-based organizations.

Under a business development unit, center faculty and staff provide consultation services to hospitals, health care systems, and community-based organizations, including senior living communities that aspire to offer patient-centered care that incorporates integrative therapies and healing practices. Consultation services are also provided to a wide range of organizations that focus on employee well-being, leadership development, and organizational culture change.

A core strategy for educating the public appears on a webpage, "Taking Charge of Your Health & Wellbeing." The website (http://www.takingcharge.csh.umn.edu/) attracts more than 250,000 unique visitors a month who want to explore healing practices, learn how to more effectively navigate the health care system, and develop a personal plan for health and well-being. Additionally, the center offers lectures throughout the year that are open to the public, and offers extensive mindfulness-based courses.

Over the past five years, much of my work has focused on advancing well-being. *Well-being* is a state of being in balance or alignment in the body, mind, and spirit. In this state, we feel content; connected to purpose, people, and community; peaceful but energized; and resilient and safe. In short, we are flourishing. I truly believe that the societal transformation needed in the United States and around the world goes well beyond health care and needs to encompass not just a shift from disease to health, but a shift to the broader notion of well-being.

At a personal level, well-being is certainly affected by our health, but it is also heavily impacted by other factors illustrated in the Wellbeing Model, as shown in Figure 8.1 (Kreitzer, 2014b). Other determinants of well-being include our sense of purpose and meaning in life, the quality of our relationships, the vitality of the community in which

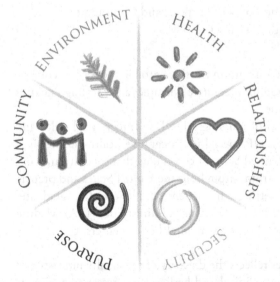

FIGURE 8.1 The Wellbeing Model.

we live, our environment, and our perception of safety and security. When any of these factors are compromised, our personal well-being is affected. And these same factors also influence the well-being of our organizations and communities. I see our role as nurses as helping people restore and improve capacity in all aspects of their lives and supporting them in attaining their full potential.

I have been deeply gratified by the interest that is being shown in the Wellbeing Model. It has been used to assess and document strengths in a standardized tool used internationally (Monsen, Peters, Schlesner, Vanderboom, Holland, 2015) and as an organizing framework within care settings such as The Waters senior living communities (http://www.thewatersseniorliving.com). It is also an integral concept within the work emerging on integrative nursing.

The inspiration for my work in integrative nursing came from nurses, literally, around the world, who told stories about their yearning to practice nursing in a different way. Although the historical legacy of nursing is deeply rooted in a tradition of caring and healing and it is that essence that attracts millions of women and men to enter our noble profession, the lived reality of many who receive nursing care and who practice nursing is quite different. I coedited the book *Integrative Nursing* in 2014 with my colleague Dr. Mary Koithan, and we were very fortunate to attract more than 70 nurse colleagues as contributors.

Integrative nursing is defined as "a way of being-knowing-doing that advances the health and wellbeing of persons, families and communities through caring and healing relationships" (Kreitzer & Koithan, 2014, p. 4). The six principles of integrative nursing (Koithan, 2014), as seen in Table 8.1, are consistent and aligned with major nursing theories; they provide practical and unambiguous guidance that can both shape and direct the care of patient populations across clinical settings. Although not intended in any way to replace nursing theory, the integrative nursing principles complement various theoretical paradigms and can be used concurrently.

In the short time since publication, the textbook has been adopted into graduate and undergraduate nursing curricula and is being used as the practice model in a growing number of hospitals. More than 250 nurses from 12 different countries attended the first International Integrative Nursing Symposium in May 2015 in Reykjavik, Iceland.

TABLE 8.1　**Six Principles of Integrative Nursing**

1. Human beings are whole systems inseparable from their environments.

2. Human beings have the innate capacity for health and well-being.

3. Nature has healing and restorative properties that contribute to health and well-being.

4. Integrative nursing is person centered and relationship based.

5. Integrative nursing is informed by evidence and uses the full range of therapeutic modalities to support/augment the healing process, moving from least intensive/invasive to more, depending on need and context.

6. Integrative nursing focuses on the health and well-being of caregivers as well as those they serve.

■ MORAL/ETHICAL FOUNDATION

Nursing has been the cornerstone of my work and the lens through which I have pro-vided leadership. When the center began, our mission was to transform health care, and my sense was that in order to do that, it was critical to provide relevant education to health professionals and to generate research that demonstrated the safety and efficacy of integrative approaches. Without a doubt that was important, but over time, I became convinced that perhaps an even more important task was empowering people to take charge of their own health and well-being. Although the center is still very engaged in the business of transforming health care, we describe our mission today as advancing the health and well-being of people, organizations, and communities.

There are definitely core values and themes that are woven throughout my career and the major accomplishments that I have highlighted in this chapter. In creating the Center for Spirituality & Healing, designing new care models, and advancing the prin-ciples of integrative nursing and the Wellbeing Model, I have had a strong preference for whole person/whole systems thinking that is nonhierarchical, empowering, innova-tive, and aligned with broader strategic objectives. I also deeply value stewardship of resources—whether that is time, money, or people. Over the course of 20 years, the Center for Spirituality & Healing has never had a budget deficit, and when I work with organizations, my goal is always to cocreate with them care models that will meet needs and be sustainable over time.

■ VISION

Nursing is exquisitely well positioned to provide leadership as the health care system, as we know it, disintegrates and as new forms and possibilities emerge. Health care in many ways is at a crossroads. The issues of rising costs, shortages of nurses and other health care providers, patients who are dissatisfied, poor outcomes, and disengaged care providers are global in nature. Addressing these issues requires a systems approach that will not be easy or fast. Integrative nursing provides a whole person/whole systems approach that addresses the needs of patients and their families who are demanding care that is comprehensive, coordinated, and attentive to the whole person—body, mind, and spirit. Integrative nursing also engages nurses who yearn to practice in a way that is aligned with their personal values and the passion that ignited their call to a nursing career. It may be an effective strategy in buffering stress and attenuating the impact of burnout that is costly and takes a significant toll on patients, families, and caregivers. Health care today is a team-based endeavor, and nurses with the skills of integrative nursing are well positioned to be partners in delivering integrated health care.

I wish that earlier in my career I knew about the concept of gentle action. As articu-lated by David Peat (2005), *gentle action* is the use of grassroots efforts and collective intelligence to focus many small coordinated efforts on the best point of leverage within a given system. Three guiding principles inform the practice:

- Small changes can have large effects.
- Turbulent systems may be very sensitive to change. Stable ones are highly resistant.
- There is great power in small, collaborative, and highly coordinated actions.

Understanding these principles, the chaos in the current health care systems gives us an excellent window of opportunity to advance innovative thinking and new approaches to care and healing. We live in a world of turbulence. Our role as nurses is to understand how we can use these dynamics to be agents of social change and transformation. We should never underestimate the impact of small changes and the power of nurses who work collaboratively and in coordination to change the world.

■ REFLECTIONS

1. *Who are the role models that inspire me?*
2. *How do I see the principles of integrative nursing shaping my practice and the way I think about my practice?*
3. *Have I created a personal plan for my own health and well-being?*
4. *What issue am I passionate about in which gentle action could be strategically applied?*
5. *How does whole person/whole systems thinking expand how I consider my role as a nurse leader?*

■ REFERENCES

Koithan, M. (2014). Concepts and principles of integrative nursing. In M. J. Kreitzer & M. Koithan (Eds.), *Integrative nursing* (pp. 3–16). New York, NY: Oxford University Press.

Kreitzer, M. J. (2014a). Whole systems healing: A new leadership path. In M. J. Kreitzer & M. Koithan (Eds.), *Integrative nursing* (pp. 47–55). New York, NY: Oxford University Press.

Kreitzer, M. J. (2014b). Advancing wellbeing in people, organizations, and communities. In M. J. Kreitzer & M. Koithan (Eds.), *Integrative nursing* (pp. 125–136). New York, NY: Oxford University Press.

Kreitzer, M. J., & Koithan, M. (Eds.). (2014). *Integrative nursing*. New York, NY: Oxford University Press.

Monsen, K. A., Peters, J., Schlesner, S., Vanderboom, C., & Holland, D. (2015). The gap in big data: Getting to wellbeing, strengths, and a whole-person perspective. *Global Advances in Health and Medicine, 4*(3), 31–39.

Peat, D. (2005). *Gentle action: Bringing creative change to a turbulent world*. Pari, Italy: Pari Publishing.

Wagner, D. (1980). The proletarianization of nursing in the United States, 1932–1946. *International Journal of Health Services, 10*(2), 271–290.

CHAPTER NINE

Holistic and Aware: Pioneering Change With Heart, Head, and Hands

Carla Mariano

> **NURSE**. One Who Through
>
> Heart   Head   Hands
> (Caring)   (Knowledge)   (Skill)
> Gives to Others
> <u>N</u>urturance for healing:
>   Where one is
> <u>U</u>nderstood through being heard and connected;
>   And
> <u>R</u>evered in all his or her humanness;
>   To feel
> <u>S</u>afe and Special: unique, important, loved;
>   Becoming
> <u>E</u>mpowered to grow & find meaning & be.
>   —Mariano (2010, p. 25)

■ WHY NURSING?

I grew up in a small town in Connecticut. As a child, I was not drawn to nursing, but to music and teaching. My parents were in the health field—dentistry and nursing—and many of their friends and colleagues were in similar areas. I was socialized at an early age

125

to the idea of nursing as a career choice and it became an unstated (and often stated) expectation that nursing would be my path. As education was highly valued in my family, a college degree was the other expectation. So, one could say I fell into nursing rather than chose it.

As is true of many other nurses, I was a family caretaker. I was the only girl of four children and spent much of my childhood caring for two younger brothers. This imbued me with a strong sense of responsibility. During community crises (e.g., floods and flu outbreaks), my parents volunteered to assist in community health activities, such as giving immunizations. I learned early on the importance of service and interconnectedness.

■ EARLY IMPRESSIONS

As a college student, I attended the University of Connecticut (UConn) School of Nursing. I studied nursing and minored in philosophy to take the edge off the hard sciences. The UConn program provided a formidable foundation in nursing, especially the psychosocial aspects. After completing the first two years at the Storrs campus, I was introduced to the clinical portion of the program. This was by far the most challenging. Actual responsibility for the care of patients was a frightening realization and a daunting task. I was beset by the constant fear that I would injure, harm, or cause the death of a person. I found most of my clinical experiences uncomfortable and only relaxed when I was talking with patients and not "doing" something. The clinical experience in psychiatric nursing truly interested and excited me and seemed to give me a reason for pursuing nursing.

Following graduation from my BSN program, I worked at Newington Veterans Administration (VA) hospital in orthopedics/neurology and the emergency department on the weekends. I witnessed the many debilitating physical and emotional challenges that veterans faced. It gave me an even greater appreciation for the need people have to be listened to and understood. Although overwhelmed with technical tasks and medical treatments, I soon earned the reputation of the "talking nurse." I was even reprimanded for spending too much time talking with the patients and not completing my nursing duties on time.

But hearing peoples' stories—allowing them to share their concerns, fears, pain, and hopes—reduced the patients' anxiety and made them more amenable to treatments. It also gave meaning to my work. I especially enjoyed when I could talk with the veterans in the shower room during the lonely, nighttime, and nightmare-ridden hours.

It soon became obvious that my path lay not in medical–surgical practice but in psychiatric mental health nursing. I accepted a position at the Institute of Living in Hartford, where I felt validated and happy and where my skills and propensities were a better fit. There I was given the nickname the "whistling nurse," as I exuded joy in my newfound passion. I knew that to manifest this passion, I had to further my education.

My journey then took me to New York City to pursue my master's degree in psychiatric/mental health nursing and nursing education at Teachers College, Columbia University. It was an exciting time in New York City—especially at Columbia. Student strikes were a weekly occurrence, with classes often interrupted. And the psychiatric/mental health nursing program at Teachers College was, in and of itself, stimulating and innovative. We were introduced to the new field of community mental health, family and group therapy, the latest interpersonal and social theories of psychiatry, and a broad range of clinical settings. I also became acquainted with learning and educational theories and the role of the nurse educator. I had found my niche at last.

■ PROFESSIONAL EVOLUTION/CONTRIBUTION

Throughout my career, I have been fortunate to be in the right place at the right time. There are truly no accidents in the universe. I consider myself to be eclectic—interested in many things and in many ways. So, my contributions have not focused on any one area. I have been presented with many opportunities and because of my eclectic nature, many of them interested me. I am thankful that I was guided and had the inherent wisdom to take advantage of what was put before me.

I began my teaching career at the State University of New York Downstate Medical Center, College of Nursing, in the early 1970s. Here my interest in interdisciplinarity was cultivated. As an academic medical center, nursing was an integral player and many of the nursing faculty had joint appointments as staff at the University Hospital. I was fortunate to work with Dean Audrey J. Conley, who encouraged originality and innovation and new ways of approaching health professional education. We collaborated with the medical school faculty on elective courses and team-based methods of patient care and introduced a mobile van for community health. In addition to teaching, I worked in partnership with a psychiatric resident and midwife to develop a bereavement clinic for parents who had a stillbirth. Prior to this initiative, mothers were not shown their babies, and they often developed strange ideas about what happened to their babies after birth. Allowing the mothers to view their babies and providing counseling sessions during and following hospitalization facilitated a healthier grieving process for both parents, as well as a more realistic account of the event. It also helped staff in dealing with this difficult situation. This experience gave me a great appreciation for crisis intervention and the importance of an interdisciplinary perspective.

I returned to Teachers College, Columbia, to attain my doctorate in nursing education. Following receipt of my EdD, I was recruited to the University of Southern Maine (USM) in Portland as the associate dean in the School of Nursing. In that role, I developed the first master of nursing program in the state of Maine with a clinical focus, "Families in Crisis," as well as two functional foci, teaching and administration. I was very grateful for my background as a psychiatric/mental health nurse in my administrative role, as it taught me the importance of relationship-centered administration and transformational leadership. USM also provided further experience in interdisciplinary education through a collaborative project between nursing and social work faculty and students in a hospital with primarily elderly residents in Portland.

In the mid-1980s, I returned to New York City and accepted a faculty position in the New York University (NYU) Division of Nursing, now the Rory Meyers College of Nursing. I had the opportunity to teach with many superb faculty and also to have frequent conversations with Martha Rogers. I developed a strong appreciation for the unitary nature of human beings and the necessity of a holistic perspective. Holding many roles and being involved in numerous projects and grants, while also teaching and guiding doctoral students, gave me a true understanding of the complex faculty role. I served as director of master's and post-master's programs for several years, introducing many of the nurse practitioner programs that exist in the College of Nursing today. Furthering my interprofessional interest, I also coordinated the interdisciplinary Urban Health Care Program with nursing and medical school faculty and students. My commitment to qualitative research peaked and resulted in my developing a doctoral course in qualitative research as well as being the qualitative methodologist on numerous doctoral dissertations. I was appointed as a research associate at NYU Medical Center and a Senior Advisor at the NYU Hartford Institute of Geriatric Nursing. During the very trying period following 9/11, the World Trade Center disaster, I volunteered to provide mental health crisis intervention services to students and to clients at the St. Vincent's Mental Health Clinic. All of these experiences served to prepare me for the next chapter of my journey.

My love and passion for holism culminated in the development of the Advanced Practice Holistic Nurse Practitioner Program at NYU—the first and only program of its kind in the country. It fit well within the philosophy of the NYU Division of Nursing and was timely in the evolution of holistic nursing in the United States. After developing the program, I became the coordinator and extended my efforts to include the American Holistic Nurses Association (AHNA), where I became president-elect, president, and elder. During my tenure at the AHNA, my focus was to increase membership size and diversity, grow research, focus part of our education endeavors to influence nursing education nationally, form collaborations and partnerships within nursing and with other disciplines, and actively prepare successive leaders for the AHNA. I was also integrally involved in developing *Holistic Nursing: Scope and Standards of Practice* (first and second editions) and spearheaded the initiative that gave holistic nursing official recognition by the American Nurses Association (ANA) as a distinct specialty within the discipline of nursing (see Chapters 4 and 7 for more information on the AHNA).

It is gratifying to witness and be a part of the evolution and increased recognition and appreciation of holism and holistic nursing nationally and internationally. The relevance and validity of holistic nursing as a science, a practice, and a way of being have been confirmed in recent years. An editorial in the *Journal of Holistic Nursing* explains:

> While becoming more popular and more highly regarded, holism and holistic nursing have contributed to enhancing the human condition in many ways. . . . Holistic nursing has progressed through the development of standards, endorsement of programs, and certification of beginning and advanced practitioners. Holistic nursing's contributions to human welfare have been increasingly recognized . . . as evidenced by their current standing in health care and appreciation by society . . . . [H]olism as a perspective and holistic nursing as a response may offer the world something that counteracts the fragmentation and isolation that exists so predominantly in our society. (Cowling, 2011, p. 5)

Furthering my journey, I became a consultant to develop the bachelor of science completion program in holistic nursing at the Pacific College of Oriental Medicine, New York, New York—the first baccalaureate nursing program in a complementary and alternative medicine/complementary integrative medicine (CAM/CIM) school in the country.

I now teach in that program, as well as consult at the University of Massachusetts at Amherst to integrate holistic nursing and CIM into the nursing curriculum.

I am blessed as I continue my life's work in holism.

My numerous and varied experiences in nursing education have taught me many important lessons. Lesson 1 is *The Importance of Interdisciplinarity/Collaboration:*

> The human service professions are facing problems so complex that no *single* discipline can possibly respond to them effectively. Domestic violence, substance abuse, poverty, homelessness, adolescent pregnancy, global communicable disease, and the growing elderly population pose but a few of the crises facing society and the health professions today. Each of these crises requires a comprehensive approach and necessitates that professionals relate to many client–institutional systems as well as collaborate with many professions. The client is an integral partner in this collaboration. . . . With the complexity of modern societal and health issues, and with the knowledge explosion and concomitant escalation of specialization and fragmentation, interdisciplinary collaboration will take on ever-increasing importance in the years ahead. For cooperation among disciplines to become a generally accepted policy, there needs to be a full understanding of interdisciplinarity and what promotes or hinders it. Resocialization, training, and new skills will be required of educators, practitioners, and administrators. Most importantly, we need pre-professional and professional education where students—our future professionals—come together with various disciplines to learn principles and skills of collaboration, to explore role specificity and generality, to examine the unity of knowledge and connections among disciplines, and to develop flexibility and positive regard for one another. (Mariano, 2006, pp. 2–3)

It has been in the quietest of moments I have come to know and appreciate Lesson 2—*The Centrality of Meaning.* The greatest gift a person can receive is to be understood. It is interesting that "silent" and "listen" have the same letters. A foundation of holistic nursing practice is assisting individuals to find meaning in their experience. Despite a person's condition, the meaning that the person ascribes to his or her situation can influence the response to it. Holistic nurses pay attention to the subjective world of the individual. Holistic nurses take into account meanings such as the person's concerns in relation to health and family, finances, as well as deeper meanings related to the person's purpose in life. No matter the technology or treatment, holistic nurses attend to the human spirit as a major influence in healing. The individual's perception of meaning is related to all factors in health-wellness-disease-illness.

"Holistic nurses recognize that suffering, illness, and disease are natural components of the human condition and can teach us about ourselves, our relationships, and our universe. Every experience is valued for its meaning and lesson" (Mariano, 2016a, p. 64). When the foci are individuals' perspectives, meanings, uniqueness, and subjective lived experiences, the aim is understanding (Mariano, 2015; Hoskins & Mariano, 2004).

Lesson 3 recognizes *Holism as the Foundation of Practice and Knowledge Generation.* The American public increasingly calls for health care that is compassionate and respectful, provides a variety of options, is economically feasible, and is grounded in holistic ideals. Health care is experiencing a shift where people desire to be more actively involved in their own health decision making. They have communicated their dissatisfaction with conventional (Western allopathic) medicine and are appealing for a care system that encompasses health, quality of life, and a relationship with their providers (Mariano, 2016b). Mittelman et al. (2010) note that nurses are very well positioned to become leaders in integrative health (see Chapter 8 for more information on integrative nursing). They constitute the nation's largest group of health professionals—more than 3 million. Nightingale identified the nurse's work as helping put the patient in the best possible condition so that nature can act and self-healing may occur. Nurses extend beyond fixing or curing the disease to ease the edges of patients' suffering. They assist people to return to daily functioning, maintain their health, live with chronic illness, and/or move through the stages of dying and death. Nurses demonstrate expertise in managing symptoms, coordinating care, managing chronic disease, and facilitating health promotion. In addition to caring for people from birth to death, nurses currently administer care for communities, conduct research, lead health systems, and attend to health policy issues.

Holism is also needed as a foundation to broaden and deepen knowledge generation. Researchers today must look at alternative philosophies of science and research methodologies that are congruent with studies of humanistic and holistic occurrences. Also needed are investigations of phenomena that explore the context in which they occur and the meaning of patterns that evolve. We need approaches to interventions studies that are more holistic and that are sensitive to the *interactive* nature of the body-mind-emotion-spirit-environment. Instead of isolating the effects of one part of an intervention, we need more all-embracing interventions and more subtle instruments that measure the interactive nature of each person's biological, psychological, sociological, emotional, and spiritual patterns. "In addition, comprehensive comparative outcome studies are required to determine the usefulness, indications, and contraindications of integrative therapies. Further, researchers must evaluate these interventions for their usefulness in promoting health and wellness as well as preventing illness" (Mariano, 2016b, p. 94; Mariano, 2008).

Lesson 4 has shown me that there is always opportunity to be found amid crisis—*Crisis as an Opportunity.* Crisis is defined as the impact of any event that challenges the assumed state and forces the individual to change his view or readapt to the world, himself, or both (Parad, 1965). However, as the Chinese character for "crisis" represents, "crisis" means both "danger" and "opportunity"—a danger because it threatens to overwhelm the individual, family, or group; and an opportunity because during times of crisis, people are vulnerable and much more receptive and open to new perspectives, therapeutic influence, and help from others. This brings with it the possibility of growth and change. The Greek word for crisis is "turning point," again demonstrating the peril and the opportunity for positive resolution and growth that crises present (Mariano, 2002). Throughout my career, I have witnessed the opportunities that challenges bring to patients/clients, students, colleagues, and myself. If we can allow ourselves to be vulnerable, stay open to what our experiences have to teach us, listen and attend to our inner voice and knowing, discover the strength that lies in gentleness, let go of the outcome, and trust the universe, we can take advantage of the potential that evolves from crises (Mariano, 2004).

Again and again I have been reminded of Lesson 5, *Teaching is a Gift.* As Anna from *The King and I* stated, "By my students, I will be taught." I am honored to be a nurse educator and feel it has been a lifelong gift. Through teaching, I have been able to touch many lives and be a constant learner at the same time. I have had the privilege of partnering with and empowering students and others in our mutual path to understanding. Students have trusted me with their beliefs, aspirations, vision, enthusiasm, learning needs, and their transformation. Teaching has given me important insights about safe space and caring cultures. I have witnessed students grow and blossom into new and inventive individuals and practitioners. Additionally, I have been given the rare opportunity to share my knowledge and communicate my beliefs and values about people, the human condition, caring–healing, relationships, and the nature of nursing. Being an educator has reinforced for me the unity and connectedness of all. It embodies the concept that "there is a little bit of someone in everyone" (Mariano, 2005). Teaching has been my raison d'etre.

And for this I give thanks . . . Lesson 6—*Gratitude.* As a person, an educator, and a nurse, there are so many people and experiences in my life that I give thanks for. Many individuals have affirmed and encouraged my work and me. I am so grateful for dear relationships, friends, teachers, colleagues, students, and for the guidance of Spirit. I am grateful for all my life events—good and difficult. The people I have been fortunate to know and the experiences that I have had have truly been my teachers. My life has been filled with unique and interesting adventures—all of which have made me evolve into the person I am and am still becoming.

■ MORAL/ETHICAL FOUNDATION

My views concerning the moral and ethical foundation of nursing are articulated in an article I wrote on conscious change (Mariano, 2012) and consist of the following:

Caring. Conscious change begins with caring deeply about something. It challenges us to ask "What story am I living?" and to identify your big story. Is your story

- Serving a higher purpose?
- A work requiring something of worth? Do you see the value, contribution, and meaningfulness of your work?
- A validation and belief in the importance of your life and perception of life in terms of the greater good?
- Giving you a sense of fulfillment?
- A higher calling?
- A story you will feel glad you lived?

Conscious change requires us to spend our precious time and energy on endeavors that we are truly passionate about—and that mean something.

Openness. Conscious change necessitates our being wide-awake to opportunities—seeing every person as a teacher and every experience as a lesson. Being in the right place at the right time is not merely coincidence. It is being aware of your present experience, being vulnerable, nurturing your intuitiveness, unconditionally accepting what each moment has to offer, and taking advantage of the moment.

Nightingale. Florence Nightingale was the consummate exemplar of conscious change. As Beck (1996) states: "Nightingale saw 19th century problems and created 20th century solutions." In this day and age, we can learn much from her vision, her commitment, her strategies, and her legacy (see Chapters 4 and 18 for more information on Nightingale's legacy).

Special. Everyone is special and unique. "In the most profound sense, to be creative is to fulfill oneself as a person. Each of us gives to and receives from life something that will never be repeated" (Kneller, 1965, p. 89). Experience yourself directly—respect, honor, and appreciate yourself for the unique human being that you are, for the unique gift you offer, and for the unique vision you hold. When you are conscious of yourself, you will participate consciously in change.

Courage. The ways of the world are uncertain. Conscious change requires courage to vision outside of your comfortable zone, to take risks, to live with ambiguity, to listen to your own inner wisdom and own your mistakes—to share, to be empathic, and to play fair.

Intentional. Mindfulness and integrity are essential to conscious change. Mindfully considering all options (and the implications of each) before making final choices discourages premature decision making and/or the adopting of self-serving agendas.

Optimism. You determine what your world is like. You are the passage through which your life opens up. How you perceive an event or challenge determines how you will respond to it. If problems are viewed as opportunities to grow and improve, rather than obstacles to be feared and avoided, change can be approached with an attitude of possibility versus doom.

Unknowing. Unknowing that leads to reflection and contemplation provides the foundation for conscious change. Robert Boostrom's (2001) counsel is most appropriate: Become aware of "for granteds" and ask, "How, why, when, where, what?" Look at what is to be seen, pay attention to the ordinary, and then see again. Ask, "What about, what if, what else?" Know what you do not know, look for patterns, pay attention, be thoughtful, be open, and be willing. Finally, keep a beginner's mind: "In the Beginner's mind there are many possibilities; in the expert's mind there are few. When we have no thought of achievement, no thought of self, we are true beginners. Then we can learn something" (Suzuki, 1983, pp. 21–22).

Sense of community/unity. Margaret Mead once said: "Never underestimate the power of a small group of committed people to change the world." Conscious change agents are consensus builders, facilitating a resolute collective to achieve the necessary change and advance the work.

Commitment and compassion. Conscious change requires an understanding that everything is connected and interdependent. Therefore, we must use all the ingredients of our lives to commit no harm—treating the world and all its creatures with loving care; performing actions that benefit individuals, families, society, and the natural world; and acting for the well-being of all. As conscious change agents, we honor ourselves as instruments of healing.

Humility. True humility involves knowing ourselves—knowing the limits of our knowledge, power, and understanding; knowing our strengths and understanding when we need help or resources; and knowing when and how to say no. Humility encourages us to laugh a lot, and to trust our spirit and the universe.

Accountability. Conscious change agents are accountable for both the outcomes/results of the change, as well as the process by which that change occurs. And importantly, they are accountable for and own who they are, what they do, and how they do it. Accountability for one's actions and approach fosters self-accountability in others and models dependability and trustworthiness. (pp. 18–20)

Nonattachment. To effect change consciously requires nonattachment to opinions and outcomes. It necessitates understanding things as they are, deep listening and deep seeing, and not investing our ego in our views. Letting go—not clinging to ideas, beliefs, things, or relationships that no longer serve us—makes room to receive what is next offered. Nonattachment can assist our changing with discernment and ease.

Groundedness. Groundedness creates an atmosphere of well-being during times of change. Change is endless; therefore, a sense of balance is crucial, providing for

- Experimentation and creativity within an atmosphere of safety
- Innovation while recognizing the past
- Vision with authentic dialogue and input from all stakeholders
- "Right" decision/action within context

Empowerment. Conscious change is a transformational process. It empowers others to have confidence in their inherent knowledge, wisdom, and abilities. By encountering all beings with respect and dignity, recognizing the potential of everyone, facilitating the contributions of all, and acknowledging or rewarding people for their contributions, we encourage broad participation in needed change that can be owned and embraced by all.

■ VISION

My vision for nursing is articulated in a statement produced by the Task Force on Values, Knowledge, Skills, and Attitudes of the Integrated Healthcare Policy Consortium's (IHPC) National Education Dialogue, which I chaired (Mariano, 2013). The task force sought to identify a set of core values, knowledge, skills, and attitudes necessary for all health care professional students (Mariano, 2016b, 2013). These core values are shown in Table 9.1.

I see these core values as a vision for the future of nurses and nursing. I also see challenges and opportunities, in particular for holistic nursing, in the upcoming years (Mariano, 2016b, 2013). These can be seen in Table 9.2.

TABLE 9.1 **Integrated Health Care Policy Consortium Core Values for All Health Care Professional Students**

Core Values
• Wholeness and healing—interconnectedness of all people and things with healing as an innate capacity of every individual
• Clients/patients/families as the center of practice
• Practice as a combined art and science
• Self-care of the practitioner and commitment to self-reflection, personal growth, and healing
• Interdisciplinary collaboration and integration embracing the breadth and depth of diverse health care systems and collaboration with all disciplines, clients, and families
• Responsibility to contribute to the improvement of the community, the environment, health promotion, health care access, and the betterment of public health
• Attitudes and behaviors of all participants in health care demonstrating respect for self and others, humility, and authentic, open, and courageous communication

TABLE 9.2 **Future Challenges and Opportunities for Nurses and Nursing**

Education

- Integration of holistic philosophy, content, and practices into nursing curricula nationally and staff development programs
- Recognition, support, and legitimization of holistic integrative nursing practice in accreditation, regulation, licensure, and credentialing processes

Research

- Identification and description of outcomes of holistic therapies/interventions, relationships, and environments
- Focus on whole systems research and wellness, health promotion, and illness prevention
- Funding nurses for CAM/CIM and wholeness research
- Dissemination of nursing research findings to broader audiences, including other health disciplines and public media

Practice

- Influencing and changing the health care system to a more holistic, humanistic orientation
- Development of caring cultures within health care delivery models and systems
- Collaboration with diverse health care disciplines to advance holistic health care
- Improvement of the nursing shortage through incorporation of self-care and stress management practices for nurses and improvement of health care environments

(continued)

TABLE 9.2   **Future Challenges and Opportunities for Nurses and Nursing (*continued*)**

Policy

- Coverage and reimbursement for holistic nursing practices and services
- Education of the public about the array of health care alternatives and providers
- Increased focus on wellness, health promotion, access, and affordability of health care for all populations
- Care of the environment and the planet

CAM, complementary and alternative medicine; CIM, complementary integrative medicine.

By developing theoretical and empirical knowledge as well as caring and healing approaches, nurses will advance holistic nursing practice and education and contribute significantly to the formalization and credibility of this work. They will lead the profession in research, the development of educational models, and the integration of a more holistic approach to nursing practice and health care.

I conclude with the words of Dr. Jean Watson:

> Our work—nursing—is a calling, not only to serve but to deepen our humanity. It is a spiritual practice. . . . The tasks of *Nursing* are the tasks of *Humanity:* healing and relationship with self, others, the planet; developing a deeper understanding of human suffering; expanding and evolving an understanding of life itself; deepening an understanding of death and the sacred cycle. . . . We must revisit the foundations of our work. Caring is an ethic—it forces us to pay attention. Pause and realize that this one moment with this one person is the reason we are here at this time on this planet. When we touch their body, we touch their mind, heart, and soul. When we connect with another's humanity, even for a brief moment, we have purpose in our life and work. (Watson, 2010)

■ REFLECTIONS

1. *What is my vision of a caring, healing, holistic health care system?*
2. *What are my beliefs, values, and assumptions about my contributions as a nurse and other disciplines' contributions to the health of society?*
3. *What opportunities have I created for myself out of crises?*
4. *What people and experiences in my professional and personal life am I grateful for?*
5. *What gives meaning to my practice?*

■ REFERENCES

Beck, D. (1996). *The flame of Florence Nightingale's legacy.* Scutari, Istanbul: United Nations Human Settlements Summit.

Boostrom, R. (2001). *Developing creative and critical thinking: An integrative approach.* New York, NY: Glencoe/McGraw-Hill.

Cowling, W. R., III. (2011). Holism as a sociopolitical enterprise. *Journal of Holistic Nursing, 29*(1), 5–6.

Hoskins, C., & Mariano, C. (2004). *Developing and understanding research: Quantitative and qualitative methods.* New York, NY: Springer Publishing Company.

Kneller, G. (1965). *The art and science of creativity.* New York, NY: Holt, Rinehart, & Winston.

Mariano, C. (2002). Crisis theory and intervention: A critical component of nursing education. *Journal of the New York State Nurses Association, 3*(1), 19–24.

Mariano, C. (2004). The holistic heart—A pathway to healing. *Beginnings, 24*(3), 8–9.

Mariano, C. (2005). Caring cultures. *Beginnings, 25*(5), 8–9.

Mariano, C. (2006). The case for interdisciplinary collaboration. *Beginnings, 26*(4), 2–3.

Mariano, C. (2008). Contributions to holism through critique of theory and research. *Beginnings, 28*(2), 12, 26–27.

Mariano, C. (2010). Nurse. *Beginnings, 30*(2), 25.

Mariano, C. (2012). Conscious change: A Zen perspective. *Beginnings, 32*(2), 18–20.

Mariano, C. (2013). Holistic nursing. In *Clinicians' and educators' desk reference on the licensed complementary and alternative healthcare professions* (2nd ed., pp. 179–186). Seattle, WA: ACCAHC.

Mariano, C. (2015). Holistic integrative therapies in palliative care. In M. Matzo & D. Sherman (Eds.), *Palliative care nursing quality care to the end of life* (4th ed., pp. 235–265). New York, NY: Springer Publishing Company.

Mariano, C. (2016a). Holistic nursing: Scope and standards of practice. In B. M. Dossey & L. Keegan (Eds.), *Holistic nursing: A handbook for practice* (7th ed., pp. 53–76). Burlington, MA: Jones & Bartlett.

Mariano, C. (2016b). Current trends and issues in holistic nursing. In B. M. Dossey & L. Keegan (Eds.), *Holistic nursing: A handbook for practice* (7th ed., pp. 77–100). Burlington, MA: Jones & Bartlett.

Mittelman, M., Alperson, S., Arcari, P., Donnelly, G., Ford, L., Koithan, M., & Kreitzer, M. J. (2010). Nursing and integrative health care. *Alternative Therapies, 16*(5), 74–84.

Parad, H. (Ed.). (1965). *Crisis intervention select readings.* New York, NY: Family Service Association of America.

Suzuki, S. (1983). *Zen mind, beginner's mind.* New York, NY: Weatherhill.

Watson, J. (2010). *Human caring and holistic healing: The path of heart and spirit.* American Holistic Nurses Association Annual Conference, Colorado Springs, CO.

CHAPTER TEN

Accountable and Interprofessional: Owning the Breadth of the Nursing Role

Margaret L. McClure

Nursing has continually raised its educational ceiling without ever raising the floor.

—McClure (1976a, p. 101)

■ WHY NURSING?

It is often said that all of life is a process of becoming. Certainly, that has been my experience in being a nurse. This chapter represents an attempt to share the genesis and growth of many of my ideas about nursing, including the context in which they were formed and the individuals and events that helped to shape them and to shape my practice.

The first question to address, then, is this: What does it mean to practice? I once had a patient say to me that he would be much happier if his doctors would stop talking about "practicing," as it made him feel that that they were not quite up to the job at hand and that he was their guinea pig. His comment forced me to examine what professional practice entails. In this effort, it was helpful that I entered nursing with a brief (and unimpressive) background in music. To the musician, practice means to continually study and reflect on one's own performance in order to achieve, and/or improve on, desired outcomes.

It seems to me that is the identical definition that should apply to all professional practice, regardless of discipline. In other words, true professionals take an analytical approach to their work, acquiring the habits of study and self-reflection on an ongoing basis so that they continually learn from their successes and failures. I have tried to adopt this approach in my own work and to persuade others to do the same.

As we look back, every one of us can point to both people and experiences that provided us with the materials on which to build our careers. For me, this process started very early because my mother was a nurse. She was also a wife and a mother during the years when no wife or mother worked outside the home. Then along came World War II, and any nurse who could not enlist in the armed forces was expected to work in the civilian world. My mother immediately took a position on the night shift in our community hospital. At the conclusion of the war, she simply refused to return to the role of a housewife.

As my sister and I matured, our mother often told us that we could be whatever we wanted to be as long as we did not go into nursing. Her reasons were "Poor pay, awful hours, and hard work." Yet we both noted that she seemed to love caring for patients and often came home with intriguing tales of her work life. So, of course, we both went into nursing. And, like my mother, I always practiced in acute care hospitals where, for me, the intensity and the pace seemed to fit my temperament perfectly.

The second person who influenced my career immensely appeared in my first year of nursing school. I was a student in a hospital-based diploma program, which meant that I had a great deal of clinical experience. As it happened, there was an enormous upheaval in the institution. Things were not going well for the school of nursing or for the hospital nursing service. As a result, the two responsible directors were dismissed and replaced by a new leader who was given responsibility for both the school and the hospital. The change that resulted was palpable. Rigid rules for students were modified and new faculty was hired. More important, patient care standards in the hospital began to improve so markedly that even a first-year student could appreciate them. What an eye-opener that was! In fact, that experience influenced my entire career. I realized then that competent, committed, caring leadership is the key factor in determining the quality of patient care. And I wanted to play that leadership role.

■ EARLY IMPRESSIONS

My career as an RN began with a very rewarding tour of active duty in the Army Nurse Corps, followed by the pursuit of baccalaureate and master's credentials. During those years, I kept returning to the hospital where I had trained, specifically to work in progressively more responsible positions and to experience mentorship from the nurse leader who had influenced me while a student. It was during my last position at that hospital that an incident occurred that caused me to return to school once more.

We had a patient who was a senior executive for a large corporation. Following his discharge, he contacted the hospital administrator stating that he would like to help the institution become more efficient in its care delivery. To accomplish this, he offered the pro bono services of his company's organizational development group. The proposal was for a team to conduct a study that would result in cost savings. Of course, because nursing was the largest and most visible department, it was chosen for the focus of this work.

Since my mentor and I were the only master's prepared nurses in the institution, it fell to us to review the research plan and either approve it or suggest changes to the methodology. The interesting thing is that both of us sensed there were problems with the design, but we were hard-pressed to identify exactly what changes were needed, and in the end, we did approve it.

The study was completed and the findings were anything but helpful. The conclusions could be summarized in one sentence: The appropriate staff for each nursing unit, on each shift, was determined to be one RN assisted by one nurse's aide for every six patients. Needless to say, this represented a considerable decrease in RN staffing and a significant danger to patients! And because we had been given the opportunity to approve the methodology in advance of the data collection, it was difficult to refute the findings. Fortunately, we did prevail, but at a considerable cost to our credibility.

This experience made it clear to me that nurses in administrative positions need to have preparation in research design and methodology. In most health care settings, nursing departments represent the greatest share of budget dollars, making them always vulnerable to redesign efforts. As a consequence, nurse leaders must be prepared to actively participate in such efforts in order to ensure that such studies are well designed. Fortunately, my alma mater, Teachers College, Columbia University, offered a doctoral program with a major entitled Research in Nursing Service Administration, and I returned to school posthaste. This decision was aided considerably by a federal grant that made it possible for me to pursue my studies full-time.

■ PROFESSIONAL EVOLUTION/CONTRIBUTION

During the years in my former position, I was puzzled by an issue that became a significant question for me: We had managed to decrease the RN turnover rate at the hospital rather substantially, but we had made so many changes in the environment that we were never sure exactly what factors had been responsible for this positive change. As a result, for my doctoral dissertation, I wanted to study the reasons that staff nurses remain in their positions. However, as I began to review the literature on the topic, I was stunned to learn that there were virtually no studies on the subject of retention, either in nursing or in any other field. In addition, I began to fear that my own quest for such answers could, in fact, cause resignations among my subjects. As a result, I settled for doing an exploratory study on the reasons for hospital staff nurse resignations. The outcomes can be briefly summarized as follows: Voluntary RN job-related turnover is most often connected to a feeling of alienation. Specifically, two subsets of alienation, namely, powerlessness and normlessness (i.e., lack of fair play), were found to be the basis of resignation among my subjects (McClure, 1972). These findings provided principles that I have used every day of my working life since, proving that your second-favorite study topic can be almost as valuable as your first. I would also suggest that the findings quite likely apply to turnover in any professional field.

During doctoral study, I also began to deliberate about the need for a definition of nursing, one that could spell out the responsibilities that nurses have to patients in such a way as to create a sound basis for decisions that are made in practice settings. In particular, I wanted to create a model that could be used to guide and justify staffing decisions. The result is a contribution of which I am particularly proud, as it has proven useful to so many other aspects of our work, from basic nursing education to nursing informatics.

The role of the nurse involves two distinct, complementary subsets, one being that of "caregiver" and the other that of "integrator." In examining the *caregiver subset*, it is immediately apparent that it comprises the most familiar portions of our work and, in fact, involves meeting patient needs in relation to the following:

1. Dependency: Hygiene, nutrition, elimination, ambulation, and so forth.
2. Comfort: For nursing, this particular function has a unique centrality. Although other health care disciplines have tangential interests here, nurses are expected to focus on both the physical and psychological comfort of patients (and their families) as a major portion of their concern.
3. Education: The educational responsibility is one that expert nurses take on, almost unconsciously, as they deliver care on a day-to-day basis. In fact, most nurses actually do this, giving numerous pieces of advice related to self-care and coping, as they perform other tasks and functions. Also, as efforts intensify to make patients and families increasingly self-reliant, this aspect of our role will become more and more vital.
4. Therapies: This category represents an enormous spectrum of care components, including medications, intravenous fluid administration, and myriad other technological interventions. It is indeed this aspect of our work that has most added to the complexity of our lives, creating untold assets and liabilities for patients and nurses alike. Thus, although we know, for example, that chemotherapy can promote an extension of life and even cure certain diseases, we also know that these treatments are often dangerous and can have deleterious consequences if errors in judgment or protocol occur. Technology, then, is a double-edged sword that has clearly become central to the high error rate that has been reported in recent years.
5. Monitoring/surveillance: It is in this final category that the true mettle of the expert nurse is displayed, because this function involves collecting, interpreting, and acting upon data. In other words, signs and symptoms must be understood in such a way that even the most subtle changes in the patient's condition are detected early and appropriate action taken. It is also important to understand that every single interaction with a patient involves monitoring. As a result, all of the other functions mentioned earlier provide opportunities for observations that cue the nurse as to whether patients are following their normal course or whether, instead, they are deviating from the norm and require intervention, either by the nurse or by another professional. The knowledge component required for this responsibility is extraordinary and certainly not appreciated by patients and physicians—or even by nurses themselves. One of the trickiest aspects of this monitoring function is the fact that it is not passive. It is not merely a matter of noting data and conditions, but rather of using those data wisely and well. There is the responsibility to act, or to see that others act, based on the information at hand. This implies that the nurse possesses the knowledge and judgment to understand the interventions needed. Further, when the required actions are beyond the nurse's scope of practice, then there is the added responsibility of convincing others to respond appropriately, a responsibility that often leads to interpersonal and interdisciplinary conflict.

From the preceding text, it should be obvious that as one moves down the list of caregiver functions, the amount of educational preparation required increases. This, of course, is the reason that assistive-level personnel must be deployed wisely and well. It is also the reason that nursing education standards must be raised.

The *integrator subset* of the nurse's role is less obvious and therefore less clearly understood. The term was created by two organizational theorists (Lawrence & Lorsch, 1967) who taught us a great deal about how organizations actually work. They demonstrated that complex organizations are composed of a large number of specialized departments, each of which functions as an entity unto itself. In so doing, these departments develop their own rules, regulations, norms, and cultures; they also contribute output that is required and used by the larger organization.

These scholars discovered that, because of this departmental specialization, all such organizations create a role that they termed the *integrator*. The integrator's responsibility is to take the work (output) from the various departments and bring it together in such a way that a product is developed and delivered to the customer.

Clearly, hospitals are an example of complex organizations in health care. They have endless numbers of specialized departments, each with its own subcultures whose output must be coordinated and combined to create the product known as patient care. It is also clear that patient care delivery systems have always had an integrator, namely, the professional nurse. Lawrence and Lorsch (1967) indicated that this is not a formal or acknowledged position; rather, it is one that arises at the point of greatest knowledge related to the product. Nurses act as the integrators because they alone know, on a moment-to-moment basis, what is going on with the patient and what services are required. (This means that both routine and emergent processes are involved.) As a result, they are the only providers who *can* function as integrators. I would suggest that this is exactly what the distinguished physician, Lewis Thomas, was observing when he wrote his classic statement: "One thing the nurses do is to hold the place together. . . . My discovery, as a patient . . . is that the institution is held together, glued together, enabled to function as an organism, by the nurses and by nobody else" (1983, p. 67). Although the glue analogy has been used by many of our colleagues over the years, my own analogy for the integrator role is that of orchestra conductor. Nurses have so many responsibilities that seem akin to that of a maestro. They are the folks who call for the social workers, physical therapists, wound specialists, physicians, laboratory technicians, maintenance workers, and security guards— in fact, everyone required to meet patients' needs. Although many of these specialists have their own routines and often see patients without such bidding, it is the nurses who most frequently call on them—and they are expected to respond, just as the oboe player is expected to respond to the baton of the conductor. It is also possible to see the attending physician as the soloist, the artist whom the patient actually paid to see, but who is heavily dependent on the conductor for a satisfactory or, better yet, excellent performance.

In understanding the integrator role, it becomes quite clear that the nurse is the leader of the health care team, including professionals and nonprofessionals. Because that leadership is usually carried out unconsciously by nurses, and without any real recognition on the part of other members of the team, this critical role actually goes unnoticed. I should also emphasize that this leadership by nurses is a fact of life in all health care settings, not just in hospitals. A very interesting phenomenon—and the reason for my chapter title.

The model mentioned in the preceding text was first published decades ago (McClure, 1988), but it has withstood the test of time, having been presented at numerous conferences and consultations, involving nurse administrators, educators, and informatics specialists. It continues to evolve as my own insights and observations continue to inform the subject.

Following doctoral study, I accepted my first position as a nurse executive. It was an exciting and challenging time, both for me and for the institution. The hospital was large and staffed with an interesting mix of very experienced diploma school nurses and new graduates, most of whom came to us from associate degree programs. I had no former experience with the latter, but had learned a great deal about their programs at Teachers College, where the idea for community college education for nurses had been born. This initial exposure led me to become conscious of our need to elevate the standards for nursing education, an awareness that quickly grew into a passion that remains to this day. Why? Because I found real, everyday patient care problems that could be traced to well-meaning practitioners who were simply inadequately educated for the complex job that is nursing.

As a result of these problems, I became a great proponent of the necessity for baccalaureate education for entry into the practice of nursing and vowed to get involved in changing our educational standards. A group called the Deans and Directors of Greater New York was forming at that time; as the name suggests, it was composed of the deans of baccalaureate and higher degree programs and their counterparts in nursing service administration. We soon began efforts to introduce legislation that would change the New York State licensure law as follows: Starting in 1985, all candidates for the RN would be required to have graduated from a BSN program and all candidates for the LPN would be required to have graduated from an ADN program.

This effort received a great deal of attention at that time, both in New York State and across the nation, and many of us, including such notable leaders as Claire Fagin and Cathryne Welch, spent countless hours endeavoring to get this legislation passed (McClure, 1976b). And we failed miserably. Just as well. Looking back, there were serious flaws in the plan. But I have remained committed to this fundamental idea: *Professional nursing requires at least a baccalaureate degree for safe and effective practice.*

One educational project, to which I have made a significant contribution, is noteworthy in this regard. In the early 1990s, Brenda Cleary and I cochaired the Committee on the Preparation of the Workforce for the American Academy of Nursing (AAN). Our deliberations highlighted an innovation that had been introduced in Oregon called the Oregon Consortium for Nursing Education. This project involved the implementation of a statewide model of seamless nursing education between the community colleges and the baccalaureate programs. It was attractive in that it offered students entering community college the option of dual enrollment into the ADN and the BSN programs at the same time. This was not simple because it required identical admission standards and curriculum changes for both types of schools. The goal, of course, was to encourage community college students to immediately continue their studies at the university level upon completion of the associate's degree requirements (Tanner, Gubrud-Howe, & Shores, 2008).

Cleary and I decided to apply for a Partners Investing in Nursing (PIN) grant being offered at the time by the Robert Wood Johnson Foundation (RWJF), the aim of which was to encourage small, local foundations to fund nursing projects. In order to obtain such a grant, the local foundation was expected to contribute 50% of the monetary support needed for the project. I was on the advisory board of the new Jonas Center for Nursing Excellence, a foundation, which, at that time, was focused on supporting nursing projects within New York City. Cleary and I approached them about assisting us in developing an adaptation of the Oregon model at two sites, one in New York City and the other in Ashville, North Carolina. The idea was that we would demonstrate that the model could be successful in both urban and rural settings. We named the project Regional Increase in Baccalaureate Nurses (RIBN). It should be noted that we were greatly assisted in the application process by Marilyn DeLuca, the former executive director of the Jonas Center. Fortunately, both foundations responded favorably to our proposal, so we began the work at Hunter College and Queensborough Community College in New York and at Western Carolina University and Asheville-Buncombe Technical Community College in Ashville.

As had been the experience in Oregon, the RIBN project required an enormous amount of academic and administrative effort to get it off the ground. This was accomplished through rather herculean efforts on the part of our colleagues in the four schools involved. Thanks to them, there has been success in implementing the changes and among graduating students from both baccalaureate programs (Hall, Causey, Johnson, & Hayes, 2012). The progress in North Carolina is especially noteworthy, as there has been great enthusiasm for RIBN across the state. It should be noted that the state has 58 community colleges and they are gradually all coming on board. In fact, a goal has been set to have all North Carolina community colleges offering RIBN by 2016. The uptake in New York has been slower, but progress is definitely being made within the City College of New York system.

The outcomes of RIBN have been exceptional. The funding ended some time ago, but the program lives on and, I hope, will become a model for others across the country.

Of course, my largest research endeavor and greatest contribution has been the work that I have been privileged to do in relation to the American Nurses Credentialing Center (ANCC) Magnet Recognition Program®. It actually came about as a result of the national nursing shortage that the United States was experiencing in the late 1970s. I was a fellow in AAN, which was not yet a decade old at that point. The organization had been formed by the American Nurses Association (ANA) with the explicit mission "to generate, synthesize and disseminate nursing knowledge in such a way as to make it available to inform health policy." Clearly, the shortage qualified as a serious policy issue and, because the shortage was most severe in hospitals, the AAN appointed a Task Force on Nursing Practice in Hospitals. I was fortunate to serve as chair of the task force and even more fortunate to have three highly qualified and energetic members appointed with me. They were:

- Muriel A. Poulin, EdD, professor/chair of the program in nursing administration, Boston University
- Margaret D. Sovie, PhD, associate dean for nursing practice, University of Rochester
- Mabel Wandelt, PhD, professor and director, Center for Health Care Research and Evaluation, University of Texas at Austin

Professor Wandelt was chosen for the task force because she had published a very useful study regarding nursing turnover among Texas hospitals. One vital insight that she shared with us at our very first meeting was her observation that although the institutions in her study were facing serious shortages due to excessive rates of resignations, there were occasionally neighboring hospitals that were actually experiencing great success in their recruitment and retention efforts. Of course, she was curious as to the cause of their differences.

From this single observation, the idea for the original Magnet® Hospital research emerged. Having shared with the group my earlier foray into the literature regarding the matter, the task force determined that an exploration of the reasons that nurses are attracted to and retained in hospital settings was badly needed and was the most critical contribution the AAN could make toward solving the national nursing shortage.

We spent a number of meetings creating a research proposal that was eventually approved by the AAN Governing Council, in spite of the fact that the organization had never undertaken such a project. They, like us, assumed that we would be able to secure outside funding for the work, due to the high degree of national attention the shortage was receiving in both the professional and lay press. Unfortunately, no major funding was ever secured, in spite of many applications being submitted to various organizations and agencies.

Undaunted, the task force members committed to the value of the research proceeded with the study. Both the AAN and the ANA deserve a great deal of credit for the support they gave to our travel in relation to the data collection; the remainder of the work was supported primarily by the task force members themselves, with great assistance from the University of Texas School of Nursing, especially their dean at the time, Billie Brown. We also received vital support from the deans of the schools of nursing that served as hosts for our data collection sites across the country. They provided space, meals, graduate students to assist us, and moral support. We could not have managed without them.

The original research was published in 1983 as *Magnet Hospitals: Attraction and Retention of Professional Nurses* (McClure, Poulin, Sovie, & Wandelt, 1983). For the task force, this was an exciting time, marred only by the fact that the ANA, in publishing the book, neglected to list the task force members as authors. In fact, our names did not appear anywhere in the original publication! And that was not our only issue. As expected, it had taken more than two years for the study to be published, and by that time, the shortage had abated somewhat; as a result, we were concerned that it would not attract the attention we believed it deserved.

Fortunately, building on the foundation we had laid, a number of other researchers, most notably Kramer and Schmalenberg (2002) and Aiken (2002), continued to study our sample hospitals, adding incrementally to our knowledge of these practice settings. Moreover, thanks especially to Linda Aiken, the later studies brought us evidence that Magnet Hospitals create positive outcomes for patients as well as for nurses. It is undoubtedly because of their early efforts that the ANA decided to create the Magnet Recognition Program, under the auspices of ANCC.

I was appointed to serve on the early Magnet Hospital Commission, the group charged with overseeing the Magnet program and developing the standards for the application process (Urden & Monarch, 2002). Today, the Magnet Hospital designation has become the gold standard for excellence in patient care, with hundreds of institutions, including many from abroad, seeking to achieve this distinction. I should add that it is quite rewarding to realize that all of the major findings from the original study still form the basis for today's standards.

Although the task force that conducted the study strongly believed that our findings would make a valuable contribution to the field, I feel quite comfortable in stating that none of us, in our wildest dreams, could have hoped for the outcome it has achieved. The impact the program has made on both the quality of patient care and the quality of nurses' work lives has proven to be extraordinary.

■ MORAL/ETHICAL FOUNDATION

The nature of a profession is that it must have a strong ethical and moral foundation. In fact, in many, a rite of passage at the completion of one's basic education involves a formal declaration or pledge that spells out the components of that foundation, the Hippocratic oath taken by physicians being the best known.

Nursing is no exception. In reality, the practice of nursing probably requires greater attention to this foundation, simply because there are innumerable opportunities that expose the most personal information and/or assets of patients, and this exposure frequently occurs when they are highly vulnerable due to either their physical or emotional state. Integrity, then, is essential for every member of the profession. Although this statement may seem self-evident on its face, there are real complications that arise in relation to ensuring such integrity.

Those of us in administrative positions have a major role to play in creating an environment that is safe for patients in this regard—and there are several areas that require our very careful attention. First, of course, our hiring practices must be designed in such a way as to provide the best possible screening of all candidates applying for nursing department positions, including nursing attendants and unit secretaries. Second, every effort must be made to see that checks and balances are in place: for example, adequate, competent supervision, policies and procedures designed to protect both patients and staff, and, perhaps most important, clear lines of authority available to individuals who need to report unethical behaviors on the part of others.

A noteworthy topic in the recent safety literature related to ethical practice is the importance of a "just culture" in the handling of clinical errors. Integrity is encouraged—in fact, it thrives—in situations where human error is acknowledged as such and the individual involved is not subject to blaming behavior under the guise of "accountability." Such an approach creates an environment in which staff members feel safe in reporting their errors, which, in turn, opens the possibility for future error prevention to be explored through a systems focus (Duthie, 2015).

From an organizational standpoint, it is most important that the corporate culture be one that actively rewards integrity in practice, regardless of profession or discipline. In other words, high ethical standards must be maintained throughout the institution. I have had the amazing good fortune to serve in senior management positions where this was the case. The three CEOs with whom I worked were principled decision makers, never afraid to tackle unethical incidents head-on. Such an environment enables excellence in patient care and may, in fact, be the most significant underlying component of Magnet Hospitals.

■ VISION

Our health care delivery system is headed for rather radical change, driven by the tsunami of baby boomers who are achieving senior citizen status at an alarming rate. And those in the population who are ahead of this curve are living much longer, a function of the success of health care advances and healthier lifestyles in recent years—it is a costly problem. The United States, like all developed countries, is therefore facing the unpleasant task of rationing the amount of care that citizens will receive in the future, forcing consumers, even now, to become more self-reliant. It is simply a financial matter. As a result, more care delivery will move into the community and nurses will need to follow—and manage—that migration.

It seems quite likely that the role of the nurse will remain the same, except that the caregiver portion of the role will decline and the integrator portion will greatly increase. As a consequence, there will be great demand for nurses prepared to serve as case managers for individuals or families, and this will result in business models involving either independent or interprofessional team practice, or a mixture of both. In any case, the need will be for highly qualified RNs who are able to function quite independently, making judgments and referrals in ways not heretofore experienced.

To meet these new practice models, the educational standards for nursing will inevitably have to change. It should also be noted that our long delay in addressing this issue has the potential to create adverse effects on patients across the nation. It is probably safe to predict that change will come, and it will come quickly, because health care employers and other stakeholders will force the issue. We are already seeing pressures build: As reimbursement systems shift to a pay-for-performance mode, the evidence that nurses' educational preparation makes a difference is increasingly accepted as fact. That is clearly the reason that so many institutions are giving preference to baccalaureate-prepared nurses or are requiring that new hires agree to complete their BSN within a particular time frame, most commonly five years.

It is instructive to understand the history of community colleges in the United States in order to appreciate our own history. The system was actually formed by a federal law following World War II. It was one piece of legislation designed to be a companion to the well-known G.I. Bill, and its purpose was to offer job training to returning veterans; the highlights were as follows:

- A national network of educational programs, federally funded, with little or no cost to students
- State owned and state controlled
- Designed to offer technical/vocational training to students *who could not otherwise attend college*
- Open enrollment, requiring only a high-school diploma or General Educational Development (GED) test for admission.

In other words, the community colleges were developed to essentially offer a two-year extension of high schools. They were never intended to serve as the early years of a baccalaureate education (Bailey, Smith, & Jenkins, 2015).

It is evident from the preceding text that the decision to develop nursing programs within these new community college settings was a mistake from the outset. The action was apparently taken with the good intention of moving nursing education out of the apprentice-type training that diploma schools were offering and into mainstream higher education (Mildred L. Montag, class lecture, Teachers College, Columbia University, 1970). Instead, it has created a situation in which the demands of practice have steadily exceeded the educational preparation of the majority of our colleagues. Yet we have been blocked in our many and persistent efforts to raise our entry standards by political pressures on state legislatures, exerted by community college presidents reluctant to lose a major revenue source. The result is that we are in the unique position of continually raising our educational ceiling without ever raising the floor.

To be fair, the knowledge base for nursing has changed dramatically in the years since World War II. It should be noted, however, that no other comparable occupation pursued the community college route initially—not teachers, not social workers, not physical therapists; no other profession—only nursing. In the very near future, job market pressures will force the community colleges to retool in order to continue to offer nursing programs, a change that has been resisted by far too many for far too long.

The other educational issue to be addressed is that of the preparation of nurse practitioners. Several movements are underway that will be argued but finally resolved: The first is the degree that should be required (i.e., master versus doctor of nursing practice); the second is the amount of clinical training needed. Both will be subject to heated debate. In order to meet this goal, however, we will need to collect more and better evidence related to this entire area of responsibility so that our decisions are well informed and made in the best interests of all concerned.

In spite of these educational issues, I believe the future for nursing, and, therefore, for patients, is bright. The 21st century has brought new and exciting opportunities to members of our profession: More qualified applicants than ever are seeking admission to schools of nursing and the public has a growing awareness of the important role that we play in patient care. Many health care influentials are beginning to recognize that the bulk of primary care will be delivered by nurses in the coming years. Moreover, interprofessional teams are gradually becoming a reality rather than an unfulfilled dream. All of these changes will necessitate our developing substantial numbers of nurses ready and able to give leadership in a variety of settings across the nation.

It is, indeed, our time. *Carpe diem*—seize the day!

■ REFLECTIONS

1. *It has been noted that the bedside professional nurse is the "glue" or "orchestrator" that maintains the integrity of patient care and procures optimal outcomes for patients and families. How do I view the implications of this privilege and accountability? What analogy would I use to describe this full-spectrum leadership duty and why?*

2. *How do I understand my roles as both caregiver and integrator? What are the biggest obstacles to successfully implementing these responsibilities? What are my solutions?*

3. *Consider the ever-evolving complexity of nursing care. What are my opinions regarding the educational requirement for RNs? What level of degree preparation do I believe would provide the soundest, safest, and most appropriate level of care for patients? Consult the literature to support the argument.*

4. *Read more about the model of the Magnet Recognition Program at http://www.nursecredentialing.org/Magnet. Which principles does my institution thrive at and which ones is it struggling to meet? Reflecting on my role, regardless of position, how do I help to promote or maintain these principles in practice?*

5. *What training or education am I planning to pursue in order that I continue to play a pivotal and meaningful role in the transition of patient care from institutional to community-based practice? How do I envision a broadened scope of nursing to evolve in this process?*

■ REFERENCES

Aiken, L. H. (2002). Superior outcomes for Magnet hospitals: The evidence base. In M. L. McClure & A. S. Hinshaw (Eds.), *Magnet hospitals revisited* (pp. 61–82). Washington, DC: American Nurses Association.

Bailey, T. R., Smith, S. S., & Jenkins, D. (2015). *Redesigning America's community colleges.* Cambridge, MA: Harvard University Press.

Duthie, E. A. (2015). Accountability: Challenges to getting it right. *Journal of Patient Safety* (ePub ahead of print, April 7, 2015).

Hall, V. P., Causey, B., Johnson, M., & Hayes, P. (2012). The RIBN initiative: A new effort to increase the number of baccalaureate nurses in North Carolina. *Journal of Professional Nursing, 28*(6), 377–380.

Kramer, M., & Schmalenberg, C. (2002). Staff nurses identify essentials of magnetism. In M. L. McClure & A. S. Hinshaw (Eds.), *Magnet hospitals revisited* (pp. 25–60). Washington, DC: American Nurses Association.

Lawrence, P. R., & Lorsch, J. W. (1967). *Organization and environment.* Boston, MA: Harvard Graduate School of Business Administration.

McClure, M. L. (1972). *The reasons for hospital staff nurse resignations* (Unpublished doctoral dissertation). Teachers College, Columbia University.

McClure, M. (1976a). Can we bring order out of the chaos in nursing education? *American Journal of Nursing, 76*(1), 101.

McClure, M. (1976b). Entry into professional practice: The New York proposal. *Journal of Nursing Administration, 6*(5), 12–17. Reprinted in N. L. Chaska, (1978), *The nursing profession: Views through the mist.* New York, NY: McGraw-Hill.

McClure, M. (1988). Nursing administration in the twenty-first century. In M. K. Stull & S. Pinkerton (Eds.), *Current strategies for nursing administrators* (pp. 80–87). Rockville, MD: Aspen.

McClure, M., Poulin, M. A., Sovie, M. D., & Wandelt, M. A. (1983). *Magnet hospitals: Attraction and retention of professional nurses.* Washington, DC: American Nurses Association.

Tanner, C. A., Gubrud-Howe, P., & Shores, L. (2008). The Oregon consortium for nursing education: A response to the nursing shortage. *Policy, Politics, and Nursing Practice, 9*(3), 203–209.

Thomas, L. (1983). *The youngest science: Notes of a medicine-watcher.* New York, NY: Viking.

Urden, L. D., & Monarch, K. (2002). The ANCC Magnet recognition program: Converting research findings into action. In M. L. McClure & A. S. Hinshaw (Eds.), *Magnet hospitals revisited* (pp. 103–116). Washington, DC: American Nurses Association.

CHAPTER ELEVEN

Ethical and Economical: Calling the Profession to Social Justice

Donna M. Nickitas

Nurses cannot be silent and must . . . articulat[e] clearly the injustices caused by lack of access and the inequities, inefficiencies, and brokenness of our health care delivery system. By changing the world with words, I can tell the truth and encourage my colleagues to act to promote social and economic justice.
                                                              —Nickitas (2008, p. 141)

■ WHY NURSING?

I knew at an early age that I wanted to be an RN. Although no one in my immediate family was a health professional and I did not know any nurses, I knew I wanted to be a nurse. As I grew up in a loving family whose members respected and cared for one another, I recognized the importance of caring for others. When I decided at the age of 14 to become a nurse, I had the full support of my parents and siblings. I was one of the first members of my family to pursue a college education. With my family's encouragement, I understood that if one worked hard, persevered, and was determined, one could achieve anything. Indeed, all I had to do was look around at my own family to understand how values and drive shape who and what one is.

As a young girl growing up in a traditional Italian household, I learned the cultural values of family, faith, and food. Sitting at the kitchen table, surrounded by parents, grandparents, family, and friends, I learned everything about life and living. In the heat of the kitchen, as the meal fragrantly simmered, my family debated world affairs, religion, politics, and the economy. Little did I know that these conversations would frame and influence my perspectives on equality, equity, and social justice, but they did.

My parents instilled in me a strong sense of self-advocacy and activism. If one wants to make the world a better place, start by making oneself a responsible citizen. My father worked extremely hard, often working two jobs to care for his family. I witnessed his strong work ethic and followed his example. As a young girl, I was studious and focused my full waking hours on my schoolwork and extracurricular activities. By the time I finished grammar school and went off to high school, I had become interested in civil rights, women's rights, and equality. Although I was too young to march or even protest against the injustices suffered by people of color and women, I knew that I could use my voice in other venues. I joined student government, community service clubs, and the high-school yearbook committee. It was in these organizations that I recognized how to influence others and make a difference in the public sphere.

My Catholic elementary and high-school education taught me about human dignity and emphasized respect, concern, and care for others. These values framed my perspective toward how I interacted with the world around me. During the summer of my freshman year of high school, when I was 14, and still too young to obtain employment, I became a Red Cross volunteer or candy striper as we were known. I was placed at St. Vincent Medical Center in lower Manhattan, New York, where I had daily interactions with nurses and nursing students. These observations of hospital acute care nursing convinced me beyond a shadow of doubt that nursing was my calling.

The very next summer, I applied to become a Vincenteen—this was a program for students of high-school age who wanted to be nursing assistants. I was accepted into the program and employed every summer at St. Vincent's until I graduated high school. It was this experience that drew me deep into the throes of the nursing profession. This program had a profound impact on my perceptions of what a nurse was, as well as the moral and ethical responsibilities of being a professional. At the time, I witnessed the activities of acute care nursing without fully appreciating the real impact nurses have on the health and well-being of others. Being a Vincenteen provided me with a basic understanding of how nursing worked. I knew that being a nurse would allow me to make a difference to individuals, families, communities, as well as the profession at large. My dream was to become "just like Florence Nightingale."

I wanted to be a social activist, change the world, and make a difference. I believed that being a nurse would give me a real sense of purpose. I would learn to leverage the love and support of my family and community to serve society as a whole. When I entered nursing school, I chose community service projects and other voluntary opportunities to address issues of social justice: food banks, clothing drives, and visiting the homebound. My commitment toward equity, equality, and social justice would eventually provide a solid footing for my service to the profession. I learned early in my nursing career that professional nursing was more than clinical practice and involved important areas that were essential to the status of the profession, such as the need for advanced education, licensure issues, scope of practice, and health care policy. I learned that nurses were engaged in frontline health care but could also be involved in economic, political, and policy debates around issues of health and health care. I recognized that if I wanted to participate in these debates, I would need to be informed and educated about the affairs impacting my workplace, community, and profession.

I knew that being and becoming a nurse would heighten my advocacy and activism toward improving the health and well-being of others. I understood that serving society and doing public good was a moral imperative of nursing. Moreover, I also appreciated how my core values of family, faith, respect, and preserving the dignity of others aligned me with the values and ethics of nursing. For me, nursing is and has always been a call to action and a call to social justice.

Those early days as a Vincenteen were invaluable. In those days, I became astute in observing and appreciating the staff nurses and nursing students as teachers. They made quite an impression on me and my decision to pursue nursing as a career. They were excellent role models. And, as I reflect on those early days, I realize now as a nurse educator, I am that nurse, acting as role model—fulfilling my destiny to influence and prepare the next generation of nurse scientists and leaders.

■ EARLY IMPRESSIONS

Some of my earliest observations as a nurse involved recognizing just how complicated the health care delivery system in the United States was, with all its regulations, laws, and policies. I was intrigued by the many overall facets of health care and the need to understand health and public policy. I quickly learned that, regardless of the health care workplace (hospitals, nursing homes, community-based agencies, ambulatory clinics, or schools), nurses must recognize that health care and health care delivery are severely regulated and under constant financial pressure.

In my early days as a staff nurse on the front line of care, I saw how nurses often bore the brunt of complying with the demands of internal and external regulatory forces, including, but not limited to, the State Department of Health and the Joint Commission on Accreditation of Healthcare Organizations (JCAHO). As I became more experienced, I realized that when nursing units were understaffed, the demand for productivity increased. However, nurses in general were not equipped for identifying, acknowledging, and managing the larger institutional, social, political, and economic forces that impacted their profession and work productivity. In other words, nurses on the front line of care were often unaware of the external forces and policies that were relevant to their daily activities and professional lives.

To be a clinically competent nurse meant that I had to ready myself to know exactly how health and public policy were connected to the delivery of care. My view of nursing care delivery was changing and I needed to alter my impressions of how health care was regulated, financed, and monitored to assess quality outcomes and performance. I was moving away from the microlevel of nursing clinical practice at the bedside to the macrolevel of understanding health care at the institutional and governmental levels (regulation, costs, and quality). This macrolevel included expanding my understanding of the opportunities and constraints that confront the nursing profession in a larger perspective. Achieving improved health care quality and performance requires that nurses participate in the processes that address barriers to care; screen for low health literacy and personal and cultural preferences; eliminate disparities in the quality of care for minorities, the poor, the aged, and the mentally ill; and provide quality care for the chronically ill through coordinated, interdisciplinary care.

I knew that nurses were being constrained by their state legislatures and unable to practice to the fullest scope or extent of their education and training. For equity in health care to be entirely realized and experienced, these issues around scope of practice and equity at the macrolevel required that I engage in the policy process. For me, policy making is a dynamic, interactive process. I learned to understand that the government dictates the response of health care providers. In other cases, health providers dictate the response of government. By developing a more nuanced understanding of the ways policy shapes the health care system, I developed a working knowledge of health care delivery and gained the necessary tools needed to influence health care decisions. I was ready to move from observing changes in my profession to actively participating as a change agent.

I wanted to change nurses' views on practice issues at both the micro- and macrolevels. My goal was to participate in both the private and public spheres of policy at the local, regional, and national levels. I wanted a seat at the table so that I could use my voice and assist other nurses in finding their voices as well—collectively, we could influence health and public policy. Given nurses' role as caregivers, I came to realize how nurses bring a unique perspective to policy making. For nurses to truly make a difference and influence the regulatory, financial, and quality outcomes of patient care, they have to be engaged. This is essential if nurses are to advance the nation's health in order for good health to flourish across all demographics, where every individual has the opportunity to be as healthy as possible and where everyone has access to affordable, quality health care. I wanted to be a nurse leader and activist participating fully in influencing health and nursing care. This participation allowed me to address the issues of equity, equality, and leadership and align them with the historical roots and fabric of professional nursing. These issues of equity, equality, and social justice framed my vision, interests, and passions of nursing.

As I reflect upon the early impressions that sparked my interests and passions in nursing, I realize that those same passions are still relevant today, including increasing access to care and improving quality by such actions as reducing medical errors, promoting health and wellness, and improving efficiency and reducing costs. Like my fellow nurse colleagues, I understand that our health care system is broken and needs complete, comprehensive reform to assure that future generations may enjoy a delivery system that will ensure their health and well-being.

Since the passage of the Patient Protection and Affordable Care Act (ACA) in 2010, there has been more governmental oversight for increased quality through wellness and preventive care initiatives and greater efforts made to reduce costs through payment reform. There is no better time to be a nurse than now. However, nurses must exercise their clinical judgment, political acumen, and leadership skills to make important and much-needed changes that further increase access to and improve the quality and affordability of health care.

From my early days as a Red Cross volunteer, I learned that nursing is not a spectator sport, and that advancing the nation's health means being involved in professional nursing on multiple levels: public and private; professional and personal; regional, national, and international; and academic and nonacademic. So now, as a chief academic administrator, nurse educator, and researcher, I aim to strengthen the academic productivity and overall excellence of future nurse scholars by providing them with ongoing research mentorship and leadership development.

■ PROFESSIONAL EVOLUTION/CONTRIBUTION

I continue to contribute to the nursing profession through my leadership, scholarship, and service. As my leadership capacity expanded from my days as a young staff nurse, I realized that frontline nursing care was not working for me. I yearned for new and different opportunities to influence nursing and health care. I joined the United States Air Force (USAF) Nurse Corps. After completing my BSN, I pursued 3 years of active-duty nursing and then an additional 15 years as a nurse reservist. My military nursing experience provided a solid foundation in leadership and management. As an officer and a nurse, I had the combined ability to advance my clinical skills while leading others. I never wielded any responsibility or authority that was beyond my positioned rank. In other words, my scope of authority and accountability aligned with my rank as a lieutenant, captain, or major. During my military nursing career, I would learn important lessons about teamwork, effective communication, and human and fiscal resource management.

The rules, regulations, and discipline of the USAF were not very different from the moral and ethical responsibilities of being a professional nurse. I fully knew the boundaries and expectations of being a professional nurse, so those of a military officer were not completely alien. Moreover, I came to appreciate and honor my military service—it was the best training for my future positions as a nurse leader. I mastered the art of managing human resources by learning and respecting how to work with a diverse workforce, including leading and following a command and understanding control structures between officers and enlisted personnel. You are not a leader unless you have followers and you can only learn leadership by following astute and superior leaders. The military creates and builds unique opportunities for leadership development and I was fortunate enough to step up and take charge as a young officer in the USAF Nurse Corps.

After three years of active duty, I entered New York University (NYU) as a full-time graduate student under the G.I. bill. While at NYU, I majored in nursing education and was exposed to Martha Rogers's Science of Unitary Human Beings. This was the first time I actually realized the importance of nursing science and the implications of theory-guided practice. Through the exposure to models and theories of nursing focused on human existence and universal energy, I began to realize the importance of nursing research as another aspect of nursing. Until this time, I had not fully understood the different philosophies and theories of nursing and how they had advanced nursing practice. Because the entire nursing curriculum at NYU integrated Rogers's theory within the coursework, I became fully indoctrinated by the time I graduated. I began to understand how my perspective of nursing was changing and my worldview expanding into one with a greater understanding that "the purpose of nurses is to promote health and well-being for all persons wherever they are. Thus, the art of nursing is the creative use of the science of nursing for human betterment" (Rogers, 1992, p. 28).

As my appreciation for the art and science of nursing matured, I came to recognize how nursing was developing outside the traditional biomedical model and creating its own models to build new visions of nursing knowledge, practice, and research. After I completed my graduate degree, I was anxious to return to clinical practice rather than enter a career in nursing education. I accepted a position in nursing administration as a clinical director in maternal–child nursing at a large public academic medical center. It was during this time that my early commitments to equity, equality, and social justice came full circle. This large urban public hospital served all the people of New York City, regardless of their ability to pay. This population was composed mostly of individuals who either had health insurance through Medicare or Medicaid or were uninsured and underserved.

Caring for individuals, families, and communities who were exposed to health care inequities had a profound impact on my purpose as a nurse. Addressing the social determinants of health (SDH), as well as other factors such as poverty, unequal access to health care, lack of education, stigma, and racism, impacted my understanding of public health and the overall health of populations. I knew that I had to learn how best to understand and recognize the effects of poverty, economic inequities, stress, social exclusions, and job insecurity within populations, especially among those who are medically underserved and the most vulnerable. The integration of caring at the macrolevel of the health system required me to develop a caring perspective that aligned with population health. This macrolevel integration of health outcomes, disease burden, and behavioral and physiological factors became an overriding reality of providing health care at an underresourced public hospital. At the forefront of such a system, I was charged with the goals of improving health outcomes and reducing health disparities.

As a nurse administrator responsible for the health care needs of women and children, I was challenged to ask, "Where do nurses fit in the care value equation and how will nurses improve overall population health, achieve better experience, and lower cost?" We know today that "the variation in nursing resources provided to each patient is essentially unknown and there is no alignment among nursing direct-care time and costs, billing for nursing services, and payment for care" (Welton & Harper, 2015, p. 14). My administrative responsibility was to define what constituted the components of nursing care value and how best to cost out nursing services wherever nursing care occurred. It was, indeed, challenging to integrate these financial considerations and determine nurse staffing that would sufficiently address the health disparities and care needs of the women and children under my services.

I had no technology or software that could pull these analytics together. I had to quickly master the fundamentals of population health for these women and children, as well as health care finance. I had a moral and ethical obligation to understand the key SDH and seek effective ways to distribute resources for this special population in order to meet their health care needs. This meant addressing care gaps and avoiding service duplication. None of the mechanisms to achieve the aforementioned was available in the early 1980s: no diagnosis-related groups (DRGs), clinical guidelines, or tracking length of stay. At that time, much of nursing care was focused on the acute care phase and discharge planning. There was very little attention on addressing health disparities at the individual patient level. If health disparities were addressed at all, it was in the domain of social work and not nursing.

With the adoption of the ACA, there was a resurgence of interest in measures that address the SDH and how to improve health status (Mahony & Jones, 2013). In fact, Title IV of the ACA mandates improved disease prevention in public health systems and increased access to preventive services and provisions for healthier communities, with recognition and attention to SDH (ACA, 2010). The World Health Organization (WHO) writes that these SDH are "These inequities in health, avoidable health inequalities, arise because of the conditions in which people are born, grow, live, work, and age, and the systems put in place to deal with illness. The conditions in which people live and die are, in turn, shaped by political, social, and economic forces" (2008, para 2). The ACA has provided unique opportunities for nurses to create models of care that improve the public's health, including provisions that improve access to care and quality while controlling costs.

The more I understood how the SDH impacted women and children, the more I began to see the links between the universal need for reducing high-cost preventable hospitalizations and greater access to primary population health care. The economic and human suffering caused by poor access to primary care for women and children, an under-served and vulnerable population, was deeply disturbing. It became abundantly clear that my ability to improve and impact the long-term overall health and well-being of the women and children under my care would be a daunting task. For me to have a greater impact, I knew I would have to leave nursing administration and the acute care hospital. I began to understand that targeted application of preventive services, based on unique patient history and evidence-based practice, was going to be the most cost-effective way to promote health and prevent disease—not episodic acute care. Hospital nursing care was centered on acute illnesses and I was beginning to shift my nursing perspectives toward a greater focus on health promotion and disease prevention. It was time to go.

I left hospital nursing administration after four years for nursing education, where I have been for the last 32. I jumped with great enthusiasm to teach and prepare future nurses with the opportunity to understand and improve health disparities and health care equality. I believed that education was the one way that I could influence the next genera-tion of nurses to understand how clinical practice is derived from regulations, laws, and policies, all of which are within the domain of government. Nurses have a responsibility to learn about government and regulatory agencies, as well as how these bodies influence professional nursing, health care, and public policies.

As a nurse educator, I could demonstrate how nurses could lead and advocate for the profession and for their patients. For example, the simple lesson of having students understand the importance of using their collective voice through participation in gov-ernment and governance was a challenge I was up for. To make the lessons more realistic, I encouraged students to become active in school governance by serving on college or school nursing standard committees or even running for elected positions as officers in their chapter of the student nursing association, at either the local or state levels. In fact, at one point I was appointed the faculty liaison to the school's chapter of the National Student Nurses Association just so I could drive the lesson home. These outside-the-classroom civic lessons were instrumental in demonstrating that becoming a change agent goes way beyond the knowledge and skills needed for clinical practice and includes being fully informed and educated about the democratic process, participation, and ser-vice to the profession.

To be successful in leading change in nursing and health care, nurses must know firsthand how to tip the levers for change through advocacy and action. As the largest segment of the health care workforce in the United States, nurses are the professionals who spend the most time providing direct care to patients. They play an essential role in advancing the nation's health (Nickitas, 2016). Armed with the full knowledge and appreciation of the contribution that nurses provide to health care, and to society overall, I have sought to model the way so that others may learn. My professional evolution and contributions are focused on ways in which nurses can lead change to improve health and health care, driving economic and social policies that effectively promote the health of the nation.

When I obtained my PhD, I realized this was a key component in my professional development and transformation as a nurse leader. I was fortunate enough in my early career to have mentorship, leadership development, a network of lifelong colleagues, and financial support to pursue nursing as a career. I had the capacity to put evidence-based, innovative ideas for systemic change into practice, education, and research. I wanted to inspire the next generation of nurses. I have learned to leverage a productive academic career and have inspired future nurse scholars to reach their greatest potential as leaders in science, policy, innovation, practice, and education. Over the course of my 32 years as a nurse educator, I have educated thousands of nurses and mentored and developed nurse scientists who are finding solutions to pressing health care issues and developing new and innovative models of nursing care. These professional nurses and nurse leaders are committed to long-term careers that advance science and discovery, strengthen nursing education, and bring transformational change to nursing and health care. I know that I am building my career legacy and living my destiny as a nurse leader and educator.

Today, I am advancing the recommendation given by the Institute of Medicine (IOM) report, *The Future of Nursing: Leading Change, Advancing Health* (2011), to double the number of nurses in the United States with doctoral degrees by building a well-prepared cadre of researchers, leaders, and practitioners. Currently, less than 1% of the nursing workforce has a PhD in nursing or a related field, and a large proportion of nurses are nearing retirement. Nurses with doctorates are needed to educate future generations of nurses. To get the right numbers, there must be competitive salary and benefit packages available so that highly qualified academic and clinical nurse faculty are recruited and retained (Nickitas & Feeg, 2011).

Doctorally prepared nurses are well positioned to lead change and advance health care in America. They stand ready to conduct research that becomes the basis for improvements in nursing science and advanced practice. Therefore, by investing in more PhD education, I am preparing nurses who will, over time, help replenish our desperately needed supply of nurse scientists and educators. My life's work within nursing has been to build a legacy of advocacy and activism through my scholarship, research, service, and academic leadership.

Nursing care is a critical factor in care delivery and nurses have a pivotal role in meeting the evolving health needs of individuals, families, and communities in coordinating that care. The effective coordination of health care is essential to speed recovery, economize on resources, and enhance patient satisfaction. Importantly, nurses have an innate ability to work closely with patients and family caregivers to encourage them and to help patients understand their treatment so they may play an active role in patients' care. Care transition and coordination are vital contributions that nurses make to care delivery.

Today, nurses are expected to deliver care across different settings, increase both patient and provider satisfaction, reduce hospitalizations, and enhance cost savings (Naylor et al., 2013). In order to accomplish this expectation, nurses must be ready to step up to the challenge to identify and quantify their economic and social value. There are increasing opportunities to practice to the full extent of a professional nursing license

(IOM, 2011) and impact health as never before. The economics of care for populations is supported and embedded in the ACA, where prevention and wellness as well as improvement in quality and health system performance are measured and evaluated. The long-term objective of health is to leverage nursing practice to places where people live, work, and play to improve quality and safety and reduce costs in health care.

Our nation's health care system is facing significant challenges. I want to be in a position to prepare a new generation of nurse leaders who can engage in knowledge and scientific discovery, successfully maneuver in health and public policy, create new innovative care delivery models, and be present in the boardrooms of health care. The nurses of tomorrow must be prepared to develop science through research and scholarship, to engage in policy decision making and discovery through innovation, and be prepared to lead and influence change. These are substantial skills that must be mentored and nurtured by nurse leaders in science, education, innovation, policy, and health care. I have an obligation and a moral imperative to create internal and external professional networks with other nurses, health care professionals, policy makers, and other stakeholders who will bring about real transformational change in health and health care delivery.

From its beginning, *nursing* was defined as having "charge of the personal health of somebody . . . and what nursing has to do . . . is to put the patient in the best condition for nature to act upon him" (Nightingale, 1860, p. 126). This early definition of nursing represents how strategic Nightingale was in her thinking about the importance of the nurse's observational skills and the impact of the environment on health. Nightingale clearly recognized health promotion and health maintenance as important responsibilities of nursing (see Chapters 4 and 18 for more information on Nightingale's legacy).

I know that my view of nursing has evolved over time but has been strongly influenced by health care policy. As a health professional, I have become more acutely aware of how health policy impacts nurses and patients, whether that policy is created through governmental actions, institutional decision making, or organizational standards. Thus, health policies create a framework that can facilitate or impede the delivery of health care services, and nurses' engagement in the process of policy development is central to creating a health care system that meets the needs of both nurses and the populations they serve.

I have been instrumental in educating and informing nurses about the importance of political activism and a commitment to policy development. I have taught undergraduate, graduate, and doctoral students how to assume broader leadership roles on behalf of the public as well as the nursing profession. However, much of my early teaching at the master's level was dedicated to preparing nurse managers for the administration and leadership of health care organizations. I have found plenty of opportunities to weave the lessons of the "three Ps"—policy, politics, and power—into education regarding the expansive roles and responsibilities of nurse leaders. I wanted other nurses to appreciate how health policy influences multiple health care delivery issues, including health disparities, cultural sensitivity, ethics, the internationalization of health care concerns, access to care, quality of care, health care financing, and issues of equity and social justice in the delivery of health care.

I have advocated for health care policy that addresses issues of social justice and equity in health care as I realized that nurses are potent influencers in policy formation. We have the capacity to analyze the policy process and the ability to engage in politically competent action. Professional nurses must be seen as leaders in the practice arena and provide a critical interface between practice, research, and policy. Policy makers need to understand the role of nursing to make the best decisions. With this goal in mind, nurses must work with key policy makers to promote crucial conversations about economic and social policies that can reduce costs and effectively promote the health of communities. The profession is well positioned to play a leadership role in helping the government address the $2.7 trillion spent on health care annually (Hartman, Martin, Benson, Catlin, & The National Health Expenditure Accounts Team, 2013).

■ MORAL/ETHICAL FOUNDATION

Keep your thoughts positive, because your thoughts become your words. Keep your words positive, because your words become your behavior. Keep your behavior positive, because your behavior becomes your habits. Keep your habits positive, because your habits become your values. Keep your values positive, because your values become your destiny. (Gandhi, n.d.)

Reflecting on the words of Gandhi, I am reminded of my humanity and why I have been called to be a nurse. Each day I have an opportunity to use my thoughts, words, behaviors, habits, and values to make a difference in the lives of others. Gandhi reminds us that our values shape who we are and how we live in the world. For me, my values have shaped my moral and ethical foundation in nursing education, practice, and research. As I reflect on the core values of professional nursing—human dignity, autonomy, altruism, and social justice—I realize how much Gandhi's words help me to uphold nursing's code of ethics to protect and serve society with honesty, integrity, and trust.

The American Nurses Association (ANA) declared 2015 as the Year of Ethics. This was in recognition of the newly revised *Code of Ethics for Nurses with Intepretive Statements* issued by the ANA (2015), known as "The Code." The Code can be a tool for nurses and patients to hold people accountable for ethical practice. It is important for nurses to understand and appreciate their ethical code of conduct, as they are confronted every day with ethical dilemmas when they bear witness to health care practices that endanger the lives of others. Nurses often have to choose between being silent and experiencing the moral distress of knowing that they are not living up to their professional responsibilities by being outspoken advocates for ethical practice. It is not easy to address ethical dilemmas when you witness them. However, the Code for nurses provides a framework to be responsive and responsible in their professional actions and behaviors.

Ethical dilemmas exist across all aspects of professional nursing; I have had plenty, including academic dishonesty and cheating. I knew that I had a responsibility to uncover, openly discuss, and condemn dishonesty and cheating with my students. This ability to be transparent about what I witness in the classroom was not easy. The reality is that discussing this dilemma with my students may not guarantee that this situation will change or improve, but it has been an important lesson for me to advocate for ethical practice. I have been able to weather the storm and distress of these dilemmas because nursing's ethics ground my actions and behaviors. Nurses have an ethical and legal obligation to recognize and address ethical malfeasance in education, practice, and research.

There exists an inherent imbalance within the health care system that favors and rewards specialty care over primary and preventative care. This imbalance is economically and socially unjust. Nurses know firsthand that efficient, high-value care cannot be achieved without fundamental change in provider choice and payment. Together, nursing's economic and social value can be framed within a primary public health care perspective that addresses the SDH and prevents health conditions among individuals and families in underserved, vulnerable communities. This economic and social value framework is a moral/ethical obligation of the profession and is aligned with the WHO's (2008) call to reduce health disparities as well as with the IOM's (2011) integration of primary public health, where *health* is a shared goal of population health improvement and community engagement to define and address population health needs.

Nurses have strong historical roots in advocacy and action, which include determining how best to distribute resources to populations (Nickitas, 2016). Public health nurses continue to contribute strategically in population-based efforts to enhance care. They use data to influence public policy and have a rich heritage of using such data to improve health outcomes (McBride, 1993). This practice dates back to Florence Nightingale, who demonstrated the relationship between data and improvement in care through statistical analysis and graphic representation (Goldwater & Zusy, 1990). Knowing how to use measurable metrics to drive improvements in health will fundamentally reshape how care is delivered, including the evolution toward value-based payments that increase quality at lower costs.

■ VISION

As I reflect upon my vision for the future of nurses and nursing, I think about the incredible capacity nurses have to lead health care and public policy. Nurses play an essential role in supporting and realizing the vision for health care in the United States and globally. They stand ready to ensure that the nursing profession receives the knowledge, data, and evidence needed to transform practice, education, and leadership through timely research, knowledge development, and evidence-based practice. I envision a future where nurses have the opportunity to secure positions on influential committees, commissions, and boards. Nurses maintain all of the essential knowledge, skills, and attributes to become qualified board members, and yet they remain underrepresented on governing boards; data from 2011 reveal that only 6% of board members are nurses (Wilson Pecci, 2014).

Skills and attributes alone will not be sufficient to gain board access. Nurses will need strategic insight on board function and responsibility, including board acumen regarding finance, legal, ethical, safety, and quality issues. The unique characteristics and values that nurses bring to the boardroom can heighten the awareness of how to curb costs without compromising patient safety and clinical quality. Nurses on boards have the necessary clinical expertise and possess the critical business skills that hospital boards require, such as firsthand knowledge of health care delivery, management, informatics, technology, and evidence-based practice expertise, along with an awareness of effective employee retention strategies.

When nurses are fully represented on key boards and commissions, organizations can rest assured that questions on access, quality, and safety are being addressed. It is my belief that hospital boards and influential committees must be balanced with a diversity of skills, background, and knowledge. Nurses have the prerequisite knowledge and responsiveness to secure a seat at the table. It is my hope that each and every U.S. hospital boardroom will have at least one nurse director or trustee. Where are the nurse directors and trustees? Why have hospital governing boards not valued the clinical expertise of nursing? It is no longer appropriate for the CEO, chief of staff, and vice president of medical affairs to be the only voting board members. Nurses are a hospital's most valuable asset and, as such, must actively secure an invitation to the table. Nurses must learn to lobby effectively for committees, commissions, and hospital board appointments to ensure that they have a nurse as director or trustee. Nurses must volunteer themselves or ask a colleague to serve on a board or influential committee.

The only sure way to increase nursing's influence on health policy and quality improvement is by securing seats at these tables. Nurses can no longer wait to be "asked to participate"; they must actively recruit and ask others to assist them in gaining access to circles of influence. Nurses are well positioned to drive strategies that affect cost, quality, and safety because they confront these issues every day. They must learn to reach across the aisle to colleagues in all types of public and private organizational and health care settings. It does not matter if your workplace is the bedside or boardroom, classroom or clinic, or executive suite or the dean's office; each of us is confronted with meeting the daily challenges and priorities of nursing. Day after day, we are reminded of the need to increase the supply and competencies of RNs, expand nursing faculty, promote diversity in the profession, and, last but not least, enhance access to nursing education in rural and underserved areas. The future of nursing and health care delivery requires ongoing strategic planning and the formation of nurse faculty–nurse executive partnerships.

Nurses have an obligation to stay informed, be diligent, and be prepared to carry the dialogue of health care reform beyond the issues of affordability, individual choice, and competition in coverage. For example, nurses can critically analyze health policy proposals, health policies, and related issues from the perspective of consumers, nursing, other health professions, and other stakeholders in policy and public forums, as well as influence policy makers through active participation on committees, boards, or task forces at the institutional, local, state, regional, national, and/or international levels to improve health care delivery and outcomes.

I wish I had understood earlier in my career the importance of how policy—all types of policy—influenced my professional knowledge and my development. It was not until I completed graduate school that I realized how academia, practice, and research are all driven by policy, rules, and regulation. As a novice nurse, I was never really informed about the large role government has in health care. Today, with the passage of the ACA, nurses recognize the importance of knowing how legislation provides access, coverage, and protection to the public.

Being a nurse requires stamina, courage, confidence, and intelligence . . . and much more. The "more" comes with the time you take as you grow and develop from a novice to an expert, pursue an advanced degree, and become board certified or credentialed in your chosen specialty area. I have been a nurse for more than 41 years and would never have imagined that my career would have offered such diversity in terms of positions, opportunities, and contributions. I have devoted my career toward advocating for social justice, equity, and equality in a variety of spheres: public and private; practice and education; at institutional and community levels; and locally, regionally, nationally, and internationally through my leadership, scholarship, and service. As a nurse editor, I use my words to debate and discuss issues of the day important to nurses, nursing, and health care.

With the passage of the ACA and the publication of the IOM report (2011), I know that the nursing profession is on the way to becoming fully embodied. Nurses now are involved in a new vision in building a culture of health that recognizes and addresses the SDH and their present-day contributions to prevention and health promotion efforts. They are developing new programs and implementing bold policies to improve health across the life cycle. Today, the nation understands the importance of primary care that is preventive, patient centered, coordinated, and interprofessional.

Nurses are at the forefront of services offering new models for integrating prevention and health care. They are consistently reaching out to people in need, providing home visits in inner-city high-rises, public libraries, barbershops, and beauty salons. At more than 3 million strong in the United States, nurses are vital to the integrity of the American health care system. I know that nurses have an extensive presence in acute care hospitals, but they also have an extensive community presence. Now, through transitional care and care management, nurses are taking full advantage of their skill sets to build bridges between families, health care settings, and the community resources people need to become and remain healthy. How is the next generation of nurses going to be empowered to adapt to these diverse roles and settings?

As a nurse educator, if I and my fellow nurse faculty colleagues are to be responsive and responsible for educating the workforce, we must consider health issues within a larger context, one that includes the SDH. This holistic view of health also serves nurses well in public and community health departments, where nurse leaders are making and implementing policies that support population health. So, what I would like nurses and society at large to know that I did not know earlier in my own career was that when they hear the word *nurse*, it does not refer to a person in a white uniform with a cap on his or her head in a hospital but, rather, to profoundly capable clinicians, academics, and policy advocates who serve people across the continuum of care in the community and hospital, at multiple levels, and in multidimensional ways. I want to ensure that the next generation of nurses is fully prepared to improve the health of communities and individuals across the life span, through their presence in hospitals, homes, schools, and other vital places where people gather to play, work, worship, and live.

Finally, I offer this advice to new graduate nurses and to nurses in transition: Always stay enthusiastic about why you selected nursing as your profession. Keep that excitement and energy. Keep the passion that you had on the very first day of nursing school. Keep up the Code; make sure your code of conduct sustains integrity and follow your ethical principles. Do not get stuck in the mundane and deceptive cadence of, "This is what I need to do in order to get my job done." Do more than that. Just keeping doing your best. Follow the words of Mahatma Gandhi that I mentioned earlier:

Keep your thoughts positive, because your thoughts become your words. Keep your words positive, because your words become your behavior. Keep your behavior positive, because your behavior becomes your habits. Keep your habits positive, because your habits become your values. Keep your values positive, because your values become your destiny.

If you do this, you will create a career legacy that will be both personally and professionally satisfying. I can promise you that! In my own career, I am still developing as a professional to this day and continuing to create my destiny as I write these words.

■ REFLECTIONS

1. *How do I best represent my values and voice within the nursing profession? In other words, how do I model and manifest what I believe contemporary nursing to be?*
2. *What challenges and/or opportunities can I advocate for on behalf of patients, families, and populations to improve their health?*
3. *What motivates me as a professional nurse? What is my personal and professional moral/ ethical foundation? How does my moral and ethical conduct align with my motivation?*
4. *What is my professional nursing legacy? What do I want to be known for as a nurse? What will my contributions to the profession be?*
5. *Create an action plan to become more involved in health policy. What issues am I most passionate about? Which organizations are doing the kind of advocacy work I would like to be involved in?*

■ REFERENCES

Affordable Care Act. (2010). *Read the act.* Retrieved from http://www.hhs.gov/healthcare/rights/law/index.html

American Nurses Association. (2015). *Code of ethics with interpretive statements.* Silver Spring, MD: Nursebooks.org.

Gandhi, M. (n.d.). Notable quotes. Retrieved from http://www.notable-quotes.com/g/gandhi_mahatma.html

Goldwater, M. & Zusty, M. (1990). *Prescription for nurse effective political action.* St. Louis, MO: Mosby-Year Book.

Hartman, M., Martin, A. B., Benson, J., Catlin, A., & National Health Expenditure Accounts Team. (2013). National health spending in 2011: Overall growth remains low, but some payers and services show signs of acceleration. *Health Affairs, 32*(1), 87–99. doi:10.1377/hlthaff.2012.1206

Institute of Medicine. (2011). *The future of nursing: Leading change, advancing health.* Washington, DC: National Academies Press.

Mahony, D., & Jones, E. J. (2013). Social determinants of health in nursing education, research, and health policy. *Nursing Science Quarterly, 26*(3), 280–284. doi:10.1177/0894318413489186

McBride, M. (1993). *From the president: On being opportunistic.* Nursing Outlook, 41, 275–276.

Naylor, M. D., Bowles, K. H., McCauley, K. M., Maccoy, M. C., Maislin, G., Pauly, M. V., & Krakauer, R. (2013). High-value transitional care: Translation of research into practice. *Journal of Evaluation in Clinical Practice, 19*(5), 727–733. doi:10.1111/j.1365-2753.2011.01659.x

Nickitas, D. M. (2008). Changing the world with words. *Nursing Economic$, 26*(3), 141.

Nickitas, D. M. (2016). Economics and populations primary care. In S. B. Lewenson & M. Truglio-Londrigan (Eds.), *Caring for populations* (pp. 75–87). Burlington, MA: Jones & Bartlett Learning.

Nickitas, D. M., & Feeg, V. (2011). Doubling the number of nurses with a doctorate by 2020: Predicting the right number or getting it right? *Nursing Economics, 29*(3), 109–125.

Nightingale, F. (1860). *Notes on nursing: What it is, and what it is not.* New York, NY: D. Appleton & Co.

Rogers, M. E. (1992). Nursing and the space age. *Nursing Science Quarterly, 5*, 27–34.

Welton, J. M., & Harper, E. M. (2015). Nursing care value-based financial models. *Nursing Economic$, 33*(1), 14–25.

Wilson Pecci, A. (2014). No nurses on your hospital board? Why not? *Health Leaders Media.* Retrieved from http://www.healthleadersmedia.com/nurse-leaders/no-nurses-your-hospital-board-why-not#

World Health Organization. (2008). *Commision on Social Determinants of Health final report: Closing the gap in a generation: Health equity through action on the social determinants of health.* Retrieved from http://apps.who.int/iris/bitstream/10665/43943/1/9789241563703_eng.pdf

CHAPTER TWELVE

Transformed and in Service: Creating the Future Through Renewal

Daniel J. Pesut

Personally and professionally, I believe reflection is a means of renewal. My logic goes something like this: as self is renewed, commitments to service come forward more easily. Renewed commitments to service require attention to mindfulness and reflective practice. Mindful reflective practice begets questions that support inquiry. Such inquiry guides knowledge work and evidence-based care giving. Care giving supports society as knowledge, values, and service intersect. Knowledgeable people and especially knowledgeable nurses provide care that society needs. Creating a caring society is the spirit work of nursing. Creating a caring society starts with nurses caring for themselves and becoming, through reflection, more conscious and intentional in their being, thinking, feeling, doing, and acting. Reflection is a form of "inner work" that results in the energy for engaging in "outer service." Reflection in-and-on action supports meaning-making and purpose management in one's professional life.

—Pesut (2005, p. 1)

■ WHY NURSING?

Why did I become a nurse? I became a nurse because of a commitment to service and caring. I responded to an invitation to explore nursing after it became clear to me that the priesthood was not going to be a path for which I was destined or called. As fate would have it, one of my first jobs was working as an orderly at a nursing home. The year was 1972, and I had just spent six years in the seminary and decided that a vocation to the priesthood was not the right life path. Interesting is the fact that the evening charge nurse at that nursing home, Frank McIlmail, had also decided that a vocation to the Alexian Brothers religious order was not the life path for him. Perhaps it was the similarities in our life stories that served as a foundation for our friendship.

I worked side by side with both Frank and his wife, Judy (who was also an RN), at the nursing home. I believe they recognized I had an aptitude for service and could see things in me I could not see in myself. Friendship, admiration, and respect developed. One day, Frank and Judy asked if I had ever considered a career in nursing. They also suggested that a career as an Army nurse might be a way forward for me. So I responded to the invitation and began to explore the Army student nurse program and nursing as a career. I changed majors from psychology to nursing. I had to take some additional sciences including chemistry, microbiology, and anatomy and physiology. I liked what I was learning and realized that I had an aptitude for caring and service, a life path that was consistent with my gifts and talents. I was accepted into the Army student nurse program, commissioned as a first lieutenant in 1975, served in the Army Nurse Corps for three years, and was in the active reserve for three additional years, where I completed my service as a captain.

I am grateful for the care, attention, advice, friendship, wisdom, and guidance that Frank and Judy provided. I went on to develop an extraordinary career in nursing. Clinical research related to volitional psychosomatic self-regulation gave way to educational research interest in creative thinking, metacognition, and clinical reasoning. Administrative and professional service contributions evolved and developed through time. Eventually, I became president of the Honor Society of Nursing, Sigma Theta Tau International (STTI; 2003–2005). I have had a rich, rewarding 39-year career in nursing and appreciate the fact that being and becoming a nurse activated and sustained my curiosity, creativity, and courage and enabled me to use my strengths and values in a purpose-driven way.

■ EARLY IMPRESSIONS

I entered the Army Nurse Corps toward the tail end of the Vietnam War. I believed that it was important to serve the country, but only if I could do it in a healing–restoring mode, as opposed to a wounding–destructive one. So my intention and vision was to be a healing force in service to a greater good. I am not sure I realized what a nurse really did or all the dimensions of nursing at the time, but I soon learned, through experience, the power of presence, the value of creative thinking, the influence of positive relationships, and how to help patients access their own internal coping and healing capacities.

My first duty station was Brooke Army Medical Center Institute for Surgical Research (ISR) in San Antonio, Texas. I began my career taking care of burn patients and mastered the clinical skill set to care for them. I was not, however, prepared to deal with the patients' emotional or psychological responses to painful debridement procedures, loss of limbs, disfigurement, and painful dressing changes. I also witnessed and marveled at the degree of psychosocial trauma that so many of the patients' families experienced. I was determined to gain more knowledge related to the psychiatric mental health aspects of burn victims, their family members, and health care providers who worked in this specialty area. Because I did not believe I had the knowledge to work with the psychiatric aspects of burn trauma patients, I went back to school. I believe the future happens at the intersection of knowledge and service; if you have the knowledge, you can provide the service.

So I enrolled in a graduate program at the University of Texas Health Science Center School of Nursing and earned a master's degree in psychiatric mental health nursing while working full-time on active duty as a nurse at the Brooke Army Medical Center Burn Unit. One of the deals I struck with my head nurse was that I would work permanent nights and evenings in order to attend school during the day. The fact is that I loved working the evening shift because I was the person in charge and there was more time to talk with patients. The pace of the evening was less hectic than the day shift with its routines, rounds, and endless menu of treatment procedures. I completed the master's degree program in 18 months and had new knowledge, skills, and abilities, and developed the systems-thinking mindset of a clinical nurse specialist.

Equipped with new knowledge, skills, and abilities, I created the first psychiatric clinical nurse specialist position at the burn unit and worked with patients, families, and staff. My clinical experiences with burn care prompted my curiosity about patient self-regulation and coping strategies. I began to ask patients what they did and how they coped with the traumatic treatments that were inflicted on them. I was surprised by what they shared, and this clinical experience prompted my clinical interest in self-regulation research. I wanted to know more about how patients engaged or did not engage their own self-regulation capacities. I was also curious to see if self-regulation strategies could be taught to patients to speed recovery.

■ PROFESSIONAL EVOLUTION/CONTRIBUTION

During the course of my professional career, I have been interested in how the creative process supports personal and professional development, enhances reasoning, and provides a foundation for future thinking. I appreciate the fact that nursing demands curiosity, creativity, and courage. Is it not interesting that the root of the word *curiosity* comes from the Latin *cura*, which means *to care*? Curiosity is a desire to know or learn. Caring and curiosity go hand in hand. If one is curious, he or she is eager to acquire information or knowledge. A desire to learn and know and acquire information about clinical issues that matter enables one to care more effectively. Curiosity by itself is not going to be enough to be successful in a nursing career. Curiosity coupled with creativity and courage can lead to innovations in caring.

Fundamentally, I believe it is vital to challenge and support nurses as they explore the creative process in terms of creating meaningful care plans, generating novel solutions to complex challenges, and planning for the future, as well as helping to support thinking, feeling, and doing. It is in the development of creative thinking skills that people renew commitments to themselves and the people they serve and promote the value of nursing in the world. Creativity is the foundation for clinical research and scholarship in nursing.

Creative thinking skills are vital in the conceptualization of a problem, the development of a line of research, the delivery and dissemination of technology, and the management of human resources (Pesut, 1990). Scientific research activity presupposes creative thinking skills and abilities. Despite the essential role of creative thinking in the development of discipline, some perceive the creative process as a mysterious, magical, and mystical phenomenon. I have come to understand that there is an essential dynamic in the creative process that makes it less mysterious, less mystical, and more tangible. It is a dynamic that nurses manage every day. The essence of creative thinking and creativity is appreciating how opposite or discordant qualities can be reconciled and managed. My career in nursing has provided me a training ground for negotiating and developing paradoxical and polarity management leadership skills (Lavine, 2014; Johnson, 1996), and one of my many professional missions has been to challenge, educate, and support the development of creativity in myself and others.

For example, one of my frustrations with nursing in the mid-1970s was the professional focus on problems rather than solutions. In essence, the old nursing process model was a problem-solving model—assess, plan, implement, and evaluate (APIE). A great deal of time was spent on assessment and defining the problem space. Little attention was given to the idea or notion of outcomes in this early nursing process model. Over time, APIE evolved and gave way to another iteration that involved the notion of diagnosis. At the time, the idea that nurses did any diagnosis was radical! The next-generation nursing process now involved five steps or stages rather than four. APIE developed into assess, diagnose, plan, implement, and evaluate (ADPIE). What troubled me about this was the missing link related to outcomes. Based on my clinical experiences, I realized that outcomes were often the opposite of problems, and if one were to be creative, one would hold the problem and outcome together in the same framework or mental model.

For every nursing diagnosis (problem), there is a nursing outcome (solution). Early in my career, I would observe that nurses would declare or define outcomes as the negative definition of the problem state. For example, "no pain" would be the outcome associated with a diagnosis of "pain." This just did not make sense to me, as it did not support any movement forward to a well-formed outcome, which should be stated in positive terms. So in my mind, if pain is the problem, comfort and pain control is the outcome. This set the stage for me to think about problems and outcomes in a different way and I realized that creative thinking is a core nursing skill to support a patient's transition from a problem state to a desired outcome state.

Creative thinking involves appreciating the contrast between figure and ground, foreground and background, and seeing both at the same time. Polarities exist in every situation. Imagination fuels creative thinking as one oscillates back and forth between problems and solutions, barriers and facilitators, risks and benefits, darkness and light, accepting and rejecting, admitting and denying, allowing and controlling, and healing and irritating. Nurses are constantly called upon to negotiate the tensions that exist between fear and aspiration, scarcity and abundance, compliance and commitment, regret and hope, tolerance and prejudice, unifying and dividing, valuing and exploiting, and illness and health.

Kelso and Engstrom (2006) propose the use of the tilde (~) as a new symbol to represent the complementary nature of paired phenomena. They note that reconciliation of opposed aspects is easier said than done. They provide people with ways to deal with polarization and reconciliation through the creation of a new vocabulary, symbolic representation system, philosophy, and science that help people gain insight into the coordinated pattern dynamics. For example, nursing is a profession that is full of polarities, paradoxes, and complementary natures: life ~ death, pain ~ comfort, nursing ~ negligence, abnormal ~ normal, acceptance ~ rejection, conscious ~ unconscious, dynamic ~ static, expert ~ novice, feeling ~ thinking, mind ~ body, object ~ subject, self ~ other, individual ~ group, passive ~ aggressive, learning ~ forgetting, individual ~ team, work ~ play, defensive ~ offensive, good ~ evil, grief ~ joy, love ~ hate, order ~ disorder.

The dictionary tells us the opposite of nursing is negligence. Nurses are the moral agents and advocates who manage the tension between negligence and nursing on a daily basis. Nurses manage several paradoxes that require sensitivity and insight into the complementary nature of phenomena. Kelso and Engstrom define *complementary nature* as "a set of mutually dependent principles responsible for the genesis, existence and evolution of the universe relating to or suggestive of complementing, completing, or perfecting relationships and being complemented in return" (2006, p. 39).

Thinking of things as contrary or opposite often leads to polarized debate and discourse about either/or, right/wrong thinking and reasoning. Rather than filter and frame the world in terms of duality or contraries, Kelso and Engstrom (2006) argue that contraries are really complementary pairs contained within a greater whole and that valuing the complementary nature of phenomena allows for the reconciliation of opposites, leads to insight, creativity, and understanding, and represents a self-organizing coordination dynamic. In essence, our brains are wired to discern the complementary nature of experience. Complementary pairs are dynamic, and reconciliation leads to a harmonizing and bringing together of that which has previously been considered incommensurate. What I realized is that polarities exist in every situation and reflecting on polarity dynamics has helped me appreciate and value the different stances people take in light of competing commitments.

According to Christopher Johns (2000), the powerful, reflective self is born as one embraces commitment, contradiction, conflict, challenge and support, catharsis, creation, connection, caring, congruence, and constructing personal knowing in practice. *Commitment* involves a belief in oneself and in the value of practice. Commitment requires openness, curiosity, and a willingness to challenge norms and the status quo. *Contradiction* requires negotiation of the tensions that exist between the ideals and the realities of practice. *Conflict* involves managing the tensions that exist between competing commitments and using that tension and energy to create new options. Such conflict can be helpful if challenges are linked with support. *Catharsis* involves working through negative feelings. *Creation* involves holding the tension of contradictions and opposites long enough for something new to emerge from the tension.

Connection involves linking new insights with past learning, bringing past learning to new situations, and connecting the dots associated with pattern recognition and intuition. *Caring* is the energy that fuels desirable practice as an everyday reality. *Congruence* requires alignment of thoughts, feelings, and actions and is facilitated through reflective practice (see Chapter 22 for more information on reflective practice). *Constructing personal knowing* in practice involves spinning and weaving the threads of personal knowledge along with theory to construct knowledge that builds nursing intelligence and scholarship. In terms of scholarship, I think the following quote is constructive: "Identities change in practice as we start doing new things (crafting experiments), interacting with different people (shifting connections), and reinterpreting our life stories through the lens of emerging possibilities (making sense)" (Ibarra, 2003, p. 16).

Barry Johnson (1996) makes a distinction between problems to solve and polarities to manage. Polarity management and polarity leadership (Johnson, 1996;

Wesorick, 2014) support the development of creative systems thinking and community dialogue because polarity management and polarity leadership help people uncover the multiple dimensions, the upsides, and the downsides of polarized stances. When people have different stances on an issue and rely on each other through time, it is important to consider the benefits polarity management has to offer. In many polarized situations, there is a tension between fear and values and problems and principles. Each party in a polarity is likely to have strong beliefs and emotions about its stance. A skilled nurse leader helps unpack the upsides and downsides of each polarized stance in light of two other, often tacit, polarities that are both the greater purpose and the deepest fear. Creating dialogue about the fears and values as well as the greater purposes and deepest fears people harbor in regard to polarized issues is revealing and useful. Mapping polarities is often beneficial in groups so that people come to understand and appreciate the larger frames of reference that are revealed as one acknowledges the deepest fears and greater purposes associated with issues of change, growth, and transformation.

There is an art and science to framing and reframing (Pesut, 1991). I appreciate how the lessons I have learned in my nursing career have enriched my being, thinking, and doing and my development of paradoxical leadership skills. For example, when I am upset or angry at someone or a situation or think that he or she is controlling and/or stubborn, I realize that I have to ask myself, "What in me is being triggered to feel this way? Am I projecting my own anger or stubbornness onto that person? How am I responsible for what is happening to me?" I have come to realize the importance of exploring what it is about that other person that activates issues within me, that requires me to attend to the management of my own emotions and state of consciousness. Elsewhere, I have written about the value and importance of doing both "golden" and "dark" shadow work for personal and professional transformation (Pesut, 2013a).

Cultivation of a polarity management leadership skill set is worth the investment because these skills contribute to nurses' success in organizations (Pesut, 2007; Moody, Horton-Deutsch, & Pesut, 2007). What was not working for me early in my career were the restrictions I saw and experienced when people focused on one aspect of a very complex and complicated situation. I wanted to move beyond situations where people identified the one "right" way to do something, because I could see many ways to approach a situation that could contribute a creative solution. For example, strictly adhering to visiting hour rules and regulations with burn patients made absolutely no sense to me, so I would often find creative ways to flex the rules and enable family members to see patients to provide support and comfort. Such situations often helped the family and the rest of the nursing staff on the unit, as we would know that patients had people close by, providing care and surveillance.

I wanted to find a way to move beyond "either/or" thinking and help people process and develop a "both/and" mindset. As people struggle with the polarities and paradoxes of issues, new insights emerge and creative solutions find their way to the conversation. Creativity and the development of an innovative mindset are what I most want to cultivate in nursing colleagues (Pesut, 2013b, 2013c). As a result of my nursing career, I believe I have come to accept, differentiate, and integrate many aspects of myself and others in a more integral and holistic way (Pesut, 2012a, 2012b, 2012c, 2012d).

When my military service commitment was complete, I accepted a teaching position at the University of Michigan School of Nursing. At Michigan, I teamed up with mentor and colleague, Dr. Jean Wood, and we began a series of investigations related to volitional psychosomatic self-regulation. Recall that during my early nursing career I would ask burn patients what they did inside their heads while the staff performed painful wet to dry dressing changes. I wanted to satisfy my curiosity and see if there were patterns in what people did to help themselves feel better or get better during a recovery episode. My mentor, Jean Wood, was also interested in this self-regulatory mental phenomenon. So we teamed up and developed a number of studies (Wood & Pesut, 1981; Massey & Pesut, 1991; Pesut & Massey, 1992). From these early studies and patient interviews, we developed categories of self-regulation strategies and eventually created an instrument, the Carolina Self-Regulation Inventory (Massey & Pesut, 1991). Norms were established for the inventory. Several PhD students have used the instrument to measure and correlate self-regulation with self-efficacy, weight loss, pain management, and exercise in adolescents. Dr. Wood and I were pioneers in the area of self-regulation and self-management in the early 1980s.

I realized that an academic career best reinforced my strengths, values, skill sets, interests, and aspirations. I enrolled for a PhD in the clinical science program at the University of Michigan and graduated in 1984. By this time, given my teaching experiences, I became focused on self-regulation of student learning and was especially interested in metacognition. My PhD dissertation, *Metacognition: The Self-Regulation of Creative Thought in Nursing* (Pesut, 1984), set the stage for future research, development, and testing of teaching ~ learning innovations that investigated the nature of clinical reasoning skills in nursing (Pesut & Herman, 1992; Pesut & Herman, 1998, 1999; Kuiper & Pesut, 2004).

I believe I am best known for my work in clinical reasoning and nursing education, graduate education in psychiatric mental health nursing, futures thinking, and leadership development in nursing. An invitation to teach clinical reasoning in an undergraduate program at the University of South Carolina resulted in the development of a teaching – learning innovation with colleague Joanne Herman: the Outcome-Present-State Test (OPT) Model of Reflective Clinical Reasoning (OPT model). The clinical thinking of nurses has changed over time and we noted three generations of nursing process evolution and development. We created the OPT model (Pesut & Herman, 1998, 1999) and proposed it as a third generation of nursing process focused on outcome specification and the significance of clinical judgments. I was again able to relate my early interest in juxtaposing problems – outcomes into a meta-model that would guide and support the development of clinical reasoning skills in students and clinicians.

The OPT model has gained national and international reputation. Nurse educators in the United States and in many countries such as Spain, Italy, Iceland, Brazil, Mexico, Taiwan, Thailand, and China have adopted and are using the OPT model. The original book, published in 1999, was translated into Mandarin in 2007. I have worked with a research team to evaluate the teaching ~ learning strategies associated with the model and its impact on student thinking and reasoning. After the OPT Model of Reflective Clinical Reasoning was developed, my research interests shifted from clinical research to research in nursing education. While refining and developing the OPT model, there was the concurrent evolution and development of nursing knowledge classification systems such as the North American Nursing Diagnosis Association (NANDA), Nursing Intervention Classification (NIC), and Nursing Outcome Classification (NOC). The OPT model provides a structure for the use of these nursing classification systems. Research shifted to investigate student use of the OPT and the effect the model had on the development of clinical reasoning skills (Kautz, Kuiper, Pesut, & Dannekar, 2005; Kautz, Kuiper, Pesut & Williams, 2006; Kuiper, Pesut, & Kautz, 2009; Pesut 2004a, 2004b, 2006, 2008).

At Indiana University, my educational research focused on the redesign, development, and evaluation of a graduate program in nursing administration using Problem-Based Learning (PBL) methods (Baker, Pesut, McDaniel, & Fisher, 2007; Baker, McDaniel, Pesut, & Fisher, 2007). As a teacher, one of the most important things I do is help people self-regulate and manage their own creativity and thinking processes. I challenge students to "think about their thinking" and provide strategies and structures for them to build on what they already know through assimilation as they develop and construct new knowledge through accommodation.

With an eye to the future, I believe another significant contribution was authoring a featured column titled "Future Think" (Pesut, 2002a, 2002b, 2002c), which appeared in *Nursing Outlook*, the official journal of the American Academy of Nursing. Over a 5-year period, these 36 editorial think pieces challenged and sensitized members of the profession to reflect on future trends and ponder the nursing consequences of the trends and issues. I continue to prompt reflections through the *Meta-Reflections Blog*, sponsored by the Honor Society of Nursing, STTI.

Some of my most significant contributions to the nursing profession are related to service. I consider my presidency and the years of service on the STTI Board of Directors the highlight of my nursing career (McBride, 2004; Tahan, 2004). While serving on the board of directors of STTI (1997–2005), I was troubled by professional tensions that I experienced and witnessed. I became concerned about an emerging discourse of regret and burnout among nurses in the field. It occurred to me that these individuals were not doing a very good job of taking care of themselves or developing the leadership resilience to withstand the extraordinary stress and pressure nurses experience (Allison-Napolitano & Pesut, 2015).

I began to study the works of Dr. Frederick Hudson (1999), who devoted his life to the study of self-renewal in human growth and development. Dr. Hudson was attracted to this area of study because he was troubled by the decline of confidence and hope he witnessed as people aged. He cites five reasons for such decline. First, he notes, we often get lost in yesterday's decisions and become trapped by those decisions and the choices and consequences that follow. Feeling trapped, we become risk averse. Second, he notes, we are often betrayed by our expectations. Maturity forces us to negotiate youthful expectations with life experience. Third, social systems that once protected us are destabilizing. Fourth, we are inundated by information and random choices and experience a sense of being overwhelmed. Finally, he notes that people are bewildered by complex change because of the disruptions it creates. Thus, we become defensive and resist change to protect ourselves. The combined result of these forces triggers disillusionment and discontent and creates a dialogue of "regret" rather than conversations of "hope."

I have witnessed some nurses give way to the harmful effects of these experienced realities. Some nurses feel victimized, trapped, and burdened by bureaucracies. Social systems that were once protective of nurses and nursing care are destabilizing. Information overload burdens nearly everyone. To some degree, nurses have become disillusioned and defensive, rather than inspired and hopeful about the future. Conversations of regret, rather than hope, center on the theme that things today are not the way they once were or that it is necessary to do more with less. Like Dr. Hudson, I was troubled by what I witnessed. Creating the future through renewal requires awareness, conversation, and action. Yet another polarity emerged for me: How do you help nurses move from a state of burnout and resignation to one of professional engagement, resilience, and renewal?

Every president of STTI crafts a call to action. My presidential call to action for the two-year term (2003–2005) of my Honor Society presidency was "Create the Future through Renewal" (Pesut, 2004c, 2004d). It was a theme that resonated with the membership and focused on self-care, professional development, and a future time orientation. I am humbled that an international award was created in my name, the Daniel J. Pesut Spirit of Renewal Award. This award is given at the STTI convention every two years. I believe professional renewal is vital and my vision was, and continues to be, about finding methods to best inspire people to appreciate value and act in creative ways to realize their full potential. Supporting people in the development of their leadership knowledge, skills, and abilities is important for several reasons, and the quote that begins this chapter best represents my vision-logic related to renewal, reflective practice, and overcoming nursing's challenges to create a caring society.

■ MORAL/ETHICAL FOUNDATION

In terms of moral and ethical foundations, I have come to admire and appreciate the work of Christopher Peterson and Martin Seligman (2004). These scholars have done a masterful job of defining and categorizing character strengths and virtues (Peterson & Park, 2009). Given my propensity for reflection and renewal, meditating on the virtues over and through time has enriched my own understanding, personal development, and nursing practice. The universal virtues that Peterson and Seligman (2004) have defined and classified are wisdom, courage, humanity, justice, temperance, and transcendence. Based on an analysis of history and different cultures, the six virtues identified are valued by moral philosophers and religious leaders throughout the world, and I think they are very consistent with the foundations of nursing practice.

I happen to know that my top 12 character strengths are creativity, ingenuity, originality, fairness, equity, justice, judgment, critical thinking, open-mindedness, wisdom (perspective), self-control, and self-regulation. Interested readers may want to discover their own character strengths and virtues by visiting the Values in Action (VIA) Institute on Character and taking the VIA survey (www.viasurvey.org). Knowing what my most highly valued virtues and character strengths are enables me to manage my professional purpose with positive intentions. Having knowledge of my virtues and strengths informs my nursing practice and provides a foundation for the work that I do as an educator, consultant, coach, and psychiatric mental health nurse.

For many years now, I have been a champion of strengths-based leadership. In fact, in nearly every leadership course I teach, I invite the students to learn about their top five signature strengths (Rath & Conchie, 2008). For example, I am a very *strategic* person, who is invested in *learning, connection,* and *achievement,* and I am an *activator* or *catalyst* for getting things done. Once students discern their strengths, I invite them to reflect and write a paper that describes and explains how their strengths can help them establish trust, compassion, stability, and hope in relationships and people with whom they work. Knowing oneself and intentionally learning about one's character and strengths is the best way to bring virtue ethics to nursing practice.

■ VISION

In his book, *The Spark, the Flame, and the Torch: Inspire Self, Inspire Others, Inspire the World*, Lance Secretan (2010) explains that the essence of leadership is mastery, chemistry, and delivery. *Mastery* requires that people bring learning to the foreground. *Chemistry* involves attention to relationships and deep empathy that awakens inspiration aimed at self and others. *Delivery* answers the question, "Whom are we serving?" Such service requires deep listening in order to discern if people's needs have been met. Building on the notions of polarity, paradox, oppositional tensions, virtues, and strengths, Secretan (2010) cleverly asks people to identify the two most threatening things in the world from their experience and perspective. He calls these "terra-threats" (Secretan, 2010, p. 44). He then asks people to consider the opposite or antidote to the terra-threats and he calls these "terra-fixes" (Secretan, 2010, p. 45). As people consider the threats and fixes, they come to realize that resolving the threats with fixes is an invitation to a personal or professional calling, a spark that can be tended and developed into a flame or torch.

Working through and reflecting on the complementary nature of the threat ~ fix is a spark that deserves attention in terms of every nurse's destiny, calling, and character. I would invite every nurse to create a "why-be-do" statement (http://www.secretan.com/tools/forums/why-be-do_forum) and use it as a blueprint for building a set of leadership skills around a powerful purpose and vision for the future. Once a person has determined his or her "why-be-do" statement, he or she can continue to build on the development of the leadership skill set by getting clear on the talents, strengths, and character assets that support his or her personal and professional sense of self and contribution to the world. Knowing one's character virtues (Peterson & Seligman, 2004) and strengths (Rath & Conchie, 2008) also supports one's destiny, calling, and success.

In order to create the future through reflection, transformation, and renewal, each nurse must take responsibility for doing the inner work required to evolve his or her own consciousness, activate character strengths and virtues, confront personal shadows, heal old wounds, and become self-authoring and self-transforming. Psychologist Robert Kegan (1994) notes that personal and professional transformation takes place as we realize the complexity of subject ~ object relationships. As we grow and develop, we realize differences between self and other; the "me" and "not me." We evolve from self-consciousness to "self ~ other" consciousness. Developmentally, we progress to another level of consciousness he calls "we" or the "socialized mind." Most people's growth and development become arrested at this third level of consciousness. With experience, and as we learn the hidden curriculum of daily life, we grow into fourth-order consciousness that requires the development of a powerful reflective self.

Achievement of fourth-order consciousness results in what Kegan calls a "self-authoring mind" (Kegan, 1994, p. 302). Intentional personal and professional renewal requires this self-authoring mind. Self-authoring individuals view work, school, parenting, therapy, intimate relationships, and citizenship differently than those who operate at the third level of the socialized mind. Kegan (1994) observes that individuals who have arrived at fourth-order consciousness both invent and have a personal passion for their own work, are self-directed and self-correcting, and are inner directed; they do not rely on or wait for others or authorities to prescribe what they do or how they choose to engage in their work. These individuals take initiative and responsibility for what happens to them. They appreciate how systems function and understand the dynamic nature of how individual contributions work toward greater purposes in the context of an organizational whole. Fourth-order consciousness in an educational setting is manifested by self-direction, the exercise of critical and creative systems, and complexity thinking that supports reflection and appreciation of the influence of self, culture, and milieu in the context of personal values and beliefs as well as organizational purposes and goals (Kegan, 1994).

Kegan argues that professional growth and development in a postmodern society may require a fifth order of consciousness or "self-transforming mind." At this level, people integrate polarities and contradictions in their own behavior as they develop and appreciate complexity thinking and engage in the really hard work of psychological and spiritual integration (Richo, 1991). Perhaps it is through the lens of the self-transforming mind that we see how the fifth-order consciousness is interrelated with Ken Wilber's (2007) integral vision.

Fifth-order consciousness or the self-transforming mind supports advanced renewal work. Becoming aware of these levels is a stimulus for conversation and action-oriented development. In fact, the way we talk can transform the way we work (Kegan & Lahey, 2001) if we understand the complexity advantage (Kelly & Allison, 1999). Fourth- and fifth-order consciousness states are things to strive for in the service of renewal and creating a preferred future. As we become more conscious of ourselves and where we are developmentally in meeting daily demands, service to others is enhanced. I believe my nursing career has fueled the development of my consciousness and helped me integrate inner and outer contradictions into appreciating the wisdom of renewal (Pesut, 2008) and valuing a more integral perspective (Pesut, 2012c). My hope for the future is that nurses throughout the world continue to do the inner work that supports the evolution and development of their consciousness, because service to others is enhanced when we ourselves are whole (Pesut, 2001, 2013a, 2015). The power and force of nursing are achieved as each nurse acknowledges his or her needs, strengths, and talents, and uses them to master the complexity leadership skill set that is required to create a 21st-century health care system.

■ REFLECTIONS

1. *What called me to the nursing profession? Was it an intentional choice I made, or was I invited and ordained by the community to consider nursing as a vocation?*
2. *Am I struggling with a polarity or paradox in my life? Consider exploring the polarity with the Squares Technique developed by Leslie Temple-Thurston (2000); http://www.corelight .org/resources/marriage-of-spirit/chapters/chapter-eleven*

3. *How does reflection in and on action support meaning-making and purpose management in my personal and professional life?*
4. *How do I attend to my personal and professional renewal needs?*
5. *To what degree do I believe that the spirit work of nursing is to create a caring society?*

■ REFERENCES

Allison-Napolitano, E., & Pesut, D. J. (2015). *Bounce forward: The extraordinary resilience of nurse leadership.* Silver Springs, MD: American Nurses Association.

Baker, C., McDaniel, A., Pesut, D., & Fisher, M. (2007). Learning skills profiles of master's students in nursing administration: Assessing the impact of problem-based learning. *Nursing Education Perspectives, 28*(4), 190–195.

Baker, C., Pesut, D., McDaniel, A., & Fisher, M. (2007). Evaluating the impact of problem-based learning on learning styles of master's students in nursing administration. *Journal of Professional Nursing, 23*(4), 214–219.

The Honor Society of Nursing, Sigma Theta Tau International. (2003–2005). *Scholarship of reflective practice resource paper (Foreword).* Indianapolis, IN: Sigma Theta Tau.

Hudson, F. (1999). *The adult years: Mastering the art of self-renewal.* San Francisco, CA: Jossey-Bass.

Ibarra, H. (2003). *Unconventional strategies: Working identity for reinventing your career.* Cambridge, MA: Harvard Business Press.

Johns, C. (2000). *Becoming a reflective practitioner.* London, UK: Blackwell Science.

Johnson, B. (1996). *Polarity management: Identifying and managing unsolvable problems.* Amherst, MA: HRD Press.

Kautz, D. D., Kuiper, R. A., Pesut, D. J., Knight-Brown, P., & Daneker, D. (2005). Promoting clinical reasoning in undergraduate nursing students: Application and evaluation of the Outcome Present State Test (OPT) model of clinical reasoning. *International Journal of Nursing Education Scholarship, 2*(1). doi:10.2202/1548-923X.1052

Kautz, D. D., Kuiper, R. A., Pesut, D. J., & Williams, R. L. (2006). Using NANDA, NIC, and NOC (NNN) language for clinical reasoning with the Outcome-Present State-Test (OPT) Model. *International Journal for Nursing Terminologies and Classifications, 17*(3), 129–138.

Kegan, R. (1994). *In over our heads: The mental demands of modern life.* Cambridge, MA: Harvard University Press.

Kegan, R., & Lahey, L. (2001). *How the way we talk can change the way we work: Seven languages for transformation.* San Francisco, CA: Jossey-Bass.

Kelly, S., & Allison, M. A. (1999). *The complexity advantage. How the science of complexity can help your business achieve peak performance.* New York, NY: Business Week Books/McGraw Hill.

Kelso, J., & Engstrom, D. (2006). *The complementary nature.* Cambridge, MA: MIT Press.

Kuiper, R., & Pesut, D. (2004). Promoting cognitive and metacognitive reflective learning skills in nursing practice: Self-regulated learning theory. *Journal of Advanced Nursing, 45*(4), 381–391.

Kuiper, R., Pesut, D., & Kautz, D. (2009). Promoting the self-regulation of clinical reasoning skills in nursing students. *The Open Nursing Journal, 3,* 76–85.

Lavine, M. (2014). Paradoxical leadership and the competing values framework. *Journal of Applied Behavioral Science, 50*(2), 189–205.

Massey, J., & Pesut, D. (1991). Self-regulation strategies of adults. *Western Journal of Nursing Research, 13*(5), 640–647.

McBride, A. (2004). Daniel J. Pesut: Gentleman, creative leader. *Reflections on Nursing Leadership, 30*(1), 16–23.

Moody, R., Horton-Deutsch, S., & Pesut, D. J. (2007). Appreciative inquiry for leading in complex systems: Supporting the transformation of academic nursing culture. *Journal of Nursing Education, 46*(7), 319–324.

Pesut, D. J. (1984). *Metacognition: The self-regulation of creative thought in nursing.* Ann Arbor, MI: University of Michigan.

Pesut, D. J. (1990). Creative thinking as a self-regulatory metacognitive process: A model for education, training, and further research. *Journal of Creative Behavior, 24*(2), 105–110.

Pesut, D. J. (1991). The art, science, and techniques of reframing in psychiatric mental health nursing. *Issues in Mental Health Nursing, 12*(1), 9–18.

Pesut, D. J. (2001). Healing into the future: Recreating the profession of nursing through inner work. In N. Chaska (Ed.), *The nursing profession: Tomorrow and beyond* (pp. 853–865). Thousand Oaks, CA: Sage.

Pesut, D. J. (2002a). Awakening social capital. *Nursing Outlook, 50,* 87–88.

Pesut, D. J. (2002b). Generativity. *Nursing Outlook, 50,* 49.

Pesut, D. J. (2002c). On renewal. *Nursing Outlook, 50,* 135.

Pesut, D. J. (2004a). Epilogue: Toward the future. In L. Haynes, H. Butcher, & T. Boese (Eds.), *Nursing in contemporary society: Issues, trends, and transitions to practice* (pp. 453–457). New Jersey, NJ: Prentice Hall.

Pesut, D. J. (2004b). Reflective clinical reasoning: The development of practical intelligence as a source of power. In L. Haynes, H. Butcher, & T. Boese (Eds.), *Nursing in contemporary society: Issues, trends, and transitions to practice* (pp. 146–162). Upper Saddle River, NJ: Prentice Hall.

Pesut, D. J. (2004c). Create the future through renewal: Presidential call to action. *Reflections on Nursing Leadership, 30*(1), 24–25.

Pesut, D. J. (2004d). The work of belonging (Invited editorial). *Journal of Nursing Scholarship, 36*(1), 2.

Pesut, D. J. (2005). Foreword to *The scholarship of reflective practice* (resource paper). Retrieved from https://www.nursingsociety.org/docs/default-source/position-papers/resource_reflective.pdf?sfvrsn=4

Pesut, D. J. (2006). 21st century nursing knowledge work: Reasoning into the future. In C. Weaver, C. W. Delaney, P. Weber, & R. Carr (Eds.), *Nursing and informatics for the 21st century: An international look at practice, trends and the future* (pp. 13–23). Chicago, IL: Health Care Information and Management Systems Society (HIMSS).

Pesut, D. J. (2007). Leadership: How to achieve success in nursing organizations. In C. O'Lynn & R. Tranbarger (Eds.), *Men in nursing: History, challenges and opportunities* (pp. 153–168). New York, NY: Springer.

Pesut, D. J. (2008). The wisdom of renewal. *American Nurse Today, 3*(7), 34–36.

Pesut, D. J. (2012a). Transforming inquiry and action in interdisciplinary health professions education: A blueprint for action. *Interdisciplinary Studies Journal, 1*(4), 53–63.

Pesut, D. (2012b). Self-renewal. In H. R. Feldman, R. Alexander, M. J. Greenberg, M. Jaffee-Ruiz, A. McBride, M. McClure, & T. D. Smith (Eds.), *Nursing leadership: A concise encyclopedia* (pp. 337–338). New York, NY: Springer.

Pesut, D. J. (2012c). An introduction to integral philosophy and theory: Implications for quality and safety. In G. Sherwood & S. Horton-Deutsch (Eds.), *Reflective practice: A framework for engaging learners in education and practice* (pp. 247–264). Indianapolis, IN: Sigma Theta Tau International Press.

Pesut, D. J. (2012d). Reflecting as a team: Issues to consider in interprofessional practice. In G. Sherwood & S. Horton-Deutsch (Eds.), *Reflective practice: A framework for engaging learners in education and practice* (pp. 265–282). Indianapolis, IN: Sigma Theta Tau International Press.

Pesut, D. J. (2013a). Evolving awareness. In C. Coleman (Ed.), *Man up: A practical guide for men in nursing* (pp. 181–202). Indianapolis, IN: Sigma Theta Tau International Press.

Pesut, D. J. (2013b). Creativity and innovation: Thought and action. *Creative Nursing, 19*(3), 164–165.

Pesut, D. J. (2013c). The innovation equation: Building creativity and risk taking in your organization by Jacqueline Byrd and Chris Brown. *Creative Nursing, 19*(3), 114–121.

Pesut, D. J. (2015). Avoiding derailment: Leadership strategies for identity, reputation and legacy management. In J. Daly, S. Speedy, & D. Jackson (Eds.), *Leadership & nursing contemporary perspectives* (2nd ed., pp. 251–261). Chatswood, New South Wales, Australia: Churchill Livingston.

Pesut, D. J., & Herman, J. (1992). Metacognitive skills in diagnostic reasoning: Making the implicit explicit. *International Journal of Nursing Terminologies and Classifications, 3*(4), 148–154.

Pesut, D. J., & Herman, J. (1998). OPT transformation of the nursing process for contemporary nursing practice. *Nursing Outlook, 46*(1), 29–36.

Pesut, D. J., & Herman, J. (1999). *Clinical reasoning: The art and science of critical and creative thinking.* New York, NY: Delmar.

Pesut, D. J., & Massey, J. (1992). Self-management of recovery: Implications for nursing practice. *Journal of the American Academy of Nurse Practitioners, 4*(2), 58–62.

Peterson, C., & Park, N. (2009). Classifying and measuring strengths of character. In S. J. Lopez & C. R. Snyder (Eds.), *Oxford handbook of positive psychology* (2nd ed., pp. 25–33). New York, NY: Oxford University Press.

Peterson, C., & Seligman, M. E. P. (2004). *Character strengths and virtues: A handbook and classification.* Washington, DC: American Psychological Association, and New York, NY: Oxford University Press.

Rath, T., & Conchie, B. (2008). *Strengths based leadership.* New York, NY: Gallup Press.

Richo, D. (1991). *How to be an adult.* New York, NY: Paulist Press.

Secretan, L. (2010). *The spark, the flame, and the torch: Inspire self, inspire others, inspire the world.* Caledon, Ontario, Canada: The Secretan Center.

Tahan, H. (2004). Leader to watch: Daniel J. Pesut, APRN BC FAAN. *Nurse Leader, 2*(3), 10–14.

Temple-Thurston, L. (2000). *The marriage of spirit: Enlightened living in today's world.* Santa Fe, NM: Core Light.

Wesorick, B. L. (2014). Polarity thinking: An essential skill for those leading interprofessional integration. *Journal of Interprofessional Healthcare, 1*(1), 12.

Wilber, K. (2007). *The integral vision: A very short introduction to the revolutionary integral approach to life, God, the universe, and everything.* Boston, MA: Shambhala.

Wood, D. J., & Pesut, D. J. (1981). Self-regulatory mental phenomenon and patient recovery. *Western Journal of Research in Nursing, 3*(3), 263–271.

CHAPTER THIRTEEN

Sacred and Transpersonal: Realizing Self in Truth, Goodness, and Beauty

Janet Quinn

In this age of modern technology, we are provided with a seemingly inexhaustible array of gadgets, machines, chemotherapeutic agents, and other tools for nursing intervention. . . . Yet, there is another tool . . . that has, perhaps, the greatest potential for helping/healing. That tool is . . . our own "self."
—Quinn (1981, p. 201)

■ WHY NURSING?

Green. Yellow. Red. Green. Yellow. Red. Green. Yellow. Red. A rhythmic dance of traffic lights reflecting on the wall of my hospital room lulled 11-year-old me into restless sleep. Lonely and frightened, kept in isolation, I found their predictability soothing company as my young body struggled to heal from very serious pneumonia. It was the first experience of nurses that provided me with examples of what I aspired to be, and what I did not. "When I am a nurse," I vowed, "I will be like the nice one who comes and sits and talks to me, not the mean one who doesn't care and never smiles."

For as long as I can remember, I wanted to be a nurse. I did not receive any pressure in this direction as a young girl, despite the era in which I grew up. In fact, it was the opposite. As I grew old enough to start pursuing my dream of becoming a nurse by first being a candy striper, I was encouraged by my parents to consider medicine instead. "You're a smart girl, you could be a doctor. Why do you want to be *just* a nurse?" There it was, the "*just* a nurse" phrase. Although I appreciated the break with the prevailing stereotypes about what girls and women could and could not do, I nevertheless found the question perplexing—could they not see that these were two entirely different paths? "I want to be *with* the patients, not just passing through or talking from the doorway looking at the chart," I responded, with a hint of irritation, as if it were so obvious that the question need never be asked again. But of course it was, and is, and the phrase "*just* a nurse" is uttered even by nurses themselves, which always breaks my heart. "I'm *just* a nurse," as if being a nurse is some lesser thing, some inferior thing, something that you would only do if you were not "smart enough to be a doctor."

I persisted in my call, despite the advice, and in time went to the Hunter-Bellevue School of Nursing at Hunter College, joining one of the first BSN classes there. I worked all the way through the program, first as a nurse's aide, and then as a licensed practical nurse (LPN) when I had completed enough nursing courses to pass the LPN boards. My examples of the kind of nurse I wanted to be, and the one I did not want to be, continued to accumulate. But unfortunately, so did the evidence that nursing's profoundly beautiful and caring work carried very little status with it, and an identity of "*just* a nurse" worked its way into my psyche.

I remember vividly one such instance. As an LPN on a medical–surgical unit, I had been assigned a patient to care for who was described as "stably unstable." I found her in a miserable heap in the middle of the bed. Her sheets were damp with sweat. Her skin was pale, cool, and clammy. Her vital signs were erratic and this was, apparently, "just how it was." I took my time. I talked with her. I opened the blinds so she could see outside. I listened to her story as I gave her a warm bed bath and rubbed her back. I soaked her feet in a basin of warm water and applied powder between her toes. Of course, I changed the sheets, repositioned her, and rechecked her vital signs. When I was done, she was sitting up in bed, smiling, pink-cheeked, vital signs normal.

The physicians arrived just then to make rounds. I stepped away from the bedside, in the familiar deference. The attending physician began describing the patient's symptoms and touched her arm as he was explaining to the group that the patient's skin was always clammy. But he pulled away, stopped mid-sentence, feeling her warm skin. He touched her again, in disbelief, all along her arm. After numerous other observations, he was thoroughly perplexed at her improved and stable condition. The patient offered that she "had a very good nurse today," glancing in my direction.

The physicians turned in a group to go, the attending one still shaking his head in puzzlement. "Well then," he chuckled over his shoulder as they were leaving, "it must have been all that TLC." And they exited the room, laughing. Laughing! Laughing at his clever joke. Laughing at even the thought that good nursing, authentic caring, time, and presence could actually make such a difference. Laughing when, really, a bowed head and a moment of silence in the presence of mystery would have been more appropriate. My face turned hot and scarlet. I was after all, *just* a nurse, *just* a nurse. I am not the first nurse to notice this. As Florence Nightingale noted, "Would you do nothing, then, in cholera, fever, etc.?—so deep-rooted and universal is the conviction that to give medicine is to be doing something, or rather everything; to give air, warmth, cleanliness, etc., is to do nothing." Nightingale was clear in her delineation between medicine and nursing: "The reply is . . . that the exact value of particular remedies and modes of treatment is by no means ascertained, while there is universal experience as to the extreme importance of careful nursing in determining the issue of the disease" (Nightingale, 1860/1969, p. 9).

■ EARLY IMPRESSIONS

I graduated from the Hunter–Bellevue School of Nursing in 1972 and spent the summer with my recently relocated family in Northridge, California. I began work in a busy emergency department (ED), which was the receiving ED for the entire San Fernando Valley. I loved the pace, the challenge, and the raucous good times our 3 to 11 p.m. shift shared after work. After passing the state boards, I returned to New York and worked in a medical intensive care unit (ICU).

Initially, I loved working in the ICU. Nurses were, by and large, respected for their knowledge and experience, especially by the new medical students who rotated through each semester. But bit by bit, my enchantment began to wear off, and the underbelly began to become more apparent. I found the work intensely interesting, and the learning process unending, but something was missing, and something was hurting.

I began to notice that although the nurses were often technically brilliant, many were not present for patients. Whether it was a form of self-protection or the result of too much to do and too little time, I do not know. The physicians were no better and often worse. Most appalling to me were the times when a semicomatose or unconscious patient would be left lying utterly naked in the big open room that was the ICU, covered only by tubes and dressings, as procedures were performed and often observed by the circle of students around the bed. I remember being horrified to witness this reduction of a human being to the status of an "it," instead of a "thou," stripped of humanity and dignity along with clothing and sheets.

And then one day, it happened. I became that nurse. The nurse I said I would never be. The nurse who left the patient exposed, just trying to get the job done, the one who was highly competent technically and had forgotten, even for just that moment, the most basic human, moral stance. My heart broke in that moment of awareness. I knew I needed to leave the ICU and to either find another way or leave nursing for good. Without knowing what I would do next, I resigned. Soon after, I found a position as a medical–surgical nursing instructor in a diploma nursing program and discovered that I loved teaching. The next year, I started graduate school at New York University (NYU) and life began all over again.

■ PROFESSIONAL EVOLUTION/CONTRIBUTION

I was unprepared for the radical shift in paradigm that studying with Martha Rogers would require. The study, reading, writing, and discussions with faculty and colleagues were profoundly mind-expanding and formative for all my future work. In addition to the most cutting-edge nursing literature, I was also exposed to the seminal ideas of Carl Rogers, Sidney Jourard, Laurence Le Shan, Abraham Maslow, Rollo May, and Milton Mayeroff, among so many others. I was increasingly drawn toward the exploration of "the farther reaches of human nature" as Maslow (1971) called it, and especially to the powerful role that the actual person/self of the nurse could play in healing.

In *The Transparent Self,* psychologist Sidney Jourard writes that

professional training [of nurses and doctors] encourages graduates to wear a professional mask, to limit their behavior to the range that proclaims their professional status. . . . Patients are exposed not to *human beings* who have expertise, but to "experts" who are dehumanized and dehumanizing. . . . [This] cannot be health-engendering, either for the patient or the professional. (Jourard, 1971, p.178, emphasis in original)

My own experience was reflected back to me in the words. I submitted my first paper for publication during my final semester, which I called "The 'Self' in Nursing Practice" (Quinn, 1975). Reviewers found "much of the theory not new," and the paper was rejected.

My studies at NYU eventually brought me to a new course entitled "Frontiers of Nursing," in which Dr. Dolores Krieger would be teaching therapeutic touch (TT) for the first time. I struggled with the content for many weeks and nearly dropped the class before my own experience, as a recipient of TT, blew open my heart and mind. I pursued learning TT in earnest, completed the course, and graduated. Just a few months later, my mother was diagnosed with metastatic colon cancer and I moved to California to take care of her at home until she died six months later.

Throughout my mother's illness, I used TT to help with managing her pain and other symptoms with unexpected success. There were many experiences I shared with my mother, during TT and at other times, that did not fit conventional models of "reality" but that were easily understood using Rogers's framework (1970, 1990), among other emerging understandings of human nature and consciousness. I will share just one incident because it informed the rest of my life and my career.

One day I was sitting by my mother's bed. She was in a deep sleep, as she had been for days, slipping further and further away. Whether it was out of boredom or curiosity I do not remember, but I decided to try to administer TT to her without moving in my chair. I decided to simply follow the steps of TT only in my mind, visualizing myself going through the motions. I first centered myself, made the intention to be an instrument for healing, and then began the treatment in my mind's eye, remaining still, as I had been. Suddenly my mother's eyes fluttered open and she turned her head toward me. "You make it so much easier," she said, looking directly into my eyes. Then she smiled softly and went back to sleep. Those were the last words she spoke to me.

After my mother's death, I found myself in a true existential crisis. I could either accept that all the experiences I had and that we shared were "real," which meant that my old, mechanistic worldview was essentially and finally shattered, or I had to deny my own reality, rationalize it away, and label the experiences as "nothing more" than an interesting, but essentially meaningless, string of stunning coincidences, anomalies, and anecdotes. I chose the former and soon began doctoral studies at NYU with one intention: to learn how to do research so that I could study TT scientifically. I wanted to deepen my understanding of consciousness, healing, and what was happening in TT. It was also my hope that I could help to demonstrate the efficacy, if not the mechanism, of TT in language and methods acceptable to the mainstream health care system and thus bring this gentle healing art, literally, into the hands of every nurse who wanted to learn it.

Returning to NYU, my mind and conceptual frameworks continued to expand. During this time, I published my first book chapters (Quinn, 1979a, 1981) and a paper in the *American Journal of Nursing* called "One Nurse's Evolution as a Healer" (Quinn, 1979b). These earliest publications began framing several areas of inquiry, scholarship, and practice that would inform and direct the path of my evolving career: namely, healing as a distinct construct from curing, and the farther reaches of the therapeutic/healing relationship, including the self in nursing practice.

In or around 1976, I had started teaching a new course at the Hunter–Bellevue School of Nursing entitled "Alternative Forms of Healthcare," which I continued teaching when I returned from California. There was minimal but growing literature in nursing about these therapies, including TT, though many nurses experienced rejection or even ridicule when trying to bring the interventions into their work. This was long before the 1993 *New England Journal of Medicine* paper that showed for the first time how much money people were paying for "alternative therapies" out of pocket (Eisenberg et al., 1993). After that paper, alternative therapies, previously dismissed as worthless at best and fraudulent quackery at worst, suddenly became mainstream. But nursing's early contribution to the development and use of these caring-healing modalities remained virtually invisible as medical schools and hospitals set up new centers for complementary and alternative medicine (CAM), employing a host of "alternative practitioners," sans nurses.

My doctoral dissertation, completed in 1982, was titled *An Investigation of the Effects of Therapeutic Touch, Done Without Physical Contact, on the State Anxiety of Hospitalized Cardiovascular Patients.* The focus of the study was on *mechanisms* of action rather than *outcomes*, with a goal of contributing to the development and testing of a comprehensive theory to explain, describe, and predict about the phenomenon of TT.

This was the first study in the field to use a mimic treatment to control for the effects of presence, suggestion, and the placebo and Hawthorne effects. The control treatment consisted of having nurses who were not TT practitioners mimic the movements of TT. To control for the variable of healing intention in the mimic, nurses did the process known as "serial sevens," counting backward from 100 by sevens while they went through the movements of TT. Prior to commencing the study, it was found that a panel of naïve observers were unable to distinguish between mimic and TT treatments, thus the mimic/sham was validated as a control for the real intervention (Quinn, 1984a).

Soon after graduation, I was recruited to become the head of the department of medical–surgical nursing at the University of South Carolina College of Nursing in Columbia, South Carolina. We created a new clinical major in the graduate program with two advanced nurse training grants from the U.S. Department of Health and Human Services. It was both exhilarating and shocking to me to get the grant, the first for which I was the principal investigator.

During the same time period, I was working toward getting new investigator funding to continue my research in TT. Virtually everyone I asked advised against that plan. "Do some *normal*, noncontroversial research and get your track record established, and then you can study what you want." I almost went that way, until the day when a student or a colleague, I cannot remember which, said, "If you're not going to study TT, who is?" I wrote the grant to take the next step in developing and testing an explanatory theory for TT and received what was the first federal funding to study TT. *Therapeutic Touch and Anxiety in Pre-op Cardiac Patients* was funded for three years by the U.S. Department of Health and Human Services, Division of Nursing Research, in 1984 (Quinn, 1989a).

In 1987, I received a summer research fellowship award from the Medical University of South Carolina to explore *Immunologic Correlates of Hands-on-Healing*. This provided the laboratory and the expertise for conducting a small pilot study, funded by the Institute of Noetic Sciences, entitled *Psychophysiologic Correlates of Hands-on-Healing*. The study was conducted within a unitary framework and so both the "healers" and the "healees" were studied. Selected immunological and psychological measures were taken and then the data were examined for patterns of response within and between the participants, including between healers and healees. There were several very interesting findings with implications for future research (Quinn & Strelkauskas, 1993). Particularly fascinating to me was the observation that healer–healee pairs estimated how much time had elapsed during any particular treatment session in a shared response pattern. If one overestimated, the other did as well. In another session, the same pair might underestimate amount of time and so on. So, it was not a fixed response pattern. Because perception of time passing is an indicator of states of consciousness, I reasoned that this might be a measure of the resonance/synchronization of consciousness/energy fields between healers and healees (Quinn, 1992b).

As the research unfolded, I continued to write about TT with a particular focus on framing a research agenda that might be useful in advancing the science (Quinn, 1984b, 1986a, 1986b, 1988, 1989b). I also continued to respond to invitations to speak about TT research and/or practice around the country and in Canada and eventually around the world. Consultation activities also grew during this time, including being the outside reader for master's and doctoral work on TT at a variety of universities. Grappling with the question of appropriate research methods for TT research, I developed a schema for deciding whether descriptive or experimental methods were appropriate for a given research question. This became the foundation for a book chapter entitled "Quantitative Methods: Descriptive and Experimental" (Quinn, 1986c).

I began to participate in interdisciplinary panels and think tanks focused on how research could be done on complementary and alternative therapies, like TT, and on the broader constructs of the nature of healing and the inner mechanisms of the healing response, a focus defined by Brendan O'Regan at the Institute of Noetic Sciences. These conferences stimulated work that was eventually published as a book chapter (Quinn, 1989c) and a journal article entitled "On Healing, Wholeness and the Haelan Effect" (Quinn, 1989d), in which I first proposed that healing is the emergence of right relationship at/between/among any one or more complex and multidimensional levels of the whole person. Healing, at whatever level, does not require curing, impacts the whole body-mind-spirit, and is the manifestation of the intrinsic capacity for self-healing that I call the *Haelan effect* or the *Haelan response*.

During one conference trip, I had the very good fortune to meet Dr. Jean Watson (see Chapter 16), who had recently inaugurated the Center for Human Caring (CHC) at the University of Colorado. It was love at first sight. We thoroughly enjoyed comparing our theories and seeing the deep congruence between her caring concepts and my work in healing. Shortly after this meeting, Jean invited me to join the faculty at the CHC and I exuberantly accepted.

The CHC created and offered a variety of programs and projects, among them a focused care for the caregivers program and the Human Caring Certificate Program, in which I taught until it ended in 2011. We were successful in obtaining significant funding from the U.S. Department of Health and Human Services, Division of Advanced Nurse Training, for the Denver Nursing Project in Human Caring (DNPHC). This was a stunningly beautiful exemplar of what caring theory–guided nursing practice could offer to a community in desperate need. The DNPHC was a nurse-managed center for people living with HIV/AIDS (before the introduction of antiretroviral drugs), offering the full range of caring–healing modalities and case management in a homelike, community-based setting.

It was through the work at DNPHC and my previous study that my own model for a clinical practice evolved in 1991, which I called HaelanWork™: Integrative Healing for Body, Mind, and Spirit. HaelanWork is an integrated approach to healing rather than a specific intervention or set of treatments. It was also designed in response to what I believed to be dangerously misguided notions that were being called "holistic" or "new age." The fundamental assumptions of HaelanWork are:

1. We are not *responsible for* our illnesses but we are called to be *responsive to* them.
2. *All* curing and healing emerge from within our own unique body-mind-spirit, at times assisted by medicines, surgery, and/or other therapies, but not due to them.
3. Acknowledging that as whole people, we are body, mind, and spirit, and that spirit is always about mystery unfolding, we also acknowledge that our healing is fundamentally mysterious, beyond our control and manipulation, yet *open to our conscious participation and intention.*

The teaching, speaking, research, writing, and practice of TT also continued, and in 1992, the CHC and I published the first volume of a teaching videotape series entitled *Therapeutic Touch: Healing Through Human Energy Fields* with the National League for Nursing. This first volume, *Theory and Research*, was followed by Volume II, *The Method*, and Volume III, *Clinical Applications*. The final product in the series was produced in 1996. *Therapeutic Touch: A Video Home Study Course for Family Caregivers* evolved out of my deep desire to help other people "make it so much easier" for their loved ones who were in need of help/healing. Some years ago, through a funded project, I had seen that it was entirely possible to teach lay people, in this case, senior citizens, how to do TT for each other with wonderful effects for both the healers and the healees (Quinn, 1992a, 1992b).

The work in TT did not proceed without its critics, both within and outside of the discipline. The most vociferous waged a relentless campaign of attack and misinformation, beginning around 1991, which culminated in two levels of review at the University of Colorado Health Sciences Center, where a colleague and I were teaching TT. The Committee on Therapeutic Touch, which included three basic scientists from within the university and two external nurse researchers, was appointed by the chancellor on the recommendation of the first reviewers.

When I was summoned to meet with the committee, I felt like I imagined Galileo must have felt. Having been worn down by the years of assault (so many "war stories" could be told here), I had some time earlier shifted from fighting to surrendering to what was, reminding myself frequently that I needed to "let go of the outcome," because I was not in control of it. One day, on the treadmill trying to move the heavy energy, a new impulse suddenly arose and I knew exactly what I needed to do. Only in hindsight would I recognize that I had been trying to let go of the outcome before I had fully discerned and completed right action in right timing.

I intended to refocus the discussion from the anticipated critique and defense of the energy field hypothesis to what was really at stake in even the existence of the committee. I developed a paper (Quinn, 1994) that I hoped would frame the issues correctly, respond to the misinformation with facts, justify the right of researchers to derive and test hypotheses from axiomatic statements that might not (yet) be testable, and most fundamentally, give the committee the information it needed to protect the nursing faculty's academic freedom. This they did, issuing their conclusions and recommendations in July of 1994.

The report opened with a thorough discussion of academic freedom as it is defined and developed in the Laws of the Regents, concluding that there was no evidence of any activities that would warrant abridging the rights of the nursing faculty body to define its focus or to design and teach its curriculum. In fact, they wrote:

> Therefore, the creation of special committees to respond to public criticism of activities such as the teaching of TT should not be used as the instrument of interference or pressure. This committee thus wishes to make explicit that the teaching of TT is protected by the academic freedom set forth by the Regents. Furthermore, the regularly constituted bodies within the School of Nursing that review curriculum content and clinical practice are fully adequate to perform these functions, without interference or pressure from within or without the University. (Claman, 1994, p. 4)

The committee noted, as have I and virtually all TT researchers, that the scientific basis/mechanism for TT was not yet established satisfactorily and that more data on efficacy were required to establish TT as a unique healing modality. More importantly, they also noted that we had not gone beyond the data or misrepresented the current state of the science in any of our course materials, brochures, or publications. Very helpful suggestions for future research were offered in the last part of the report and the faculty were encouraged to pursue them: "With these considerations in mind, the Committee believes that the School of Nursing could establish Therapeutic Touch as a beneficial adjunct treatment to work along with regular medical and nursing care" (Claman, 1994, p.10). TT at the University of Colorado had survived the assault.

However, if I am to be totally honest here—and why bother being anything else?— I have to say that something in me did not. Fortunately, a local foundation head with a deep interest in consciousness and healing had been watching the unfolding from a distance and asked to meet with me soon after the University of Colorado committee released its findings. The result was a leadership award, offered through the Institute for the Study of Subtle Energy and Energy Medicine, that allowed me to take a six-month paid leave from the university, explicitly to *not do*, but to rest, recover, and renew. It felt like a miracle and exactly what was needed. I am forever grateful.

Following the end of the leave, I reduced my commitment at the university to allow for more time for *nondoing*, something I had grown to prize during my time apart. I also wanted more time for consulting, speaking, writing, private practice, and spiritual development. In 1997, prompted by the observation that so many of the issues that arose in my private practice were essentially spiritual, I began a training program to learn spiritual direction, and fell in love all over again. Being a companion to people as they engage with their deepest, most intimate interiority is an extraordinary privilege and true delight. After completing the program, I added spiritual direction to the services I offered in my practice and also began teaching and writing more about the spiritual dimensions of health and healing.

Today, in addition to consulting, speaking, and writing about integrative nursing, spirituality, healing, and so forth (e.g., Quinn, 2014a, 2014b, 2014c; 2016), I continue to have an active practice in InterSpiritual Spiritual Direction/Guidance, where I companion people from any, or no, faith tradition. I found myself once again relying on knowledge gained from my time with Martha Rogers and all the years of study since, in being open to trying this very intimate work by phone and Skype when I was asked. It works incredibly well. There is no separation in unity and so I have the privilege of working with people all over the world.

■ MORAL/ETHICAL FOUNDATION

Sidney Jourard (1971) writes, "Nursing is a special case of loving" (p. 207). Truth. Goodness. Beauty. Striving to serve these three provides the moral and ethical ground for my life and my work. Earlier in this chapter, I told the story of my mother's last words to me: *You make it so much easier.* This was an exquisite moment of truth, unfolded from goodness, and profoundly beautiful. I still remember the immense impact of those words. It was as though her utterance was a final blessing, a benediction and affirmation that all I had done to care for her over the six months of her illness and dying was not only enough but exactly what had been needed. My mother reconfirmed that once she had passed, or at least that is how it seemed to me when she came to me in a dream three nights after her death.

In the days following her passing, I was left with one niggling concern and it was about whether I had medicated her adequately near the end; whether my perspectives/biases about consciousness during dying had allowed her to suffer or struggle more than might have been necessary. The worry created an agitation of my spirit. In the dream, I saw my mother, who appeared immeasurably large. I put my question to her, telling her that I had been so worried. She said immediately, exuberantly, "No, no, you did everything right! Don't worry! I am so happy, I am so happy!" She was all radiant light and love and the joy was beyond oceanic.

When I awoke, I was completely at peace. I had not failed in fulfilling my sacred trust. This knowing filled my entire being—body-mind-spirit—with a deep sense of satisfaction and profound equanimity, even in the midst of my grief. I had a most extraordinary sense of having completed some singular purpose or mission—some would say karma—for my life. I wrote in my journal several months later that, "Whatever else I achieve in my life will be icing; *this* was the cake. My life has mattered."

I had succeeded in making the way easier for my mother in her final passage, not just a little easier, but *so much* easier, she had said. Nightingale (1860/1969) guides us that our work is to "put the patient in the best condition for Nature to act on him" (p. 133)—in other words, to make it easier for nature to heal. In the end, what else is it that we are trying to do as nurses? Is this not what we want for all in our care? And is this not a fine moral/ethical foundation for nursing practice: the willingness to bring the fullness of our limited, imperfect humanity into the service of life, to make the way easier for all beings? I often refer to this approach to life and work as *the most beautiful way of the healer*. Anthropologist/shaman Angeles Arrien writes that the one who is called to the way of the healer is the one who "pays attention to what has heart and meaning" (Arrien, 1993, p. 49).

The healer seeks truth, aligns with goodness/love, and creates sublime beauty in acts of selfless compassion that ease the way for others. The American Nurses Association's (ANA; 2015) *Code of Ethics for Nurses With Interpretive Statements* states in Provision 1: "The nurse practices with compassion and respect for the inherent dignity, worth, and unique attributes of every person" (p. 1). There it is, in the first ten words of our code of ethics—we are called to practice with compassion. We are called to be nurse-healers.

Through our compassion, called "love" by Nightingale, Jourard, Watson, and others, and all of our being, doing, and knowing as nurses, we make it easier: easier for persons, communities, and our planet to remain healthy; and easier for healing to emerge and for dying to unfold with grace, dignity, and the least amount of pain possible. (See Chapter 20 for more on nursing as love in action.) We seek relentlessly to ease suffering and to support growth and development. We do our absolute best to meet despair with hope and triumph with genuine joy. We continue to seek truth at so many levels, including the use of all ways of knowing and educating ourselves so that we can bring the richness and possibility of best evidence into the service of healing. We meet one person after the next with the profound goodness and beauty of an open mind and heart that says, "Yes, I see you, I hear you, and I am here for you. I am your nurse. You matter to me." Can you think of anything more true, good, and beautiful than this?

And so, with Nightingale, I encourage every nurse to "strive to awaken the divine spirit of love in yourself, to awaken it in doing your present work, however you may have erred in the past" (Nightingale, as cited by Calabria & Macrae, 1994, p. 96). I encourage this not just because it serves others, but because it is in this one movement that our own hearts and deepest selves can be fulfilled. And it is not just the spirit of ordinary love I speak of, but the spirit of *selfless* love.

> Selfless love is the highest expression of human nature that has not been obscured and distorted by the manipulations of the ego. Selfless love opens an inner door that renders self-importance, and hence fear, inoperative. It allows us to give joyfully and to receive gratefully. (Ricard, 2003, p. 144)

Yet encouragement is not enough. Nurses need and deserve active help to do this. If compassion is an ethical requirement for professional practice, then helping nurses to learn the skills that can allow them to become competent in this capacity is what the profession owes the nurse. Nursing education, new nurse orientations, nursing practice environments, and professional organizations must, to be in moral/ethical integrity and to ensure that patients are treated with compassion, assist nurses in connecting with, understanding, living from, and caring for the compassionate self that is the nurse-healer. A role cannot provide caring, compassion, and love. Only a whole person, a whole healed/healing/wounded healer self, can do that: the self in nursing practice. The fullness of this potentiality has yet to be achieved in health care, but remains as a light, an archetype of inspiration, drawing us ever closer to the deep heart of truth, goodness, and beauty that is nursing.

■ VISION

In 1989 I wrote:

> There is an enormous amount of dialogue today about how to fix the health-care system. . . . I suggest that perhaps there is nothing to fix, since there *is* no *healthcare* system. What is required is something entirely new, with a new focus, a new consciousness, and very different practitioners. (Quinn, 1989d, p. 555)

My work for more than three decades has been dedicated to the creation of what I have called a true *healing health care system*, one that values caring and healing of the whole person as much as the curing of diseases, and where all people have access to the full range of both healing and curing modalities. It would be holistic and integrative, and I think we may finally be on the verge of it.

All that does not work and that is not sustainable in the current *sick-cure system* has become painfully clear. The evolving national conversation, the new laws, and the political positioning and punditry are all signs that the status quo is quaking. The discourse is happening. The search for something very different is on and nurses have been called to be at the table and are essential to the dialogue (Robert Wood Johnson Foundation, 2010).

Part of the conversation is the growing multidisciplinary focus on caring, relationship-/patient-centered care, and integrative approaches. Dr. Jean Watson's pioneering work of caring theory/science and the continuous unfolding of her Carative/Caritas/Love processes offer clear direction here, as they have for decades (Watson, 2005, 2008, 2012; see Table 16.1 for a list of the 10 Caritas Processes™). Across disciplines, papers on integrative practice are being published, centers of excellence are being created, and new textbooks are emerging (Kreitzer & Koithan, 2014). Principles of integrative nursing have been articulated by a collaborative of holistic/integrative nurses and explicated by Koithan (2014). These principles hold that human beings are body-mind-spirit inseparable from the environment, with the innate capacity for health and well-being that can be assisted by being in nature and enhanced/supported through person-centered, relationship-based nursing care using the full range of evidence-informed modalities, beginning with the least intensive/invasive therapies. Finally, integrative nursing focuses on the health and well-being of caregivers as well as those they serve (Koithan, 2014).

Thus, a true healing health care system, an integrative caring/healing health care system, would also be healing for nurses and other health professionals, not fragmenting, disempowering, or, at times, even life-threatening/soul-killing. Over the years, different models for such healing environments have emerged. One model is what I have called *Habitats for Healing* (Quinn, 2002).

Habitats for Healing are defined as "environments which allow a context of caring for the purpose of healing that may include curing" (Quinn, 2002, p. 11). The key defining characteristics of a Habitat for Healing, on a nursing unit level in any setting, inpatient or outpatient, institutional or community, are autonomy of the nursing staff, a holistic/integrative, caring/healing/relationship-centered framework that guides practice, and the integration of caring-healing modalities into regular nursing care.

Perhaps most importantly, nurses in such work environments are seen and acknowledged as nurse-healers. They are supported in bringing the fullness of their authentic selves into caring and healing relationships with self and others and in using the complete skill sets that they possesses, including all of nursing's ways of knowing, being, and doing (Quinn, 2000, 2014b, 2014c; Quinn, Smith, Ritenbaugh, Swanson, & Watson, 2003). Nurses would be encouraged to practice radical self-care, and they would be offered opportunities to learn skills, such as centering and mindfulness, that would allow them to be fully and truly compassionate while remaining vital and energized rather than depleted and burned out (see, for example, nurse Jerome Stone's work at http://www .mindingthebedside.com). This is an essential ethical component. Provision 5 of the ANA Code of Ethics states, "The nurse owes the same duties to self as to others, including the responsibility to promote health and safety, preserve wholeness of character and integrity, maintain competence, and continue personal and professional growth" (ANA, 2015, p. 19).

In a Habitat for Healing, nurses have the opportunity to discover, or recover/ reclaim, their knowing of self as healer. As a result, they might regularly have deep satisfaction from their work that leaves them happy and fulfilled, at peace, and well beyond any self-limiting or dispiriting inner stories of being "*just* a nurse."

The essence of my own personal vision and deep heartfelt wish is this: I want to make the way easier for nurses who work so hard and give so much every day in the service of life and healing. They are my heroes. The work of nurses is sacred, holy work, a spiritual practice of the highest order (Nightingale, 1860/1994). It is, at its best, a sublime manifestation of the true, the good, and the beautiful, more than worthy of being loved, honored, cherished, and supported. Every nurse is more than worthy of being loved, honored, cherished, and supported.

In a truly integrative, caring/healing health care system, a Habitat for Healing, the way would be made easier—easier for patients, families, and communities to remain whole and to heal, in all the cycles and seasons of life, including dying, and easier for nurses to fulfill the depth of their calling to be of genuine, skillful, compassionate, loving service while thriving themselves. Nightingale said it would take 150 years—are we there yet?

■ REFLECTIONS

1. *What is present right now in my body-mind-spirit as I complete my reading of this chapter?*
2. *How do truth, goodness, and beauty speak to me in my life?*
3. *In what ways can I reintroduce the sacred back into my nursing practice?*
4. *What do I notice in my body-mind-spirit when I consider Nightingale's advice to "awaken the divine spirit of love" in my work?*
5. *What do I imagine it would it be like to work in a Habitat for Healing? What would be the difference from my current situation that I would most look forward to?*

■ REFERENCES

American Nurses Association. (2015). *Code of ethics for nurses with interpretive statements*. Washington, DC: Author.

Arrien, A. (1993). *The four-fold way: Walking the paths of the warrior, teacher, healer and visionary*. New York, NY: HarperOne.

Calabria, M., & Macrae, J. (Eds.). (1994). *Suggestions for thought by Florence Nightingale: Selections and commentaries.* Philadelphia, PA: University of Pennsylvania Press.

Claman, H. (1994). *Report of the chancellor's committee on therapeutic touch (CCTT)* [Internal document]. Denver, CO: University of Colorado Health Sciences Center.

Eisenberg, D. M., Kessler, R. C., Foster, C., Norlock, F. E., Calkins, D. R., & Delbanco, T. L. (1993). Unconventional medicine in the United States—Prevalence, costs, and patterns of use. *New England Journal of Medicine, 328*(4), 246–252

Jourard, S. M. (1971). *The transparent self.* New York, NY: D. Van Nostrand.

Koithan, M. (2014). Concepts and principles of integrative nursing. In M. J. Kreitzer & M. Koithan (Eds.), *Integrative nursing* (pp. 3–16). New York, NY: Oxford University Press.

Kreitzer, M. J., & Koithan, M (Eds.). (2014). *Integrative nursing.* New York, NY: Oxford University Press.

Maslow, A. H. (1971). *The farther reaches of human nature.* New York, NY: Viking Press.

Nightingale, F. (1860/1969). *Notes on nursing: What it is and what it is not* (1st American ed.). New York, NY: D. Appleton & Co.

Quinn, J. (1975). *The self in nursing practice* (Unpublished manuscript).

Quinn, J. (1979a). A guide to nursing assessment. In G. Molnar & S. Kennedy (Eds.), *Current practice in nursing care of the adult* (pp. 3–18). St. Louis, MI: C.V. Mosby.

Quinn, J. (1979b). One nurse's evolution as a healer. *American Journal of Nursing, 79*(4), 662–664.

Quinn, J. (1981). Client care and nurse involvement in a holistic framework. In D. Krieger (Ed.), *Foundations of holistic health nursing* (pp. 197–210). Philadelphia, PA: J. B. Lippincott.

Quinn, J. (1982). *An investigation of the effects of therapeutic touch, done without physical contact, on the state anxiety of hospitalized cardiovascular patients* (Doctoral dissertation [Dissertation Abstracts International]). New York University, Ann Arbor, MI.

Quinn, J. (1984a). Therapeutic Touch as energy exchange: Testing the theory. *Advances in Nursing Science, 6*(2), 42–49.

Quinn, J. (1984b). The healing arts in modern health care. *The American Theosophist, 72*(5), 198–203.

Quinn, J. (1986a). In search of holistic research: The impossible dream? *Search, 10*(1), 1–2.

Quinn, J. (1986b). Therapeutic Touch: Report of research in progress. *Research in Parapsychology, 27*(3), 287–303.

Quinn, J. (1986c). Quantitative methods: Descriptive and experimental. In P. Moccia (Ed.), *New approaches to theory development* (pp. 57–73). New York, NY: National League for Nursing.

Quinn, J. (1988). Building a body of knowledge: Research on Therapeutic Touch 1974–1988. *Journal of Holistic Nursing, 6*(1), 6–16.

Quinn, J. (1989a). Therapeutic Touch as energy exchange: Replication and extension. *Nursing Science Quarterly, 2*(2), 79–87

Quinn, J. (1989b). Future directions for therapeutic touch research. *Journal of Holistic Nursing, 7*(1), 19–26.

Quinn, J. (1989c). Healing: The emergence of right relationship. In R. Carlson & B. Shield (Eds.), *Healers on healing* (pp. 139–144). Los Angeles, CA: J.P. Tarcher.

Quinn, J. (1989d). On healing, wholeness and the Haelan effect. *Nursing and Health Care, 10*(10), 553–556.

Quinn, J. (1992a). The senior's therapeutic touch education program. *Holistic Nursing Practice, 7*(1), 32–37.

Quinn, J. (1992b). Holding sacred space: The nurse as healing environment. *Holistic Nursing Practice, 6*(4), 26–36.

Quinn, J. (1994). *Therapeutic Touch as a healing art in nursing: An analysis of its discipline-specific content and academic relevance* (Unpublished manuscript). Prepared for the Chancellor's Committee on Therapeutic Touch, University of Colorado Health Sciences Center, Denver, CO.

Quinn, J. (2000). The self as healer: Reflections from a nurse's journey. *AACN Clinical Issues: Advanced Practice in Acute and Critical Care, 11*(1), 17–26.

Quinn, J. (2002). Revisioning the nursing shortage: A call to caring and healing the Health care system. *Frontiers of Health Services Management, 19*(2), 3–21.

Quinn, J. (2014a). Integrative nursing care of the human spirit. In M. J. Kreitzer & M. Koithan (Eds.), *Integrative nursing* (pp. 314–330). New York, NY: Oxford University Press.

Quinn, J. (2014b). The integrated nurse: Way of the healer. In M. J. Kreitzer & M. Koithan (Eds.), *Integrative nursing* (pp. 33–46). New York, NY: Oxford University Press.

Quinn, J. (2014c). The integrated nurse: Wholeness, self-discovery, and self-care. In M. J. Kreitzer & M. Koithan (Eds.), *Integrative nursing* (pp. 17–32). New York, NY: Oxford University Press.

Quinn, J. (2016). Transpersonal human caring and healing. In B. M. Dossey & L. Keegan (Eds.), *Holistic nursing: A handbook for practice* (7th ed., pp. 101–110). Burlington, MA: Jones & Bartlett Learning.

Quinn, J., Smith, M., Ritenbaugh, C., Swanson, K., & Watson, M. J. (2003). Research guidelines for assessing the impact of the healing relationship in clinical nursing. In W. B. Jonas & R. A. Chez (Eds.), *Definitions and Standards in Healing Research, Alternative Therapies in Health and Medicine, Special Supplement, 9*(3), A65–A79.

Quinn, J., & Strelkauskas, A. J. (1993). Psychoimmunologic effects of therapeutic touch on practitioners and recently bereaved recipients: A pilot study. *Advances in Nursing Science, 15*(4), 13–26.

Ricard, M. (2003). *Happiness: A guide to developing life's most important skill.* New York, NY: Little, Brown.

Robert Wood Johnson Foundation. (2010). *Nursing leadership from bedside to boardroom: Opinion leaders' perceptions.* Survey by Gallup for RWJ. Retrieved from http://www.rwjf.org/pr/product.jsp?id=54488

Rogers, M. (1970). *An introduction to the theoretical basis of nursing.* Philadelphia, PA: F. A. Davis.

Rogers, M. E. (1990). Nursing: Science of unitary, irreducible, human beings: Update 1990. In E. A. M. Barrett (Ed.), *Visions of Rogers' science-based nursing* (pp. 5–11). New York, NY: National League for Nursing.

Watson, J. (2005). *Caring science as sacred science.* Philadelphia, PA: F. A. Davis.

Watson, J. (2008). *Nursing: The philosophy and science of caring* (Rev. ed.). Boulder, CO: University Press of Colorado.

Watson, J. (2012). *Human caring science* (2nd ed.). Sudbury, MA: Jones & Bartlett.

CHAPTER FOURTEEN

Healed and Healing: Advancing Nursing Knowledge of Healing Through Caring

Marlaine C. Smith

Nursing is the study of human health and healing through caring (Smith,1994a, p. 50). *From the unitary perspective, healing can be conceptualized as awakening to one's authentic Nature, awareness of integrality, and unfolding of integral human-universe patterning* (Smith, 2002, p. 7). *Healing might be described as remembering wholeness, awakening to the essential nature of human being-becoming . . . grasping our interconnectedness with all that is. This happens through a shift in consciousness, which can be evolutionary or revolutionary. It happens as we discover and cocreate meaning (recognizing pattern) and care and are cared for* (Smith's section of Cowling, Smith, and Watson, 2008, E45).

■ WHY NURSING?

Although I did not grow up with an abiding desire to be a nurse in my early years, my essence and experiences created the rich soil from which the passion for nursing emerged. I was raised in a small industrial town, Turtle Creek, on the outskirts of Pittsburgh, Pennsylvania, the older of two children in an Italian American family. We were a working-class family; my father was a laborer and my mother cared for us at home. Both of them had a variety of part-time jobs and, although we lived modestly, we had enough. For some time, both my grandmothers and my grandfather lived on our street, as did my aunt, uncle, and cousins. So, for better or worse, I was surrounded by family.

As second-generation Italian Americans, my parents emphasized the importance of education and hard work to "make it" in this country. We were encouraged to acculturate because of the discrimination that Italian immigrants experienced. Although my father and grandparents spoke Italian, we never learned the language, something that I regret today. Both of my parents were strong, loving, and giving people who exquisitely cared for their children and were kind to others. From them I learned the damage that marginalization and discrimination can have on families and the importance of education and caring for others.

I was a shy, introverted child, comfortable spending long periods of time alone in my room, thinking . . . writing poetry . . . drawing . . . imagining. I had a rich inner life and a very close relationship with the Holy, talking with and praying to both the masculine and feminine images of God the Father and the Blessed Mother from a very young age, and I had what might be labeled as mystical or pan-dimensional experiences.

I was bright, labeled by others as "brainy." In the 1950s, this did not engender popularity for a girl, and often my peers teased me. I tried to hide any intellectual gifts so as to fit in with others, sometimes even purposefully missing questions on tests so that I would not always get As. My parents set high standards and, from a very young age, my sights were set on attending college. As valedictorian of my class of about 200, my guidance counselor encouraged me to pursue a career in medicine. The message to me was that nursing was not worthy of my potential. Perhaps the pressure to hide my intellect and the message that nursing, as women's work, was a nonintellectual pursuit led me to become a proud feminist.

But along the way, I had some formative experiences that led me to a career in nursing. When I was about 6 years old, my mother was diagnosed with rheumatoid arthritis. It was quite severe and I remember that she was often in bed for days with flare-ups. Although my father assumed the role of primary caretaker, I became acutely aware of the devastation of pain and suffering on individuals and families. As an avid reader, some of the popular nursing books, like the *Cherry Ames* series, were part of my collection. The romanticized images of a nursing career captivated me. At 14, I became a candy striper and, for several years, worked on weekends and some evenings in a community hospital.

I witnessed the sacred work of nursing and it captured my heart. The doctors were in and out of the patient rooms, but the nurses were there all the time, ministering to those suffering. They were strong, intelligent, capable, skilled, and caring. To me, nurses were healers, saviors, and the embodiment of the sacred feminine. I loved my candy striper role of feeding patients, talking to them and encouraging them as I transported them or delivered their trays, reading to them, playing with the children, and just being there. The hospital felt like home and I saw meaningful work within it. By the time I was 16, I knew what my life's work would be and never wavered from that certainty.

When it was time to start applying for postsecondary education, I thought I had to choose between nursing and attending college. In the late 1960s, diploma education was the primary path to a nursing career, especially in Pennsylvania, and I was not aware of baccalaureate nursing education. When I discovered that there were collegiate nursing programs, I was elated and became clear about my path. I would get a BSN. With my continuing commitment to Catholicism, I applied to Duquesne University in Pittsburgh, founded by the Holy Ghost (now Spiritan) fathers.

My baccalaureate nursing education contributed significantly to the nurse and person I am today. Unlike many current programs, I was admitted to nursing in my freshman year and introduced to the discipline and profession of nursing from my first semester in college. I found the curriculum to be very challenging. My first clinical nursing course, Fundamentals of Nursing, was taught in my sophomore year by Dr. Rosemarie Parse, and I was inspired by her as a role model. She was brilliant, a doctorally prepared nurse, who challenged us intellectually and ethically. The way she introduced me to nursing shaped how I envision it to this day. Although nursing theories were not prominent at the time, she organized her course around a conceptual framework based on Maslow's hierarchy of needs. I came to think about nursing as a discipline, with its own emerging body of knowledge separate from medicine, and as a scholarly pursuit. At that time, Duquesne was an international center for existential-phenomenological philosophy and psychology, and I was introduced to thought leaders such as Heidegger, Sartre, Merleau-Ponty, Tillich, Kierkegaard, Van Kaam, Colaizzi, and Giorgi in my philosophy and psychology courses. These ideas permeated Dr. Parse's nursing course and so I learned to honor personhood, human experience, freedom of choice, and caring as important guiding principles for nursing practice.

One particular patient experience will be with me forever. As a sophomore in my first clinical experience, I was assigned to Mr. McCray. His diagnosis was pulmonary fibrosis and he was admitted for symptoms of dyspnea and heart failure. He knew very little about his disease and its implications for his life and was frightened by the progressing symptoms. We established a close relationship over my 3 days on the unit. The hospital was situated right next to Duquesne's campus, so on the Friday night after my week in clinical, I walked to the hospital to visit him. When I entered his room, I could see that he was in trouble, struggling to breathe, and cyanotic. I immediately notified the staff and they came in and called a code. Mr. McCray reached for my hand and I saw the terror in his eyes as they intubated him. Shortly afterwards, he died. The staff called his wife to come in and they asked me to inform her that her husband had died. To this day, I can see her walking into the waiting room . . . I hear myself telling her what happened . . . I feel myself holding her as she sobbed and crumbled in my arms. This taught me that relationship is central to our work and that a caring presence can promote healing even in the darkest hours of our lives.

■ EARLY IMPRESSIONS

My early experiences as a nurse informed my future career direction. My first positions were in a large 40-bed medical–surgical unit at a teaching hospital, a long-term care facility, and floating to a variety of units in a rural community hospital. I learned that those in my care shared common human experiences, regardless of where I encountered them, and that nurses needed to focus on what the person was experiencing rather than the disease process. In other words, I shifted the diagnosis, prognosis, treatments, surgical procedures, and medications to the background, and the person's experience moved to the foreground—and that was the focus of my caring.

I discovered the rampant and toxic "anti-intellectualism" present in nursing. Most of the staff had been educated in diploma programs and they made every effort to prove that some whippersnapper with a college degree did not make a "good nurse." Also during this time, I recognized that families are just as important as the person in the bed; they, too, are my "clients." I realized that our health care systems are focused on treating disease rather than promoting health. Finally, I learned that labels are limiting and that the relationship between the person (family) and the nurse can be life-altering for all involved.

I experienced such a relationship with Rita when I was a novice nurse working on a busy medical–surgical floor. This story was shared as an exemplar in another article that I coauthored (Hines, Wardell, Engebretson, Zahourek, & Smith, 2015). Rita was a 44-year-old mother of three who was on the unit after a subarachnoid hemorrhage. She could not move, had a tracheostomy, and, although her eyes opened and moved around, she could not communicate in any other way. All the nurses on the unit avoided caring for Rita. She was "total care" and some of the nurses referred to her as a "vegetable." Everyone assumed that she was not responsive because of the extensiveness of her brain damage. One day I was assigned to care for Rita. Her care was complex for me as a novice. I began my assessment and morning care with intention. I talked with Rita throughout her care, explaining what I was doing, sharing events of the day, and commenting on the photos of her daughters. She seemed to focus and, in her eyes, I perceived an understanding, but I questioned my perceptions. The charge nurse came in and scolded me for taking too much time in the room and told me to hurry up, that I was late with a dressing change in another room and the doctor was arriving any minute.

After attending to my other patients, I returned to Rita to finish her care, and turned on the radio as I brushed her hair and teeth and applied some cream to her face. Rita's eyes turned toward the radio when a new song came on. I said, "Rita, do you know the name of this song?" She mouthed the words, "Carolina Moon," as tears streamed down her face. I cried too and held her hands to my face. She was in there all this time and none of us had taken the time to connect with her.

> Everyone saw her as . . . a "vegetable" . . . less than human. In some way, I felt she was resurrected through the loving care that I gave her that day. . . . I was committed to be the nurse I wanted to be, and I've always been grateful for the lesson she gave me. (Hines et al., 2015, p. 39)

I wanted to attend graduate school but was not sure about what area of nursing I would pursue. Because of my desire to extricate myself from the medical model and pursue a more autonomous practice, I decided to get my MPH with a concentration in public health nursing at the University of Pittsburgh. Although studying a more population-focused approach to health and disease was interesting, I missed the connection to my discipline. I could not find nursing knowledge in my curriculum, so after completing my first year, I coenrolled in the University of Pittsburgh's School of Nursing to pursue my master's in nursing with a clinical focus in oncology and a functional focus in education. My first nursing course was with Sr. Rosemary Donley and my thirst was quenched with our discussion of nursing theories. Through my studies in oncology nursing, I was introduced to the emerging field of healing through mind–body and energy therapies such as relaxation, breathing, and guided imagery, integrating them into the care of patients and families. This led me to study an array of complementary therapies including therapeutic touch (TT), aromatherapy, Jin Shin, and Reiki.

After completing my MPH, I accepted a position at Duquesne University as an assistant professor. Dr. Rosemarie Parse, the dean of the school of nursing at the time, was developing her Theory of Man Living-Health (now Humanbecoming), a synthesis of Rogers's Science of Unitary Man (now Unitary Human Beings), and tenets of existential phenomenology. Parse formed Discovery International, an organization that held international nursing theory conferences, attracting attendees from all over the world. I quickly became grounded in philosophical and theoretical thinking and learned phenomenological methods of inquiry.

At the time, it was challenging to find PhD programs in nursing in the Pittsburgh area. Dr. Parse encouraged me and several other faculty to pursue our doctorates at New York University. So, when I was about 30 years old, three colleagues and I made weekly commutes to New York, leaving early in the morning and returning late at night for three classes in 1 day. I had classes with Martha Rogers, Dolores Krieger, and other doctoral students like Elizabeth Barrett, Richard Cowling (see Chapter 3), Martha Alligood, and Janet Quinn (see Chapter 13). All were exploring concepts within the Science of Unitary Human Beings (SUHB). It was the most thrilling educational experience of my life and it changed me forever. We were reading books like *Flatland, The Dancing Wu Li Masters, The Tao of Physics, FutureScience: Forbidden Science of the 21st-Century*, and *Stalking the Wild Pendulum*. Our classes were alive with fascinating dialogue about constructs like time, aging, mystical experience, creativity, imagination, and energy within the context of the SUHB. In the evenings, we met at coffee shops in Greenwich Village to continue our lively discussions. This was an amazingly rich environment for fostering the growth of nursing science and it set me on the path that I have continued to pursue to this day.

■ PROFESSIONAL EVOLUTION/CONTRIBUTION

A significant portion of my scholarship has been focused on writing about philosophical and metatheoretical issues within the discipline. From the late 1980s through the 1990s, I was a regular columnist for *Nursing Science Quarterly (NSQ)*. Dr. Rosemarie Parse, the editor of *NSQ*, was a generous mentor, and I will always be grateful to her for this opportunity. I am proud of those pieces, and in revisiting them for this chapter, I found that many have stood the test of time. The column started out with the title of "Practice Applications," and in one series I described the applications of several nursing theories (Orem's Self-Care Deficit Theory, Roy's Adaptation Model, King's Theory of Goal Attainment, and Newman's System's Model; Smith, 1988a, 1988b, 1989a, 1989b). The intent of those columns was to bring nursing theory to life through practice stories that students or practicing nurses could relate to.

Other columns that I wrote for *NSQ* tackled provocative questions within the discipline: Does nursing practice generate theory or is it guided by theory (Smith, 1990)? What is the influence of existential-phenomenological thought on the evolution of nursing theories (Smith, 1991)? What is the distinctiveness of nursing knowledge (Smith, 1992b)? What are the possibilities for nursing practice for the next millennium (Smith, 1994b)? Are Carper's ways (patterns) of knowing a logical structure for nursing's emerging epistemology (Smith, 1992a)? What is the core knowledge for advanced practice nursing (Smith, 1995)? Through these columns, I honed my skills of critique and argumentation. I learned to analyze issues, state my positions, and support them with logical rationales.

For example, during this time, I challenged Benner's view of nurses being the frontline developers of nursing theory. I argued that every practicing nurse comes to practice with some conceptual framework guiding practice, and without a nursing perspective, that framework is often the medical model. My position was that nursing is a distinct discipline and that it is important to value and clearly articulate nursing's unique perspective when working within interdisciplinary teams. I asserted that all knowing is personal knowing because we filter all sources of knowledge (empirical, ethical, metaphysical, and aesthetic) through a personal interpretive lens. I took the position that the work of advanced practice nurses needed to be grounded in nursing, rather than medical, knowledge.

In several other articles written for *NSQ*, I tackled other contemporary concerns. For example, in a point–counterpoint format, a colleague addressed concern about a perceived lack of attention to the "body" in unitary theories, and I explained the perspective of the "body" as a manifestation of the human energy field (Smith, 1991). Having learned phenomenological methods from Colaizzi and students of Giorgi, I was concerned about a misinterpretation of phenomenology due to the accompanying lack of a systematic, rigorous, auditable process in phenomenological research, and wrote a piece that clarified some aspects of phenomenology (Smith, 1989c).

There are several other papers in this category of which I am proud. One is a chapter in a book that contained a compilation of papers presented at a nursing philosophy conference in Banff. The paper was called "Arriving at a Philosophy of Nursing: Discovering? Constructing? Evolving?" In the paper, I laid out my perspective of nursing as a discipline, a science, and an art. I defined the discipline of nursing as "the study of human health and healing through caring" (Smith, 1994a, p. 50), and I described my model of the structure of the discipline of nursing, explicating relationships among the metaparadigm, paradigms, grand theories/conceptual models, middle range theories, and research and practice traditions of grand theories/conceptual models. I have referenced this chapter in several of my later writings about nursing theories (Smith & Parker, 2010, 2015a, 2015b; Smith, 2008, 2014). In Smith and Liehr's *Middle Range Theory for Nursing*, I contributed a chapter (Smith, 2003, 2008, 2014) articulating criteria and an approach to evaluating middle range theories. Last, but certainly not least, I coauthored a paper (Newman, Smith, Dexheimer-Pharris, & Jones, 2008) in which we revisited the focus of the discipline and redefined it as *relationship*: with *health* as the intent of the relationship, *caring* as the nature of the relationship, *consciousness* as the informational pattern of the relationship, *mutual process* as the way in which the relationship unfolds, *patterning* as the evolving configuration of the relationship, *presence* as the resonance of the relationship, and *meaning* as the importance of the relationship.

Several other key articles contained perspectives on nursing ontology and epistemology; they appeared in obscure sources and so may not be well known. One was a paper on knowledge development for the health sciences that I delivered at a conference of sports and exercise scientists (Smith, 1998). In it, I identified four epistemological paradigms for the health sciences and the stances that they encourage: empirical-analytic, with the stance of "radical objectivity"; phenomenological-hermeneutic as "radical subjectivity"; critical-poststructural as "radical contextualism"; and unitary-integrative as "radical integration." The final paradigm reflected tenets of complexity science. In another chapter on holistic knowing (Smith, 2009), I identified foundations of a holistic epistemology and offered four concepts that elucidated them: pattern seeing, resonant relating, caring consciousness, and integral synopsis. Another piece focused on reconciling outcomes research within the acausal unitary worldview. This was an important epistemological piece for those researchers struggling to study the outcomes of interventions that they were framing within the unitary-transformative paradigm (Smith & Reeder, 1998). An article (Smith & McCarthy, 2010) calling for educational programs in nursing to go beyond the American Association of Colleges of Nursing (AACN) essentials for baccalaureate, master's, and DNP education to include more philosophical and theoretical nursing knowledge was influential in shaping nursing curricula.

Finally, a 2009 article that I coauthored with Kagan and Chinn (Kagan, Smith, Cowling, & Chinn, 2009) uncovered the theoretical and philosophical assumptions that underpinned the *Nursing Manifesto* written by Cowling, Chinn, and Hagedorn (2000). We asserted an emancipatory process of knowledge development that emerged in the document that could advance praxis directed toward social justice. Two of the three books I have coedited (Smith & Parker, 2015b; Parker & Smith, 2010; Kagan, Smith, & Chinn, 2014) focus on nursing theories and their accessibility for nursing practice and on philosophies of emancipatory nursing and social justice. So, this work on analyzing and critiquing the critical issues within the discipline of nursing and offering my perspective on the ontology, epistemology, ethics, and praxis of the discipline of nursing has been an important contribution to the literature.

In the early 1990s, the Center for Human Caring (CHC) at the University of Colorado School of Nursing started to offer massage therapy for inpatients at the University Hospital. As the requests for massage therapy increased, I recognized an important responsibility to evaluate this program. In partnership with the nurse educator at the hospital and the massage therapists offering the treatments, I designed an evaluation study to capture the patients' and staff's perspectives of the program. The results of the descriptive and qualitative portion of the evaluation study (Smith, Stallings, Wilner, & Burrelle, 1999) revealed that the most frequently identified benefits were increased relaxation, a sense of well-being, positive mood change, greater energy, increased participation in treatment, and faster recovery. The study supported the value of this hospital-based massage therapy program and uncovered areas for future study. It was the foundation of my research career in investigating the healing outcomes of touch.

Following that study, a nurse administrator at the Denver Veterans Administration Medical Center approached me about conducting a study of massage therapy. A nurse massage therapist had been offering treatments to veterans on the oncology unit and both the administrator and nurse massage therapist were noticing that the patients receiving massage seemed to do better. We designed a study to examine the effects of therapeutic massage on the outcomes of pain, subjective sleep quality, symptom distress, and anxiety in hospitalized persons with cancer receiving radiation or chemotherapy. Patients on the oncology unit were assigned to receive massage or the control condition, nurse interaction. The same nurse massage therapist provided both massage and interaction. Valid and reliable instruments were used to measure the outcome variables. Pain, sleep quality, symptom distress, and anxiety improved from baseline for those receiving therapeutic massage and only anxiety improved for the group receiving nurse interaction. Sleep improved only slightly for those receiving massage, but deteriorated significantly for those in the control group. The findings supported the potential of massage as a nursing intervention for hospitalized cancer patients receiving chemotherapy or radiation therapy (Smith, Kemp, Hemphill, & Vojir, 2002).

Meanwhile, practitioners at the University of Colorado Hospital were offering TT to patients on the bone marrow transplant unit. The staff was noticing that those patients who received TT were engrafting more quickly than other patients. They suggested a research study to look into this and contacted me, so my next study was an investigation of the effects of TT and massage therapy on the outcomes of engraftment time, complications, and perceived benefits of therapy. This randomized clinical trial (RCT) enrolled participants into one of three groups who received the interventions of (a) TT, (b) massage therapy, and (c) a "friendly visit," an attention control, where patients were visited by a lay volunteer who chatted with them. A significantly lower score for central nervous system complications or neurological complications was noted for those who received massage therapy compared with the control, but no other differences were found for other complications. Patients' perception of the benefits of therapy was significantly higher for those who received massage as compared to the control group, and the rating of comfort was higher in those receiving both massage and TT. There were no significant differences among the three groups in time for engraftment (Smith, Reeder, Daniel, Baramee, & Hageman, 2003).

After three studies, I was prepared to submit a study for National Institutes of Health (NIH) funding. The final study that I conducted was a multisite RCT of massage therapy and simple touch for outcomes of pain, symptom distress, and quality of life for persons with advanced cancer enrolled in hospices (Kutner et al., 2008). My coprincipal investigator on the study was Dr. Jean Kutner, a renowned specialist in palliative care. We assembled a large team of researchers, therapists, volunteers, data collectors, and coordinators. I learned so much about what it takes to conduct a multisite RCT. Participants receiving massage had less pain and better mood right after massage than those receiving simple touch, but there were no differences between the two groups on the sustained measurements of the outcomes. The improvements in both groups on the sustained measures of pain and symptom distress suggested potential benefits of simple touch and attention for patients with advanced cancer. This study affirms the value of caring intention and touch in facilitating healing outcomes.

In 1988, I moved from Pennsylvania to accept a position at the University of Colorado School of Nursing where Dr. Jean Watson was dean (see Chapter 16). Dr. Watson, a truly visionary leader, was creating an international center for the development of caring science. I think of my time there as "Camelot," alive with idealism that attracted leading nursing scholars such as Peggy Chinn, Sally Gadow, and Janet Quinn, and nurtured doctoral students like Kristen Swanson, Karen Miller, and Maureen Keefe. Dr. Watson invited artists, poets, and scientists to explore the mysteries of relationship, caring, health, and healing. Practice leaders were implementing caring-based practice models in their hospitals. The school of nursing housed the CHC with faculty associates and a Denver Nursing Project in Human Caring, a nurse-managed center for persons with HIV/AIDS. I brought my grounding in unitary science to the study of caring and this integration became a prominent thread in my scholarship.

Several key pieces reflected my work in this area. On a sabbatical assignment in 1998, I studied with Margaret Newman and Richard Cowling, intrigued by their work on recognizing and appreciating pattern as a path to healing. During this time, I systematically examined the literature within the SUHB and caring science for intersections that helped me articulate caring with this conceptual system. I was motivated by the critique in the literature by several scholars, including Martha Rogers, that caring was ubiquitous and nonsubstantive and, therefore, should not be considered a central and defining attribute of the discipline of nursing. In addition, I appreciated the perspective that concepts such as caring have multiple meanings depending on the theoretical perspective from which they are viewed. I presented the paper "Caring and the Science of Unitary Human Beings" at the Society of Rogerian Scholars Conference and then published it (Smith, 1999). In it, I identified five constitutive meanings of *caring* within the context of the SUHB: manifesting intentions, appreciating pattern, attuning to dynamic flow, experiencing the Infinite, and inviting creative emergence. These either were named concepts within the SUHB such as Cowling's (1993) "appreciating pattern," or were synthesized constitutive meanings based on my analysis. In another article coauthored with Dr. Watson (Watson & Smith, 2002), we examined the discourses in unitary and caring sciences, especially from Watson's Theory of Human Caring, and offered ways to explicitly language caring from the perspective of SUHB postulates and principles. In 2007, I was on a panel with Richard Cowling, Margaret Newman, and Jean Watson at the International Association for Human Caring. That panel discussion was published, and my individual contributions were represented there (Cowling, Smith, & Watson, 2008, E44–48). The five constitutive meanings of caring were expanded by adding "ontological competencies" for each one (Watson, 1999). Since that time, this work has evolved into a middle range Theory of Unitary Caring (Smith, 2010, 2015).

Several pieces of work focused specifically on the phenomenon of healing. After studying Joseph Campbell's work on myths, I presented and published a paper on healing using the metaphor of the myth of the hero's journey (Smith, 2002). In it, I argued that myth was an epistemic form within the unitary-transformative paradigm, a path toward pan-dimensional understanding, and I defined healing from the perspective of this paradigm. At the invitation of the Samueli Institute, I joined a group of four scholars to discuss guidelines for studying healing in nursing (Quinn, Smith, Ritenbaugh, Swanson, & Watson, 2003). That paper included a systematic review of theoretical and empirical work on healing, an elucidation of the difficulties in studying healing, and recommendations for future research.

After considerable theorizing about healing, I was eager to study it empirically. My final work in this area occurred from 2009 through 2014 when I joined a group of five researchers to study healing in holistic nurses. We selected holistic nurses because they could understand our intended meaning of healing and would be invested in the research. We analyzed, separately, stories of personal healing (Smith, Zahourek, Enzman-Hines, Engebretson, & Wardell, 2013) and those of healing another (Hines et al., 2015). In both studies, participants described a meaningful connection with another; the reciprocal nature of healing; profound, ineffable experiences that accompanied healing; and gratitude for the experience.

■ MORAL/ETHICAL FOUNDATION

My moral/ethical foundation is fused with and evident in the work that I have cited and briefly described. Perhaps the most coherent and comprehensive explication of this foundation is reflected in the *Nursing Manifesto* (Cowling et al., 2000; Kagan et al., 2009). My core values are consistent with the "Ideals and Principles" articulated in that document. I believe that nurses, as the healing environment for persons served, must attend to their own spiritual development. The grounding for all my actions comes from a solid connection to this center that often provides tacit guidance for my actions before I can even analyze or language a rationale. This intuitive sense has served me well.

I believe that persons are whole and complete, and that each of us is unique and equally worthy of dignity and respect without discrimination related to sex, race, ethnicity, religion, sexual orientation, education, income, or social standing. I believe that choices based on individual values need to be honored and supported when they do not cause harm and that each of us on life's journey knows our own way deep within us. I believe that love and caring are what matters most in this world, and it is my responsibility as a person and nurse to be loving and caring in my relationships as best I can. I believe that all people should have equal access to quality health care. And I believe that peace begins with me.

We are privileged to be nurses. We enter the lives of those we serve, often at the most vulnerable times of their lives. It is important to understand the sacredness of the nursing covenant with the public and the influence that nurses have on lives. I am so grateful for the portrayal of nurses and nursing in two recent media pieces. The first one is the documentary, *The American Nurse*, and the second is the PBS television series, *Call the Midwife*. Both so beautifully reveal the moral–ethical foundation of professional nursing. Nurses are called to care. Watson refers to it a "moral imperative." We are called to care equally for victims and perpetrators of crime; for the wealthiest and the poorest; and for those who disrespect us and those who extoll our virtues. We are called to care . . . period.

It is important to see the value, worth, and beauty of each person, to look at each person through "God's eyes." Virginia Henderson reminded us to "get into the skin" of the person for whom we care. Understanding and valuing each person's experience becomes the seeds of compassion. We recognize our own humanness in the face of the other and we are moved to compassion. Although a compassionate response may be to relieve pain or fear and to provide comfort, at times it may be to journey with the other, bear witness to the pain, to assist in birthing new ways of being within a situation, or to be authentically present with the other.

Acknowledging the agency, or freedom, of the other is essential. Rather than approaching anyone from a paternalistic stance of "knowing what is best" or "having the answer," I approach nursing, teaching, and leading as a partnership, characterized by mutual engagement to achieve shared goals. In this partnership, I do not have all the answers. I listen deeply with my heart to what is most important to the other and together we explore how to achieve those hopes and dreams.

Social justice is very important to me. I am committed to dismantling the inequalities of our world, our nation, and our health care system. Health is a human right and each person has a right to access quality health care. I am committed to eliminating structures that are barriers to equality and social justice.

■ VISION

Envisioning the future is an active process. It is exercising our imagination to cocreate a preferred future. From the point of view of unitary science, imagining, dreaming, and envisioning are ways of participating knowingly in the process of change. Intentions are energetic blueprints for one's hopes and dreams. As I thought about what I envision for the future of nursing, I considered the current stream of becoming or what we are seeing in process right now, and then I colored it with my own preferred future. There are four future dimensions that I will comment on: advancing caring knowledge within the discipline of nursing; creating structures that nurture nursing praxis; preparing the next generation of nurse scholars and leaders; and transforming environments toward peace and social justice.

In my envisioned future, there is no question that the discipline of nursing is defined clearly with caring as a focus. Nursing is the study of human health and healing through caring. Relationship is central to the study of nursing as we examine caring relationships that facilitate health and healing. The metaparadigm of person, environment, health, and nursing is outdated and should be replaced. It was an early attempt in our history to define nursing. Now we have matured to embrace deeper, integrative definitional statements of the discipline. We find this direction for the discipline in our nursing journals, nursing curricula, and policy statements. The development of caring knowledge is emerging systematically, with defined areas of inquiry to be pursued. Caring is a substantive area that is a broad umbrella for focused areas of research and theory development. PhD programs focus on the development of caring science. For example, the doctoral program at the Christine E. Lynn College of Nursing at Florida Atlantic University prepares graduates who will advance caring science in any of four focus areas: holistic health, healthy aging, health equity, and transforming practice environments. Questions are emerging from these areas of caring science that move the science forward. We discover opportunities for funding caring science both within the NIH and beyond. Additional grand and middle range theories are emerging from these inquiries. A new generation of young scientists will begin their research career in their 20s instead of their 40s and 50s. Caring science evolves through multiple methods based on multiple epistemologies.

Nursing praxis is simultaneous caring-based reflection and action directed toward the goals of human health and healing. Nurses study and learn to practice from a variety of nursing theories. Some health care systems embrace a particular theoretical perspective. New structures for health care delivery emerge. There is a shift to population-focused care delivered through accountable care organizations, embracing goals of keeping people healthy and providing an appropriate level of care with a primary care focus on health and well-being, to specialty care and acute care, and to community-based long-term care that is more frequently delivered in the home with all the support needed. These structures beg for nursing practice from a caring-based perspective. Every family will have a nurse who will be responsible for coordinating the care delivered. These nurses will come to know the family and respond to calls for nursing as they negotiate the vicissitudes of life, provide counsel related to dilemmas such as managing life with a chronic illness, aid in making decisions about long-term care, and sort out the best practices related to discipline for a child. The family nurse has a relationship with the family that focuses on promoting health, well-being, and quality of life. Interprofessional teams honor the expertise of the nurse in human caring, holistic health, and promoting well-being. They are the recognized experts in this sphere of praxis. Health care organizations are healing environments that incorporate sunlight, music, and gardens and offer an array of caring–healing modalities such as heart-focused breathing, guided imagery, aromatherapy, and TT. From birthing centers to hospices, nurses integrate all that we know about healing and well-being into creating spaces for healing. Technology is used to advance health and the humanization of care. From person-centered documentation systems; to the use of robots; to sensors that quickly signal when help is needed; to the use of telehealth for assessment, communication, and education; and to the development of apps and social media for social support, inspiration, and wellness, technology is an indispensable tool for extending caring.

Entry-level professional nursing occurs at the graduate level, consistent with all other health professionals. Besides our current schools of nursing, there are structures to support continuing learning that will bridge the practice–education divide. Institutes such as the Watson Caring Science Institute and the Anne Boykin Institute for the Advancement of Caring in Nursing offer colloquia, conferences, programs, and academies to engage nurses in continuing learning about the burgeoning work in caring science. Nursing students learn nursing from nursing situations or stories, contextualizing knowledge rather than teaching facts. Caring praxis is infused in simulation and professional practice labs. Students learn and practice the skills of leadership, advocacy, political activism, and community-based practice. Nursing students are engaged in preparing themselves as instruments for healing. In an effort to fine-tune this instrument, nursing students develop the ontological competencies through meditation or other spiritual practices and reflective exercises.

In my vision, caring values guide health policy. Nursing is engaged in reflection and action directed at transforming the world. The profession must "speak truth to power" to promote health equity, social justice, and peace. The *Nursing Manifesto* and *The Institute Report* of the Fetzer Institute say it clearly:

> We are opposed to all forms of oppression, including that based on gender, race, ethnicity, nationality, sexual identity, physical abilities, economic status, or any other attribute seen as "difference". . . . We believe that nurses are particularly attuned to the needs for social justice throughout the world, given their connection to humans in times of personal change and challenge. (Cowling, Chinn, & Hagedorn, 2000)
>
> If we understand our common work as fundamentally unifying the inner life of mind and spirit and the outer life of service, we must inhabit and do our work with a deeper vision that focuses our attention on the world that is nearest to us, the world within our own hearts. Within the world of being, we discover, again and again, that our common work is to support each other in the deepest, most sacred part of our own selves. This work of being leads us repeatedly into the world of action and service, where our energies can contribute to those cultural trends that are renewing the relationship between the interior and exterior dimensions of life. (Lehman, as cited in Cowling et al., 2000)

We no longer see the paternalistic practices that have thwarted the advancement of nursing and the health of those we serve. We flip the paradigm so that health professionals ask individuals, families, and communities what they want for their care, and we pursue that earnestly, as best we can, in partnership. Finally, caring extends to the environment, to Gaia, our mother earth, as we engage in practices that respect all the gifts she has given us.

I am so grateful to Billy Rosa for this opportunity to reflect on my life and my work. I have never done this before and it has been a gift to me. I can only hope that it is worth something to those reading this.

■ REFLECTIONS

1. *How does Smith's definition of the discipline of nursing as "the study of human health and healing through caring" relate to my own conceptualization of the nursing discipline's focus?*
2. *Do I agree that advanced practice nurses need to practice from a nursing philosophic and theoretic perspective? Why or why not? And, if so, how might this differentiate nurse practitioner practice from physician and physician assistant practice?*
3. *How have nursing philosophy and theory informed my practice? How should students be introduced to philosophical and theoretical ideas in the discipline?*
4. *In the Kutner et al. (2008) publication "Massage Therapy Versus Simple Touch to Improve Pain and Mood in Patients With Advanced Cancer," the researchers found that simple touch and massage therapy were effective in improving pain and symptom distress in persons enrolled in hospice with advanced cancer. They concluded that simple touch alone was beneficial to patients. Knowing this, what evidence-based practice guidelines would I implement on an oncology unit or hospice setting?*
5. *A nurse centers herself before entering Mr. Gray's room, and during her handwashing ritual, she affirms her desire to be a healing presence for him. What concept in unitary caring is reflected in this example? How might this be applicable to my daily practice setting?*

■ REFERENCES

Cowling, W. R. (1993). Unitary knowing in nursing practice. *Nursing Science Quarterly, 6*, 201–207.

Cowling, W. R., Chinn, P. L., & Hagedorn, S. (2000, April 30). *A nursing manifesto: A call to conscience and action*. Retrieved from https://nursemanifest.com/a-nursing-manifesto-a-call-to-conscience-and-action/

Cowling, W. R., Smith, M. C., & Watson, J. (2008). The power of wholeness, consciousness & caring: A dialogue on nursing science, art and healing. *Advances in Nursing Science, 31*(1), E41–E51.

Hines, M. E., Wardell, D. W., Engebretson, J., Zahourek, R., & Smith, M. C. (2015). Holistic nurses' stories of healing of another. *Journal of Holistic Nursing, 33*(1), 27–45.

Kagan, P. N., Smith, M. C., & Chinn, P. L. (eds.). (2014). *Philosophies and practices of emancipatory nursing*. New York, NY: Routledge.

Kagan, P. N., Smith, M. C., Cowling, W. R., & Chinn, P. L. (2009). A nursing manifesto: An emancipatory call for knowledge development, conscience and praxis. *Nursing Philosophy, 11*, 67–84.

Kutner, J. S., Smith, M. C., Corbin, M. D., Hemphill, L., Benton, K., Mellis, K., . . . Fairclough, D. (2008). Massage therapy versus simple touch to improve pain and mood in patients with advanced cancer. *Annals of Internal Medicine, 149*(6), 369–380.

Newman, M. A., Smith, M. C., Dexheimer-Pharris, M., & Jones, D. (2008). The focus of the discipline of nursing revisited. *Advances in Nursing Science, 31*(1), E16–E27.

Quinn, J. F., Smith, M. C., Ritenbaugh, C., Swanson, K., & Watson, M. J. (2003). Research guidelines for assessing the impact of the healing relationship in clinical nursing. *Alternative Therapies in Health and Medicine, 9*(3), A65–A79.

Smith, M. C. (1988a). King's theory in practice. *Nursing Science Quarterly*, *1*(4), 145–146.

Smith, M. C. (1988b). Theory-based practice using Roy's adaptation model. *Nursing Science Quarterly*, *1*(3), 97–98.

Smith, M. C. (1989a). An application of Neuman systems model to practice. *Nursing Science Quarterly*, *2*(3), 116–117.

Smith, M. C. (1989b). Applying Orem's theory in practice. *Nursing Science Quarterly*, *2*(4), 160–161.

Smith, M. C. (1989c). Facts about phenomenology in nursing. *Nursing Science Quarterly*, *2*(1), 13–16.

Smith, M. C. (1990). Nursing practice: Guided by or generating nursing theory. *Nursing Science Quarterly*, *3*(4), 147–148.

Smith, M. C. (1991). Existential-phenomenology in nursing: A discussion of differences. *Nursing Science Quarterly*, *4*(1), 5–7.

Smith, M. C. (1992a). Is all knowing personal knowing? *Nursing Science Quarterly*, *5*(1), 2–3.

Smith, M. C. (1992b). The distinctiveness of nursing knowledge. *Nursing Science Quarterly*, *5*(4), 148–150.

Smith, M. C. (1994a). Arriving at a philosophy of nursing: Discovering? Constructing? Evolving? In J. Kikuchi & H. Simmons (Eds.), *Developing a philosophy of nursing* (pp. 43–60). Thousand Oaks, CA: Sage.

Smith, M. C. (1994b). Beyond the threshold: Nursing practice in the next millennium. *Nursing Science Quarterly*, *2*(1), 6–7.

Smith, M. C. (1995). The core of advanced nursing practice. *Nursing Science Quarterly*, *8*(1), 2–3.

Smith, M. C. (1998). Knowledge development for the health sciences in the 21st century. *Journal of Sport and Exercise Psychology*, *20*, S128–S144.

Smith, M. C. (1999). Caring and the Science of Unitary Human Beings. *Advances in Nursing Science*, *21*(4), 14–28.

Smith, M. C. (2002). Health, healing and the myth of the hero journey. *Advances in Nursing Science*, *24*(4), 1–13.

Smith, M. C. (2003). Evaluation of middle range nursing theory for the discipline of nursing. In M. J. Smith & P. Liehr (Eds.), *Middle range theories in nursing* (pp. 189–205). New York, NY: Springer.

Smith, M. C. (2008). Disciplinary perspectives linked to middle-range theory. In M. J. Smith & P. Liehr (Eds.), *Middle range theories in nursing* (pp. 1–11). New York, NY: Springer.

Smith, M. C. (2009). Holistic knowing. In R. Locsin & M. Purnell (Eds.), *The unbearable weight of knowing* (pp. 135–152). New York, NY: Springer.

Smith, M. C. (2010). Caring. In J. Fitzpatrick (Ed.), *Encyclopedia for nursing research* (pp. 37–39). New York, NY: Springer.

Smith, M. C. (2014). Disciplinary perspectives linked to middle range theory. In M. J. Smith & P. Liehr (Eds.), *Middle range theories in nursing* (pp. 3–14). New York, NY: Springer.

Smith, M. C. (2015). Marlaine Smith's theory of unitary caring. In M. C. Smith & M. E. Parker (Eds.), *Nursing theories and nursing practice* (4th ed., pp. 509–519). Philadelphia, PA: FA Davis.

Smith, M. C., Kemp, J., Hemphill, L., & Vojir, C. (2002). Outcomes of massage therapy for cancer patients. *Journal of Nursing Scholarship*, *34*(3), 257–262.

Smith, M. C., & McCarthy, M. P. (2010). Disciplinary knowledge in nursing education: Going beyond the blueprints. *Nursing Outlook*, *58*(1), 44–51.

Smith, M. C., & Parker, M. E. (2010). Nursing theory in the discipline of nursing. In M. Parker & M. C. Smith (Eds.), *Nursing theories and nursing practice* (pp. 3–15). Philadelphia, PA: F.A. Davis.

Smith, M. C., & Parker, M. E. (2015a). Nursing theory and the discipline of nursing. In M. C. Smith & M. E. Parker (Eds), *Nursing theories and nursing practice* (4th ed., pp. 3–18). Philadelphia, PA: F.A. Davis.

Smith, M. C., & Parker, M. E (Eds.). (2015b). *Nursing theories and nursing practice* (4th ed.). Philadelphia, PA: F.A. Davis.

Smith, M. C., & Reeder, F. (1998). Clinical outcomes research and Rogerian science: Strange or emergent bedfellows? *Visions: The Journal of Rogerian Nursing Science*, *6*(1), 27–38.

Smith, M. C., Reeder, F., Daniel, L., Baramee, J., & Hageman, J. (2003). Outcomes of touch therapies during bone marrow transplant. *Alternative Therapies in Health and Medicine, 9*(1), 40–49.

Smith, M. C., Stallings, M. A., Wilner, S., & Burrelle, M. (1999). Benefits of massage therapy for hospitalized patients: A descriptive and qualitative evaluation. *Alternative Therapies in Health and Medicine, 5*(4), 64–71.

Smith, M. C., Zahourek, R., Enzman-Hines, M., Engebretson, J., & Wardell, D. (2013). Holistic nurses' stories of personal healing. *Journal of Holistic Nursing, 13*(3), 173–187. doi:10.1177/089810113477254

Watson, J. (1999). *Postmodern nursing and beyond.* Edinburgh, Scotland: Churchill Livingstone.

Watson, M. J., & Smith, M. C. (2002). Caring science and the Science of Unitary Human Beings: A transtheoretical discourse for nursing knowledge development. *Journal of Advanced Nursing, 37*(5), 452–461.

CHAPTER FIFTEEN

Unafraid and Confident: Empowering the Staff Nurse With Fearless Moral Courage

Laura Gasparis Vonfrolio

Stand up for what is right, each and every time, even if you stand alone.
— Laura Gasparis Vonfrolio
(personal communication, November 15, 2015)

■ WHY NURSING?

When I reflect upon my childhood, I realize that I always enjoyed helping people. I particularly remember caring for my 80-year-old grandmother. I was only a teenager, yet mature enough to provide total care for a great woman who had suffered a stroke. I felt such a sense of giving and accomplishment. I felt empowered to be able to affect a person's well-being and make a difference, a big difference at that. It was such a natural progression to seek a career in nursing.

I had mixed emotions about nursing school—not the content but the delivery. We were treated like children. I remember the first day, when the professor said to us, "Look around you, for only half of you will pass." What a way to greet a class! The cranky old witch, face distorted by misery and grief, untouched by human hands—man or woman—lived up to her threat. Clinical rotations were terrifying and, at the same time, fascinating! I had an insatiable appetite to learn all that I could. And I did!

While working full-time as a staff nurse, I went on to do my bachelor's and then master's degree. I continued on to my doctorate in nursing while working as a staff nurse part-time and began teaching as an adjunct instructor, later being promoted to a tenured assistant professor of nursing. I cannot say I enjoyed the last degree. The course of study was so removed from bedside nursing. It took 10 years, but I finally finished my PhD in 1992. At that time, there were very few doctorally prepared nurses. It was a degree that I worked so hard for, yet the hospital I worked for eventually sent out a memo stating that if nurses obtained a doctorate degree, they were not allowed to be addressed as "doctor," as this would be too confusing for the patients. Nothing like getting a pat on the back for an accomplishment! Only in nursing would you see this!

■ EARLY IMPRESSIONS

Unafraid and confident, the title of this chapter, pretty much sums it up for me. In a nutshell, my 43-year career in nursing has been filled with moments of wonder, joy, conflict, frustrations, and lots of vocalizations—which I might add, are not welcomed in this profession, especially if you are working as a staff nurse (Roberts, 1994). I always remember the following quote by Bernard M. Baruch: "Be who you are and say what you feel, because those who mind don't matter, and those who matter don't mind."

Throughout this chapter, I refer to and reference hospital staff nurses, the largest group of nurses, who in my opinion are a leaderless, overworked, and underappreciated group. Why leaderless? I do not know of a single nursing administrator who, through legislation, has ended mandatory overtime or provided protection for those nurses who blow the whistle. I do not know of a nursing administrator who has put forth legislation for safe nurse:patient ratios. Thus to me, the hospital staff nurse, the backbone of the health care setting, has not been adequately or appropriately represented. No one has stood up for us, represented us, cheered us on in a public forum, or helped advocate for us and our patients. Yet, as hospital staff nurses, we are involved in patient care and in every conceivable aspect of life and death (Ulrich, Lavandero, Woods, & Early, 2014).

We work tirelessly around the clock, around the calendar, and on all shifts, including holidays and weekends. Despite this, we are undervalued, subject to the most ancient and pernicious stereotypical behavior, and treated with cavalier indifference or crass condescension (McHugh & Ma, 2014). Most bedside nurses exclaim, "I am fed up and I'm not going to take it anymore!" Everyone has their figurative "bottom line," the point beyond which they cannot be pushed. In the bedside staff nursing community, the bottom line has been consistently flexible, ever accommodating to the indignities of insults and shabby treatment, which few others would abide. Nurses' compensation is simply not equitable and recognition of their invaluable contributions is woefully inadequate (Gordon, 1995). Unfortunately, across the country, nurses are expressing their grievances quite dramatically—they are leaving nursing (Flinkman, Isopahkala-Bouret, & Salantera, 2013; Barlow & Zangaro, 2010) . . . a statement of epic proportions.

I am not angry with America for displacing the recognition and compensation that nurses deserve to other professions. We as nurses have not bothered to explain our practice to each other, let alone the public. We have just kept working—working cheaper, longer, and harder (Schmalenberg & Kramer, 2009). America needs to know why we are worth preserving and why we are so needed at the bedside.

I hold nursing administration accountable. I am angry that our so-called nurse leaders, also known as nurse administrators, place bedside nurses in unsafe patient care situations. The current nurse:patient ratios in most hospitals are simply not conducive to safe patient care. I am angry that our so-called nurse leaders float staff nurses to areas outside their area of expertise, thus jeopardizing and compromising patient safety

(Frith, Anderson, Tseng, & Fong, 2012). I am angry, as my career comes to an end, that the plight of the staff nurse has changed only minimally and insufficiently (Cho et al., 2009).

I can honestly say I put all my energies toward the insurmountable effort of trying to make changes. Maybe, as small as they were, I did. Through lecturing to nurses in every state to publishing a nursing magazine, *REVOLUTION—The Journal of Nurse Empowerment*, to unionizing the staff nurses at my hospital and other hospitals, to organizing the Nurses March on D.C. in 1995, where 35,000 nurses marched down Pennsylvania Avenue, to appearing on TV shows such as *Nightline* with Ted Koppel and *Good Morning America*, to attempting to attain legislation for safe nurse:patient ratios, to publishing books such as *Nurse Abuse: Impact and Resolution* and *25 Stupid Things Nurses Do to Self-Destruct*—I have tried. And my inner voice recites a quote by Edward Everett Hale: "I am only one, but I am one. I cannot do everything, but I can do something. And because I cannot do everything, I will not refuse to do the something that I can do."

■ PROFESSIONAL EVOLUTION/CONTRIBUTION

It all started at the United States Public Health Service Hospital. I was a young nurse, floored by the treatment—or should I say the mistreatment—of nurses by some physicians and nursing administration. Back in the early 1970s, experimentation was allowed on patients without their consent in government hospitals. I was taking care of a 95-year-old female patient who was on a ventilator. She was very with it, alert and oriented, and a very special patient. A doctor came by to give her an intravenous injection, something he had concocted, as he felt it would get patients off of the ventilator faster. I had never seen it work. As a matter of fact, *all* the patients who had received this medication had died.

So I spoke to my patient to let her know that I thought this was not a good medication to take. When he went to give her the injection, she waved her hands as if to say "no." She was pushing him away. I stepped in and told him that she did not want the injection. He proceeded to hold down her arm to inject her. I put my hand on his and said "No." He then swung back his arm, elbowed me in the stomach, and knocked the wind out of me! Being a black belt in karate, I chopped him—twice! He went down, unconscious. The patient was ecstatic. She was on a ventilator, but her actions and facial features said, "Attagirl!"

Later that day, I was terminated. I made a call to the police to press charges of assault and battery, but the police have no jurisdiction on government property. It was that moment that thrust my nursing career into action—to stand up for what is right, no matter the cost, even if it meant loss of employment.

Two weeks later, the patient was discharged from the hospital. I got in touch with her and off we traveled on a Greyhound bus to Washington, DC. We went to the U.S. Department of Health and Human Services (HHS) and to the U.S. Department of Health, Education, and Welfare (HEW). We filled out forms and met with department heads. Our voices were clearly heard as, after their investigation, it was found that this physician was from a foreign country and had forged his medical license.

My inner voice recites a quote by Martin Luther King, Jr.: "There comes a time when one must take a position that is neither safe, nor politic, nor popular, but he must take it because conscience tells him it is right."

Soon after the loss of my first job, I continued to work as a critical care nurse at a local 400-bed hospital. The working conditions were terrible and unsafe. Short-staffing, floating, and frequent mandatory overtime were a daily occurrence. The straw that broke the camel's back was when a nurse supervisor mandated a nurse, who was eight months pregnant, to work another shift. The nurse had just finished working 3 p.m. to 11 p.m. and was expected to continue working from 11 p.m. to 7 a.m. As she stood there with swollen ankles and total exhaustion, she explained her concern for patient safety. She went on to say that her husband would be leaving for work at 6 a.m. and she needed to be there for her two other children. The nurse supervisor demanded that she stay and threatened her with termination if she refused. "That's it!" I said to myself.

Thus, I went on to unionize the hospital with a contract that prohibited mandatory overtime. I might add that I was fired in April 1989 for doing so, but sought legal action and won my position back at the hospital in November of that same year. Interestingly, the phrase "One door shuts and another door opens" holds true. After getting fired from this hospital, I received a call from the dean of a nursing program to teach. I started as an adjunct instructor and within four years, advanced to a position of tenured professor. During the time after I was fired, I also formed a company called Education Enterprises, in addition to teaching at the college and working part-time as a staff nurse. I began traveling around the country offering critical care seminars and would lecture each month to more than 2,000 nurses. I spoke to the attendees in almost every state and they all had the same message: frustrated and powerless.

My inner voice spoke a quote from Albert Einstein: "Life is like a bicycle. To keep your balance, one must keep moving." I was disheartened to see nurses so discouraged. I often saw how it would foster horizontal violence among nurses—that is, nurses fighting among themselves. Criticism, shaming behaviors, and impatience among colleagues were common occurrences.

I also longed to read those articles that exposed the feelings I was having about nursing: the frustrations and the powerlessness. At the time, there were many articles on nursing burnout. The blame was on the nurses themselves. The articles preached, "Work smarter, not harder." They got it all wrong! No, it was not us! It was the horrendous work assignments not conducive to safe patient care. Not one nursing journal exposed the truths about being a nurse in a hospital setting. No discussion about nurse:patient ratios found in nursing journals, no discussions about short-staffing and what to do about it (Reiter, Harless, Pink, & Mark, 2010). No discussion about blowing the whistle on incompetent doctors; about hostile work environments; about floating to areas outside our expertise and how to end it. No discussion about mandatory overtime and ways to obliterate it.

So I decided to start a 132-page, full-color nursing publication called *REVOLU-TION—The Journal of Nurse Empowerment*. This journal was about turning the status quo in nursing upside down, challenging the "establishment" that was responsible for our working conditions, both inside and outside the world of nursing, and blazing new trails. It was about those articles that made our voices in nursing audible. Our journal issues covered sexism on the job; a look at the patriarchal systems in hospitals; war stories—all about the real stuff that goes on in the clinical areas with commentaries that hit hard at the people who want to keep you " in your place"; exposing occupational hazards; legislative updates—which got legislators to write and call to bring about change in the major nursing issues; and setting up shop—a section devoted to nurse entrepreneurs, using their nursing backgrounds to expand their horizons. It was a fabulous journal. I had many nurse "leaders" laugh at the idea. One nurse editor squawked and said, "Oh my, aren't we setting our goals a little too high." And again, my inner voice spoke: "Never give up on what you really want to do. The person with big dreams is more powerful than the one with all the facts" (author unknown).

In 1994, my refereed journal, *REVOLUTION*, won the gold at the *Folio Magazine* awards. Those individuals who cast doubt on this endeavor soon received a bronzed copy of our award. When I first started the peer-reviewed journal, I worked hard to get $275,000 in advertising dollars. Many of the advertisements were from health care recruitment agencies, and hospital supply and pharmaceutical companies. The first edition was published with articles on unionization, nurse empowerment strategies, and legislative updates regarding health care. I started to receive notifications from my advertisers stating that they had received calls and letters from hospitals that threatened not to buy their products if they continued to advertise in *REVOLUTION*. Many advertisers requested that they be allowed to read the editorial content before going to print. Well, I did not think so! I was not going to be silenced. I refunded all $275,000 back to all advertisers with a short letter clearly stating that no one would dictate my editorial content. The quarterly journal had more than 50,000 paid subscribers and ran a course of 9 years, from 1991 through 1999. I passed the journal onto the California Nurses Association, a few years after their split from the American Nurses Association (ANA), knowing that they would continue the message of empowerment.

The proudest moments in my nursing career have always been saving a life or easing a patient's pain, taking exceptional care of a loved one so near death. The *most* life-changing moment was the Nurses March on Washington, March 31, 1995, when more than 35,000 nurses from every state showed up to march from the Capitol to the White House, followed by meetings with their state representatives. A spectacular day, which took more than a year to organize and orchestrate.

Obtaining the permits from the Capitol police, White House police, park police, and the Washington, DC, police department were the biggest hurdles. Not to mention arranging for the staging, sound system, porta-potties, and congressional speakers (how terrible, I put them after the porta-potties!). Marketing the event to nurses throughout the United States was a never-ending adventure. I would like to add that I received no support whatsoever from any professional journals or professional associations. The nursing journals refused to place a paid ad for the Nurses March on DC, as they said it would offend the hospital advertisers in their journal. The professional organizations said that their philosophy was not in line with the cause of the march. The only support I received in terms of promotion, not financial assistance, was from unions, such as 1199, Communications Workers of America (CWA), Service Employees International Union (SEIU), and American Federation of Labor and Congress of Industrial Organizations (AFL-CIO). Once the ANA found out about the response I'd received, they let their members know via their newsletters about hotel room booking information.

Throughout the planning period for the Nurses March on DC, I worked with Congressman Major Owens (D-Brooklyn) to draft a bill for nurse:patient ratios (Worth, 1998). My staff and I set up meetings with senators from each state so that the marching nurses could meet with them after the event. The nurses were given the opportunity to discuss the necessity of this important bill with the senators of their state.

It was a truly life-changing event for me and all the nurses who attended that day. How do I put into words the feeling of 35,000 nurses descending upon Washington, DC with a cause, a mission, and a vision of being able to provide safe nursing care? The nurses came by car, bus, plane, and train. We all gathered at the Capitol, up the stairs, around the terraces, packed throughout the courtyard. It was a Friday, 10 a.m., and Congress was still in session. I could have died then and my mission would have been complete. The sight, feeling, and power of nurses sticking together is unforgettable. There were speeches by congressmen and senators, presidents of labor unions, staff nurses, and myself. After the speeches, the song "Ain't No Stopping Us Now" by Ashford and Simpson was played. We danced and then began our march of a mile and a half from the Capitol to the White House, down Pennsylvannia Avenue, 35,000 strong. For a momentous event in nursing, you can view the Nurses March on DC, Laura Gasparis Vonfrolio at https://www.youtube.com/watch?v=tHe6ERV9mQo.

The biggest disgrace bears repeating: Nowhere in our so-called professional journals did you read about the march, let alone the legislation to ensure patient safety. Nowhere. More than 35,000 nurses descend upon Washington, DC, to present Congress with a bill for safe staffing, and not one nursing journal features an article on this historic event. Based on their lack of response, support, and participation, the perspectives of professional organizations and journals regarding nurses was made loud and clear: Keep them silent, keep them uninformed, then control them.

■ MORAL/ETHICAL FOUNDATION

I recently received an e-mail from one of my nursing students who graduated almost 15 years ago. She wrote, "I always keep your ethical approach of nursing in my daily practice." What a fabulous compliment! I was thrilled to know that I had such an influence during student teaching. Throughout my entire life and professional career, I have always strived to make ethical decisions using moral courage—very often, at the risk of standing alone.

Nurses, by the very essence of their practice, find themselves in situations that compromise their ethical beliefs. On a daily basis, nurses struggle and are faced with ethical challenges. Whether it be birth complications, end-of-life scenarios, staffing issues that prevent safe patient care—or anything and everything in between—nurses need a formidable foundation of moral courage.

Moral courage is described as the commitment to stand up and act upon one's ethical beliefs—an essential virtue for all health care professionals (Clancy, 2003; Day, 2007; Lachman, 2007). I believe that when you are dealing with ethical issues, it is moral courage that will guide you through the process of following your ethical beliefs. It is moral courage that pushes you to strive to do the right thing, even when others will not agree with or support you.

When you are faced with an ethical dilemma, follow your heart. Keep in mind your real purpose in caring for patients. Your passion for making a difference in their lives is your goal. The process involves *commitment*, which is the desire to make the right choice regardless of the consequences for you. Following commitment is *consciousness*, the awareness to be consistent in applying your moral courage to make ethical decisions each and every time.

Throughout my nursing career, I have been labeled a troublemaker and repeatedly told that I have a bad attitude—all for speaking up against unsafe patient environments. I wear those titles with honor. I remember a situation that reinforced my commitment to speak out for my patients. I had been fired from a hospital for being vocal; you know, for showing signs of a mouth, a mind, and a brain—something that is often punished in the nursing world for those nurses working at the bedside. Years later, this director of nursing was a patient in the intensive care unit (ICU) where I was working. She was critically ill. Her husband approached me and asked if I would be his wife's nurse. I asked him, "Are you sure? Your wife fired me three years ago." I was perplexed. He told me that she was frightened and she told him that if I was her nurse, she knew that I would always do the right thing, no matter the outcome. Moral courage. She wanted me at her bedside. Thank heavens, I do not hold grudges!

Another situation, which ended with my suspension from a hospital, took place on a maternity floor. I had just become the staff development instructor for the evening shift at a large teaching hospital. I made my rounds introducing myself. Critical care has always been my area of expertise. I cautiously walked onto the maternity floor, feeling inadequate, for I knew little about the alterations in health that affect obstetrical patients. As I walked down the hallway, I heard a woman calling out in pain. I looked in, saw that she was in labor, and immediately ran to the nurses' station to summon help. I was told that she was a "salting." Whatever that meant, I knew I had to go back to that patient's room. I was terrified, as I had never assisted with a birth. She delivered a baby boy. The child was cyanotic and appeared not to be breathing. Outside the room in the hallway was a code cart. I grabbed it, took out an airway and ambu bag, and proceeded to resuscitate the baby. I suctioned the baby's mouth and in no time, the baby's color improved. I was so proud. The medical troops and some of the staff nurses finally entered the room. The physician read me the riot act. "This was a salting—the baby was to be a stillborn, you were not supposed to resuscitate." The baby's condition improved and he survived. I, however, got suspended from the hospital, as this child was not supposed to be resuscitated. If I had it to do over, I would resuscitate again and again and again.

From that moment on, I pushed forward. I made an appointment to speak with Mayor Edward Koch in New York City and then met with Governor Hugh Carey in Albany, New York. Moral courage—full throttle ahead! I told my story to newspapers and anyone else who would listen. Within a month, the hospital stopped all abortions using saline amniocentesis. My only regret looking back is that I did not keep the name of the baby so that I could be in touch with this precious life.

And so in closing, I hold on to this quote from Andre Gide: "Be faithful to that which exists within yourself."

■ VISION

A voice in my head says, "Difficult things take a long time . . . impossible things take a little longer" (author unknown).

Let us talk about academia. Nursing schools have failed to address the crucial issues that affect the very modus operandi of the nursing profession. Nursing schools fail to include in their curricula the tools essential to cope with or survive the rigors nurses must endure daily. Academia has failed to include in curricula those subjects that would allow the nurse's individuality to swim, not sink, in the bureaucratic setting. Along with clinical knowledge, nursing schools must include those courses that teach nurses how to secure a safe patient care environment. Politics, implementing legislation, and unionization must be included in the nursing curriculum.

Let us also not forget about clinical competence. What kind of experience does a nursing student have when given only one patient? Clinical instructors must prepare the student nurse for the real world. When I was teaching clinical, I would give my students three, four, or five patients each. The initial main focus was planning of care. I would have them jot down the nursing priorities, such as nursing assessment, vital signs, medication administration, feeding, dressing changes, suctioning, documentation, teaching, and so forth. The students would have to put the approximate time needed for each of the activities and interventions and then add the time up. This would give one an indication of the time needed to take care of a particular patient. If I gave them five patients and they calculated the nursing care time to exceed the time for their shift, they would tell me that they were unable to provide adequate, safe nursing care, and the assignment would have to be changed. You see, preparing them for the real world and giving them knowledge to enforce safe patient care. For decades now, we as nurses have been writing up care plans, but have left out the most important focus: the time needed to implement and render patient care.

Another idea to consider is that nursing care is such a marketable skill. I often wonder why nurses do not band together and form corporations. That is, all the nurses of labor and delivery form a corporation and market their services to the hospital. All the nurses of the emergency department form a corporation and market their services to the hospital. This should be possible to implement for all the specialty units within any medical center. A business model such as this would foster nursing independence, autonomy, opportunity to invest as a corporation in a 401(K) retirement plan and health care insurance. It would take all control away from hospital administration and place it in the hands of the bedside nurse.

Another brainstorm I have as the progression of education continues: Why not a law degree? A nurse is taught in nursing school to be a patient advocate, but often it is very difficult to advocate what is in the patient's best interest when working in a hospital setting. Ask any staff nurse working at the bedside what happens when one vocalizes about short-staffing, floating to areas outside their expertise, and mandatory overtime. You are labeled a troublemaker or told you have a negative attitude. The wrath of hell will come down upon you, especially during your performance-based evaluations. It would be much easier and less of a battle if a nurse had a law degree. It gives the staff nurse a power base. The degree would also enhance the nurse's ability to advocate for safe health care policies and help to inform lawmakers on important issues within the health care system. Nurse attorneys can advocate for policies that directly affect nursing interests to provide a safe patient environment.

Can you imagine a physician having a temper tantrum and verbally assaulting you in a condescending manner knowing that you are an attorney? How about nursing administration placing you in an unsafe patient care environment knowing that you are an attorney? How about calling a physician at 4 a.m. asking him to come in for a patient—you know he would be right there—if you were an attorney? Just something to think about!

I hope that I have imparted a theme throughout this chapter in the book and this chapter in my life journey. It is important for nurses to be fearless in following their dreams, their ethics, and their morals. Surround yourself with like-minded colleagues, ones who will encourage you and believe in you. In times of setbacks or failures, keep moving forward. In addition, be sure to make yourself an expert in whatever path you choose and do not fear calling upon experts in other disciplines to help you actualize your goals.

The future of nursing can be resolved if we invoke the philosophy of "Nurse—heal thyself." It is time to turn our full attention not to the image we have, but to the substance that we have. Nursing must take a hard and critical look at itself, acknowledge its flaws, and then embark on revolutionary measures of change in order to cultivate and develop a new type of effective and courageous nurse leader. Some of these changes have already begun. It is up to us—the bedside nurses of America—to see that the momentum continues.

In closing, I propose a Nurse's Bill of Rights, found in Table 15.1.

TABLE 15.1 **A Nurse's Bill of Rights**

1. Nursing warrants fair and equitable compensation and retirement benefits as is given to other professions with comparable education, expertise, and responsibility.

2. It is nursing's privilege to consider and implement collective bargaining in order to secure and resolve the issue of comparable worth.

3. Nurses must have the right to refuse reassignment to patient care areas foreign to their specialty of practice, for nurses must be regarded as unique practitioners. Nurses are not interchangeable.

4. Nurses must be respected and valued by colleagues as integral and vital members of the health care team, their assessments and recommendations considered essential in formulating the strategies of patient care.

5. Nurses employed in a bureaucratic institution are entitled to the respect of and support from administration regarding issues concerning the delivery of patient care.

6. Nurses must be able to actively participate in formulating policies that directly affect them and patient care.

7. Employers are obligated to establish an environment in which nurses are actively involved in determining the standards of practice necessary for implementing quality patient care.

8. Employers must provide an adequate amount of ancillary services to abolish time spent in non-nursing duties.

9. Nurses must be guaranteed a technologically efficient atmosphere in which to function, enabling them to maximize the time spent delivering direct patient care.

10. An effective mechanism of disciplinary action must be established in which nurses, as patient advocates, may report professional incompetence and situations that compromise patient care.

■ REFLECTIONS

1. *When the author described bucking the status quo by unionizing hospitals, did it remind me of something I have thought about doing in my own life? Did that thought motivate me? Scare me? Make me say to myself, "I could never do that" or "I think I'm going to try that"? If it scared me, why? Was it something from my childhood, someone who discouraged me, a failure from the past I do not want to repeat? Or was it more practical, such as risking losing my job and income? Or was it simply not simpatico with my style or personality? By delving into our inner lives, we can learn more about ourselves than we could in 20 physics classes!*

2. *When the author discussed standing up to physicians, was it "too extreme or unrealistic" to take seriously? Or did it represent a new way of looking at the world we now live in and the legal protections it affords professionals—whistle-blowers—who do speak up?*

3. *If someone injected me with "truth serum" or if I had a blackboard to write on and no one to judge me, what would I list as the top three things I would like to achieve/accomplish in the next 5 years? In the next 10 years?*

4. *What are the factors, constraints, and systems that prevent me from creating a safe patient care environment? How can I change them? Can I band together with fellow nurses? Write an article? Meet with my representatives? What needs to happen before I change it?*

5. *What education can I propose to academic institutions that would address real-world coping and survival within the nursing profession? What do I know now that I wish I had known as a new nurse? How will I go about ensuring the preparedness and well-being of other new nurses during their transition into professional nursing?*

■ REFERENCES

Barlow, K. M., & Zangaro, G. A. (2010). Meta-analysis of the reliability and validity of the Anticipated Turnover Scale across studies of registered nurses in the United States. *Journal of Nursing Management, 18*(7), 862–873. doi:10.1111/j.1365-2834.2010.01171.x

Cho, S., June, K., Kim, Y., Cho, Y., Yoo, C., & Sung, Y. (2009). Nurse staffing: Quality of nursing care and nurse job outcomes in intensive care units. *Journal of Clinical Nursing, 18*(12), 1729–1737. doi:10.1111/j.1365-2702.2008.02721.x

Clancy, T. (2003). Courage and today's nurse leader. *Nursing Administration Quarterly, 27*(2), 128–132.

Day, L. (2007). Courage as a virtue necessary to good nursing practice. *American Journal of Critical Care, 16*(6), 613–616.

Flinkman, M., Isopahkala-Bouret, U., & Salantera, S. (2013). Young registered nurses' intention to leave the profession and professional turnover in early career: A qualitative case study. *ISNR Nursing.* doi:10.11552013/916061

Frith, K., Anderson, E. F., Tseng, F., & Fong, E. (2012). Nurse staffing is an important strategy to prevent medication errors in community hospitals. *Nursing Economics, 30*(5), 288–292.

Gordon, S. (1995). Voices from the frontlines: Nurses speak out! *REVOLUTION—The Journal of Nurse Empowerment, 5*(1), 24–30.

Lachman, V. (2007). Moral courage: A virtue in need of development? *MEDSURG Nursing, 16*(2), 131–133.

McHugh, M., & Ma, C. (2014). Wage, work environment, and staffing: Effects on nurse outcomes. *Policy, Politics, & Nursing Practice, 15*(3–4), 72–80. doi:10.1177/1527154414546868

Reiter, K., Harless, D. W., Pink, G. H., & Mark, B. (2010). Minimum nurse staffing legislation and the financial performance of California hospitals. *Health Services Research and Educational Trust.* doi:10.1111/j.1475-6773.2011.01356.x

Roberts, S. (1994). Oppressed group behavior: Implications for nursing. *REVOLUTION—The Journal of Nurse Empowerment, 4*(3), 28–34.

Schmalenberg, C., & Kramer, M. (2009). Perception of adequacy of staffing. *Critical Care Nurse, 29*(5), 65–71.

Ulrich, B., Lavandero, R., Woods, D., & Early, S. (2014). Critical care nurse work environments 2013: A status report. *Critical Care Nurse, 34*(4), 64–79.

Worth, M. (1998). Word from Washington: The campaign for patient safety HR 1191. *REVOLUTION—The Journal of Nurse Empowerment, 8*(2), 76–77.

CHAPTER SIXTEEN

Caring and Compassionate: Unveiling the Heart of Humanity

Jean Watson

Nursing's social, moral, professional, and scientific contributions to human kind and society lie in its commitment to sustain and advance human caring values, ethics, philosophies, knowledge, practice, and ideals through theory, caring praxis models, education, and research (Watson, 2012, p. 43). *This model of nursing is not for every nurse. It is an invitation to nurses who seek a deeper dimension of their work . . . [It is] ultimately about translating a deep ethic, an authentic value system . . . into living and breathing models of caring and healing in the world* (Watson, 2008, pp. 195–197).

■ WHY NURSING?

I do not really know, "Why nursing?" Yet of course, at some deep level, I think I know, "why nursing." But maybe not.

Was it because of my early moments and memories as a young child, when a friend of an older sister had a seizure at our home, and I both witnessed and experienced my childlike helplessness and also my desire to help or to do something?

"Why nursing?" Maybe because it was an inner unknown calling that I only later caught up with.

Maybe "Why nursing?" because it became the only practical and realistic option, against the limited options of a girl who, at 16 years of age, suddenly lost her father to a heart attack and thus was detoured from her plans to study English literature at a university where she had already been accepted.

■ EARLY IMPRESSIONS

So, I entered nursing school in Roanoke, Virginia, with reluctance and disappoint-ment—only to both accept and critique my learning experience at Lewis Gale School of Nursing. It was there that I first experienced the power of both the absence and the presence of human caring. Classroom education and training were dominated by medi-cal diagnosis and professional/distant medical–nursing interventions. There was never any attention to the human dimensions, only the objective medical–professional clinical phenomenon and related tasks.

However, behind the medical–clinical scenarios were my lived experiences with patients and families and an almost unconscious caring culture within the clinical nurs-ing wards.

Nevertheless, I felt inadequate and uneducated and somewhat uncomfortable that I was not being *educated*, but rather trained in medical institutional protocols and clinical priorities. There was no attention, concepts, philosophies, theories, or inspired visions of patient care—only medical-dominated thinking.

It was only later, during my psychiatric–mental health rotation, which was at Spring Grove State Hospital in Maryland, that my spirit was awakened to some new possibilities for nursing. It was there that I witnessed and experienced interdisciplinary teams. It was there that I was invited to use my intuition and my natural interpersonal approaches to respond human-to-human to patients. It was there that I was exposed to group therapy and group dynamics. It was there, in psychiatric nursing, that for the first time, I was exposed to human behavior and theories and philosophies of humanity and personality.

It was there that I was offered a relational worldview, allowing for ambiguity, curios-ity, paradox, creativity, diverse interpretations, unknowns, mystery, and exploration—all in a shared quest, seeking to better understand the dynamic human phenomenon. This relativist focus was in direct contrast to the dominant absolutist worldview of clinical–medical science, which restricted my creativity and expanded thinking.

It was there in psychiatric nursing that I found my way to imagine a new possibility for myself in nursing—that is, connecting with humans and human behavior, human phenomena—realizing that nurses could and do experience and deeply touch and are touched by the lives of others. I began to recognize that we can never know the subjective inner life world of others, but can be open to connecting human-to-human with others, realizing that one person's level of humanity reflects on us all.

In this growing insight, I appreciated that there are universal vicissitudes, yet diverse longings of humanity. Every human has longings to be understood, to be seen, and to be heard, beyond medical diagnosis and treatment regime. It was with that understanding that I was awakened to the reality of suffering and inner healing beyond body–physical focus.

It was there, in an inpatient, acute admission unit in a state-run hospital, that I personally experienced and witnessed a deeply depressed, nearly catatonic patient recover; it was there that I received his feedback about my being with him; there, stand-ing beside him every day, often in silence or one-way conversation; there, where I spoke about what he may be feeling and how isolated he must be.

It was there that I was able to see him discharged and say to me what my presence had meant to him, when he was not able to speak and was frozen in his mental depres-sion. It was there that I awakened to the beauty and the mystery, that we never know how we are touching the life of a patient. It was there that I became committed to *seeing* nursing very differently for myself and helping others to realize a new vision and new importance of nursing, beyond medicine.

It was there that I was inspired as a nursing student to get my doctorate degree—a dream and inspiration, which led me forward in my vision, passion, and commitment to nursing as the human caring profession, the one that touches the inner life world of others, in ways that we can never know. It was there that I appreciated nursing as a unique gift to humanity, beyond anything we have been taught.

This visionary guide from my psychiatric student nursing experience led me, years later, as a new faculty member at the University of Colorado, to give voice and language to nursing, beyond medicine. My first book, *Nursing: The Philosophy and Science of Caring* (and its reprints and new editions and more than 20 other books that followed; see Watson, 2015) was written as my way of giving voice and language to the core phenomenon and focus of nursing and nursing's covenant with humanity: to develop knowledge and practices to sustain human caring as its moral/ethical foundation.

■ PROFESSIONAL EVOLUTION/CONTRIBUTION

I ask myself as you may ask yourself: What is this moral, visionary map that has inspired and inspirited this so-called leadership—my writing, teaching, speaking, administering, living, being, becoming, evolution in my life, and work in the world? What is the essence of this conversation I am having not with you, but with myself? As I ask myself these rhetorical, philosophical questions about my life and my life's work at this point in my career, I discover new truths about myself and my own motivations—truths and motivations that were lying dormant in my subconscious. These remembrances are now activated for this essay as I attempt to recapture my conversation and dialogue with and for others for this book chapter on leadership.

My journey as an "identified leader" in nursing has taken me, and continues to take me, into the heart of nursing—the soul of nursing, the sacred dimensions of nursing—to be more specific. It is to learn to embody that timeless, essential core of nursing that embraces, as its very foundation, humanity itself—and to acknowledge that the heart of nursing is ultimately about preserving humanity, sustaining human caring when it is threatened, and preserving human dignity, our own and others' very humanness. Nursing engages in the life-death journey-dance of living/being/becoming/dying and participating in the sacred circle of birthing-living-suffering-playing-loving as the very fabric of human existence—honoring the deeply human-to-human connections, the synchronicities, the unknowns, the complexities, and the crazy, zany, paradoxical, mystical mystery. It depends on realizing that everything is in some universal divine order for our life and believing that, somehow, beyond what we think we control, we are drawn to that which is life-giving/life-receiving for our soul—our purpose, our destiny, our soul's code journey, and our raison d'etre, for self-other-community-society-Planet Earth-the Universe-the great unknown. This work consists of cultivating a deeply authentic caring–healing practice referred to as *Caritas*, which integrates caring and the deep source of love, helping self and others to engage and commit to creating/becoming the Caritas field, which is the tipping point for transforming both self and system.

Writing the treatise on nursing as the philosophy and science of caring became the origin of all other acts, in that in attempting to more fully actualize the Nightingale vision of nursing, my first work led me, through my diverse academic roles at the University of Colorado, toward greater depths of scholarship, teaching, writing, research, increasingly diverse positions, and leadership responsibilities. These positions have ranged from and included department head, director of doctoral program, academic associate dean to school of nursing dean, distinguished professor, and have led to visiting professorships, Kellogg and Fulbright awards, and invited keynotes around the nation and world. From that background, I began implementing, consulting, and teaching the model of caring-healing in a variety of ways as a professional practice guide and as a curricular–pedagogical guide, and having it serve as a deeper level of personal–professional ethos in education, practice, research, policy, and administrative leadership. This focus was on making *Caritas Connections* between caring-love-healing-peace in my personal–professional life and work.

The core of caring theory is the *transpersonal caring moment* and language of 10 Caritas Processes™—considered universals of human caring. The 10 Caritas Processes™ (Watson, 1979/2008, 2012) are the foundation and structure of the caring theory and guide all the integration, translation, and implementation of the theory and science of human caring; they can be found in Table 16.1.

The Center for Human Caring (CHC), which was created with my guidance and vision at the University of Colorado School of Nursing in the 1980s, became a source

TABLE 16.1 **The 10 Caritas Processes**™

---

1. Sustaining humanistic altruistic values—through the practice of loving kindness, compassion, and equanimity with self/other.

2. Enabling faith/hope/belief system through authentic presence (honoring subjective inner, lifeworld of self/other.

3. Being sensitive to self and others—cultivating own spiritual practices—beyond ego to transpersonal presence.

4. Developing and sustaining loving, trusting–caring relationships.

5. Allowing for expression of positive and negative feelings—authentically listening to another person's story.

6. Creatively problem solving—toward "solution seeking" through caring process; full use of self and artistry of caring–healing practices—use of all ways of knowing/being/doing/ becoming.

7. Engaging in transpersonal teaching-learning within context of caring relation—staying within other's frame of reference—shift toward coaching model for health/wellness/ wholeness/well-being.

8. Creating a healing environment at all levels—attending to subtle environment of energetic authentic caring presence ("becoming the environment").

9. Reverentially assisting with basic human needs as sacred acts—touching mind-body-spirit of other—preserving and sustaining human dignity.

10. Opening to existential–spiritual, mysterious unknowns—allowing for miracles.

Adapted from Watson, 1979/2008, 2012.

of creative change, transformative educational-pedagogical-theory-guided clinical and academic-scholarly practices, as well as interdisciplinary, intellectual, and clinical demonstration projects for experimenting/implementing caring theory-guided practice models. It was a source of innovation for critiquing and developing caring science knowledge and its intersection with philosophy, ethics, arts, humanities, and new forms of healing practices for nursing education and health care practices. As such, it served somewhat as a research and development center for ontologically and empirically validating and affirming caring philosophy and ethics within a caring science context for education, practice, and research. The center served as a symbol and exemplar for nursing and nurses around the world and as a site where scholars and practitioners visited and learned during its decade of activities and continuing programs. For more information on CHC as an exemplar of "ontological design caring projects," see Watson (1999, reprinted 2011).

In the mid to late 1980s, during another period of acute national nursing shortage, our public university school envisioned nursing for the 21st century when the school would be 100 years old. As dean of nursing at the time, collaborative and creative intellectual and financial partnerships were created between the school and clinical agencies, as well as private foundations, even in the presence of those who were skeptical. Thus, against tremendous political odds and oftentimes limited support, partnerships were formed, and collaborative relationships within and without resulted in the University of Colorado developing a professional clinical doctorate program (ND), the first publicly supported university in the United States to do so.

The formal planning and implementing of the program allowed for a decade of change: moving from the vision to the awarding of the degree, with formal collaborative clinical partners in the community and state. This program laid the foundation of the latest national unified clinical practice doctorate (DNP). Although the DNP is the national standard degree for advanced practice nursing, the ND program was unique in that it built upon the history of the nurse practitioner program at the University of Colorado, but emphasized a mature *nursing qua nursing* disciplinary focus on caring-healing-health-wholeness and new advanced modalities and practice roles and creative possibilities, in and out of conventional institutions and settings.

More recently, I have led and collaborated on the creation of new professional caring theory-guided practice models and Caring-Healing Nursing Units, including the Attending Nurse Caring Model™. Because of the continuing crises of nursing shortage, retention, and advancement of clinical nursing, and the incentives for hospitals to achieve Magnet® recognition, increasing numbers of hospitals and clinical agencies are introducing caring philosophies and caring theory. This effort seems to serve as one of the criteria to restore, retain, and encourage the advancement of nurses and nursing. There is a parallel phenomenon in nursing education, with the rise of advanced practice, with attention to holistic caring and healing and desire for new forms of curricula and pedagogies.

Thus, my recent scholarship has expanded to more formally include caring theory-guided activities and educational–practice directions within the caring science foundation. The clinical activities range from using caring theory as a philosophical–ethical guide to restore the heart of nursing practices, to more formal use of the Caritas Processes™ as a middle range theory format, to including language of the phenomenon of caring, to introducing caring language into computerized documentation systems and outcomes studies. Other early initiatives included creating "Nightingale Units" in veterans hospitals and, later, experimental professional practice transformative caring–healing units, including healing environments for nurses and patients/families alike.

In 2008, the nonprofit Watson Caring Science Institute (WCSI) was created to continue the mission of transforming nursing and health care. The Caritas Coach Education Program was developed and introduced in 2008, and currently more than 320 Caritas Coaches work as experts in human caring across hospitals and clinical settings nationally and internationally.

Caritas Coaches help to translate the philosophy, values, language, culture, knowledge, and skills throughout conventional cultures of biomedical science and sick-care approaches. They invite and educate others into authentically living caring theory/Caritas in practice situations and personal/professional life. This direction represents a movement toward caring science organizations adhering to new forms of authentic evidence and new criteria; the shift is toward intentional, evolved, conscious approaches attending directly to the whole person's/family's caring–healing needs. This shift goes beyond medical–treatment/institutional–system responsibilities, making oneself directly accountable for repatterning outdated institutional industrial sick-care practices to person-centered healing care, providing system, community, and societal leadership for new standards of authentic caring-healing and health for all.

Partnerships with inter/national Caring Science Affiliates of WCSI are generating Caritas nursing models and practices around the world. These exemplary organizations meet new criteria for new authentic standards of human caring and healing. The affiliates are creating forums in the teaching and practice worlds, which are uniting personal practices of caring and healing with deep personal work, at ontological-ethical-epistemological-methodological-praxis levels.

This Caritas fieldwork is now being generated privately and publicly in educational and clinical settings around the globe, wherever others are inclined to engage at the deep level of self-practice. This is an invitation and skill I am cultivating wherever I am speaking, consulting, or practicing. The goal is to create a new way of *being* human, *becoming* the Caritas one wishes to have in one's own life. Thus, others are invited to join in a global agenda of uniting one's personal practice with professional practice, knowing the personal is the professional. It is the nurse's consciousness, intentionality, and energetic field pattern of caring and love that becomes the transformative source for change.

In summary, my so-called leadership has evolved from within, leading by following my inner passion, heart-centered vision, and ethical ideals of acknowledging and honoring that nurses hold a moral covenant with humanity to sustain human caring, health, and wholeness with dignity and informed moral compassion.

■ MORAL/ETHICAL FOUNDATION

This essential sacred core of caring and healing and humanity offers the moral and philosophical-values foundation for the discipline of nursing and true health care; it differs from, and even transcends, conventional nursing science and conventional nursing–medical practices. It is this dimension of wisdom traditions and new unitary worldviews that called me to write, to give language to caring science, to acknowledge and honor and make visible this invisible phenomenon of human caring, the essence of nursing and health care, this vision, motivated by energy and passion and the promise of love—the greatest source of all healing. It is this return to source that allows us to connect with our shared humanity. Reminder: At ground zero, there is ultimately one heart—one world—in our vast universe. It is my desire to somehow serve humankind and the survival of Mother Earth through my work in caring science.

This heart-rendering focus of nursing has offered me energy and inspiration and a moral foundation for myself, as well as the discipline of nursing, transcending the passing fads and fashions of the profession, along with the public politics at a given point in time. This essential sacred core of nursing continues to inspire and motivate me to give voice and language to the phenomenon and moral practices of human caring-healing-health-wholeness, transcending conforming trends, mindsets, and the medical system's naiveté regarding *health*—aka medical/sick/cure technological life-saving models for medical body–physical treatments, protocols, commercial medical–pharmaceutical economics, and costly technological interventions.

The practice of heart-centered loving-kindness, equanimity, human caring, and healing for self and other is one of the greatest gifts we personally and professionally can offer to self and other and our world, especially when humanity and our Planetary Earth survival are in despair, turmoil, and conflict from within and without, facing existential–spiritual environmental crises of living/dying/changing/growing/evolving/becoming/ needing to transcend and transform outdated minds and mindsets.

The human–sacred dimension of nursing is the bedrock and the moral motivation, which sets the value's frame and serves as the moral map, vision, guide, and prophetic mentor into our future. This timeless bedrock becomes especially precious at this time between modern and postmodern eras, especially when other aspects of our lives and practices and profession seem to have gone awry and are experiencing a deathbed of sorts for this time.

It is here in the light–dark places of humanity, addressing, celebrating, and honoring the human spirit, that nursing lives and grows and evolves into its maturity as a caring–healing health profession. This place of maturing for this now space, between paradigms, centuries, and worldviews, is propelled by nursing's past heritage, traditions, wisdoms, and insights through the ages. This comes not from us, but through us today, from our ancestors across time and space and national/cultural/religious/geographic/ political boundaries, uniting nursing as a moral, values-guided discipline and profession around the globe.

It is this deeply human foundation of the discipline of nursing, which has sustained, guided, inspired, and inspirited me to be/become/evolve—with and for humanity—in my own way. I have merely followed the ancient story—the Aboriginal song line of nursing—and my own inner voice and vision of what nursing is, that has not yet actualized for itself or for society. This pursuit and passion of human–divine existence is what has motivated and energized my human spirit, my work, my life, and my career.

■ VISION

Time and time again, I have sought to bring forth an inspired voice of core values related to perennial issues: What does it mean to be caring, to sustain humanity?

What does it mean to offer hope, language, vision, and informed action where bureaucracy and economic priorities are dominant? How does nursing transform caring practices from inside out for self and system?

What does it mean and how are we to make visible what has been invisible for hundreds of years? Caring theory along with a new worldview of science is one way forward. Right now, this moment is a critical turning point for nursing—a crossroads—and a decisive awakening if we/it are to survive.

From where I happened to be, in different positions, at different points in time, I have pursued an opening of the human spirit, artistry of being human, creativity, appealing to our human heart and the heart of nursing, and holding a vision of new possibilities, where others may have conformed, been discouraged, dispirited, or detoured from the bigger vision and purpose of why we are here—transcending positions, politics, titles, and credentials.

It is easy to be pulled toward conformity or the status quo, to "fit in," to be "normal," to gain "acceptance" by the dominant worldview framework. Thus, nursing often has pursued conforming to "what is" and identifying with the dominant paradigm, rather than sustaining its timeless dimensions and envisioning "what might be," within its own foundation and moral map that runs through time as a river of timeless gifts for humanity itself.

However, we are still in a physical plane place and space in time, between our individual and collective human consciousness evolution and awakening, in which we still have to learn about ourselves and our own power *with*, not *force over* another person, another nation, another culture, another nationality, and another's values and subjective life world, beliefs, devotions, faiths, practices—which, for them, sustains their humanity and their relation with the infinite, in some way, beyond our limited judgment. And on it goes.

At this point, we can and must hold an inspired vision for nursing and humanity–planet survival into this millennium. We have reached a new era in human history. Nursing, in its maturing role, adhering to its disciplinary caring core foundation and values, can and is helping to craft a new world order and moral community. When the universal energy of love—of caring, healing, wholeness, connectedness, and compassionate human service honors the evolving human spirit and infinite field of creativity and visionary moral ideals for humanity, nursing is then contributing to healing of self, other, society, the planet Earth . . . the very universe.

How lofty these ideas and ideals are. But simultaneously how true and how inspiring to be one among many nursing and enlightened leaders shedding light on these truths as a basis for sustaining nursing, humanity, and our Mother Earth—honoring this ancient and noble profession for its survival across time and space.

So, in being asked to write about or offer a conversation about my journey of leadership in nursing, I digress to the most primal, basic foundation of my motivation, inner power, intelligent heart, intuition, wisdom, and strength. Thus, the moral and visionary compass for my journey comes not from the head, but from the heart; it consists of me following the story line, the ancient archetypal song line already laid out from our ancestors, our visionaries from the past, but nevertheless, a story line, an indigenous song line, needing to be picked up again for this postmodern time, reconstructed anew, in order to navigate through the troubled times of the 21st century and a new millennium for human history.

I believe we are creating a revised story line to remind us how to navigate into and through the 21st century, when everything we knew, worked for, and tried to accomplish with the rise in our medical technology and science is dissolving before our very eyes as we move through time and space. This time and space is that which Martha Rogers intuited with her prescience, whereby the nonphysical reality becomes more real than the physical, and whereby energy is the metaphor for healing and treatments, and the human spirit and energetic consciousness of caring and connectedness reunite us and nursing across time and geographic boundaries, perennial wisdom traditions, and knowledge, into a new era for global human–Earth health and healing traditions and practices.

■ REFLECTIONS

1. *What will nursing be? How will nursing be defined/redefined when the systems that have stood behind it, defined it, and largely controlled its caring–healing practices are no longer there? What will nursing then become? What does nursing want to be/become when free and no longer defined in relation to conventional medical-technical science models?*
2. *How can nursing theory assist me in shifting from a medical–clinical professional practice orientation toward caring–healing professional models to serve humanity?*
3. *What is the relation between and among a leader's vision, passion, and authentic motivation and transformative outcomes?*
4. *What are the ethical–philosophical differences that I can identify between medical science and caring science?*
5. *In what ways do I connect with the human spirit and the consciousness of caring and connectedness throughout the day in my personal–professional life?*

■ REFERENCES

Watson, J. (1979). *Nursing: The philosophy and science of caring.* Boston, MA: Little, Brown. Reprinted (1988) Boulder, CO: University Press of Colorado; New revised edition (2008), *Nursing: The philosophy and science of caring.* Boulder, CO: University Press of Colorado.

Watson, J. (1999, reprinted 2011). *Postmodern nursing and beyond.* New York, NY: Elsevier/Boulder, CO: WCSI.

Watson, J. (2012). *Human caring science* (2nd ed.). Sudbury, MA: Jones & Bartlett.

Watson, J. (2015). *Full CV and list of all publications.* Retrieved from https://www.watsoncaringscience .org/wp-content/uploads/2016/03/JeanPDFrevmarch3CV2016JeanWatson.pdf

PART II

Building the Inroads

Evolving and Redefining: Forging the Path Toward Transformation of Self and System

Veda L. Andrus and Marie M. Shanahan

As architects of change . . ., seeing the big picture and utilizing "out-of-the-box" thinking allows for innovative co-participative strategic actions. . . . The visionary leader is often a catalyst for innovation, working with imagination, insight, and boldness through a partnership approach with other nurse colleagues and in concert with the multi-disciplinary team.

—Andrus and Shanahan (2016, p. 598)

■ WHY NURSING?

Veda L. Andrus

Nursing was not a career I had ever consciously considered when I was in high school. I enjoyed the sciences, especially biology, and wanted to study medicine in college; however, in the 1960s, girls became homemakers, librarians, secretaries, or nurses. The guidance counselor told me I could not become a physician, so I became a nurse.

When I entered nursing school, I excelled in courses such as microbiology, anatomy and physiology, pathophysiology, and pharmacology. Then, upon beginning clinical rotations where I could interact with people-patients who needed not only scientific expertise but also kindness and caring, I knew I had found my calling as a nurse. What a gift to bring together my love of science and my desire to care for people in need! I could see, even at this early stage of my career, that it was the nurses, not the physicians, who developed meaningful relationships with patients and found fulfillment in bringing together the science and art of nursing practice.

In retrospect, after now dedicating myself for 42 years to the nursing profession, I see this as divine intervention and am grateful, with no regrets, to have become a nurse. In recent years, I learned that I come from a family where women were chemists, dentists, and nurses. My mother, though not a nurse by profession, was a role model of caretaking and kindness. She instilled in me qualities that have been core to my nursing career and key to our noble profession.

Marie M. Shanahan

I do not have a strong recollection of wanting to become a nurse as a child, although there is a picture of my four-year-old self dressed as a nurse, complete with navy blue cape, white cap, and medicine tote. As the oldest of four children, caring for my siblings was a natural role for me in my family. My grandparents lived with us and I cared for them as well. I did not challenge this role, as it seemed like it was a given. My childhood friends who were also firstborn females assumed similar duties in their family structure. Today when I speak to nurses, I always ask, "Were you the caregiver in your family growing up?" Consistently, I receive the same response; the majority answer, "Yes." Often, our birth order or circumstances place us in the caregiving role early on. It certainly did for me. The upside is that I learned to handle responsibility at an early age. Being responsible, having empathy for others, and being part of a team are all qualities I learned from my family. I also learned that caring for others was an expectation.

During my high-school years, my grandfather and grandmother suffered with cardiovascular disease and colon cancer. My exposure to hospitals and nursing care grew during their illnesses. But it was the care my grandmother received in her last month of life that drew me to choose nursing as a career. She was cared for by a cadre of nurses from all different ethnic backgrounds, of all ages, and both genders. What this diverse group had in common was empathy and kindness toward her and my family. They helped her maintain her dignity, cleaning and feeding her when she could not do it for herself. They worked hard to manage her pain while also attending to our fears and sorrow. I knew nothing about their technical skills at the time, but I knew they were helping her and us through one of life's most important transitions. I knew I could trust them to get it right. And they did.

After that experience, I felt I was being directed on a spiritual path to become a nurse. I applied to one school, was accepted immediately, and eventually assigned to work on the floor with the same nurses who cared for my grandmother and family.

I did not know much about nursing when I started nursing school, but I think I had a romantic notion of what nurses did and followed my heart to take on the task of learning how to be a "good" nurse. As early as nine years of age, my grandmother would tell me I had healing abilities. I had several instances of precognition and she referred to it as "the sight"—an old-school Irish sensibility about one's ability to intuitively know things. I could sense personal energy and hidden emotions in others. My mother, being a first-generation American with a college degree, discouraged these conversations. But my grandmother understood what I was experiencing and helped validate my experiences and encouraged me to "respect my gifts." The support and context she provided me later proved invaluable in my career, as I learned to read energy fields and trust my gut.

■ EARLY IMPRESSIONS

Veda L. Andrus

I was fortunate to have had three undergraduate nursing instructors who sparked clarity that nursing was the right career path for me. Two nursing fundamentals instructors were warm, inviting, and caring and listened to student needs and concerns, a true demonstration of the artistry of nursing practice. Equally important was a medical–surgical instructor in my junior year who was a progressive and inspiring out-of-the-box thinker who embodied all of what I wanted to become as a nurse and as a human being: visionary, nonconformist, and a change agent. She demonstrated expert clinical skills along with caring and compassion, a wonderful blend of science and artistry. Her approach to nursing inspired me to excel as a student nurse (being a mentor for other nursing students in my junior and senior years) and to become a role model for my own students (reminding them of the importance of the art and science of nursing practice). Unfortunately, probably due to her broad-minded teaching style, her faculty contract was not renewed after one year. I was blessed to be her student and will always think of her as my mentor and inspiration.

I recall being a nurse's aide in high school and thoroughly enjoying anticipating people's needs: bringing an evening cup of coffee to a gentleman before being asked, providing a blanket to an elderly woman when I knew she often felt chilled. My early years as an RN (1974–1977) were spent as a nurse practitioner (NP), first in family practice and later in college health. I went directly from a BSN program into an MSN program, where I created my clinical practicum to rotate through a wide array of medical specialties (cardiology, dermatology, urology, gastroenterology, etc.) in the outpatient department of the University of Arizona Medical Center. I gained many important skills that informed my practice as an NP. These were the days prior to advanced practice roles and NP certification. I was part of an early movement of nurses who informed the next stages of development of the NP role we see today.

The quality of the relationship I had with people-patients was always important to me. When I had succumbed to the limitations of the conventional medical model with short scheduled appointment times, while knowing that additional time would have provided the needed quality care, I acknowledged I had lost the heart and soul of my nursing practice. I left the nursing profession and worked in the natural foods industry, studied nutrition and biochemistry, experienced many healing modalities, and became a master herbalist. Throughout the following six years, I gathered valuable skills and had many remarkable opportunities that have informed the past 32 years of my career as a holistic nursing educator.

I moved to Massachusetts from New Mexico in 1983 and within three days of my arrival, I was handed a catalogue of Omega Institute for Holistic Studies, announcing a weekend workshop for "nurses in transition." It was beginning the following day and there was still an opening for registration. I attended the program along with 44 other nurses of like mind and vision—my spirit was filled with a deep sense of knowing that I was not alone and that other nurses were seeking meaningful relationships in their nursing practice. I knew I had found my nursing heart once again.

My focus in nursing care revolves around the importance of *making connections* and *building relationships*. It is the *quality* of the relationship that is important, not the *quantity* of time spent with another person. Practicing mindful presence and being a healing environment are core elements of holistic nursing practice. I feel this has gotten lost in health care today where tasks and technology rule—where information overload, interruptions and distractions, compassion fatigue, burnout, nurse fatigue, and moral distress/moral residue impact a nurse's ability to be a therapeutic presence within the work environment; where *doing* takes precedence over *being*; and where *accomplishing* takes precedence over *the process of building and healing relationships*. The shift to include the artistry of nursing practice is what I have worked hard to model and inform and what I have contributed at the grassroots level of nursing and health care practices. I have never lost my passion or commitment to my work in nursing and see it as an avenue to influence the healing and transformation of the nursing profession, the health care system, and our world.

My early image and experience of a nurse was (and still is) an integration of a highly competent, intelligent, skilled practitioner, with a kind, caring, and compassionate heart. As one of the early NPs, I started (and have continued) my career as a visionary leader and a maverick, pushing the edges to evolve and redefine the potential of nursing as a spiritual practice by guiding-encouraging my students to explore and actualize their full creative potential as holistic nurses and amazing, full-hearted human beings.

Marie M. Shanahan

I attended a hospital-based diploma program, which placed heavy emphasis on clinical competence and assuming professional responsibility. As students, we were expected to perform nursing tasks correctly and assist the registered nursing staff with their regular duties. We quickly learned the rules and our place in the pecking order. As novices, it was important to master the tasks and observe and learn from others whenever we had the opportunity to do so. I remember the excitement I felt when I was allowed to observe a complex dressing or accompany my patient to a procedure. I also remember the emphasis that was placed on the patient's psychosocial well-being. It was very important for us to *know* our patients and be present for them.

My first assignment as a freshman student was to talk to my patient. Awkwardly, I tried to make conversation with a woman who was scheduled for a cholecystectomy. She was miserable from the prep and the last thing she wanted to do was talk to a scared newbie. After five minutes of peppering her with questions and receiving monosyllables in return, I left the room defeated. My instructor listened to my excuses, nodded her head in sympathy, and then sent me back in to sit quietly by my patient's bedside for the remainder of my shift. Inside, I was groaning. I wanted to be where the action was, not sitting quietly. Surely, there was a bed to be changed or a patient to transport or a procedure to observe. I did not have an epiphany that day, but in time that would come. I was clearly a novice interested in mastering the tasks. It would take some time before I would learn that *being with* a patient was as important as *doing for* (or to) a patient. It would take a while before I would be as competent, compassionate, and confident as the nurses who cared for my grandmother and inspired me to enter the profession.

Working my way through nursing school as a nurse's aide gave me a solid clinical foundation. When I was not studying or sleeping, I was working on every clinical unit in the hospital. Upon graduation, I was hired on the evening shift in the medical intensive care unit (ICU). The nurses in that unit were sharp, at the top of their game, and wonderful mentors. I yearned to be like them. They took me under their wing and positively influenced my skills, knowledge, and opinions about nursing. I loved my time there. I learned an incredible amount from these talented professionals. Though I was by far the youngest and least experienced, they treated me with respect and were eager to teach me. In retrospect, they did the wisest thing they could do: Without fanfare and with great patience, they helped me become the type of team member they needed me to be. In the ICU, it is imperative that nurses work as a strong team and be comfortable relying on each other. Anything can change in a moment, often without notice, and the team must be able to think and execute accurately as a cohesive crew. Without ever voicing it, they were modeling for me how to train and pattern a new nurse toward becoming a competent, skilled, and reliable colleague. This early lesson greatly influenced how I felt about my responsibility to welcome new nurses into the profession and encourage them to grow and learn.

In this same ICU I had another formative experience. I was caring for a gentleman over a 10-day period and he had improved enough to be transferred to the step-down unit. We had grown fond of each other and had an easy rapport. The evening I arrived for my shift, he was sitting in a chair, intravenous (IV) pump next to him, with his belongings packed. At report I was told he was waiting for the transport team and would soon be headed to the next unit. I remember making a mental note at the time of the proximity of the emergency equipment to his room as I prepared to enter his room, greet him, and wish him well. However, upon entering his room, I had an immediate sense of discomfort. I felt anxious suddenly though I had no logical reason to do so. His monitor displayed a normal cardiac rhythm and his blood pressure (BP) was within normal range, yet I could not shake a feeling of hyperalertness, as if I was waiting for something to happen. We greeted each other warmly and he seemed happy and ready to be leaving for his next step on the journey. I did a brief assessment, checked his pulse, and then took the chair next to his. As I sat next to him, I sensed something and I could tell he did too. Very softly, I said to him, "Would you mind getting back into bed?" He nodded and silently I helped him to the bed. As I was doing so, I noticed my charge nurse glancing at me through the glass door. She held my glance for a couple of seconds and then looked away. I wondered at the time if she thought I was mistaken and was getting the wrong person back to bed. I settled my patient in his bed and went to find her to explain my actions, though I did not have any clinical findings to back up my concerns. I had to be honest and said simply, "Something is not quite right, though I can't put my finger on it." She nodded and said, "That's OK, we'll keep an eye on him." Within 15 minutes, his BP dropped, he became diaphoretic, and was rapidly declining. He was in full-blown septic shock. We eventually had to code him and he made it.

Several days later when he was stable, we talked and he thanked me and said I saved his life. I was too young and overwhelmed by the events and how they came about to process his gratitude. I was not sure what to do with this new experience and my part in it. I had always been somewhat psychic as a child, but precognition had no place in the complex technical and pharmacologic world of ICU. Or did it? When I finally told my fellow nurses what I had experienced, they validated my feelings. "It is nurse's intuition," they told me, and they used it all the time. That evening they shared many of their own stories and helped me reframe my experience so that I could appreciate my natural instinct and begin to see it as a valuable tool, not an odd personal trait.

Later when I studied Martha Rogers's Science of Unitary Human Beings, I found the language and framework that helped me understand my experience on an intellectual level. As Rogers explained, the patient and I were in an unspoken mutual process of energy exchange that was ongoing and constantly changing (Manhart Barrett, 1990). When his subtle energy field, which I had become sensitive to because of our relationship, began to make subtle changes, my field picked up the changes and registered them as discomfort and alarm. Well before the changes manifested in his physical field as visible symptoms, they were already in process in his biochemical and subtle energy fields. As I received those early signals from his field, through mutual exchange of our energies, I began to subconsciously acknowledge that they were early signs of trouble. In response, he noted my concern and followed my direction based on the trust and understanding we had previously established with each other. Hence, I began to prepare for the code before I had any tangible evidence that it would happen, and he acquiesced to my request though I had not fully explained my reasons.

Martha Rogers, always ahead of her time, helped me to understand intuition in a way that made sense to me, though that understanding was still far from being accepted by the nursing profession and the medical field. That would take years to happen. But that day with my patient was the beginning of viewing nursing with new eyes. I believe that experience shaped my unique perspective of care and led me to being open to the path of holistic nursing. I am so very grateful that I had wonderful mentors and one amazing patient as my teachers.

I honed my skills in that ICU and eventually was invited to be part of a start-up of a relatively new field of critical care, hemodialysis for end-stage renal disease. It had all the prestige and challenge of the ICU and the close working relationships with physicians that I enjoyed, but there were also two other aspects that attracted me to it: I would have greater autonomy in the care of the patient and I would be able to develop more long-term relationships with my patients. In truth, though I loved working in the ICU, once I had mastered the technical skills, I began to become uneasy with how often patients—as *people*—were somehow lost in the process of saving their lives. I had witnessed one too many scenarios where interns and residents used patient treatments as practice sessions. If a patient was not likely to make it, unfortunately, he or she became the recipient of unnecessary procedures as MDs-in-training jockeyed for the opportunity to place a tube or insert a line. I knew they needed to learn, but I was conflicted about the methodology.

My move to hemodialysis, with its life-extending focus, seemed like a way to build the types of relationships I was missing in the fast-paced, often tragic environment of critical care. I stayed in the field of nephrology for 18 years. I wore many hats: staff nurse, educator, manager, and, eventually, administrator. Each time I switched roles, I anticipated that I would be able to make changes. I envisioned advancements that would bring about more autonomy and better working conditions for nurses, improve outcomes for patients, and humanize the health care experience for all. I was becoming increasingly concerned with the trends in health care, as the business and customer model overtook the bio-psycho-social model I had learned and practiced.

I had "grown up" in the era when physicians practiced to cure patients and nurses practiced to care for the patient's body, mind, and spirit. This new wave in health care was turning everything upside down. Consultants were cutting budgets, withdrawing resources, and restructuring work processes. We were told to work smarter, not harder, at the same time that nurses were being laid off and patients were being discharged earlier and sicker. The age of redesign and reengineering of health care had arrived and it was not pretty. As an administrator, I was expected to participate in this process and sell it to my managers and staff. If someone raised a concern, it was often viewed as a complaint and he or she was labeled as not being a "team player." It was a difficult time for everyone and people suffered. As nurses, we were not prepared for the speed and depth of the changes. We knew patient care was suffering and we voiced our concerns. But, unfortunately, we did not have the evidence to support our concerns and they were often dismissed as the complaints of change resisters.

I was becoming disillusioned with the profession I loved and feared that the direction it was heading would destroy the essence of nursing. I began to look to other avenues that were aligned with how I saw health and healing. I had begun a yoga practice and was tentatively exploring meditation, vegetarianism, and energy healing modalities. I took a Reiki course and found that the healing techniques I was learning brought me and others great comfort and relief from physical, emotional, and spiritual distress. I began to meet with RNs, MDs, and others who were also exploring a new field known as alternative health and medicine. In those days, the pond was small and it was exciting and daring to pursue this knowledge. Mainstream medicine was far from accepting anything new (or ancient for that matter) that did not fit within the allopathic paradigm. Those of us who did follow this path were often subjected to criticism for suggesting that the mind and the body could work together to heal a person. Without the many studies that are in place now to support the mind–body connection and integrative therapies, we could only trust our instincts, work together, and envision a more open and receptive future.

■ PROFESSIONAL EVOLUTION/CONTRIBUTION

Veda L. Andrus

The contribution I have made and continue to make to the nursing profession is simple: I plant seeds of possibility. What am I most proud of? My students—how they have embodied what they have learned and know from within and how they have stepped beyond limitation to change nursing practice at the grassroots. Role modeling a way of being that inherently holds the key to transform lives and transform the culture of nursing and health care: This is my life's work. How fortunate I am to have found my calling, my meaning, and purpose.

Some time ago, I was invited to become the Northeast regional director for the American Holistic Nurses Association (AHNA) by Charlotte (Charlie) McGuire. I recall attending my first board of directors meeting in Telluride, Colorado, when a board member raised the idea that the AHNA needed to develop a holistic nursing certificate program and asked if anyone would be willing to initiate and direct the process. I had what I fondly call an "out-of-body experience" where, without conscious awareness, my hand shot up, volunteering for what has become my life's work in nursing. I was fortunate to access a small group of holistically minded nurses to collaborate in the development of the Certificate Program in Holistic Nursing, which became the cornerstone program for my first company, Seeds and Bridges Center for Holistic Nursing Education. I served as president and CEO of Seeds and Bridges for 17 years and closed the company in 2000 to begin a new adventure with Marie Shanahan in the establishment of our current company, The BirchTree Center for Healthcare Transformation, for which I serve as the vice president for education and program development.

After serving as the Northeast regional director, I served as the AHNA president (1991–1993) and international director (1993–1995). During my two-year tenure as international director, I was selected by the Citizen Ambassador Program of People to People International to be the delegation leader for the first holistic nursing delegation to China and Mongolia.

The core of my work centers around informing culture change within nursing and health care, one nurse at a time. I have been blessed with the opportunity to meet thousands of remarkable nurses who are early adopters, each yearning to fulfill his or her calling in nursing by contributing to the healing journey and well-being of the people in his or her care. For many, their health care organization is not ready to engage in changing the culture to become a caring–healing environment; therefore, they become the change agent, the light-bearer, the seed planter within their organization. This can be a lonely experience and so the building of a supportive community of program graduates is crucial for success.

Over the past 15 years, my partner Marie Shanahan and I have presented our work within health care organizations that are themselves early adopters, ready to create a caring, compassionate culture and a healing environment for patients and their families, and for care providers who work within the organization. Healing health care and healing nursing through mutual respect, kindness, and inclusive collaboration: This is the work I had envisioned many years ago, finally coming to fruition.

The broader nature of my life's work is to contribute to a more kind, just, and compassionate world. As Gandhi reminds us: "Be the change you wish to see in the world." I reflect on this every day, knowing that my influence, as an educator and role model, is critical—and not to underestimate how powerful one person's contribution can be.

Marie M. Shanahan

My path in nursing has always been influenced by listening to my inner guidance. It has led me to become an entrepreneur and found a business based on holistic health principles. I chose this path because I saw a need to provide nurses with this type of education. My colleague Dr. Veda Andrus and I began The BirchTree Center for Healthcare Transformation in 2000. Together we developed the Integrative Healing Arts Certificate Program (IHAP), our cornerstone program. The IHAP teaches nurses the art and science of holistic nursing practice. It also prepares nurses with the necessary skills, knowledge, and experience to be transformational leaders and compassionate agents of change. In addition, it is a pathway to national board certification in holistic nursing.

Being an entrepreneur has not always been the easiest professional choice. The learning curve was initially quite steep. However, it has provided me with the avenue to express my creativity and bring my vision of service to fruition. A quote by Parker Palmer (2000), referring to vocation, sums it up for me. He says vocation is "where your deep gladness meets the world's great need" (p. 16). I see my work as a nurse entrepreneur as a mix of purpose and passion.

One of my ongoing professional passions is promoting self-care and renewal in nursing practice. The AHNA lists *Holistic Nurse Self-Care* as one of their five core values (Helming, Barrere, Avino, & Shields, 2014, p. 13). I think it is important that all nursing specialties and membership associations include nurse self-care and renewal as an essential aspect of practice. I firmly believe that attention to one's own being and addressing one's own needs strengthens one's capacity to be a healthy role model, competent clinician, and compassionate practitioner. In my experience, nurse self-care is integral with excellent nursing practice. I have been teaching a course called "Caring for Self, Caring for Others" to nurses for 15 years. With a handful of exceptions, nurses have shared with me that they did not receive formal education on how to care for themselves as health care professionals when faced with stressful work situations. Nor are they receiving this important information in their current academic settings, employee orientations, or work environments. The lack of inclusion of self-care in nursing curriculum and continuing education has left a void in our professional preparation and development. Without teaching nurses the value of self-care and renewal, we are not preparing them sufficiently for the stressors of the workplace. This failure to adequately prepare nurses leads to burnout, performance issues, and demoralization of nurses. Furthermore, we have exacerbated the situation by increasing nurse workloads, decreasing clinical resources, and diminishing the autonomy of frontline nursing personnel.

I see this as one of the most important issues in nursing today: promoting and supporting the capacity for resilience, creativity, innovation, and excellence by instilling the value of self-care and renewal in nurses. As part of my 2005 graduate work, I explored the concept of self-care in nursing practice and found the concept almost nonexistent in the nursing literature. The closest related concept was burnout. Sadly, there was plenty of literature on burnout, but very little on how to prevent it. My research explored self-care practices of clinical nurses and self-perception of their therapeutic presence. Nurses' perception of their therapeutic presence increased in correlation to the frequency of their self-care practices.

Concurrent to my graduate work, I began to focus on improving the work environment as a strategy to retain nurses at the bedside. The growing nursing shortage was pointing to job dissatisfaction, specifically related to reengineering of the nursing role and poor work environment conditions. Nurses were coping with rapid role changes, advancing technology, and diminishing resources. Many nurses I knew spoke about caring as a lost value in health care. Knowing that nursing self-care promotes deeper engagement in practice and greater job satisfaction, I pursued a research study with nurse leaders at the Valley Hospital in Ridgewood, New Jersey. The project was entitled, "A Return to Caring and Healing: Enriching the Professional Practice Environment for Registered Nurses." The results showed that nurses who were taught self-care and renewal in the context of a holistic learning process and supportive work environment reported higher work satisfaction than their peers who did not receive the education. In addition, the study supported that this education helped lower nurse turnover, increase patient satisfaction, and improve safety scores. The hospital CFO identified the cost avoidance for the two-year study to be between $3 and $5 million (Christianson, Finch, Findlay, Jonas, & Choate, 2007, p. 119).

The study was significant in another way: It led to the development of The BirchTree Center Model™ (BCM), which is used today as the cornerstone philosophy of all our programs and is shown in Figure 17.1.

> The model is used within healthcare settings to re-orient the values, behaviors, actions, and group practice ethic towards healing and caring through greater awareness of shared humanity. When compassion is appropriately linked with organizational excellence, the shift in organizational identity begins. The identification of compassion as a cultural anchor linked to performance fosters the transformational change. As individuals within the organization build a capacity for personal transformation, the organization expands its capacity for sustaining cultural transformation. This results in higher performance of individuals and groups, while creating a culture of continuous, heart-centered innovation. Caring and healing are seen as valuable resources in the organization and are tied to performance indicators related to quality, safety, employee satisfaction, patient satisfaction, and cost containment. (Shanahan, 2014, p. 7)

Creating a model that links compassion with clinical excellence and organizational effectiveness has been extremely rewarding.

The practice of nursing must evolve to meet the needs of the health care consumer. Nursing today is not the same as it was 30 years ago, 10 years ago, or even 1 year ago. The profession must continue to respond to the current climate that includes complex health care needs, cutting-edge technology, Hospital Consumer Assessment of Healthcare Providers and Systems (HCAHPS) surveys, Centers for Medicare & Medicaid Services (CMS)

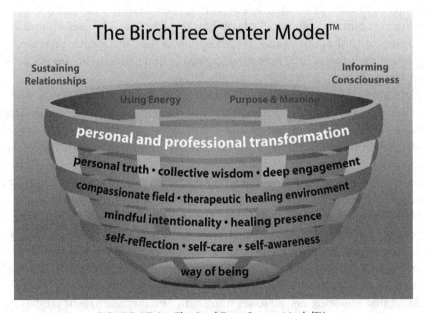

FIGURE 17.1 The BirchTree Center Model™.

reimbursement, and the demand on the part of the consumer for a context of relatedness through nurse–person engagement. Nurses must be willing and able to let go of the old adage "But we've always done it this way," stop being resistant to change, and collaboratively work together in cooperation for the highest good of the person in their care.

As more and more health care services are required within communities, nurses must become creative in a full-spectrum focus on long-term chronic care as well as health promotion, wellness, and prevention. Nurse-run centers, expanded roles for nurses (nurse navigators, nurse coaches, and nurse nutritionists), and collaboration with other health care professionals will become the norm that consumers will anticipate. These are exciting times for nurses who are visionary, ingenious, out-of-the-box thinkers.

To be able to meet these ever-growing needs, self-care practices become essential for nurses to develop the resiliency and tenacity to remain in the profession for the longevity of their career and to serve as role models for others.

■ MORAL/ETHICAL FOUNDATION

Veda L. Andrus and Marie M. Shanahan

Holistic nurses have an ethical responsibility that is guided by the American Holistic Nurses Association's *Position Statement on Holistic Nursing Ethics* (AHNA, n.d.). A strong ethical core is important to set the stage for accountability, competency, best practices, and the quality of care we safely provide for the person in our care. Note the shift in language: *person in our care* as opposed to *the patient*. The word *patient* focuses on the illness, the disease, the health care issue, whereas the word *person* views the individual as a whole, healthy human being who is currently responding to a health challenge-opportunity. This subtle shift in language helps us see the precious nature of humanity.

When coming into relationship with others, holistic nurses have a responsibility to release preconceived judgments, to view individuals with fresh eyes, acknowledging the diversity of lifestyles and life practices. Through the practices of intention setting, grounding, centering, and aligning with a kind and compassionate heart, nurses can greet others in a manner that honors the sacred nature of life. By engaging in this way, nurses become role models for others and, by extension, contribute a caring–healing ethic to our world—a world that sorely needs kindness, compassion, and caring for its healing and transformation.

The creation of a healing environment through attending to the physical–energetic environment and intentionally *becoming* a healing environment through our way of coming into relationship with others are core to nursing practice. It is our moral–ethical responsibility to become therapeutic partners in care, recognizing our competency and expert level of skills, yet understanding that the person in our care is an expert in knowing his or her own life story. Preparing ourselves through authentic presence, a quiet mind, and an open heart contributes to an environment that allows others to reflect, hear their own voice, and recognize how their story presents insight into the current chapter of their life experience. It is the artistry of becoming comfortable with silence, of listening between the sounds, which allows for an understanding of the full spectrum of information transfer possible in partnership with another human being.

■ VISION

Veda L. Andrus and Marie M. Shanahan

"The future is co-created in a collaborative manner through the recognition that *everyone is a leader* and drawing out each person's creative potential calls forth the best in people, bringing them together around a shared sense of purpose" (Andrus & Shanahan, 2016, p. 598). This exemplifies much of our vision for nursing and health care. Shifting from a dominator model to a partnership model will take time and healing, and yet it is the only way that the nursing profession can take its place at the health care decision-making table.

Nurses must find their voice, learn how to articulate their message, and come together as a powerful unified profession to be a strong force in the evolution of health care. Until we nurses can articulate what we do and how our contribution to the health and well-being of health care consumers is central to their care, until we can identify the compelling value proposition of nursing, the profession will continue to be viewed as secondary to the profession of medicine. The American Nurses Association has worked diligently to influence and change the perception of nurses—and we still have a long way to go.

A key element in the healing of nursing is to become partners with one another. This will require a shift in the culture of nursing to one in which nurses treat one another with respect and dignity, transforming the harmful patterns of lateral violence, work-place bullying, and judgmental behaviors to become kind, respectful, and compassionate toward one another. This is truly the only way to become a unified profession—one where we support each other, genuinely care for one another, and role model healthy, loving behaviors for future generations in our profession.

There is a similar need for healing between the professions of nursing and medicine. A strong collaborative partnership between the two professions could only strengthen the vision each profession has for enhancing person–provider engagement and improving the quality and safety of care provided for health care consumers. When we consider what health care could look like with true partnership, we envision a culture of deep respect, acknowledgment of unique contributions, and an enriched practice environment where loving-kindness and sincerity become the core foundation and springboard for our practice. Where "us" and "them" become "we." How powerful we can all be when we transform health care silos into becoming a united partnership for healing through genuine appreciation for our unique contributions.

We may not see the full manifestation of our vision for nursing and health care within our nursing careers; however, we take pride in knowing we have contributed to creating opportunities that have inspired and enriched the lives of our students, personally and professionally. We have been intentional in teaching nurses to be bold, courageous advocates for the advancement of the nursing profession, for their fellow nurse colleagues, and for the people in their care. We continue to encourage them to be cultural transformational agents, influencing the culture of their organizations to view everyone as a leader and facilitator of change. We remind them that *who they are*, in their beauty, wonder, and wisdom, is what is vital to create necessary change in the world.

Nursing, as a fully embodied profession, can and will be a strong, articulate, and respected voice and partner in health care transformation throughout the coming years. Nurses can and will work collaboratively as clinical leaders with reverence and dignity and with acknowledgment of the valuable contribution of each nurse colleague.

We hold sacred this vision for the future of nursing.

Our words of wisdom to nurse leaders: Listen deeply to hear your vision, keep your focus, and draw others to you who share a similar vision. Then, take off your blinders and let go of attachment to a specific outcome—the detours are the richest part of the journey.

■ REFLECTIONS

1. *Why is it important for me to engage in self-care practices? In honest reflection, have I experienced compassion fatigue, chronic exhaustion, burnout? If so, how has this impacted my nursing practice? What would my life look like if I intentionally created space for self-reflection, self-care, and resiliency building?*

2. *How will shifting the language from* patient *to* person *influence the quality of the relationships developed within my work environment? What does it mean for me to create a healing environment that nurtures these relationships?*

3. *What is the value in my viewing every person as a leader? How might that influence my work environment? The relationships within the interdisciplinary team? The culture of my organization?*

4. *What leadership skills do I contribute to my work environment? How do I role model these behaviors? What has been the impact of my leadership contribution?*

5. *What unique qualities do I, in my beauty, wonder, and wisdom, possess to transform the health care scenario? How can I use these qualities to heal my relationships with both nurses and doctors? What do I need right now to make that healing possible?*

■ REFERENCES

American Holistic Nurses Association. (n.d.). *Position on holistic nursing ethics*. Retrieved from http://www.ahna.org/Resources/Publications/Position-Statements#P2

Andrus, V., & Shanahan, M. (2016). Holistic leadership. In B. Dossey & L. Keegan (Eds.), *Holistic nursing: A handbook for practice* (7th ed., pp. 591–607). Boston, MA: Jones & Bartlett Learning.

Christianson, J., Finch, M., Findlay, B., Jonas, W., & Choate, C. G. (2007). *Re-inventing the patient experience: Strategies for hospital leaders*. Chicago, IL: Health Administration Press.

Helming, M., Barrere, C., Avino, K., & Shields, D. (2014). *Core curriculum for holistic nursing*. Boston, MA: Jones & Bartlett Learning.

Manhart Barrett, E. A. (1990). *Visions of Rogers' science-based nursing*. New York, NY: National League for Nursing.

Palmer, P. (2000). *Let your life speak: Listening for the voice of vocation*. San Francisco, CA: Jossey-Bass.

Shanahan, M. (2014). The Birchtree Center model: Transforming health care with heart! *Beginnings*, *34*(3), 6–9, 30.

CHAPTER EIGHTEEN

Artistic and Scientific: Broadening the Scope of Our 21st-Century Health Advocacy

Deva-Marie Beck

Modern nursing is at a crossroads . . . we can struggle along, as before, or determine what nursing could become. Nightingale's world needed her. Our world needs nursing. Like Nightingale, nurses can become global visionaries for the health of humanity. As we stand at our crossroads, her light can help us see.

—Beck (2005a, p. 128)

■ WHY NURSING?

Surprisingly, now looking back upon my youth, I did not want to become a nurse at all. Modeling my parents' strengths, I was into the liberal arts: music, theater, dancing, writing, crafts, and design. My father was a journalist and my mother an artist. This was what I knew. Also, one extended family member was the kind of nurse I did not like—the starched variety, very structured. I remember, as a very small child, being bothered by the way she abruptly flicked the thermometer to prepare to take my temperature and adhered to rules that seemed too strict for my liking. The deep compassion that I was later to understand as the foundation for nursing's arena (Watson, 2008) was not apparent in this earliest encounter I had with a "nurse."

Within my immediate family, our experiences with wellness and illness also deeply shaped my take on "medicine." My father contracted dengue fever during his army service in the South Pacific during World War II. He told us that he had been sick throughout the last year of the war and was posted at the Army–Air Corps Hospital at Hickam Field in Hawaii. He counted himself lucky to have "fully recovered." But, looking back,

I am not so sure he really did. After the war, he was always frail, struggling with a low vitality and vague debilitating symptoms for as long as I knew him. Doctors could not help him. His health—or lack of it—seemed an unsolvable mystery.

Then, when I was four years old, my mother gave birth to a baby who suffered from failure to thrive. My sister was limp and her muscles never gained in strength. She ate well and grew heavy but remained flaccid, never able to sit up on her own without pillows propping her. Looking back, from what is now known, this was most likely a severe form of congenital muscular dystrophy (Leyten et al., 1989). But back then, it was not clear what was wrong and what, if anything, could be done about it. Again, this was from a medical doctor's perspective. I was six when my sister died of pneumonia. For two years, I had watched my mother's struggles to provide what seemed to me to be 24/7 care. I was already skeptical of what medical doctors were capable of and questioned their lack of capability. And without more encouraging role models, I was skeptical of nurses as well.

Then, when I was nearly 16, my appendix ruptured and I was rushed for testing and emergent surgery. Peritonitis had already set into my abdominal wall. After a month of critical status in the hospital, I was told that my recovery was a miracle. I was at home for another half a year before becoming well enough to return to high school. It was during this time that I became fully aware of what both doctors and nurses could do. My surgeon had been the best and most of the nurses looked after me very, very well. But, the fortitude of my conviction—to not be a nurse myself—had not yet been softened. From this experience, I learned firsthand of the sacrifices nurses and doctors make for the sake of patients. I did not see how I could possibly make such a professional commitment. I did not yet know that I had become, even then, a *wounded healer* (Luton, 2015). In this way, I was prepared through this life experience with a certain kind of attribute that can make a nurse effective in situations requiring deep empathy. I had obtained, through my own illness and brush with death, a way of "being with" suffering that I would not have been able to previously understand or apply.

Still, it would be a number of years and take many more unexpected personal experiences before I was ready to consider becoming a nurse. I attended university, majored in theater and dance, but could not find a related job and spent several years looking for the best alternate vocation to begin my adult life. I finally discovered medical-assisting school and was surprised to find that the basics of anatomy, physiology, and pharmacology were easy for me to learn. I went on to work in hospital outpatient clinics and doctors' offices and eventually took a job as a lab and EKG technician. There, the cardiologist who watched over my work saw something in me that I had not yet known. He realized he could teach me hemodynamics and EKG interpretation, especially to understand how and why ischemic changes indicative of myocardial infarction appeared on the tracings. Then, as I arrived to provide EKGs for patients with chest pain, I found myself teaching the nurses what I had learned. It was only then I realized that if I could *teach* nurses, I could actually be one myself.

Thus, becoming a nurse was, for me, more than a childhood ideal, more than the study of the science and theory, and more than the mastery of the clinical skills and practice. It was, even then, a *calling* (Dossey, 2010), although I had come to this knowledge in roundabout ways. Even while I was a first-year nursing student, it had become a commitment to deeply address the suffering, even the inexorable suffering, of people and their unfulfilled needs.

Because of this ethical commitment, my intention and vision had already extended beyond "getting the job done" and other normal physical expectations in my first years of clinical practice. I wanted more. I defined this inner calling as an ability to impact upon the recovery and health of people through what is now known as holistic nursing (Dossey & Keegan, 2016), to become an agent of healing at emotional, mental, and even spiritual levels. I had seen these broader levels of need in my father's chronic illness, in my mother's struggles to cope with my sister's birth defects, and in my own recovery. For me, nursing became much more than taking a temperature properly or adhering to strict rules. Although, by then, I also practiced technical clinical excellence and I highly valued this skill, nursing became less about the sterility of procedure and more about the preservation and promotion of dignity and humanity.

■ EARLY IMPRESSIONS

Because I had already excelled in heart monitoring and because critical care nurses were then in short supply, I was assigned to the coronary and surgical intensive care units right out of school. As expected, it took quite a bit of discipline and time to master these skills. But, as I did so, I also saw—again—through the lens my earlier life had provided me that emotional, mental, and spiritual factors were significant in either the recovery or the decline of patients who were critically ill. I noticed that the attitudes of doctors and nurses, and their own emotional, mental, and spiritual "takes" on their essential work, were also factors in their patients' life or death.

I was then assigned to be an assistant head nurse on an oncology ward where some of the patients received aggressive chemotherapy and some were already under the auspices of palliative care. There, emotional, mental, and spiritual factors were once again fully apparent to me. Interacting with those suffering from severe cancer treatments and watching the slow dying process of others, I was even more keenly aware of what it took to become an effective nurse in this setting, including—and yet beyond—the physical components of nursing. As the months passed, I also became aware of the deep need to become an effective leader for the nurses working alongside me who were also challenged by bearing witness to and engaging with this suffering.

It was during those years that I also experienced, as nurses often do, the challenge of doing *everything* well with the limited amount of time, resources, and staffing that were provided. After many a shift, I finished knowing that I had not been able to do enough. I also knew that I was even at risk of "negligence" because too much had been assigned for me to safely handle and that my colleagues and our ward, collectively, had been assigned too much as well. The critical worldwide nursing shortage (Kingma, 2001) and its effects on patients and nurses were already becoming painfully apparent to me. I wanted to do something about this but did not yet begin to know what or how. The nursing shortage remained one of my lived experiences for many years—and I lived with it, unsatisfied.

It was also during that time that I became quite interested in the written and spoken work of authors leading in holistic health topics. I appreciated Cousins's (1979) *Anatomy of an Illness: As Perceived by the Patient*, where he told the story of his own full recovery from crippling ankylosing spondylitis using laughter as an effective antidote for his pain. Learning more about the science of holistic factors, I studied the early work of Selye (1974), the researcher who identified *stress*. I also appreciated Larry Dossey's (1989) research on the connections between spirituality and healing and Segal's (1986) discovery of the powerful role the mind can play in fighting illness, especially cancer.

Additionally, neuroscience was identifying new connections between physical health and emotional health. In 1975, endorphins were discovered to be naturally occurring neurochemicals, more powerful in pain relief than opioids like morphine (Davis, 1984). Neuroscientists were even proving that emotional experiences—for instance, particularly happy memories or deeply held beliefs in a given therapy—could become triggers of the natural release of pain-killing endorphins. It was then proven that this "emotional" pain relief could trigger the release of neurochemicals and could even actually be reversed to return the pain sensation through the administration of naloxone, the powerful antidote to opioid overdose. Also, endorphins—and the morphine-like euphoria they release when triggered—were discovered to be prevalent in the limbic brain, the neuro-epicenter of our body's ability to maintain immune strength and hormonal balance.

I became so interested in these discoveries that I independently studied numerous biomedical journals about endorphin research. Through this and my growing confidence to share what I had learned, I began to teach other nurses through workshops focused on holistic health, along with my first husband, who was also a nurse interested in these fields. From these experiences, we wrote and self-published our own book about endorphin research (Beck & Beck, 1986). Then we invested several years of our time to promote this publication and its French version (Beck & Beck, 1988), to eventually sell more than 20,000 copies in two languages.

Even though endorphins were later understood to be only one part of a complex soup of neurochemicals in our brains and bodies mixing with the powerful effects of others, including dopamine, norepinephrine, and serotonin, these early endorphin discoveries significantly changed how science now understands the dynamic interchanges between physical, emotional, and mental health, stress, and disease (Davis, 1984).

Nurses watch the effects of these neurochemical complexities every day in the recovery or failure to thrive of their patients. Also, nurses have their own neurochemicals to deal with in their individual health and in their ability to respond to the repetitive stresses of modern health care delivery. Although awareness of the holistic factors of health and disease are still growing, I still often wonder if enough is being taught to nursing students regarding the multidisciplinary theories and science that expound upon the emotional, mental, and spiritual factors of health. Is this education foundational to their clinical practice in serving their patients? The realm of neuroscience—addressing the triggers of stress and how to cope with it—is foundational to nurses' own capacities for self-care to sustain such a demanding profession (Dossey & Keegan, 2016). Do we really know and practice this?

I thoroughly explored all of these ideas and participated in early approaches to address these needs in my own community. But as I was soon to learn, a wider world of global health concerns based on what I had already discovered and experienced was on my life's horizon.

■ PROFESSIONAL EVOLUTION/CONTRIBUTION

By then I had been in clinical practice for nearly 20 years and could have been satisfied with the work I had achieved, as well as the new studies I had advanced and taught. But I began to notice changes in the world around me and found new areas of interest. When a trash-burning plant proposed to emit toxic chemicals into the clean air of my own rural neighborhood, I joined the fight to keep our town from approving it. This set me on the path of learning more about environmental science and the economic dynamics of pollution, the seeming tensions between making money and keeping our air and water clean. This was the early 1990s and the United Nations (UN) Earth Summit was soon to be convened in Rio de Janeiro in 1992 (UN, 1997). I noticed that governments were not necessarily committed to solving environmental problems but that concerned individuals acting as advocates were the conscience that kept these issues in the public eye. Ordinary people were asking and even demanding that government officials pay attention to their commitments. I wanted to learn more about this concerned citizenry, known also as "NGOs" or nongovernmental organizations (UN, 2016).

This led me, for the first time, to travel to the east coast of the United States for a conference where I met many people working on environmental concerns, as well as others working on global issues such as human rights and conflict resolution. I wanted to learn more and become actively involved myself. It was at this juncture of my own midlife crisis that my marriage also came into crisis. My husband, who was hunkering down in favor of quiet, reflective life, wanted none of this wider world. So, after several years of separation, we agreed to a friendly divorce. I moved to Washington, DC, to continue my exploration of "civil society" advocacy. This move also led to meeting new networks in Canada's capital, Ottawa, and opportunities to frequently visit and learn from new friends and NGO experiences there.

During these initial years in Washington, DC, and Ottawa, I also learned more about the worldwide needs of women and the growing empowerment of women to address these needs. In 1995, the UN Women's Summit was convened in Beijing, China, with opportunities and challenges similar to the 1992 Rio Earth Summit. Here, women's issues came to the forefront, such as the lack of rights to determine when to have sex or bear children, being forced to do heavy menial tasks like carrying wood long distances for cooking fires, disregard for the education and value of girls and even the killing of infant girls, where boys were the preferred consumers of already scarce food (UN Women, 2015).

During this same time, my own nursing practice seemed to be merely a means to an end. I lived simply and supported my travels and discoveries with short-term nursing contracts that allowed me the time to attend NGO conferences at the G-7 Economic Summit in Halifax, Nova Scotia (University of Toronto, 2014), at the World

Bank, and even the UN. I was soon called upon to share my reflections on the holistic connections between health and stress in the context of these wider issues. I joined a new team of friends, from many disciplines, who were speaking about and connecting the dots between health, stress, ecology, and economics. These endeavors expanded my take on holistic health to wider considerations, finally inclusive of emotional, mental, and spiritual health, and also addressing the broader environmental, cultural, and social concerns of humanity. I learned that *health* was globally defined, upon the founding of the World Health Organization (WHO; 1948) as "a state of complete physical, mental, and social well-being and not merely the absence of disease or infirmity."

But I had also assumed that, with all of my global discoveries, I was actually walking away from nursing. It seemed to me that I was the only nurse at any of these NGO conferences. While working part-time in clinical settings, I would sometimes share my experiences with my coworkers. They would listen politely, but almost no one could see the value of what I was learning. I remember watching a nurse colleague's eyes glaze over and even being confronted by people who told me that these broader ideas had nothing at all to do with nursing. I tended to agree.

It was just at that moment that I encountered the most significant turning point in my nursing career. By then, I had established a pilot program with new friends called "Wellness Dynamics," to further share the global holistic connections between health and related issues of economics, environment, education, society, and culture (Wright & Beck, 1996). With this program, we were encouraged to present our work at the UN in New York City, in preparation for the 1996 UN Human Settlements Programme (UNHSP, 2015), also called "Habitat II," to be convened in Istanbul, Turkey, that June. Because our presentation addressed multiple health connections in the context of this summit's theme, the "habitats" where people live, we were invited to share our work in meetings convened during the summit's International NGO Forum.

In the midst of our early planning to achieve this new project, I was asked if I knew that Florence Nightingale had begun her famous nursing work in Istanbul. "She did?" I responded, much surprised. Then, to be honest, I only had a vague memory, from first-year nursing school, that Nightingale had somehow founded modern nursing education. But I did not remember how.

However, our host of the Istanbul planning group knew all about her. She knew that Nightingale had indeed begun her famous nursing work at a Crimean War (1854–1856) barracks hospital, then called Scutari (now Selimilye) that is still standing on the Asian side of Constantinople, now Istanbul (Dossey, 2010). It was agreed that it would be a significant opportunity to honor Nightingale at this very barracks site with a special UN tribute to her during this upcoming summit. Two weeks later, this plan was confirmed. I was to collaborate in planning and cohosting this event with leading Turkish nurses and nursing educators in Istanbul.

This encounter sent me to look more closely at the significance of Nightingale's life. But I wondered whether—beyond her work to nurse war-wounded and dying soldiers and to contribute to modern nursing education—Nightingale's life had any relevance to what we were doing as concerned civil society of the then late 20th century. Would Nightingale's insights have anything to do with a UN summit focused on the quality of life in the places where people live in "human habitats?" What would she have said to the then active *global citizen* efforts to make a difference for the many global concerns at the dawn of the 21st century?

What I found was truly amazing to me. I discovered that, after her initial famous nursing work in Turkey, Nightingale had continued to focus on the critical multifactorial global health issues of her time for nearly four decades. She accomplished this in ways familiar to us now. She changed political will by interacting with government leaders across the British Empire and elsewhere. She improved the environments of both rural and urban people to sustain health, advocating for better living conditions for women, children, and the poor. She collaborated with the media, while also broadly networking through written correspondence with numerous friends and colleagues (Beck, 2005b). Today, more than 14,000 of her letters exist in collections around the world (McDonald, 2013). Calling all of her work "health nursing," she said, "Health is not only to be well, but to use well every power we have" (Nightingale, 1893, p. 289).

Much to my surprise, Nightingale thus became the very model I was looking for, as both a nurse and a civil society activist. She was, indeed, a *global citizen nurse* who had worked not only at the bedside and in nursing education, but also on the same broader issues I had come to understand and work upon myself! At the UN's International Tribute to Nightingale at Scutari that convened several months later in Istanbul, I spoke to the audience about my own renewed conviction and clarified my focus for the years to come. "Nightingale saw 19th century problems and created 20th century solutions. We see 20th century problems and we can create 21st century solutions. That's why we are here today" (Beck, 1996).

I also pondered the possibility that Florence Nightingale's legacy could well inspire the nurses of our new century to become global citizens themselves, collaborating together to advocate for global issues related to health beyond the limits of their hospital culture. I would invest several more years of time and energy to develop this idea further. During this time, I collaborated with new friends and colleagues, including several Nightingale scholars, who would also come to share this vision with me. In time, I became a Nightingale scholar myself.

Researching the previously unexamined work that Nightingale achieved near the end of her life, I wrote a doctoral dissertation to establish a stronger academic connection between the practice of nursing and Nightingale's global insights and outreach (Beck, 2002). Based on this, I then coauthored a nursing textbook that has become a new model for studying Nightingale's life and its relevance to today's nurses (Dossey, Selanders, Beck, & Attewell, 2005).

Nevertheless, something was still missing and my coauthors and I knew it. Although it was all very well and important to study Nightingale and to establish in-depth academic relevance of her work to today's challenges, we knew that research and textbooks would not, in and of themselves, achieve change. Ideas developed in books must be further developed by people working on the ground to establish sustainable improvements based on ideas. It is all about putting *theory into action,* aiming for that flawless well-oiled machine of praxis. What next?

We knew that Florence Nightingale had become widely known and loved as an inspiring, heroic figure. This is not just in the United States, Canada, and Britain; it is so also in modern China, Japan, and India, Africa and the Arab world, Turkey and the Caribbean, the South Pacific, and all the Americas. We knew this worldwide love of Nightingale had occurred for a number of reasons. She was fluent in six languages. Beyond English, she read, wrote, and spoke French, German, Italian, Latin, and Greek, and advocated for cross-cultural understanding (Dossey, 2010). She established an extensive correspondence and received into her home a wide range of people from across the world who consulted with her about how to improve and create better health conditions for their people. Through her own networking, she spread her ideas out into the wider world, essentially functioning as an international health minister and popular global health writer would today (Beck, 2005c).

Based on her own foundational experience with battlefield conditions, she drafted the British position papers presented first in a series of Geneva Conventions that directly led to establishing the International Red Cross, then the League of Nations, and, later, the UN (Dossey, 2010). Anticipating the wider interconnected concerns we readily see today, she called for better conditions for women, children, the poor and hungry, and for better education programs for marginalized people. She identified what we now call *environmental health determinants* like clean air, water, food, and houses, and *social health determinants*, such as family and community relationships, literacy, education, and employment (Beck, 2010).

In response to studying these Nightingale insights and methods to achieve these efforts, we asked ourselves, in the year 2001, "What would Nightingale have done with fax machines, e-mail, and the Internet? What kind of similar network can we build now?"

Like me, I noted that Nightingale had also maintained a vision—a calling to use her life to serve the suffering she witnessed as a nurse. So clear was her sense of intuition and connectedness that, throughout her life, Nightingale took her own stand to courageously become a health advocate from a worldview of caring for and about the needs of others. As a woman living in a world dominated by a society of men, including the paternalism displayed by doctors, she achieved a new level of concern for the sick and impoverished people of the world (Dossey, 2010). Also, she sought to remedy the causes of that suffering. Although she faced many cultural barriers stemming from the patriarchal worldview of her times, she stood within her own conviction for changes that were necessary. In doing so, she became a catalyst for an emerging worldview that created "nursing" as we know it today. As a woman, she was an agent of change who set a culture of caring in motion that still continues, even now, into the wider possibilities of the 21st century (Beck, 2013). As a nurse, Nightingale challenged other nurses and leaders on every continent to raise their standards of practical concern for humanity. For her, nursing was both personal and global, a method for establishing her public advocacy and widely communicating her knowledge, skills, and commitments.

From these Nightingale achievements, a compelling idea arose in collaboration with my visionary new colleagues—an idea that would later become the Nightingale Initiative for Global Health, often called NIGH (Beck, Dossey, & Rushton, 2013a; see Chapter 4 for more information on NIGH). In 2004, NIGH was established upon this broader Nightingale legacy to become a catalytic nurse-inspired grassroots-to-global movement of public advocacy and to increase wider concern about the priority of health. To establish this, we cocreated a new "Nightingale Declaration for A Healthy World" that begins with the words, "We the nurses and concerned citizens of the global community, hereby dedicate ourselves to achieve a healthy world" (NIGH, 2013a). As of this writing, this Declaration is known to have more than 25,000 signatories from 110 nations (see Figure 4.1).

Further, NIGH has focused on using continually emerging Internet tools to empower nurses and as many concerned citizens as possible with stronger public advocacy skills to influence the changes needed to improve overall global health. As of 2015, NIGH's outreach has evolved to include an online audience of more than 95,000 people from 146 nations and territories, many of whom are leaders representing millions more around the world. NIGH is developing a new culture: a global network of people using innovative approaches to advocate for and about global health needs through the lens of nursing.

Across this same timeline, in the year 2000, a UN Millennium Summit was convened to establish eight "Millennium Development Goals" (MDGs). Of these eight goals, three MDGs—#4, "Reduce child mortality," #5, "Improve maternal health," and #6, "Combat HIV/AIDS, TB, malaria, and other diseases"—are directly related to health and nursing. The other five goals are all social and environmental determinants of health and are concerned with poverty and hunger, education, gender equality and empowerment, environmental sustainability, and global partnerships (UN, 2015).

UN Secretary General Ban Ki Moon has noted that "health" is the common thread running through all eight UN MDGs (Beck et al., 2013a). This observation points directly to the work Nightingale achieved in her time and directly connects these goals to our Nightingalean legacy. As these UN goals are aims similar to those we work to achieve every day, nurses are, indeed, engaged in the work of global health through a wide range of grassroots endeavors (Beck et al., 2013a).

Meanwhile, starting in 2007, I also worked closely with our growing NIGH team and other collaborators to prepare for a worldwide celebration of the 2010 Florence Nightingale Centennial to commemorate her death in 1910 and celebrate her amazing life. Framing this also as the *2010 International Year of the Nurse*, we worked together to build this campaign with worldwide outreach of the aforementioned Nightingale Declaration. Based on suggestions from senior officials, we met at the UN in both New York City and Geneva, Switzerland, and dedicated the year 2010 to celebrating how nurses, themselves, are working and advocating for the eight UN MDGs.

For this, NIGH collaborated with *Nursing Spectrum* and *USA Today* to bring coverage of the 2010 Year of the Nurse and related webinars to more than 750,000 readers (Beck, Dossey, & Rushton, 2014). NIGH's team also cosponsored and presented at key 2010 Year of the Nurse events. The biggest was the *Florence Nightingale Centennial Commemorative Global Service Celebrating Nursing* at the National Cathedral in Washington, D.C. It was cosponsored by the International Honor Society of Nursing, Sigma Theta Tau International (STTI). At this commemorative, nurses overflowed the cathedral; we were all inspired and informed by nurses from across the world. The five-camera webcast of this service can still be enjoyed from the cathedral's website (National Cathedral, Washington, DC, 2010).

These celebrations were wonderful to have, and we achieved considerable appreciation for nurses and within nurses' ranks around the world. But, we also knew that the key UN MDGs we were advocating for, especially the ones connected to health and nursing, were still representing billions of people at risk. Although these MDGs became a milestone for understanding the dynamics of both local and global development (UN Economic & Social Council [ECOSOC], 2015), progress to achieve them has been inconsistent, and, in some cases, slow. This has been particularly true for one

MDG specific to health and to nursing: #5, "Improve maternal health." Although the global ratio of maternal deaths has declined by 47% since 1990, nearly 800 women and girls still die in pregnancy and childbirth each day. This means one mother perishes, on average, every 2 minutes, totaling a shocking 280,000 each year. Despite the worldwide work of identifying and advocating for the UN MDGs, these continuing tragedies still require considerable accelerated interventions, as well as stronger social and political support for women and children (WHO, 2014). And we, as nurses, know that these must include strategies to strengthen health care delivery, particularly the services of nurses and midwives in rural areas (WHO, 2015).

How would Nightingale have dealt with these concerns? Based on her life and insights, we know she would have encouraged a number of approaches, including training more people to attend to births and educating young women and girls about their own reproductive health. We also know that one of her answers would have been to mobilize public opinion to raise awareness, advocating for commitment to improved health outcomes worldwide. With this specific strategy in mind, our NIGH team created an online outreach campaign called "Daring, Caring & Sharing to Save Mothers' Lives" (NIGH, 2016) to engage nurses and midwives in "daring and caring to share" stories that could turn the prevailing tide of apathy. With online stories and social media outreach, this campaign has focused on telling this oft-untold story and championing the needs and deeds of those nurses and midwives who are already making a difference to maternal health worldwide.

It has also been clear that although the overall MDG framework has been a key tool to increase development and concern for development, the limited MDG timeframe of only 15 years is insufficient. Thus, it was recognized at the UN MDG summit convened in 2010 that a longer framework, called the *Post-2015 Agenda*, was needed. Also, at the UN Rio+20 Summit convened in the same year, ideas to establish a new set of UN Sustainable Development Goals (SDGs) to be achieved by 2030, were proposed. The combination of plans has resulted in a series of global discussions that transcend the limits of UN member governments to include members of global civil society, NGOs, philanthropic organizations, academia, and the private sector (United Nations Development Programme [UNDP], 2015).

To participate and to further build NIGH's global relevance and outreach, I have been collaborating to build a team of nurses who are serving as volunteer UN NGO representatives at the UN headquarters in New York City. Six nurses have become actively involved in the UN post-2015 agenda discussions (NIGH, 2015a). As of this writing, four represent NIGH and two represent STTI (STTI, 2014), all attending related UN briefings, programs, and meetings together. Noting the UN's mandate to generate civil society discussions beyond these meetings, they became unsatisfied with simply attending without sharing what they had learned with others. They recognized that all nurses, as participants of civil society from across the world, could also be included in the UN's online and onsite consultations about the post-2015 agenda. So, together, we began by sharing with 100 nurses at a workshop, which NIGH cohosted in New York City in April 2014. Encouraged by the feedback we received from this first consultation, we created an online global briefing called *The World Nurses Want* to further introduce the connections between nursing and the UN's MDGs and emerging UN SDGs. This online offering provides an opportunity for nurses from around the world to participate in UN- and NIGH-related online surveys (NIGH, 2014). Further, in August 2014, this team shared this work at a UN international NGO conference (Beck, 2014). Through these diverse strategies, we have demonstrated how nurses can see themselves as global advocates, broadening their health and healing worldviews, while also achieving grassroots actions. With this wider lens, we can create new meaning-making toward health, including the process of global health-making (Beck, Dossey, & Rushton, 2013b).

■ MORAL/ETHICAL FOUNDATION

My childhood had steeped me in the realm of many of the arts. My parents provided me with an artist's mindset that I did not think too much about. It was simply our way of life. This was my own natural way of defining the world around me. It was through this artists' viewpoint from my parents' perspectives that I first came to understand and define life's inherent values and meaning. It was from this particular foundation that I also came to define my personal ethics.

Much later, while in graduate school, I came across a quote that profoundly touched upon my own life experience as a nurse and gave me an "aha" that would, thereafter, help me to better understand and define the inherent values of nursing.

> The scientist, if asked whether a given experiment could be repeated with identical results, would have to say "yes"—or it wouldn't be science. . . . The artist, if asked whether an art piece could be remade with identical results, would have to say "no"—or it wouldn't be art. (Bayles & Orland, 1994, pp. 105–106)

This provided me with a new way to understand the key differences between the lens of art and the lens of science—the differences between the way an artist views the world and a scientist views the world. The scientist and the artist each sees and, therefore, defines and interacts with his or her world differently.

Perhaps my own early artist's lens had initially blocked my ability to see myself as a nurse—to define myself as a nurse and align myself with nursing's values. Over time, I would come to learn of and apply myself to the science of modern medicine and nursing. I would come to see nursing through a science lens. Here, we rely upon accuracy and standards of practice. This is particularly true in critical care settings, where lives hang in the balance of precise medicine dosages and procedures and on fine-tuned, science-based technical equipment.

But even as I mastered the science required of a critical care nurse in these settings, I noticed that there was something beyond the science that I was also applying. With each unique interaction with patients, and often with families who were coping with the tenuous situations of their loved ones, I found that to become an effective nurse, I was tapping into something more than science could provide me. Science gave me a safe practice to rely upon. But in coping with life and death every day, my sense of nursing's meaning, the values and ethical core of nursing, came from something else, although I did not define this something else as "art." During those early years of my nursing career, I had learned to apply science to my work. I came home to do my art and to be an artist. I saw myself as commuting between these two worlds.

Much later, as I continued my in-depth study of Nightingale, I was moved to learn of her own worldview on the foundations of nursing practice: "Nursing is an art: and if it is to be made an art, it requires an exclusive devotion as hard a preparation as any painter's or sculptor's work" (1871, p. 6). There it was. She had confirmed that nursing required the same commitment, practice, and dedication of any artist. She continues:

> For what is the having to do with dead canvas or dead marble, compared with having to do with the living body, the temple of God's spirit? It is one of the Fine Arts: I had almost said, the finest of Fine Arts. (1871, p. 6)

Here, Nightingale defined nursing in a profound manner, reminding us of the sacredness of our task and a way to illuminate nursing's values, beyond the daily challenges we face to get our work done, to view the ethical foundation of our practice.

Although it is true that Nightingale's 19th-century perspective predates important scientific discoveries and the scientific progress of nursing, now into the 21st century, her lens regarding the art of nursing also provides us with a heightened perspective on the timelessness of nursing's eternal service to humanity. Science gives us a measure of accuracy for the "how" we apply our work. But it does not give us the "when" we should apply scientific breakthroughs nor the "when" we should consider these breakthroughs as inappropriate, unnecessary, or inhumane. Science does not give us the moral "why" of our work. Science gives us the *means*. But we must also continually find the *meaning* of nursing. The ethical questions we often face, given the life-and-death nature of nursing's context, require us to both incorporate the "hows" of science and tap the "whens" and "whys" of something more encompassing, something beyond the limited empirical approaches of science.

Across my nursing career, my own artistic lens provided me with that "something more," even before I realized it. The science of nursing that I learned to safely apply to my patients is, indeed, both important and vital. The art of nursing, working with unique human beings who find themselves in vulnerable and deeply personal circumstances each day requires unique perspectives on their care and unique interactions with each as individuals. This knowledge was the foundation on which I built my own nursing ethics and morality. Human beings and humanity itself, the "who" and "what" I was serving, were also questions I was also answering. This was the "why" I became a nurse and the "why" I came to believe in the values of nursing practice, shaping my ethics and personal-to-global worldview accordingly.

■ VISION

Over time, and particularly over the last decade, I have more fully identified with Florence Nightingale's wider view of nursing's potential. She was a champion for the broader health of humanity and envisioned this role of nurses as well. Near the end of her career, she articulated her vision in a unique opportunity she was given to contribute to the 1893 Columbian World's Fair. Hosted in Chicago, this fair was the first international event to highlight women's contributions to human progress. Queen Victoria was fully committed to this fair and commissioned an anthology of women writers titled *Women's Mission*, as one of Britain's lasting contributions to this leading-edge idea

(Burdett-Coutts, 1893). Nightingale was thus invited to be one the featured authors. Her chapter, "Sick-Nursing and Health-Nursing," provides detail of the many possibilities for nurses and nursing that Nightingale could see based on her own long career of nearly 40 years at the time. Indeed, including and beyond her vision for the major "sick-nursing" role that nurses had since achieved across the world, Nightingale also articulated a global advocacy role for nurses. Thus, her vision for "health-nursing" reflects the work that she herself achieved to publicly call for necessary changes to improve health across the world (Nightingale, 1893).

What if today's nurses could be engaged and empowered to become champions for the broader health of humanity like Nightingale? Might our advocacy role now emerge into becoming proactive global citizens? This is a nursing role yet to be fully realized, a role as change agent at levels beyond the sickbed to making a difference at global levels. But, how would we do this? And, perhaps more to the point, why would we not do this?

Although we see ourselves as advocates for our patients, we nurses have been conditioned across many decades to remain silent about what we see and what we have accomplished. Our nursing culture has shaped us to believe in the virtues of this silent approach to respect the confidentiality and to keep what we do and think hidden. Although the discipline of medicine has no such constraints, nursing has consistently shied away from making its contributions and the theoretical foundations of its practice visible to the public (Buresh & Gordon, 2000). It is the public we seek to protect and serve, but yet it is the public who knows nothing of the truth of our profession.

In "Sick-Nursing & Health-Nursing," Nightingale specifically called for nurses' voices to be heard, reminding that "you must form public opinion" (Nightingale, 1893, p. 292). We also hear this call from others in our time, notably from nursing theorist Dr. Jean Watson:

> Caring knowledge of women and nursing [can] no longer remain hidden . . . [and that] work today, again, requires strong voices . . . courageously and convincingly conveying a new proclamation for reform in personal, public, political and social thinking and acting of our time. (Watson, 1999, p. 264; see also Chapter 16 for more on Dr. Watson's call to caring)

In my work to develop NIGH, I have often been asked, "How do we practice global nursing?" We know how to practice nursing at the bedside. We know our tasks and our tools. At the global level, we do not have a syringe to deliver medicine to the broad scope of humanity. Nor have we identified the protocols to outline a set of global tasks. My answer has been to more clearly define how we look at achieving global health.

Global health is accomplished through the application of communications at global levels. It is the worldwide advocacy of the health needs of humanity, the dissemination of care and concern for problems that still have to be solved and the identification of how solutions have been and can be achieved. What are the tasks and tools of global nursing? We are already accomplished advocates. The task of global advocacy is simply the widening of our scopes to share the value of our perspectives and the effectiveness of our practices with the more expansive world. Our tools are all around us.

In the 21st century, the sharing of information is making a significant impact on the culture of humanity. I believe that nurses can learn to participate more fully in this emerging culture. Our new global nursing tools can include communications channels such as websites, radio talk shows, letters to the editor, and newspaper human interest stories, as well as social media venues like YouTube. Through the deliberate and appropriate utilization of these blossoming communication milieus, nurses can be encouraged and trained to become media-based health promotion advocates, to create, produce, and air our ideas for the value of health in our communities and in our world. Nurses have always shared a vision with each other for healing and for health. Now we can also share this vision with everyone else.

Across my own life and nursing career, I have come to appreciate and explore the ways in which the arts can articulate this advocacy and its inherent value. In the development of NIGH, I often celebrate how I have come full circle to return to the artistic perspectives of my childhood and my parents' skills in art and journalism. I have been granted the privilege to witness how advocating through communications, and particularly multimedia arts, can inform and inspire nurses, as well as others, to consider and commit to global health concerns. For instance, through the crafting and online posting of media projects based on collections of photographs of nurses from around the world, I have discovered how videography can articulate the art of nursing and advocate for the common ground and values of nursing worldwide (NIGH, 2013b, 2015b). I have discovered how stories about global health concerns shared through the advocacy of my nursing lens can be written through the means of "citizen journalism" via the Internet. Across the rest of my productive life, I am aiming to continue this work—encompassing the nursing experiences I have had and extending what I have learned and applied in citizen journalism, media arts, and across the scope of global advocacy for health—to share these "integral" (Beck, Dossey, & Rushton, 2011) approaches, opportunities, skills, and strategies with many other nurses around the world.

Nurses are the world's largest health care workforce. The International Council of Nurses (ICN), a federation of national nursing associations from 132 out of 193 UN member states, counts our numbers as at least 16 million strong (ICN, 2013). We are consistently polled as the most trusted of professionals (Riffkin, 2014). What better voices to collectively call for what needs to happen for the sake of health at local, regional, and global levels?

The bicentenary of Nightingale's birth will be the year 2020, but we have yet to realize how to live out our broader Nightingale legacy. By providing good sick-care and advocacy for individual patient rights, we have followed in only some of Nightingale's footsteps. To fully participate in and celebrate the 2020 Nightingale Bicentenary, might we bring her broader worldview to the global community of today? Could human health become valued enough to create consensus and collaboration toward achieving a healthy world? Could nurses become the global visionaries and global change agents Nightingale envisioned for us (Nightingale, 1893)?

We can focus our collective callings for the sake of 21st-century health care and related social, ecological, and human rights issues. We can continue the practices we have established and we can also be innovative by creating new practice arenas. We can model our art and advocacy—the fulfillment and satisfaction of being nurses, of bringing health and healing to our world—broadening the scope of our 21st-century nursing practice. Nightingale passed this vision on to us: to remember who we are, what we can do, who we care for, and why. Now it is up to us to share this vision, as she did, with our world.

■ REFLECTIONS

1. *Did I always want to be a nurse? If so, do I know why? If not, when did nursing become my chosen career or "calling" and why did this change for me?*
2. *Am I able to apply the perspective of the "art of nursing" to my practice and to my nursing leadership? If so, why? If not, why not?*
3. *How might my perspectives help me to motivate students and others who are struggling to stay enthusiastic about nursing in the face of nursing's challenges?*
4. *Given the plethora of communication strategies available today, can I see myself participating in a global public advocacy role for nurses? If so, how would I go about this? What might I do to motivate others to achieve this?*
5. *To prepare for and celebrate the Nightingale Bicentenary in 2020, what steps can I take in my community today that would further my role as a proactive global citizen?*

■ REFERENCES

Bayles, D., & Orland, T. (1994). *Art and fear: Observations of the perils (and rewards) of artmaking.* Santa Barbara, CA: Capra Press.

Beck, D. M. (1996). *In the context of Habitat II: Revisiting Florence Nightingale at Scutari.* Keynote address presented at the International Tribute to Florence Nightingale, United Nations Human Settlements Summit, Istanbul (author's notes, June 4, 1996).

Beck, D. M. (2002). *Florence Nightingale's 1983 "Sick-nursing and health-nursing": Weaving a tapestry of positive health determinants for personal, community and global wellness.* (Doctoral dissertation). Ann Arbor, MI: UMI Dissertation Services.

Beck, D. M. (2005a). At the millennium crossroads: Reigniting the flame of Nightingale's legacy. In B. M. Dossey, L. Selanders, D. M. Beck, & A. Attewell (Eds.), *Florence Nightingale today: Healing, leadership, global action* (pp. 127–141). Silver Spring, MD: NursesBooks.org.

Beck, D. M. (2005b). 21st century citizenship for health: "May a better way be opened." In B. M. Dossey, L. Selanders, D. M. Beck, & A. Attewell (Eds.), *Florence Nightingale today: Healing, leadership, global action* (pp. 177–193). Silver Spring, MD: NursesBooks.org.

Beck, D. M. (2005c). Sick-nursing & health-nursing: Nightingale establishes our broad scope of practice in 1893. In B. M. Dossey, L. Selanders, D. M. Beck, & A. Attewell (Eds.), *Florence Nightingale today: Healing, leadership, global action* (pp. 151–167). Silver Spring, MD: NursesBooks.org.

Beck, D. M. (2010). Remembering Florence Nightingale's panorama: 21st century nursing—at a critical crossroads. *Journal of Holistic Nursing Practice, 28*(4), 291–301.

Beck, D. M. (2013). Empowering women and girls—empowering nurses: A narrative to discover Florence Nightingale's global citizenship legacy. In S. G. Mijares, A. Rafea, & N. Angha (Eds.), *A force such as the world has never known: Women creating change* (pp. 40–52). Toronto, ON: Innana Publications.

Beck, D. M. (2014). *A step-by-step action agenda for NGOs to promote civil society involvement in 'The World We Want' 2015 Campaign.* A panel presentation of five nurses, as UN NGO Representatives, at the 2014 International United Nations NGO Conference in New York City (panel moderator notes, August 29, 2014).

Beck, D. M., & Beck, J. (1986). *The pleasure connection: How endorphins affect our health and happiness.* San Marcos, CA: Synthesis Press.

Beck, D. M., & Beck, J. (1988). *Les endorphins: L'autogestion du bien-etre.* Village de Haute, Provence, France: Le Souffle d'Or.

Beck, D. M., Dossey, B. M., & Rushton, C. H. (2011). Integral nursing & the Nightingale Initiative for Global Health: Florence Nightingale's integral legacy for the 21st century. *Journal of Integral Theory and Practice, 6*(4), 71–94.

Beck, D. M., Dossey, B. M., & Rushton, C. H. (2013a). Building the Nightingale Initiative for Global Health—NIGH: Can we engage and empower the public voices of nurses worldwide? *Nursing Science Quarterly, 26*(4), 366–371.

Beck, D. M., Dossey, B. M., & Rushton, C. H. (2013b). Global activism, advocacy and transformation: Florence Nightingale's legacy for the 21st century. In M. J. Kreitzer & M. Koithan (Eds.), *Integrative nursing* (pp. 526–537). New York, NY: Oxford University Press.

Beck, D. M., Dossey, B. M., & Rushton, C. H. (2014). Florence Nightingale: Connecting her legacy with local-to-global health today. *Nursing Spectrum Online CE Offering.* Retrieved from http://ce.nurse.com/RCourseSearch.aspx?SearchT=598

Burdett-Coutts, A. (1893). *Women's mission: A series of congress papers of the philanthropic work of women by eminent writers.* London, UK: Sampson, Low, Marston and Co.

Buresh, B., & S. Gordon. (2000). *From silence to voice: What nurses know and must communicate to the public.* Ottawa, ON: Canadian Nurses Association.

Cousins, N. (1979). *Anatomy of an illness as perceived by the patient: Reflections on healing and regeneration.* New York, NY: Norton.

Davis, J. (1984). *Endorphins: New waves in brain chemistry.* Garden City, NY: Doubleday.

Dossey, B. M. (2010). *Florence Nightingale: Mystic, visionary, healer* [commemorative edition]. Philadelphia, PA: F.A. Davis.

Dossey, B. M., & Keegan, L (Eds.). (2016). *Holistic nursing: A handbook for practice* (7th ed.). Sudbury, MA: Jones & Bartlett Learning.

Dossey, B. M., Selanders, L., Beck, D. M., & Attewell, A. (2005). *Florence Nightingale today: Healing, leadership, global action.* Silver Spring, MD: NurseBooks.org.

Dossey, L. (1989). *Recovering the soul: A scientific and spiritual search.* London, UK: Bantam Press-Random House.

International Council of Nurses (ICN). (2013). *Members.* Retrieved from http://www.icn.ch/members/members/

Kingma, M. (2001). *The emerging global nursing shortage.* Geneva, Switzerland: International Council of Nurses.

Leyten, Q. H., Gabreels, F. J. M., Renier, W. O., Ter Laak, H. J., Sengers, R. C. A., & Mullaart, R. A. (1989). Congenital muscular dystrophy. *Journal of Pediatrics, 115*(2), 214–221.

Luton, F. (2015). Wounded healer. *Jungian Dream Analysis and Psychotherapy.* Retrieved from http://www.frithluton.com

McDonald, L. (2013). *The collected works of Florence Nightingale.* University of Guelph. Retrieved from http://www.uoguelph.ca/~cwfn/

National Cathedral, Washington, DC. (2010). *Florence Nightingale Centennial: Commemorative global service celebrating nursing.* Retrieved from http://www.nationalcathedral.org/events/Nightingale20100425.shtml#.UZ2asRw0SPE

Nightingale, F. (1871). *Una and the lion.* London, UK: Riverside Press.

Nightingale, F. (1893). Sick-nursing and health-nursing. In B. M. Dossey, L. Selanders, D. M. Beck, & A. Attewell (Eds.), *Florence Nightingale today: Healing, leadership, global action* (pp. 288–303). Silver Spring, MD: NursesBooks.org.

Nightingale Initiative for Global Health. (2013a). Nightingale Declaration for a Healthy World. Retrieved from http://www.nighvision.net/nightingale-declaration.html

Nightingale Initiative for Global Health. (2013b). Nurses & Midwives Celebrated—Via Video—atWHO's 60th.Retrieved from http://www.nighvision.net/nurses--midwives-at-whos-60th.html

Nightingale Initiative for Global Health. (2014). *The world nurses want: Nursing and the United Nations.* Retrieved from http://www.theworldnurseswant.net/learn-more.html

Nightingale Initiative for Global Health. (2015a). *Our team: NIGH's UN DPI NGO youth representatives.* Retrieved from http://www.theworldnurseswant.net/our-team.html

Nightingale Initiative for Global Health. (2015b). *At the heart of it all: Nurses & midwives for universal health care.* Retrieved from http://www.nighvision.net/with-who-mdash-a-video.html

Nightingale Initiative for Global Health. (2016). *Raising awareness for mothers' health—UN MDG #5.* Retrieved from http://www.nighvision.net/raising-awareness-for-mdg-5.html

Riffkin, R. (2014). *Americans rate nurses highest on honesty, ethical standards.* Retrieved from http://www.gallup.com/poll/180260/americans-rate-nurses-highest-honesty-ethical-standards.aspx

Segal, B. S. (1986). *Love, medicine and miracles: Lessons learned about self-healing.* New York, NY: Harper Collins.

Selye, H. (1974). *Stress without distress.* Philadelphia, PA: J.B. Lippincott.

Sigma Theta Tau International (STTI), Upsilon Chapter. (2014). *Global initiatives.* Retrieved from http://upsilon.nursingsociety.org/globalinitiativescommittee

United Nations. (1997). *United Nations conference on environment and development, 1992.* Retrieved from http://www.un.org/geninfo/bp/enviro.html

United Nations. (2015). *The United Nations millennium development goals report 2011.* Retrieved from http://www.un.org/millenniumgoals/pdf/(2011_E)%20MDG%20Report%202011_Book%20LR.pdf

United Nations. (2016). *United Nations and the rule of law.* Retrieved from https://www.un.org/ruleoflaw

United Nations Development Programme. (2015). *Post-2015 development agenda.* Retrieved from http://www.undp.org/content/undp/en/home/mdgoverview/mdg_goals/post-2015-development-agenda

United Nations Economic & Social Council. (2015). *Millennium development goals and the post-2015 development agenda.* Retrieved from http://www.un.org/en/ecosoc/about/mdg.shtml

United Nations Human Settlements Programme. (2015). *History, mandate & role in the UN system.* Retrieved from http://unhabitat.org/about-us/history-mandate-role-in-the-un-system/

United Nations Women. (2015). *United Nations Fourth Conference on Women, 1995.* Retrieved from http://www.un.org/womenwatch/daw/beijing/fwcwn.html

University of Toronto. (2014). *G-7 Halifax summit, June 15-17, 1995.* Retrieved from http://www.g8.utoronto.ca/summit/1995halifax

Watson, J. (1999). *Postmodern nursing and beyond.* Edinburgh, Scotland: Churchill Livingston.

Watson, J. (2008). *Nursing: The philosophy and science of caring* (Rev. ed.). Boulder, CO: University Press of Colorado.

World Health Organization. (2006). *Basic documents* (45th ed.), supplement. Retrieved from http://www.who.int/governance/eb/who_constitution_en.pdf

World Health Organization. (2014). *MDG 5: Improve maternal health.* Retrieved from http://www.who.int/topics/millennium_development_goals/maternal_health/en

World Health Organization. (2015). *WHO nursing & midwifery progress report 2008 to 2012.* Retrieved from http://www.who.int/hrh/nursing_midwifery/progress_report/en

Wright, J., & Beck, D. M. (1996). *Wellness dynamics: The art and science of wellness.* Ottawa, Ontario, Canada: The Wellness Foundation.

CHAPTER NINETEEN

Egoless and Interconnected: Suspending Judgment to Embrace Heart-Centered Health Care

Joseph Giovannoni

Your competence as a healer is proportional to your courage in exploring, acknowledging, and addressing your own wounding; and revisiting the validity of long-held beliefs and prejudices.
                    —Giovannoni (personal communication, June 29, 2015)

■ WHY NURSING?

I think my inclination toward nursing is probably not much different from most who are called to the profession. In a word, I wanted to help people who were suffering. The definition of *responsibility* in Hawaiian is not separate from the word *privilege*. The infusion of privilege with responsibility most readily describes my motivation to become a nurse.

This question compelled me to think about *why* I wanted to help ease others' suffering. The narrative in the following text helps to contextualize what I think it was that most impacted my journey toward this profession. Although not exhaustive, it includes experiences I feel were significantly related to this question. During this sojourn, however, I came to better understand my own motivations, the source of my fears, my own habit formations in response to trauma, and how my own five-sensory ego personality (Zukav, 1989) was formed.

I was born in the small village of Lucca, Italy, in 1945. World War II had just ended. Prior to the war, my family had a thriving shoe-making factory. This was lost due to repeated bombings, leaving my family poverty-stricken. Unemployment was rampant in Italy after the war. My father found work, but not enough to make a living wage. My mother was forced to look for work. This was a wounding for my father who, through no fault of his own, was unable to fulfill his culturally defined role as provider.

My mother worked odd jobs. One in particular happened to be providing in-home care for the ill and dying. My mother had no professional training, but her compassion and tenderness soon made this insignificant. On overnight shifts, she would take me with her. I looked forward to this because people often gave me delicious food that my parents could not afford to buy.

It was years before I realized that I had been nourished by more than food. This was my first exposure to human suffering. My mother was shepherding families through the death of their loved ones. I could see that her presence eased their suffering, but I did not have the language for what I was witnessing.

When I was about 10 years old, my father left us behind while he went to America in search of a better life. I was too young to understand why he had to leave us. The pain of his leaving was physical. My heart hurt without him. Although I was assured that he would come back for us, the months turned to years and I felt abandoned. A child does not have the capacity to see the entirety of a situation. I could not know the pain and longing of my father who had to leave or the courage of my mother who was terrified but put on a brave face for her children.

Shortly after my father left, I became very ill. The family doctor thought I had leukemia, for which there was no cure. I was so sick that I lost nearly two years of schooling. Although I eventually recovered, the memories of what it felt like to be sick and afraid and of my mother's anxiety during that time never left me.

I was 12 when I moved to America. It was a dismal experience for me. Educationally, I had not kept pace with my peers in Italy due to my illness. I did not speak English. I was placed in a third-grade classroom with eight-year-olds. It was humiliating. I believed I was stupid. I was ridiculed by the other kids. Teachers were ill-equipped to deal with the influx of immigrants and often had little patience with me. I began to think of myself as unintelligent and incompetent. I began to develop disdain for myself. I also began to have an awareness of and shame for my own cultural heritage.

I was already shy by nature. This character trait was not a problem in a small village where everyone knew me. In America, it became a disability. I had difficulty making friends. I had no interest in competitive sports, a requisite for respect and admiration in high school that continues to this day. I spent much of my time by myself and was deeply lonely.

As an adolescent, I sought approval and validation from older males who exemplified the kind of person I wanted to be: strong, confident, athletic, the traditional "John Wayne" American male. During my first year in high school, I was sexually abused twice, once by a male stranger and the other by a trusted teacher who was also a Catholic priest. These experiences compounded what was already a fractured self-image. Not only did I feel I had done something bad to bring this on myself, but I was also deeply ashamed. Brown (2010, 2012) deciphers guilt and shame. She writes that the message of guilt is "I did something bad," while the message of shame is "I am bad" (Brown, 2010, p. 42). Brown (2012) goes on to say that "childhood experiences of shame change who we are, how we think about ourselves, and our sense of self-worth" (p. 226). This perfectly describes the self-image I had constructed from these experiences of my formative years.

I now see that I was drawn to the profession of nursing because I had experienced physical and emotional suffering throughout my childhood. I had developed deep empathy for the suffering of others because I knew what it felt like. But perhaps, more importantly, I had also witnessed the healing power of compassionate care exemplified by my mother.

As a child, I thought a nurse was a servant to the physician. This is still true today in some countries. Over time, the role of nurses, especially in the United States, has changed. My impression is that the change has occurred because nursing eventually had to come of age as the sacred profession it was always meant to be, guided by its own theory and practice of human caring (Watson, 2008).

■ EARLY IMPRESSIONS

When I finished high school, I took some college entrance exams, one of which was an IQ test on which I scored less than 60. I did not fare well on any of the other tests either. I was told that college was not an option for me. However, because of my desire for knowledge, I did not let this stop me from trying.

In 1964, I was accepted into the Alexia Brothers Hospital School of Nursing. At the time, this was an all-male school. I still spoke very little English, but a benevolent religious brother recognized my potential and became a mentor to me. I prevailed, obtaining passing grades, and earned my bachelor of science in nursing. My childhood impressions of nursing expanded somewhat to include being present at the bedside and nurturing and comforting those who were ill . . . while still serving as a mere assistant to the physician.

Following this, I became an American citizen. I enlisted in the U.S. Army Nurse Corps, serving in the Vietnam campaign from 1967 to 1970, considered by some historians to be the worst years of the war. Between 1966 and 1968, the United States dropped more than 600,000 tons of bombs on North Vietnam, carpet-bombing the countryside. The Tet Offensive occurred in January of 1968 and the My Lai massacre took place three months later. No one, soldiers or officers, could proudly wear their uniforms in American communities for fear of being ridiculed. The Vietnam War was unpopular and those who served were often referred to as "baby killers," "butchers," and other cruel descriptors. This cold reception, from a country whose soldiers were willing to sacrifice their lives, was unprecedented, and often worse than the trauma of the battlefield.

As an army nurse, I witnessed the trauma that resulted from the insanity of war and the disrespect veterans received from civilians. As a nurse who treated soldiers who returned from the battlefield, I knew firsthand what the soldiers had been through. I worked intimately with them, caring for both physical *and* emotional wounds, trying to bring light to the dark aftermath of war.

Following the completion of my service, I tried my hand at a number of specialties, including medical–surgical, orthopedics, spinal cord injury, and mental health nursing.

One of my jobs entailed working with the elderly. This made an impact on me. I witnessed the indignities of aging in a society that values youth. I saw despair in those who reflected on their lives with guilt and regret. But there were some elderly who, in spite of their physical deterioration, were joyful because they reflected on their lives with equanimity and integrity and still saw value in their lives. I told myself that in my later years, I wanted to be able to reflect on my life with forgiveness, integrity, and joy.

In the early 1970s, I was focused on developing my technical skills, but I also began to take a sincere interest in the people I cared for. I wanted to know them as human beings. I learned about their lives outside of the context of their illness. I found that caring for others in this way fulfilled my need to nurture.

Being a lifelong learner, I eventually returned to college while working full-time. I received a second bachelor's degree, and then a subsequent master's degree in psychology from Roosevelt University in Chicago, Illinois, in 1977. I then studied at the Loyola University Sexual Dysfunction Clinic in Maywood, Illinois, and became a board-certified sex therapist. In 1984, I earned a master of psychiatric mental health nursing degree from the University of Hawaii at Manoa.

Afterward, I taught nursing students in a four-year diploma program and I observed that sexual health and the impact of various medical disorders on sexual functioning went unaddressed in nursing education. I felt it was important to normalize the language of sexuality so that nurses felt comfortable in addressing the patient's sexuality as part of an overall health nursing assessment. I wanted to integrate this aspect of health into the nursing curriculum. As a certified sex therapist, I had the qualifications to develop this.

My expertise in forensic nursing and the treatment of sexual abusers came about serendipitously. During graduate school, I specialized in sexology. My internship mentor was a sexologist who did not like working with child sexual abusers and so she referred them to me. I was fortunate that the literature on the treatment of sex offenders was burgeoning in the 1980s.

At the time that I received my master of science degree in mental health nursing, there was a dearth of sex therapists in Hawaii. In 1985, I developed a community-based program for people with sexual disorders. This was, to my knowledge, the first of its kind in Hawaii. My practice included group therapy, individual counseling, family sessions, and couples counseling. In 1986, I was selected to provide consultation and training specific to the treatment of sexual abusers for workers in the Hawaii State Hospital's forensic unit.

Rapists and child molesters were and are considered pariahs of society, even among convicted felons. They live in fear of being discovered. At the time, the criminal justice system offered substance abuse programs, psychiatric care, job training, education, and other services, but there were no programs for sexual abusers. They were often imprisoned at a higher rate than others whose crime carried the same sentence. For their safety, they often served out their terms in protective custody. This is essentially solitary confinement. When they were released, the problem persisted, but now they had the additional challenge of overcoming the damage caused by prison.

I felt a responsibility to help these men for two reasons: (a) Untreated, they were likely to continue engaging in a behavior that I knew, firsthand, devastated lives, and (b) I refused to judge them. The late Maya Angelou wrote, "No human being can be more human than another human being. I liberate you from my ignorance." For that reason, she refused to judge others.

However, I still lacked confidence in working with this population. I was trained to help people freely express their sexual desires as consenting adults, without the guilt or shame of the social mores they had been raised with. I had little training in how to help someone control a dangerous sexual compulsion. The Association for the Treatment of Sexual Abusers (ATSA) had just been formed and I relied on the expertise of this organization, of which I am still a member. Later, I was trained by skilled therapists and researchers such as Anna Salter (2003) and Jan Hindman (1989).

Legislation began to support specialized sex offender units in probation and parole offices. Probation officers were trained to use evidence-based, cognitive–behavioral relapse prevention methods. The literature of the day upon which these specialized units were built indicated that these were the best practices with sexual offenders. From a public safety perspective, the staples of what came to be called the "containment approach" included a partnership with the criminal justice system, frequent contact with the client's social systems (family of origin, intimate partners, employers, clergy, mental health agencies, and other treatment systems), and polygraphy. Clients signed a complete waiver of confidentiality.

■ PROFESSIONAL EVOLUTION/CONTRIBUTION

By the time my patients are clinically discharged, they must be equipped with a set of evidence-based skills they can rely on when they are in high-risk situations. These are distinct techniques that have been empirically shown to be effective if utilized. I believe I have done a good job fulfilling the State of Hawaii contracts for more than 30 years, all of which require these best practices. I am also fortunate enough to have a highly developed sense of when a client is exhibiting subtle changes in his behavior. Often, this is an indication that he is engaging in high-risk behavior. Early intervention stops the cycle of abuse and enhances public safety.

Changing myself has changed the paradigm under which I teach evidence-based skills. I wanted to allow my clients the opportunity to see themselves as innocent. It is our deepest ego-divided self, informed by our five senses, that defines our experiences and instills within us a profound sense of guilt (Zukav, 1989). This belief is often reflected in religious dogma that has us believing we are guilty of sin.

The concept of original sin has, in my opinion, contributed to humanity's collective belief that we are guilty or bad. This belief makes us prone to acting out in dehumanizing and brutal ways. We project our own self-hatred onto humans, other sentient beings, and the Earth itself—a vicious cycle that, when practicing as a nurse, is simply unacceptable. Stephen Hawking writes that humanity's lack of understanding regarding natural phenomena has resulted in self-blame; the belief that we have sinned and we are being punished by a supreme being. He says, "The human capacity for guilt is such that people can always find ways to blame themselves" (Hawking & Mlodinow, 2010, p. 31).

This fits well with my belief that projecting one's own sense of guilt onto others is a way of keeping us from looking at our own deeds. It is what allows us to judge others. This occurs on an individual level, when we harm someone close to us, and at a global level, with war and the destruction of our Earth. It is not uncommon for my patients to blame their victims and others for their poor choices. The ego's five-sensory personality is quick to judge others rather than courageously explore one's own trauma or to accept help in developing creative solutions to one's problems.

For more than 30 years, I have been working within the confines of a judicial system that focuses on guilt and is primarily punitive and fear based. Clients are always aware that prison is the only other option if they do not progress accordingly. When

I was new to this field, my therapy reflected this model. However, this always left me feeling empty. It went against my caring nature to be confrontational and punitive. I also intuitively knew that something fundamental to healing was missing. I met with probation officers weekly to discuss their probationers' progress. I began to bring in concepts such as helping clients to forgive themselves or helping them to see that their behavior was a call for love. I wanted clients to understand that their behavior was a projection of their own self-hatred and guilt and that lasting progress was not possible without self-forgiveness. But I felt unheard. Forgiving oneself does not imply that a person is not accountable for his or her actions. It is about identifying and releasing the burdensome beliefs that contribute to the poor choices we make.

As I continued to develop professionally, I could see that being confrontational did not help my clients. I fulfilled my contract but also began to incorporate principles of spirituality, human caring, and wholeness. I worked with my clients on self-forgiveness. I call this *cognitive–behavioral forgiveness*. I began to forgive myself for being judgmental and not seeing others as whole. I never stopped advocating for language about compassion and the requirement for professionals to demonstrate real care and concern about this population to be adopted as part of statewide standards for the treatment of sexual abusers. I felt unheard . . . but I did not give up.

I knew that society's punitive attempt at trying to change criminal behavior with punishment was not working. I wanted to change the paradigm. After many years of bumping up against a philosophy that I was convinced did not work without a presence of loving concern for my clients' well-being, I eventually began to experience burnout. The work was no longer fulfilling my need to help alleviate others' suffering. I began to strategize my exit. At the age of 66, I was ready to retire, sell my private practice, and return to my native Lucca to cultivate a small parcel of land I had inherited. After working with a difficult population for so many years, I felt that my pleas to enhance the treatment milieu had fallen on deaf ears.

At about this time, I attended the 2011 American Psychological Nurses Association conference. Dr. Jean Watson, founder of the Watson Caring Science Institute, was the keynote speaker (see Chapter 16). She gave a name and language to what I had been doing for so many years. She spoke about caring science and a concept called *Caritas Consciousness* and the principles this imbued. Dr. Watson also mentioned something I had never considered: Outcomes of treatment that included such practices as love and care could be measured and empirically validated. I became reinvigorated and began to see that my work as a forensic nurse practitioner was sacred. I was hungry for more knowledge in this emerging philosophy of nursing science.

Shortly after that conference, I was accepted as a doctoral candidate in nursing practice at Brandman University, part of the Chapman University system. Dr. Watson became a formal mentor to me. She convinced me that not only should compassion, love, and human caring be included in my repertoire of treatment, they should be the cornerstones of my practice.

I was fortunate enough to be able to conduct research with probation officers for my doctoral dissertation. I worked closely with them and listened to their struggles in dealing with a difficult population and the stressors of their responsibility to the community. I wanted to infuse the principles of caring science (Watson, 2008, 2012) and the 10 Caritas Processes™ (see Table 16.1). value system into their supervision repertoire).

For example, the first Caritas Process is "cultivating the practice of loving-kindness and equanimity toward self and other" (Watson, 2008, p. 47). It has been shown to lower workers' stress while promoting a professional, authentic presence, and positive human interaction with clients. I believed that it was essential for the workers to be loving to themselves and to motivate their clients to comply with supervision while remaining nonconfrontational, empathic, attentive, caring, and directive. It was my hypothesis that if these traits were incorporated into their repertoire, the workers would experience less stress and be more effective, thereby improving their own productivity and health.

My doctoral study was both quantitative and qualitative and focused on lowering the stress encountered by probation officers in their daily work (Giovannoni, McCoy, & Watson, 2015). I received my doctoral degree in nursing science in 2013. During those educational years, I embarked on a personal journey that helped me to understand that I am interconnected with everyone, including those who choose to pause or remain in darkness. I was reminded that it is the sacred role of nursing to bring the light of love where there is darkness, even into a judicial system that is based on punishment. I was ready to take on the role as a leader in this endeavor.

■ MORAL/ETHICAL FOUNDATION

I am in an unusual profession for a mental health nurse. While I am in the business of helping my clients to change their behavior, I am also committed to public safety. Philosophically, I believe people who have harmed others are given a gift when the judicial system allows them the opportunity to rehabilitate while remaining in the community. I do my very best to help my clients. If they are not receptive to my therapeutic interventions and they are acting in a way that potentially places the community at risk, I am morally bound to the safety of the community.

I am completely transparent and collaborative with the criminal justice system. I am not constrained by traditional rules of confidentiality. I require that each client sign a waiver allowing the free flow of information to and from those who are involved in supporting my client's healing: mental health practitioners, family members, intimate partners, employers, clergy, and friends. Secrecy is the birthplace of shame (Brown, 2012) and fuels sexual abuse. I teach my patients that being honest, authentically present, and understanding their subjective inner life and world experiences are necessary for their evolution as caring, compassionate human beings.

I know of no other nurses who have chosen this population for their specialty and so I do not have a natural support system that understands the struggles relative to my professional ethics. I have to remain constantly vigilant in order to maintain the integrity of my role as an advanced practice nurse and not drift into the role of a probation officer or judge.

My ethics in this role have informed my life greatly, leading me to be guided by heart-centered wisdom, mindfulness, and introspection. The heart is not just a pump that keeps blood flowing through the body. The heart informs the brain about physical and emotional sensations by connecting with the amygdala, which is the center of the brain and limbic system. The amygdala's core cells synchronize with what are called pacemaker cells that control our heart rate. The breath also plays a role in the physiology of the heart. Through mindful, deep breathing, we can change our heart rate, regulate our emotions, and act with more clarity during times of great stress (Institute of HeartMath, 2007–2011). Good leadership in nursing depends upon the ability to control stress and work-related anxiety so one is able to make decisions quickly but not impulsively.

The amygdala also plays a key role in response to events perceived by any of our five senses as threatening. Over time, it develops habit formations that cause us to behave in ways that may have been useful to us as children living in chaos or terror, but become dysfunctional for us as adults. These habit formations are based on fear. In contrast, if we are sending the amygdala messages of safety and health, the responses, even if habitual, have a tendency toward harmony.

The process of meditation, which includes focus on the breath, activates neural structures involved in attention and control of the autonomic nervous system (Lazar, et al., 2000). Agitated heart rhythms tell the amygdala we are feeling threatened. Steady, rhythmic heart rates convey to the amygdala that everything is harmonious. If we are frequently anxious or frustrated, we create a physiological habit formation in the heart that places it under prolonged strain (Chandola et al., 2008). Chronic physical and mental stress contributes to worker distress and compassion fatigue (Anewalt, 2009; Figley, 1995; Lombardo & Eyre, 2011). This, in turn, contributes to errors in the workplace (West, Tan, Habermann, Sloan, & Shanafelt, 2009). For health care professionals, errors in judgment or procedure can result in irreversible damage.

Heart-centered health care begins when we acknowledge that we live in relationship with others. It is the practice of consciously cultivating thoughts of loving-kindness toward ourselves, loved ones, colleagues, strangers, and even those we have difficulties with. This practice changes habitual patterns in our interactions with others. In fact, heart-centered health care becomes a moral/ethical obligation for nurses wishing to practice in integrity.

Many scientists are beginning to suspect that not all phenomena can be explained and that spirituality has a place alongside science. Many Eastern philosophies and religions teach us that body, mind, and spirit are one. Learned emotional responses are so strong that rational understanding is not enough to change them. In order to change maladaptive thoughts and beliefs, we must first identify what is causing them. Because the source is often early trauma, it is painful to revisit. Mindful, heart-centered breathing is a gentle practice that can help us access early memories or defining moments. Pause, be present in the moment, and focus on your breath. Breathe into your heart area and mentally repeat, "I am," and breathe out mentally repeating, "I am love."

In addition to sustaining physical life, the heart is the energy center of unconditional love. This is often referred to as the "heart chakra" in yogic philosophy (Desikachar, 1995). It is the heart that connects us emotionally and spiritually to others. The practice of mindful, heart-centered breathing helps us to separate our ego-based agendas from what is necessary for the greater good of self, patients, and staff. As a leader, the importance of equanimity during crises cannot be understated. Heart-centered breathing is always available; one does not need a special room or equipment.

As symptoms of fatigue, depression, and stress occur in health care professionals, the entire setting is affected. Most nurses bear witness to suffering on a daily basis and so become particularly susceptible to compassion fatigue, as mentioned earlier, which can be defined as "a combination of physical, emotional, and spiritual depletion associated with caring for patients in significant emotional pain and physical distress" (Lombardo & Eyre, 2011). According to Sabo (2006), compassion fatigue is a natural consequence of caring for those who are in pain, suffering, or have been traumatized.

The profession of nursing must rely upon the wisdom of the heart if it is to be informed by compassion and loving-kindness, while shielding nurses from the damage of compassion fatigue. Heart-centered wisdom transcends all boundaries and cultures (Watson, 2008). Because of this, it is not difficult to access information on how to cultivate loving-kindness.

Mindfulness involves focusing on the breath, which naturally changes the heart rate variability (HRV), the subtle variation of a heart's beat-to-beat rhythm. The HRV is still one of the most robust indicators of the health of our nervous system, our ability to recover from stressful events, and our mental and emotional states (McCraty & Shaffer, 2015; Rea, 2014).

Using voxel-based morphometries, investigators found an increase in the concentration of regional gray matter in the brains of individuals who practiced mindfulness meditation as compared to a control group that did not meditate. High concentrations of gray matter have been shown to improve learning, memory, emotional regulation, self-referential processing, and perspective taking (Hölzel et al., 2010).

When we are anxious or fearful, we become closed-minded and resistant to others' input. It is impossible to be compassionate in this state. This can lead to becoming biopassive, biostatic, or biocidic to patients and staff as a means of trying to protect oneself from environments of high stress. *Biopassive* reactions are characterized by apathy and detachment; *biostatic* responses are life-neutral; *biocidic* responses are void of care and harmful to patients (Halldorsdottir, 2013; Watson, 2008). This type of leadership creates a generalized environment of fear. I often felt there was an elephant in the room that was crushing the spirit of cooperation between colleagues at meetings I have attended, where collective wisdom should have emerged but no one was allowed to talk about it. Leaders have an opportunity to change the paradigm by embracing *biogenic* or life-giving practices and philosophies.

I believe empathy is what connects us to all of humanity and is the essential foundation for every other quality required of authenticity. *Empathy* includes respecting others' right to self-determination and honoring peoples' choices. It is not void of holding people accountable for the choices they make. Beneficence can be applied in my work as I hold my patients/clients accountable for their actions and guide them to make better choices.

I bring the humane morals of nursing to my specialty area through the practice of heart-centered breathing. My work is very stressful. In the past, I was much more reactive to my clients' behaviors and attitudes. I responded to their darkness with my own darkness. I am not perfect; however, through my commitment to this practice, I am much less reactive. I have trained myself to breathe at least three times before responding to something that, in the past, would have caused me to react negatively. Just the act of taking this time has increased my empathic understanding. When I am in touch with what my clients are mirroring in me, I connect with them authentically rather than in an authoritarian manner. Authentic connections help me to communicate in ways that create an atmosphere of safety where my clients can openly discuss frightening and painful experiences. An environment of safety is a fertile ground for change and an ethical requisite for healing work.

The practice of heart-centered breathing allows us to access our own ego's agenda as well as to connect with the core beliefs that separate us from others. Some of the more common core beliefs include, "Something is wrong with me," or, "Something is wrong with you." These beliefs are often unconscious and are not separate from the habit formations discussed earlier. They are based on fear and create a need for external control. These traits are often observed in leaders who are overbearing, micromanage, or act condescendingly toward those they supervise. It is often the case that they themselves are experiencing personal suffering that manifests in the need to overpower rather than engage in transpersonal relations with others.

As caregivers and leaders, we must be conscious of our own agendas and not allow our fears to pull us into external power struggles. Maintaining an open heart by practicing heart-centered breathing minimizes stress and facilitates healing for ourselves and the environments in which we work. Mindfulness connects us with others, promotes equanimity in our relationships, and fosters a true appreciation of collective wisdom.

An attitude of loving-kindness helps facilitate creative, collaborative solutions. This is *inclusive leadership*. It creates a workplace atmosphere of enthusiasm, pride, and self-worth. Patients/clients and their caregivers thrive in such environments. As nurse leaders, we have a responsibility to bring caring, love, and heart-centered human-to-human practices and "authentic spirit-to-spirit connections" into our personal lives and work (Watson, 2008, p. 79).

■ VISION

Much of this chapter has been a reflection of my personal journey from being ego centered to being more interconnected with others. This has been guided by Watson's (2002, 2008) work on Caritas Consciousness. Watson explains that "*Caritas* comes from the Latin word meaning to cherish, to appreciate, to give special, if not loving, attention to" (2008, p. 39).

We must be in good relations with ourselves before we can relate with loving-kindness to others. Self-care is enhanced by gratitude. We can be thankful for all of our experiences, especially the negative ones, because they become our best teachers if we listen intuitively and stay with them.

A word about forgiveness is essential to my future vision of nurses who fully embody their leadership potential. Embracing Caritas Consciousness is an act of self-love that encompasses forgiveness of self and others. Forgiveness does not excuse hurtful actions. Those who treat others with disrespect, cruelty, and abusiveness can still be held accountable for the choices they make. However, we should not overlook the power of grace and forgiveness in helping others release what is driving their hurtful behavior. In fact, this act gives us, as nurses and healers, a clean slate from which to work effectively and compassionately (Rosa, 2015). Those who can forgive themselves can also develop empathy. Empathy is the nexus of compassion. There can be no authentic caregiving or treatment without it. Judgment has no place in the helping professions.

A heart-centered leader can bring light where there is darkness. Helen Keller said, "The best and most beautiful things in the world cannot be seen or even touched—they must be felt with the heart" (Keller, n.d.). To lead others, we must be heart-centered and at peace with ourselves. Only then can we facilitate peaceful, healing environments for our patients and colleagues.

Be present and still, be heart centered, breathe in love, breathe out fear. We allow our hearts to connect with our emotional center in order to facilitate composure and acquire insight, wisdom, and understanding. As leaders, we need to open our intelligent heart, set aside our judgments, listen deeply, observe, discern, and speak truthfully what we know, while learning to create a "deeper order of possibilities." Creating this realm of possibility requires the purposeful intention to connect with our higher selves. Before entering into any critical interaction, ask, "What is my intention?" When we set intentions and embody that intentionality, all interactions become positively informed. Miracles can happen when we are mindful of what we want out of our day, our meeting, our interpersonal relationships, and even our trip to the grocery store. Picture an entire workforce of heart-centered nurses, suspending judgment and connected to a shared humanity, who create healing environments as the vanguards of empathic, compassionate human caring . . . that is my vision.

I love the heart-centered feeling that occurs when I care for others and assist them in ameliorating their suffering. My mission is to further develop my own multisensory Caritas Consciousness and to help others do the same. Once we are aware of our own innocence, we can see that the source of our being is love. It is from this awareness that we become authentically empowered and are able to generously show loving-kindness to all beings.

Compassion and love for others cannot be measured with psychological intelligence testing and academic preentrance exams. I began the journey of personal healing with obstacles along the way. Intuitively, I knew that there was more to our world than I was seeing. Professionally, I was always searching for more peaceful ways to conduct my practice. I have discovered that I have the intuitive ability to experience the world beyond the reality of the five senses that triggers my ego fears. Florence Nightingale once said, "How very little can be done under the spirit of fear." My intentionality is to focus on love and not let my work be dictated by the ego's fears.

I believe if nurses and all human service professionals were taught and made aware of the power of Caritas Consciousness, they could become peacemakers throughout the world. In a time of world crises, especially in the Middle East where Americans can be vilified, Dr. Watson invited me to join her in Jordan in 2013 where she launched the first Middle Eastern Nurses and Partners in Human Caring conference. This started with just 20 health care professionals from Palestine and Israel. In just 3 years, it has grown to 90 professionals from all over the world.

I have been a nurse for 45 years now. I have seen many advances. Nurses can, with advanced degrees, practice medicine and prescribe treatment plans, independent of physicians. I know of many patients who prefer nurse practitioners to physicians because advanced practice nurses are more interested in the patient's subjective experience and treat them as partners in their own care. Our mission as nurses has always been more human oriented than physicians. That is because nursing was created to do just that. Doctors traditionally worked with the anatomy and physiology of the body and did not have time to deal with the trauma and fear of illness. They must have seen the need, however, because the field of nursing emerged largely to work with the emotional and human side of illness.

Nursing's time has come. Nurse scholars all over the globe are engaged, conducting cutting-edge research that speaks to the healing powers of authentic human connection (Giovannoni et al., 2015; Watson, 2009). As nurses engage in more activities previously reserved for physicians, they require more technical knowledge. It would be easy to drift into the role of physician; however, we are nurses first. Nursing is, indeed, separate from medicine (Rosa, 2014). With more authority, we have the privilege and responsibility to elevate the profession of healing.

We must be vigilant in order to stay connected to our original mission as healers. We must never lose sight of the reason we were called to this service. As nurse leaders, we must also consider the vision of the 12th-century mystic and saint, Hildegard of Bingen, who called for a "marriage of science and spirituality" (Fox, 2012, p. 154). Spirituality is not religiosity. We are reminded by Watson (2008) that our work in human caring is that of a sacred dimension, "making more explicit that we dwell in mystery and the infinity of Cosmic Love as the source and depth of all of life" (p. 8). Our role as nurses and leaders is to gracefully transition from the constraining, biocidic realm of ego consciousness to the biogenic freedom and healing space of Cosmic Love—the interconnected and unitary domain of Caritas Consciousness.

■ REFLECTIONS

1. *Can I identify how my own personal ego identification prevents me from fulfilling my healing capacity as a nurse?*
2. *Can I identify times in the past when I have acted in biopassive, biocidic, and biogenic ways? What were the consequences of each experience for me, my colleagues, and my patients?*
3. *What is my own personal definition of a heart-centered leader? What is one simple way for me to start embodying that definition right now?*
4. *Is there a need for forgiveness in my personal–professional life? How can that forgiveness lead to a greater understanding of self and other?*
5. *What are accessible and realistic ways for me to integrate heart-centered breathing and a greater heart-centered awareness into my workday?*

■ REFERENCES

Anewalt, P. (2009). Fired up or burned out? Understanding the importance of professional boundaries in home health care hospice. *Home Healthcare Nurse, 27*(10), 591–597.

Brown, B. (2010). *The gifts of imperfection: Let go of who you think you're supposed to be and embrace who you are.* Center City, MN: Hazelden.

Brown, B. (2012). *Daring greatly: How the courage to be vulnerable transforms the way we live, love, parent, and lead.* New York, NY: Gotham.

Chandola, T., Britton, A., Brunner, E., Hemingway, H., Malik, M., Kumari, M., . . . Marmot, M. (2008). Work stress and coronary heart disease: What are the mechanisms? *European Heart Journal, 29*(5), 640–648. doi:http://dx.doi.org/10.1093/eurheartj/ehm584

Desikachar, T. K. V. (1995). *The heart of yoga: Developing a personal practice* (Rev. ed.). Rochester, VT: Inner Traditions International.

Figley, C. R. (1995). *Compassion fatigue: Coping with secondary traumatic stress disorder in those who treat the traumatized.* New York, NY: Brunner-Mazel.

Fox, M. (2012). *Hildegard of Bingen: A saint for our times.* Berkley, CA: Namaste.

Giovannoni, J., McCoy, K., & Watson, J. (2015). Reduce stress by cultivating the practice of loving-kindness with self and others. *International Journal of Caring Sciences, 8*(2), 325–343.

Halldorsdottir, S. (2013). Five basic models of being with another. In M. C. Smith, M. C. Turkel, & Z. R. Wolf (Eds.), *Caring and nursing classics* (pp. 201–210). New York, NY: Springer Publishing Company.

Hawking, S., & Mlodinow, L. (2010). *The grand design.* New York, NY: Bantam Books.

Hindman, J. (1989). *Just before dawn: From the shadows of tradition to new reflections in trauma assessment and treatment of sexual victims.* Alexandria, VA: Alexandria Associates.

Hölzel, B. K., Carmody, J., Vangel, M., Congleton, C., Yerramsetti, S. M., Gard, T., & Lazar, S. W. (2010). Mindfulness practice leads to increases in regional brain gray matter density. *Psychiatry Research Neuroimaging, 191*(1), 36–43.

Institute of HeartMath. (2007–2011) .When anxiety causes your brain to jam, use your heart. Retrieved from http://www.macquarieinstitute.com/company/proom/archive/encounter_journal _brain_jam.html

Keller, H. (n.d.). *BrainyQuote.* Retrieved from http://www.brainyquote.com/quotes/quotes/h/helen-kelle101301.html

Lazar, S., Bush, G., Gollub, R., Fricchione, G., Khalsa, G., & Benson, H. (2000). Functional brain mapping of the relaxation response and meditation. *NeuroReport, 11*(7), 1581–1585.

Lombardo, B., & Eyre, C. (2011). Compassion fatigue: A nurse's primer. *OJIN: The Online Journal of Issues in Nursing, 16*(1), Manuscript 3.

McCraty, R., & Shaffer, F. (2015). Heart rate variability: New perspectives on physiological mechanisms, assessment of self-regulatory capacity, and health risk. *Global Advances in Health and Medicine, 4*(1), 46–61.

Rea, S. (2014). *Tending the heart fire: Living in the flow with the pulse of life.* Boulder, CO: Sounds True.

Rosa, W. (2014). Nursing is separate from medicine: Advanced practice nursing and a transpersonal plan of care. *International Journal for Human Caring, 18*(2), 76–82.

Rosa, W. (2015). Cleaning the slate: Forgiveness as integral to personal and professional self-actualization. *Journal of Nursing and Care, 3*(6), 216. doi:10.4172/2167-1168.1000216

Sabo, B. (2006). Compassion fatigue and nursing work: Can we accurately capture the consequences of caring work? *International Journal of Nursing Practice, 12*(3), 136–142.

Salter, A. (2003). *Predators: Pedophiles, rapists and other sex offenders.* New York, NY: Basic Books.

Watson, J. (2002). Intentionality and caring-healing consciousness: A practice of tranpersonal nursing. *Holistic Nursing Practice, 16*(4), 12–19.

Watson, J. (2008). *Nursing: The philosophy and science of caring* (Rev. ed.). Boulder, CO: University Press of Colorado.

Watson, J. (2009). *Assessing and measuring caring in nursing and health sciences.* New York, NY: Springer Publishing Company.

Watson, J. (2012). *Human caring science* (2nd ed.). Sudbury, MA: Jones & Bartlett.

West, C., Tan, A., Habermann, T., Sloan, J., & Shanafelt, T. (2009). Association of resident fatigue and distress with perceived medical errors. *Journal of the American Medical Association, 302*(12), 1294–1300.

Zukav, G. (1989). *The seat of the soul.* New York, NY: Simon & Schuster.

CHAPTER TWENTY

Empathic and Unselfish: Redefining Nurse Caring as Love in Action

Marlienne Goldin

I've comforted families who were losing loved ones, but I never fully appreciated the magnitude of their loss. I came to realize that suffering is the human condition, and only love can soften its effects. I came to see that caring is love manifested.

—Goldin and Kautz (2010, p. 13)

■ WHY NURSING?

I never set out to become a nurse. My earliest recollection of a career choice occurred at around age 8. My grandmother was having a diabetic emergency and her doctor wanted her in the hospital. She was blind and due to diabetic neuropathy could not walk well. My mother called the ambulance to take her down the two flights of stairs from our Bronx apartment and transport her to the hospital. My younger brother and I hid under the table and watched the white uniformed men's legs bring the stretcher in and take my grandmother away. We were terrified at first, but my mother quickly explained how my grandmother would now get the treatment she needed at the hospital.

I decided right then and there I wanted to be the hero in the white uniform driving down the streets of New York with sirens wailing, lights blazing, bringing people to life-saving care. Fast-forward, 33 years later: I was living in New Jersey, married with a family and still interested in emergency medical services. I was an emergency medical technician (EMT) on my local volunteer ambulance corps and applying to the newly introduced New Jersey Advanced Life Support Paramedic Program. After getting accepted, I completed the yearlong didactic portion of the course at the University of Medicine and Dentistry of New Jersey. My clinical rotations were all completed at Hackensack University Medical Center. After this course, I was able to do more technical procedures and save even more people. I loved the rush of adrenaline, the sounds of sirens, and the satisfaction of a busy shift where I had made a difference. Nursing still was not even a consideration for me. In my opinion, it was boring, devoid of excitement and adventure. I thought nurses lacked autonomy and just took orders from physicians.

It was my clinical coordinator at the hospital where I was training who urged me to further develop my career and pursue a nursing degree at the local community college. I distinctly remember our conversation. "Marlienne, you'll have so many more opportunities with a nursing degree." My response was, "What, work in an MD's office? No thanks!" I finally succumbed to her urgings that I could have a greater influence in emergency medical services with a nursing license. I enrolled in the nursing program at Bergen Community College. My experience as a paramedic enabled me to breeze through much of the curriculum and I still worked at my paramedic dream job while I continued my nursing education. When I graduated and passed nursing boards, I continued to work, dividing my shifts between nursing in the emergency department (ED) and paramedicine. I soon realized that there was plenty of excitement, decision making, and autonomy working as an ED nurse.

■ EARLY IMPRESSIONS

Within a year of finishing my associate's degree, I accepted a position at St. Joseph's Hospital and Medical Center as the clinical coordinator of a mobile intensive care unit (ICU) that employed both mobile intensive care RNs and paramedics. If I had not had a nursing license, I would never have been eligible for that position. I got myself back into school and completed my BSN, realizing that education brought both knowledge and power. After the BSN, I went on to pursue my master's degree at Seton Hall University.

For the first 19 years of my career, I remained the clinical coordinator of the mobile ICU. I was able to impact emergency care in the state of New Jersey. I worked with physicians and policy makers to improve care for the sick and injured outside of the hospital. I loved my job! I had the best of both worlds . . . or so I thought. I worked with amazing ED physicians, nurses, and paramedics. When I started becoming just a little bored, I added teaching to my skills: advanced cardiac life support, pediatric advanced life support, trauma nurse core curriculum, and neonatal advanced life support. I collected instructor certifications and started teaching in the emergency medical services program at the community college.

At a friend's urging, I applied for a staff educator position at a local community hospital. During the interview, I was asked if I would consider a nurse manager position in their ICU. I knew nothing of what goes on above the floors of the ED, so I politely declined. How the nursing inpatient departments functioned was completely alien to me. Yes, I had a BSN and a master's degree in health care administration, but the inpatient departments were still a mystery. After all this time, I still remained somehow convinced that nursing was not the ultimate career for me. Despite my courteous declination, the community hospital continued to call and ask me to reconsider. After a particularly frustrating day at work, I relented and gave in. This was the real start of my nursing career, the day God smiled on me.

I became the nurse manager of a 14-bed mixed ICU in a small community hospital. It was in that ICU that I developed my awe of what nurses do and what nursing really is. I saw firsthand that nursing was so much more than I ever imagined. It was not tasks or procedures or treatments. It was not a profession or a vocation and it certainly was not a job. It was bigger than any of those things. Watching my staff interact with their patients, seeing them answering questions from patient's families, I realized nursing was not just about taking care of physical bodies. It was about touching spirits and souls. I realized that physicians, who spent only minutes at the bedside, relied heavily upon the assessments and opinions of RNs. Orders were written and treatments administered based on input from the RNs. I continued to observe and learn, developing an admiration for my nursing staff that grew daily.

The community hospital decided they would pursue the American Nurse Credentialing Center's (ANCC) Magnet® designation. Senior leadership tasked me with researching nursing theories to see which one would be the best foundation on which to build our nursing care delivery model. I reviewed many theories; some I could not relate to, some I did not even understand. I came upon Dr. Jean Watson's Theory of Human Caring (see Chapter 16). Finally, I could connect a theory to the nursing I observed every day. It was simple, applicable, and was what was so visible in nursing. I e-mailed Dr. Watson, who responded the very next day, and off I went on my pursuit of caring science knowledge.

I went out to Colorado and studied the theory from the author herself, Dr. Watson. The more I learned, the more I wanted to learn. I completed the international certification in Human Caring and Healing at the University of Colorado with renowned nurse educators Dr. Janet Quinn (see Chapter 13), who taught about the spirituality of nursing; Dr. Jurate A. Sakalys, who relayed the importance of the patient's story; and Dr. Sally Gadow, who was a master on ethics. I was hooked. Nursing and caring science became my passion. I had become determined to find out what that inner spark was that I observed every day in the ICU nurses. I wanted to know what the driver was that kept them coming back every day to care for the sick and injured. They gave so much of themselves. . . . Who gave to them? I realized one cannot keep caring for others if one is not cared for. I welcomed the privilege of caring for nurses and quickly assumed the role of being the nurses' advocate.

As I grew in nurse leadership skills, I began to take a closer look at nurse caring. What is it? How is it demonstrated? What awakens it? Can it be taught? Is it innate? My admiration and love of nursing grew steadily. The more I looked, the more questions I had. Watson (1990) and Leininger (1991) both describe caring as the essence of nursing. But as I grew personally and professionally, I understood that nursing is not *just* caring. There is so much more to it.

A host of questions kept me passionate and determined to know more. How do nurses describe what they offer their patients? Can nurse caring really be love? Is love entwined with caring science? Is it going beyond the duty to care? Is it giving freely to another? Is it placing other before self without expecting reciprocity? Love includes a variety of concepts.

Many religious perspectives affirm, in various and diverse ways, that love is at the heart of being and that the ultimate reality or ultimate purpose of things is related to love. To explore this topic, a broad range of concepts have to be included in the discussion and research: caring, agape and compassion, empathy, knowing, honesty, and ethics, among others. What part do these concepts play in nursing? Are they attributes of love?

They certainly are embedded in nursing practice. And, ultimately, what is the relationship of love to nursing? My journey was leading me from my roots of paramedicine to new heights in caring science and from the rush of adrenaline to the deeper questions of love.

■ PROFESSIONAL EVOLUTION/CONTRIBUTION

I watch nurses perform their tasks and I think to myself, "Why do they do it?" What makes nurses come to work, day after day, cleaning bodily fluids of complete strangers, attempting to alleviate suffering of people who have no relation to them? I remember once thinking that I touched more dead bodies in one week than most people see in a lifetime. Nurses care for the homeless, the addicted, the unloved, and the unwanted. I know it is not the financial reimbursement of nursing that gets them hooked. There are people who would turn down a million dollars rather than do what nurses do, see what nurses see, touch what they touch, and smell what they smell. So what is it? I believe it is human love.

Some would say love is the most important human emotion (Fredrickson, 2013). The term love is used frequently in everyday discourse, but it is difficult to define. Fromm (1956) argues that one of the problems of the English language is that we make one word express a range of emotions. The definition of *love* can range from affection to the deep feelings of intimacy. As simple as the word may sound, its true meaning has been elusive.

The term *altruism* (French, *altruisme*, derived from Latin, *alter*: "other") was coined in the 19th century by August Comte (1891) and was generally adopted as a convenient antithesis to egoism. Altruism involves the unselfish concern for other people. It involves doing things simply out of a desire to help, not because you feel obligated to out of duty, loyalty, or religious reasons. The basic principle of altruism is that man has no right to exist for his own sake, that service to others is the only justification of his existence, and that self-sacrifice is his highest moral duty, virtue, and value.

There are some who believe we were put here to serve one another. Our nursing heroes, such as Mother Teresa and Florence Nightingale, have exhibited the strength of altruistic love and are people who have dramatically changed the world for the better. I started to look at some of the origins of love, in hopes of better understanding nursing. According to *Merriam-Webster's*, altruistic love is a moral theory that regards the good of others as the end of moral action, by extension, the disposition required to take the good of others as an end in itself. The concept of altruistic love is one that challenges the spiritual person to "love your enemies" or to "love without thought of return." It is a love that flows out to others in the form of compassion, kindness, tenderness, and charitable giving. To love is to will *real* good for another. To will not what you wish for the other nor what the other wishes for, but the *real* good.

Agape love was practiced in ancient Greek society. It is selfless; it implies relating to one's neighbors and the good of all people. Agape love is unconditional love. It is a choice we make to love another person whether he or she loves us back or not. It means that we choose to love someone even if he is our enemy. Agape love is based on an ethic. It may be contrary to our every emotion. It is an act of the will. It is self-sacrificing. We care for the drug dealer with the gunshot wound the same way we care for the elderly stroke victim.

Agape enables love to be the ethical foundation when one is confronting suffering. Agape refers to "selfless love" or "charity" as it is translated in the Christian scriptures (from the Latin *caritas,* meaning "dearness"). The tradition of agape, or unconditional love, is not exclusive to any one religion. Actually, it is a major underlying principle found in religions worldwide.

Caritas love is similar. *Caritas* is a Latin word that refers to an altruistic love or loving-kindness. It has its roots in the idea of Christian charity. This is in contrast to *eros,* which refers to intimate love or romantic love. In the fifth century, St. Augustine attempted to synthesize the eros of the Greeks with the agape of Christ and then called it caritas. Augustine believed that caritas best expressed, in doctrinal form, the outpouring of love that the Holy Trinity has for us. Love is not sentimental but watchful, alert, and ready to act. Words like agape, altruism, and caritas denote a compassionate love for all human beings. Is nursing a demonstration of altruistic, agape, or caritas love? I believe it is all of these.

These questions have been the basis of my dissertation while completing my doctorate in Caring Science as Sacred Science at the Watson Caring Science Institute. In order to look forward, I had to explore the past to see where the nursing tradition I see as love in action is rooted. Looking at the origins of nursing prior to the U.S. Civil War, women family members cared for the sick in patients' homes. The responsibility for nursing the sick went beyond a woman's duty toward her children, husband, or aging parents. To fill that need, women from the community could be hired into private homes to tend the sick. After their husbands died, widows frequently turned to tending the sick as a way to support themselves. By 1890, the percentage of widows providing nursing care was more than twice that of all female occupations (Reverby, 1987).

Urban growth spurred population shifts away from the farms and into the cities. Hospitals came into being primarily to serve the working-class poor and chronically ill. Nurses were needed to care for the hospital's sick and were hired to do so, but they were no better off than domestic servants. In their off hours, they were often called upon to repair the linen or clean the wards. There was no such thing as nursing training or education. During the Civil War, a small group of upper-class women participated in war relief activities. After the war, they took up the cause of hospital reform (Donahue, 2011). Social reformers, combined with the Nightingale movement in England, brought about hospital reform in this country.

In 1873, the first Nightingale-inspired training schools were created in New York, Massachusetts, and Connecticut. It was thought that women, by their very nature of caring and nurturing, would be excellent caregivers. The nursing workforce was made up entirely of women. Altruism, sacrifice, and submission were expected and encouraged (Reverby, 1987).

Trained nursing began as a "duty to care" (Reverby, 1987, p. 202). But can one be forced to care? One can assume a duty to perform physical acts for another, such as bathing, administering medications, assisting with physical activities, and so forth, but the attribute of true caring cannot be imposed as a duty. Caring can no more be a duty than being mandated to feel joy, sadness, or love. One cannot impose a duty to assume emotions. One cannot be ordered to care.

So, what is the emotion nurses assume when they enter the profession or when they are practicing nursing? Could it be that they willingly assume the responsibility to deliver loving care to humanity? Does choosing nursing mean that one chooses a profession of love for humanity? I had found that an ethical and existential demonstration of unselfish love allows a nurse to come into right relationship with self and to live authentically, but I needed more information to understand what makes nurses care as they do, in the way they do. Eriksson (2002) put forth three basic assumptions in this regard:

- The basic motive of caring is the *caritas* motive.
- Caring implies alleviating suffering in charity, love, faith, and hope.
- Caring relationship forms the meaningful context of caring and derives its origin from the ethos of love, responsibility, and sacrifice; that is, a caritative ethic (p. 62).

Love, in a wider sense, like the unselfish agape and caritas, has been marginalized in Western culture. The love from caregiver to patient has been misunderstood. Fitzgerald (1998) formed a thesis that human agape is what makes it possible to practice holistic caring, where caring is an art as well as a science. He concluded, "Rather than ignoring the concept of love and its relationship to the everyday practices of nurses, we should be embracing it" (Fitzgerald, 1998, p. 38). I wholeheartedly agree. Nursing is directly related to caring for people and it provides a perfect opportunity to practice the art of loving. "If one wants to become a master of any art, one's whole life must be devoted to it, or at least related to it" (Fromm, 1956, p. 86).

Why is the term *love* not embraced in the nursing profession? Is it fear? Because love in nursing is misunderstood? Jacono (1993) wrote that she experienced nurses' "fear of caring" and interpreted the main reason for this as a misunderstanding about what love means (p. 193). The nurses equated the term *love* with the eros, or romantic form, not the agape. Increasing technological and bureaucratic demands on nurses in conjunction with this "fear of caring" contributes to the objectification of patients. In nursing and in the broader landscape of health care today, emphasis is on evidence-based practice. But without love, evidence-based practices hold little significance in the deeper processes of healing.

It seems the concept of love has become taboo in nursing. If we agree that to give and receive love is essential for being human, we may go further and say it is the most important of human experiences (Fromm, 1956; Maslow, 1970; Rogers, 1957). It is impossible to separate the love we need to give/receive as persons and the love we need to give/receive as nurses. With this understanding, there is no need to attach shame to the concept of love in a professional milieu. The agape ethic transforms both the nurse and the patient being cared for. Loving care is firmly rooted in the relationship between the patient and the nurse. The commitment on the part of the nurse is demonstrated by acts that sustain and increase the welfare of the patient. As the nurse finds out more about the patient, he or she finds more about himself or herself.

Psychoanalyst and social philosopher Erich Fromm (1956) believed that elements common to all forms of love are care, responsibility, respect, and knowledge. These are the attributes nurses demonstrate every day in their practice. Caring by itself is not love. One can care, but unless one has a responsibility to act on that caring, it is not love. Respect is vital; a nurse must respect and know the human being behind the disease process. The giving and receiving of love is something rooted in daily nursing and caring practice.

Fromm's textbook was one of the first books I read when I started on my caring science doctoral journey. Fromm made it so easy for me to relate the attributes of love to nursing practice. Many nursing actions and standards originated from love but are not necessarily linked to it. Stickley and Freshwater (2002) explain that there is misunderstanding around the different manifestations of love, for example, romantic love, brotherly love, and maternal love. This may cause people to find alternate ways to articulate loving as caring. Misunderstandings and confusion can lead to embarrassment and fear, which can lead to love being denied or buried. This denial interferes with nurses' ability to engage in a meaningful and healing relationship.

Philosophers and theologians for hundreds of years have examined the qualities and merits of love. Many believe that love is a healing energy. In folklore and religious texts, the power of love to heal has been an accepted fact. Love is at the center of humanity. When one practices caring, one comes in contact with the core of one's spirit. The notion of caring as an expression of love and compassion is in direct correlation with ideas that have influenced it for hundreds of years.

Is caring a demonstration of love? According to Sister Simone Roach, "Caring is the human mode of being" (Roach, 2002, p. 23). Sister Roach believes care is the fundamental and unifying force of nursing and that curing and healing cannot occur without care. Love is at the center of humanity. Caring is natural and is an expression of love. Love is not only the heart but also the force of caring.

According to Buber (1987), considering God as love enables individuals to express love in concrete actions of compassion and caring. It is the emotion that drives a nurse to want the best outcome for the patient. Love is a healing power that can alleviate pain and suffering. One day as I was watching a new nurse caring for an elderly patient, I noticed she was naturally able to form genuinely caring relationships with her patients. I asked her where she learned to build relationships like that. She answered that God bestowed unconditional love on her and the pain of that love was so exquisite that she had to give it away. She said that was the reason she chose nursing as a career. She would always be able to bestow God's love on others. That was a very powerful conversation for me. It set me to wondering about the connections between love, the self, and God.

Caring requires us to act with unconditional love for another in order to help and heal. Meyeroff (1971) suggests that to care for another person is to help him grow and actualize him- or herself. He refers to it as a process of relating to someone, which involves personal development for the one who is caring. Could it be through caring for and serving patients that nurses also become actualized? Most nurses will agree that caring for patients gives their own lives meaning. Through this lens, demonstrating love for patients promotes nurses being in right relationship with the self. And if the true and authentic self is really a reflection of God, then the love we show as nurses is the proof of God in the world.

Possibly my most significant professional evolution and contribution has been learning and sharing this: Nurses are love and the art of nursing is love in action. The idea of caring as an expression of love and compassion fits in with ideas that have influenced caring throughout history. The relationship between the nurse and patient has many components, but the main one appears to be agape, wanting what is best for the patient for the patient's sake, not for the nurse's. The nurse does not expect the patient to reciprocate. Agape love, unlike romantic love, expects nothing in return. Agape love wants the best for the other.

■ MORAL/ETHICAL FOUNDATION

Technological thinking, medicine, and the overt medicalization of practice have influenced nurses to shy away from using the word *love* to describe their work. Nursing has been so consumed by the demand for technological competencies that the ontological competencies of caring and healing have been submerged (Watson, 2002). Research has shown that nurses who are not able to practice caring become worn-down, unhappy, and hardened (Swanson, 1999).

In some instances, it is the work environment that contributes to the suppression of caring. I experienced this firsthand in my career. While interviewing for a nurse manager position, the chief nursing officer noted my interest and background in caring science. She said, "I see you've studied caring. . . . How do you make nurses care?" My immediate response was, "You don't make nurses care. You create an environment where caring can flourish."

We do not hear the term *love* used much in health care today, but we do hear nurses explaining their feelings for patients in myriad other ways. Perhaps the agape or caritas form of love denotes the feeling of today's nurses toward their patients. Does agape enable love to be the ethical foundation when one is confronting suffering? When I asked a young nurse if he loved his patients, he replied "No, not 'love.'" When asked just exactly what the feeling was he had toward his patients, he replied, "Compassion, caring, concern." He said he was more comfortable using the word "compassion" instead of "love." Has nursing adapted a language to represent its "version" of love?

Generally, *compassion* involves an emotional response to someone who is suffering and a desire to act in a caring manner. It is considered a nursing characteristic that has a major impact on the quality of care. The results of a recent study conducted by the College of Registered Nurses of Nova Scotia indicated that 89% of the public agreed nurses are either compassionate or very compassionate (Simmonds, 2013). Compassion has also been defined as "a deep awareness of the suffering of others coupled with a wish to relieve it" (Chochinov, 2007, p. 185). Compassionate care does not always require a response to suffering, but is a relational activity born out of the way we relate to other human beings when they are vulnerable. This is the nature of nurses' work. It involves noticing the patient's vulnerability, experiencing a reaction to it, and responding in a meaningful way toward the patient. There is consensus that care and compassion lie at the heart of health care.

In 1994, the Pew-Fetzer Task Force recommended that clinicians embrace relationship-centered care, which involves communicating openly with patients and practicing with a healing and caring ethic. They argued that a practitioner's self-recognition is crucial to the delivery of effective care. "If the nurse is able to develop a transpersonal caring relationship, and a climate of trust with the patient, healing will occur, and the patient's emotional needs will be addressed" (Tresolini & The Pew-Fetzer Task Force, 1994, p. 24). Compassionate care is not taking away another person's pain or suffering; it is about entering into that patient's experience, sharing the burden with him or her, and allowing the person to keep his or her independence and dignity. Understanding the subjective perceptions of patients provides insight for nurses concerning their care expectations. Compassionate caregiving means listening with full attention. It is a shift in awareness and a developed skill that guides one to be authentically present in the moment. With compassion, the care that the nurse offers is more powerful and more rewarding for both the patient and the nurse. How can compassion be nurtured in nurses? Mindful, focused attention, or as Watson (2008) refers to it, "Caritas Consciousness," enables the nurse to form a spirit-to-spirit connection with the patient (p. 78).

With the present-day emphasis on holistic nursing care, *empathy* plays an increasingly important role in morally grounded care. It prompts one to think of ways to alleviate suffering. An example of empathy: An elderly gentleman stood in the doorway of his wife's hospital room looking out toward the nurses' station, appearing distraught. When asked by a passing nurse from another floor what he needed, he replied, "Something is bothering my wife and I don't know what's wrong." The nurse went into the room and observed the barely responsive wife with her hands fidgeting in the sheets. The nurse pulled a chair up along the side of the bed and told the gentleman to sit down and talk to his wife. As soon as the patient heard her husband's voice, she extended her hands. He held them in his calmly and said to the nurse, "She needed me to hold her hand. How did you know?" There were tears in both the husband's and the nurse's eyes. Such opportunities to care are not always dramatic events; they can be simple encounters as demonstrated in the previous example. Encouraging words, expressions of sorrow, a helping hand, or simply moving a chair next to the patient's bedside are demonstrations of empathy that are integral to effective nurse caring.

Both Mayeroff (1971) and Fromm (1956) agree that *knowing* is essential to both love and caring. In order to love something, it must first be known. If it is not known, how can it be loved? In order to care, one must understand what the other needs and respond accordingly. When a nurse knows the patient, the nurse knows him directly, as a separate being—an individual. An experienced nurse can walk into a patient's room and intuition tells her or him that something is wrong; the nurse immediately checks the patient's vital signs, not because she or he can see something wrong, but because intuition tells the nurse to do so. Caring includes all forms of knowing, all related in different ways to benefit the other. The nurse cannot teach a patient effectively without having familiarity and knowledge of the patient. In this way, the nurse fulfills the responsibility or duty to meet the needs of the patient.

Knowing the other is a requisite for quality caregiving, but does not automatically result in love. Swedish nurse Estrid Rodhe wrote a textbook in 1911 in which she modeled the nursing ethics that prevailed at that time. This was one of the first nursing textbooks to be translated into Finnish. It was also the first textbook written by a nurse that focused on nursing ethics. She wrote that altruistic women with a calling to nursing had to have other personal characteristics such as faithfulness, honesty, and maturity. She believed unselfishness was the motivation behind all of nursing's efforts. According to Rodhe (as cited in Kangasniemi & Haho, 2012) and most of her contemporaries, a nurse has womanly characteristics humanized by the abilities to nurture and to cherish. Nurturing and cherishing are also attributes that have a strong connection to love. Her first idea was the altruistic ideal as an absolute value of nursing. Her second idea referred to her conception that nurses were naturally loving and possessed a natural affinity for demonstrating human love through characteristics of gentleness, pleasing voice, and so forth. Third, she proposed that nurses possess a moral basis to practice human love in nursing. Rodhe's absolute ethical basis to describe human love in nursing is altruism. She believed nurses' role was to serve others, based on the ultimate sense of Christian charity. Rodhe pointed out that nursing was more than a profession. She believed it was based on a calling and a profession of loving/caring for others.

Eriksson (2002) and Watson (2007) maintain that love is the key to growing and developing within a caring science worldview. They are among those who see love in the form of caritas as the basis for development of their theories. We know that caritas also has roots in the idea of Christian charity. Thorkildsen, Eriksson, and Raholm (2013) say love reveals the human being's connection with the whole of existence, since love is combined in the deepest core of human beings. "Love is the underlying healing power behind a nurse's duty to care" (Watson, 2003, p. 199). Kirkegaard says that this love is a holy power that can be understood as agape, a love inside the hearts of human beings. "Love is the origin of everything, and spirituality understood, love is the deepest ground of the life of the spirit" (Kierkegaard, 2009, p. 205).

The day I brought my husband home from the hospital on hospice care, I was on the receiving end of the healing power of a nurse. As we were waiting for the ambulance to transport my husband to our home, his nurse brought over the discharge papers. The nurse handed me the ambulance schedule that he had set up to take my husband to his hemodialysis treatments. I told him there would be no more hemodialysis sessions, that we were going home, and we were discontinuing all the advanced treatments. I told him my husband had enough and was tired of it all. The nurse put his papers down, looked at me, and said, "I am so sorry," as he hugged me with tears in his eyes. I will never forget the compassion, care, and love that I felt from that nurse at that moment. Ten years later, I can still feel it. At one of the worst moments of my life, he both shared my pain and lessened it. I will never forget him.

Compassion. Empathy. Knowing. Faithfulness. Honesty. Maturity. Unselfishness. Nurturing. Cherishing. . . . *Love.* This is my ethical foundation and moral keystone: love as starting ethic, love as in between, love as what remains. Within a caring science paradigm, agape refers to ethics and not religion. Love, as an ethical act, is shown in the nurse's behavior and attitude. The nurse puts the other's best interest before her or his own without expecting anything in return. When nurses are genuinely concerned for their patient's mind, body, and spirit, love is obvious and the healing potential increases.

Caring science promotes love of self. Caritas Process # 1, "Cultivating the practice of loving-kindness and equanimity toward self and other," speaks to the importance of self-care (Watson, 2008, p. 47; see Table 16.1 for a complete list of the Caritas Processes™). If the nurse keeps caring and giving of himself or herself without being renewed, he or she becomes empty and emotionally exhausted. When the nurse cares for himself or herself and enjoys work–life balance, he or she can become the Caritas nurse who promotes healing through caring, loving relationships.

■ VISION

The education of nurses requires a broad understanding of the profession; gaining the scientific knowledge, technical skills, and competence; and most importantly, developing caring relationships. The value of caring in nursing education has a long tradition in the literature. Caring is fundamental to nursing curriculum, according to the National League for Nursing (1988). Mayeroff summarizes his work on caring by writing:

> Man finds himself by finding his place, and he finds his place by finding appropriate others that need his care and that he needs to care for. Through caring, and being cared for man experiences himself as part of nature. (1971, p. 87)

If one replaces the word "man" with "a nurse," this statement could easily be describing the profession of nursing. This may be the innate call that those who enter the nursing profession hear.

There is a distinction between caring and love. "Nurse caring" goes beyond the common definition of "caring." Nurse caring is love of other manifested in action. One has only to watch a nurse working with a patient to see examples of love in his or her daily practice. Nurse caring is agape love and it is manifested in the day-to-day practice of nursing. I have been witnessing love in action every day for 31 years. Love begets love. I do not go to work every day. I go to love.

My role, as a nursing department director, is to care for nurses, support them, and remove obstacles so that they can give the care our patients deserve. I remind them that they are never just completing tasks. When they are making a bed, they are providing a smooth surface for their patient's skin. When offering a bedpan, they are assuring and preserving the patient's dignity. When they feed a patient, they are providing nourishment that the human body needs in order to heal. When they are documenting in the electronic record, they are assuring continuity of patient care. Nurses are not in the patient's environment; they do not merely attend to the patient's environment; they *are* the patient's environment. I have witnessed patients and their families take note of the nurse's facial expressions. If the nurse looks worried, the patient and their family get concerned. The nurse's presence is a primary healing component for the patient. To quote Nightingale, "Medicine removes the obstruction, nothing more, the nurse's job is to put the patient in the best condition so that nature can act upon him" (1969, p. 133).

After all my years in nursing, I can honestly say I am still in awe of the profession. I love my staff and I make sure they are aware of that. I round on my nurses first, not the patients, every morning. When I am leaving at the end of the day, I make sure I tell each one good night. Since applying Watson's caring theory in my managerial role, I have been able to take a nursing department with a 48% vacancy rate to a department with the highest nurse engagement of all the inpatient units. We have a turnover rate below 10% and the turnover we do have is all due to professional advancement. We have been able to decrease hospital-acquired infections and length of patient stay. Staff nurses are involved in research and present at national and international conferences. Patient satisfaction is at the 95 percentile. We are a work family; we celebrate together and, in times of trouble, we support each other. Nurses are not just loving of others, but are also deeply celebrated and loved.

Nurses who are cared for and appreciated provide better patient care. It is not rocket science. Nurse satisfaction results in patient satisfaction. When patients are satisfied, physicians are satisfied. Nurse leaders who practice caring for their staff reap the benefits of increased staff engagement and increased patient satisfaction. An engaged nursing staff results in better patient outcomes. What do I attribute the success of our department to? Very simply . . . it is love.

Nurses work in a sacred environment. Touching bodies, spirits, and souls is holy work. Nurses and the rest of the world need to acknowledge that the practice of nursing is the practice of love of humanity. When nurses claim love as their professional practice, they can move forward to healing the world. I believe nursing can be a force for world peace. This is my goal: to have nursing practice acknowledged as love in action. According to Watson, "Caring/Love radiates in concentric circles from self to Other, to Community, to Planet Earth, to Infinity of the Universe" (2005, p. 141).

My vision for nursing stems from my thoughts on nursing. I thought I could save lives . . . so I took a CPR course. I thought I could save even more lives . . . so I became a paramedic. I wanted to save the world . . . so I embraced nursing. I now realize, 31 years later, that only love can save the world. My vision is that nurses realize they are love in action, and in that realization, understand how magnificent is the duty they are charged with.

■ REFLECTIONS

1. *When I was first drawn to becoming a nurse, did the idea of loving others cross my mind?*
2. *What are the connections I observe between nursing and love?*
3. *How do I relate to the requirements of effective caregiving mentioned earlier: compassion, empathy, knowing, faithfulness, honesty, maturity, unselfishness, nurturing, cherishing, and love?*
4. *Do I believe nurse satisfaction leads to patient satisfaction? Why or why not? If so, how are they directly related? If not, then what role does nurse satisfaction play in effective caregiving?*
5. *In bringing to mind an experience with a patient that was meaningful to me and that I will never forget, what aspects of love were present in that exchange? Would I define that moment of nursing as love in action?*

■ REFERENCES

Buber, M. (1987). *I and thou* (R. Smith, Trans.). New York, NY: MacMillan.

Chochinov, H. M. (2007). Dignity and the essence of medicine: The A, B, C, and D of dignity in conserving care. *British Medical Journal, 335*(7612), 184–187.

Comte, A. (1891). *The catechism of positive religion*. London, UK: Trubner.

Donahue, P. M. (2011). *Nursing, the finest art: An illustrated history* (3rd ed.). Philadelphia, PA: Elsevier.

Eriksson, K. (2002). Caring science in a new key. *Nursing Science Quarterly, 15*(1), 61–65.

Fitzgerald, L. (1998). Is it possible for caring to be an expression of human agape in the 21st century? *International Journal for Human Caring, 2*(3), 32–39.

Fredrickson, B. L. (2013). *Love 2.0: Creating happiness and health in moments of connection*. New York, NY: Penguin.

Fromm, E. (1956). *The art of loving*. New York, NY: Harper & Rowe.

Goldin, M., & Kautz, D. (2010). Applying Watson's caring theory and Caritas Processes™ to ease life transitions. *International Journal of Human Caring, 14*(1), 11–14.

Jacono, B. J. (1993). Caring is loving. *Journal of Advanced Nursing, 18*(2), 192–194.

Kangasniemi, M., & Haho, A. (2012). Human love—The inner essence of nursing ethics according to Estrid Rodhe. A study using the approach of history of ideas. *Scandinavian Journal of Caring Sciences, 26*(4), 803–810.

Kierkegaard, S. (2009). *Works of love*. New York, NY: HarperCollins.

Leininger, M. M. (1991). *Culture care diversity, and universality: A theory of nursing*. New York, NY: National League for Nursing Press.

Maslow, A. (1970). *Motivation and personality* (2nd ed.). New York, NY: Harper & Row.

Mayeroff, M. (1971). *On caring*. New York, NY: HarperCollins.

National League for Nursing. (1988). *Curriculum revolution: Mandate for change*. New York, NY: National League for Nursing Press.

Nightingale, F. (1969). *Notes on nursing: What it is and what it is not* (2nd ed.). New York, NY: Dover.

Reverby, S. M. (1987). *Ordered to care: The dilemma of American nursing, 1850-1945.* New York, NY: Cambridge University Press.

Roach, M. S. (2002). *Caring, the human mode of being: A blueprint for the health professions* (2nd ed.). Ottawa, ON, Canada: CHA Press.

Rogers, C. R. (1957). The necessary and sufficient conditions of therapeutic personality change. *Journal of Consulting Psychology, 21*, 95–103.

Simmonds, A. (2013). Cultivating compassion in nursing practice. *Nursing in Focus, 14*(2), 14–15.

Stickley, T., & Freshwater, D. (2002). The art of loving and the therapeutic relationship. *Nursing Inquiry, 9*(4), 250–256.

Swanson, K. (1999). What is known about caring in nursing research: A literary meta-analysis. In A. S. Hinshaw, S. Feetham, & J. Shaver (Eds.), *Handbook of clinical nursing research* (pp. 31–60). Thousands Oaks, CA: Sage.

Tresolini, C. P., & The Pew-Fetzer Task Force. (1994). *Health professionals and relationship centered care: Report of the Pew-Fetzer Task Force on advancing psychosocial health education.* San Francisco, CA: Pew Health Commission.

Thorkildsen, K. M., Eriksson, K., & Raholm, M. B. (2013). The substance of love when encountering suffering: An interpretative research synthesis with an abductive approach. *Scandinavian Journal of Caring Sciences, 27*(2), 449–459.

Watson J. (1990). Caring knowledge and informed moral passion. *Advances in Nursing Science, 13*(1), 15–24.

Watson, J. (2002, January–March). Nursing: Seeking its source and survival. *ICUs and Nursing Web Journal, 9*, 1–7.

Watson, J. (2003). Love and the caring. Ethics of face and hand—An invitation to return to the heart and soul of nursing and our deep humanity. *Nurses Science Quarterly, 27*(3), 197–202.

Watson, J. (2005). *Caring science as sacred science.* Philadelphia, PA: F. A. Davis.

Watson J. (2007). Theoretical questions and concerns: A response from a caring science framework. *Nursing Science Quarterly, 20*(1), 13–15.

Watson, J. (2008). *Nursing: The philosophy and science of caring* (Rev. ed). Boulder, CO: University Press of Colorado.

CHAPTER TWENTY-ONE

Emancipatory and Collaborative: Learning to Lead From Beside

Marcia Hills

Caring envelops the essence of nursing. . . . Human care requires a high regard and reverence for . . . human life, and non-paternalistic values . . . related to . . . autonomy and freedom of choice. . . . [By] questioning our existing beliefs and approaches to . . . nursing, we can . . . relinquish our control as experts and become partners in enhancing human potential.
—Hartrick, Lindsey, and Hills (1994, pp. 88, 91)

■ WHY NURSING?

I grew up in an Irish/Scottish family with four brothers and a sister. My Irish Catholic father would insist that, no matter what else was going on during the week, everyone was required to be at the family dinner table at 6 p.m. on Sunday evening. Earlier in the day, he would give instructions about the topic for debate and we were each asked to prepare our "argument" to be discussed at dinner. I remember hilarious discussions, but I also learned from this experience that it was important to have a voice, to listen, and to be heard; and that being able to disagree, to argue, or defend your position had nothing to do with respect or love . . . those were givens. I know now that I learned all this despite, as a child, being shy, an observer, and very unsure of myself and who I might become.

That era, the late 1960s, saw most women who entered tertiary education pursuing a career as a nurse or an educator. As I was finishing high school, I wanted to be an educator, but all my friends entered residence-based hospital schools of nursing to become nurses. So I followed.

I enrolled in a hospital-based Catholic school of nursing, the Halifax Infirmary, in Halifax, Nova Scotia, Canada, which was run by the Sisters of Charity. I often joke that the only problem was the sisters were not so charitable. There are many stories to tell of the adversities of that experience; I often reflect on one in particular.

It was made clear to us that it was more important to be busy, for instance, by cleaning the bathroom sink, than it was to talk to patients. I recall one day I was sitting on the side of the patient's bed, holding his hand—he was so upset and I just wanted to comfort him in some way. He had just learned that his leg would have to be amputated. I could not really imagine what this news might mean to this 45-year-old man. I was distraught—how must he feel? My nursing instructor found me in this position, deeply involved in conversation, hoping to console him—wanting him to know that he was not alone and that I could feel his pain, his loss. My instructor called me out of the room and basically scolded me for being unprofessional. I was devastated! I had actually felt like the nurse I wanted to be and was totally absorbed in a caring moment with this person. This experience built my resolve to listen to my heart and my inner voice, not that of another.

Just as I was about to graduate, I met my husband, John. He was heading to England and so I decided to join. Living in a small village outside of Plymouth, I investigated working in a hospital in the city and realized I would spend all of my earned salary on transportation to and from work. So, instead of working, I spent the year reading nursing textbooks and Shakespeare. It was enjoyable, but I also soon realized I was destined to be a career woman; being at home on my own was simply not fulfilling.

■ EARLY IMPRESSIONS

Before I left for England, I had visited my family doctor and floated the idea of my coming to work for him when I returned from my trip abroad. He was interested because he and his colleagues were expanding their building with each of the three doctors to have three offices; so the idea of a "family nurse" or a "primary health care nurse" appealed to him. By the time I had returned from England, he had convinced his colleagues that the arrangement could work, so I was hired on.

Those physicians taught me a lot about a nurse's scope of practice. I was in charge of their prenatal, postnatal, and well-baby clinics. I went on hospital and home visits and deliveries. I assisted the physicians in applying and removing casts and I spent time, particularly with mothers and women, talking about their health and family issues or concerns. This experience made me appreciate the untapped scope of nurses' practices in a health, not disease, context, dealing with the normal everyday health issues that we all encounter in everyday life. Working as a member of a multidisciplinary team opened my ideas to the potential that was resting dormant in nursing: the contribution that nursing could make to health. I wanted to do more of this work, so I decided to return to school to get my baccalaureate nursing degree.

For a brief period, right after graduation and before moving to England, I had worked in adult psychiatry. I would spend my time on nights reading patients' charts and was always left with the same feeling—these people did not have a chance. Many had in common dysfunctional family upbringings full of tragic stories, mostly from an early age. I wondered: If they had had better experiences when they were younger, would they be suffering so much as adults? So, when I enrolled in my degree program, I returned to working part-time in an adolescent psychiatry unit. I was beginning to learn about resilience and began to observe this trait in youngsters. Some adolescents, even though they had lived in very difficult circumstances, had the capacity and strength to overcome great challenges. It was then that I recognized this trait in myself. This self-awareness and developing consciousness would hold me in good stead throughout my nursing career.

About this time, my husband John decided that he too wanted to go back to school. So, for a variety of reasons, we moved west to Alberta—for me to complete my nursing degree and for him to complete his law degree, which we both did. During this time, I also worked in a child psychiatry unit and taught psychiatric nursing at the University of Alberta. After graduation, we were both offered wonderful jobs in beautiful Victoria, British Columbia, so we headed even further west.

At first, living and working in Victoria felt like we were going back in time. As far as I know, the Royal Jubilee Hospital School of Nursing was, at the time, the last standing hospital-based nursing program in the country. I again taught psychiatric nursing, but with a twist. A group of four instructors was responsible for the teaching rotation, two of us on medical–surgical units and two on psychiatric units. The rotation was designed around concepts such as body image, grief, and loss. The students spent half of their psychiatric rotation on a medical–surgical unit, where they worked with people dealing with these concepts; and the other half on a psychiatric unit working with people experiencing withdrawal (usually referred to as *schizophrenia*) or anxiety (usually referred to as *neurosis*). The students spent four days in the clinical settings and had class all day on Friday.

This was a profound teaching experience for me—emancipating my students and myself from labels and diagnoses and my first real experience where faculty and students worked collaboratively rather than from a hierarchical foundation. We four faculty members felt adventurous and I told the others about an idea I was reading about in a book by Carl Rogers (1969), called "Freedom to Learn." I had also discovered Paulo Freire (1972). As a consequence, we four decided that the next year we would not lecture our students; instead, we would think of questions for discussion and we would sit in a circle and have a dialogue with them. We felt like such rebels!

That was a turning point for me, and the groundwork for my future career was established. After giving birth to our second child, I decided to return to school and pursue a master's degree, but there were no nursing graduate programs close by and going away to school was not an option with a four-year-old and an infant at home. Instead, I decided to do a master's in counseling psychology.

I decided on this course of studies because I had heard of a professor who taught in the program, Dr. Vance Peavy, an expert humanistic psychologist from whom I could learn more about Carl Rogers. It was my five years of graduate school with Vance that really prepared me for my future in nursing. I came to understand what it meant to be in a caring, respectful, authentic therapeutic relationship—how to be fully present, to put my own judgments and thoughts aside, and to truly be there for the other.

While I was completing my master's, I discovered that I wanted to be an academic, so I commenced my doctoral studies the week after completing my master's. I also maintained my interest in working with children and families and used my doctoral time to concentrate on becoming a counseling and developmental psychologist and family therapist.

■ PROFESSIONAL EVOLUTION/CONTRIBUTION

In guiding the development of this chapter, I have continually focused on the concepts of *collaboration* and *emancipation*. Though these concepts had echoed in my early nursing days, it was at this point in my career that they became a part of me and all my work. They continue to this day to represent my ideals as a nurse educator and researcher.

I have been fortunate to have held two directorships during my career, and I believe that I made my most important contributions to nursing to date while holding those positions. The first appointment was as director of the Collaborative Nursing Program of British Columbia (CNPBC) and the other was as the director of the Centre for Community Health Promotion Research at the University of Victoria (UVic).

I spoke earlier of my entry into the discipline of nursing, but my real beginning was here—when I decided, with trepidation, to reenter nursing for a second time.

My caring science journey—during which I would learn about collaboration, emancipation, and leading from beside—began in the spring of 1989. By that time, I had accepted a tenure track academic position in the university's School of Child and Youth Care (SCYC) and I was happy in the position and finding my way as an academic and family therapist. The School of Nursing was down the hall from the SCYC, the director of nursing was a friend, and we had lunch together once a week. It was, she told me, an exciting time in nursing education—the dawning of the "curriculum revolution" (National League for Nursing [NLN], 1988). Eminent American nurse scholars were involved and they had united for the cause and collaborated to write a book called *Curriculum Revolution: Mandate for Change* (NLN, 1988). At the time, I could not know the impact this revolution would have on my life.

Serendipitously, the British Columbia government was engaged in a process of mentoring colleges within the province to become degree granting, and the School of Nursing was searching for a coordinator of a nursing program to guide three colleges through the process. The director of nursing kept enticing me to apply for the position, but by then I was feeling a part of the SCYC. I had just written an article based on Patricia Benner's (1984) work as a way to transition from nursing to child and youth care and was feeling quite content (Hills, 1989). But one Friday, on our usual lunch date, the director gave me the *Curriculum Revolution* book and just asked that I read it. I read "the book" that weekend and on Monday morning, I returned to the director's office and told her that if she was serious about what was written in this book I would apply. She said she was serious, so I did apply—and I was appointed!

My "real" job as director of the CNPBC was to help three college schools of nursing in the province gain degree-granting status. However, the steering committee for the project, composed of the lead nurse administrators at the colleges and at my university, had another vision—to create an integrated four-year baccalaureate program.

At the time, UVic offered only a post-RN program (RN to BScN), with no stated plans of developing a generic baccalaureate program. And, down the road from our university was Camosun College, preparing diploma RNs (similar to an associate degree), but not one of the three chosen by the government to become baccalaureate degree granting. We saw an opportunity, once again nurtured by collaboration. What if UVic and our neighbor Camosun College became permanent collaborative partners offering a single generic program between the two institutions? It was envisaged that students would complete the early part of their programs at the college and then transfer to UVic to complete their BScN. And so, from the outset, rather than developing an independent baccalaureate program at UVic and simply mentoring the other institutions to also become degree granting, we decided to collaborate to develop a single integrated caring curriculum that would be offered across all the colleges and our university.

I could not possibly have known that everything before this point had prepared me for the five years I would spend leading the CNPBC. As leader of this endeavor, I was initially unclear what we were doing or where we were headed, but I knew the work was important and that we had to get there. The big question at the time was, "If we are not going to develop a curriculum based on the Tylerian behavioral learning theory, what would we use?" Nursing education in North America and many other parts of the world had been entrenched in a Tylerian behavioral model of education for more than 40 years (Bevis & Watson, 1989; Hills & Watson, 2011; Hills, Lindsey, Chisamore, Bassett-Smith, Abbott, & Fournier-Chalmers, 1994; NLN, 1988).

We had established a working curriculum committee composed of two representatives from each of the six participating schools of nursing plus myself, and everyone was waiting for me to provide leadership to this great innovative project. I had heard about a new book written by Dr. Em Bevis that was about to be published and I was awaiting its release. But I was also anxious for some guidance about how to develop a nursing curriculum in this new era, so I found Dr. Bevis's phone number and decided to call her. She was very enthusiastic to hear that we were going to develop a caring curriculum and I spontaneously asked her if I might "drop in" and see her when I was in the area. She lived in South Carolina and I lived in British Columbia, Canada—not really dropping-in distance, but I asked for and received permission from my director to visit Em.

Our relationship quickly developed and soon I had the great honor of having Dr. Bevis as my first nurse mentor. She was an incredible nurse educator and an amazing human being, and she instilled the greatest confidence within me. She taught me the differences between nursing and medicine and pedagogy and curriculum. Later that year, her book I had been waiting for, Bevis and Watson's (1989) *Toward a Caring Curriculum: A New Pedagogy for Nursing*, was released and we used it to guide our work in our curriculum project. Em became our primary consultant and she introduced me to her coauthor, Dr. Jean Watson (see Chapter 16) and to Dr. Chris Tanner, both of whom also became consultants to our project.

Both Chris and Jean made significant contributions to the development of this curriculum, but it would be Jean who became a life mentor and friend, and who I continue to work with to this day. We developed an amazing bond—through hardship, resilience, and love. Jean was celebrated for her contribution to our work by being granted an honorary doctorate degree at UVic in 2011.

As our curriculum work progressed with the support of these amazing women, I came to understand nursing as "the professionalization of the human capacity to care and that nurses are in the unique position to assist people in understanding their health-related experiences and to encourage them to embrace their ability to make informed health choices" (Hills & Lindsey, 1994, p. 160). I recognized caring as a moral imperative to act ethically and justly (Bevis & Watson, 1989; Hills et al., 1994). Also, I learned that nursing's domain of practice was caring for people in their experiences with health and healing—it had little to do with diagnosing diseases or curing them. This was a rude awakening for me. I was shocked to learn that I had been teaching not nursing, but medicine for more than 15 years. It is difficult to express how deeply transforming this experience was for me. Since that time, I have always taught nurses from a nursing perspective—caring for people in relation to their health and their healing experiences (Hills & Watson, 2011).

Em's textbook (Bevis & Watson, 1989) redefined *curriculum* as the interactions that occur between and among learners, clients, practitioners, and teachers with the intent that learning occur. This view shifts the focus of curriculum from design and structure to a focus on *pedagogy*. "Most curriculum development results in minimal changes of substance. . . . We switch, swap and slide content around. . . . The very repetitiveness of our curriculum development efforts should tell us that we are not changing the substance[,] only the arrangement of content" (Bevis & Watson, 1989, p. 27). This insight entirely changed our focus and our curriculum development process. The shift from a content-driven behavioral structure to a pedagogical-oriented process was challenging, to say the least.

As we progressed through that process, we were repeatedly confronting and using the term *collaboration*, and it struck me that we needed clarity and certainty about its meaning. If we were asking each other to collaborate in our work and striving to design a collaborative program, what were we really saying? One day, a colleague who was working on the project shared a definition that she had found in Webster's dictionary: "To work together as in a joint intellectual effort," but directly below it, a second definition: "To cooperate treasonably as with an enemy occupying one's country." No wonder we felt uneasy in our curriculum discussions! We were six different institutions, all with our own existing nursing program in different bureaucratic organizations, working together with the inevitable underlying feeling of "This is my territory!" As the project leader asking for—indeed, demanding collaboration—I crafted and set down the following definition of *collaboration*, which I use to this day in all of my teaching and research:

> Collaboration is the creation of a synergistic alliance that honors and utilizes each person's contribution in order to create collective wisdom and collective action. Collaboration is not synonymous with co-operation, partnership, participation or compromise. Those words do not convey the fundamental importance of being in relationship nor the depth of caring that is collaboration. Collaborators are committed to, care about and trust in each other. They recognize that despite their differences, each has unique and valuable knowledge, perspectives and experiences to contribute to the collaboration. (Hills, 1992, p. 14; Hills & Watson, 2011, p. 71)

A key strategy to move this collaboration forward was to create a shared vision. We did this, in part, by cocreating a shared philosophy for the program about our beliefs and values related to people, nursing, health, health care, nursing, and curriculum (Hills et al., 1994). We completed this with much energy, resources, and time spent on faculty development. We discussed horizontal violence and how to overcome it in our working group (Hills & Watson, 2011). We learned about each other's strengths, perspectives, and expectations and discovered that we were all committed to creating a caring curriculum with an emphasis on health promotion that used an emancipatory pedagogy.

We committed to climbing together so that we would all arrive beside each other on a plateau—not one individual at the top of a mountain.

With our philosophy and commitment to each other in place, we were ready to tackle the daunting question of what the content should be and how it should be organized. We decided to open the collaboration to our practice, professional organizations, nurses' union, and administrative nursing partners.

The curriculum team held focus groups and did a Delphi study asking three simple questions: "What will nurses need to know to practice nursing in the 21st century?" "What will nurses need to be able to do to practice nursing in the 21st century?" "How will nurses need to be (attitudes & values) to practice in the 21st century?" (Beddome et al., 1995; Hills, 1998; Hills & Lindsey, 1994; Hills et al., 1994). These investigations included more than 200 nurse administrators across the continuum of care, practicing nurses, and nurse educators in different programs in British Columbia. We conducted a thematic analysis and, to our surprise, no one identified that nurses need to know about diseases to practice nursing. Rather, all the themes reflected a need to know about themselves, people, people's experiences, health, and healing. As a result, we organized all the nursing content throughout our new curriculum within four themes: people's experience with health, people's experience with healing, people's experience with self and others, and people's experience with professional growth. We identified two variables, caring and health promotion, that permeated the entire program and we wove four critical concepts into every course: ways of knowing, personal meaning, time/transitions, and context.

The resulting curriculum structure shown in Figure 21.1 is depicted by a Celtic knot to exemplify the connection and continuing flow of the curriculum components.

Having broken free from the dominant oppressive behavioral education system, we were able to embrace an emancipatory approach to education. We investigated many theories and committed to Freire (1972) and critical social theory (Grundy, 1987). We had

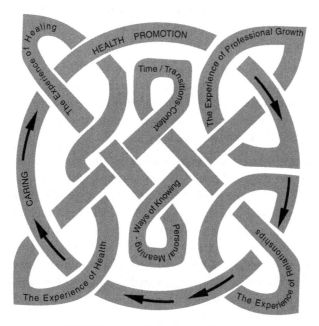

FIGURE 21.1   Celtic knot of curriculum.

previously endorsed phenomenology, and our program was definitely based in this philosophy, but we understood that, in the context in which most nursing is practiced, the hegemony is strong. Phenomenology alone would not provide the critical social reflective understanding that was needed to overcome the predominant biomedical perspective. So, as a way to create a counter-hegemony, we relied on critical social theory to open our eyes to the oppression of nursing, both in education and practice (Freire, 1972). As Shor and Freire (1987) explain,

> Even when you individually feel yourself . . . free, . . . if you are not able to use your . . . freedom to help others to be free by transforming the totality of society, then you are exercising only an individualistic attitude towards . . . freedom. . . . While individual empowerment . . . is not enough . . . it is absolutely necessary for . . . social transformation. (p. 109)

As educators, we realized that it was our responsibility to address this oppression by beginning with our own practice as nurse educators. We asked ourselves the question: How would we educate student nurses using an emancipatory pedagogy? We recognized, as Bevis and Watson (1989) explain,

> Without emancipation, education is . . . oppressive . . . an assembly line industry producing nurse-workers who . . . follow the status quo. They may make waves, but . . . stay within the rules . . . bear[ing] the inevitable stamp[s of] banality and mediocrity. Emancipatory education encourages learners to ask the unaskable . . . and be active agents in their lives and . . . work. (p. 162)

We knew that we had a steep learning curve. All the schools had "taught" in very traditional behavioral ways—using behavioral objectives—lecturing and measuring outcomes based on those objectives. We had to learn how to teach in an emancipatory pedagogy, and we did! We came to understand our relational emancipatory pedagogy as the transformation of consciousness. Unlike the banking concept of education, as shown in Figure 21.2, where the teacher is the "giver" of knowledge and the student is the "receiver," with emancipatory pedagogy, as shown in Figure 21.3,

> learning occurs at the juncture or intersection where the teacher and the student are in a caring relationship and are co-creating knowledge . . . the intersection of the complexity of caring relationships that lead to new insights, new knowledge and deeper understandings resulting in the transformation of consciousness. (Hills & Watson, 2011, p. 54)

Multiple teaching strategies exist to implement this type of pedagogy; we chose to use learning activities designed specifically for our program. In this way, we could be sure that the critical components of "caring" and "praxis" could be incorporated into every learning activity throughout the program. All faculty became involved in developing learning activities for each course. We shared these among all faculty members and in this way created a repository of learning activities across the program. The intention with all the learning activities was to encourage students to stand in their own power and knowledge. As Kahlil Gibran so eloquently stated, "If the teacher is indeed wise, [s]he does not bid you enter the house of [her] wisdom but leads you to the threshold of your own mind" (Gibran, 1923/1997, p. 18).

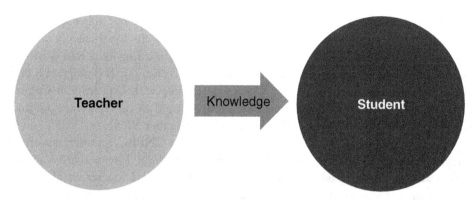

FIGURE 21.2   Banking concept of education.

My work in caring science curriculum came full circle when I joined Jean in 2009 and volunteered my time to her nonprofit organization, Watson Caring Science Institute (WCSI). As a tribute to Em and to carry her work forward, Jean and I published our book, *Creating a Caring Science Curriculum: An Emancipatory Pedagogy for Nursing* (Hills & Watson, 2011).

Working with Jean is always a delight and you never know exactly what you are in for. When she began receiving inquiries about the possibility of creating and granting a doctorate in caring science, she did what is typical of her: Generous, adventuresome, free-spirited, and gracious as always, she threw the road out in front of her, truly having no concrete idea of how it would work.

Being her colleague and friend, I volunteered to stand beside her and help her develop a nontraditional doctoral program in caring science through WCSI. Being involved in this highly creative, innovative program has been a highlight of my career. Students have the freedom to explore fascinating topics that are outside the realm of most academic institutions. For example, one student is studying love (see Chapter 20), another gratitude in

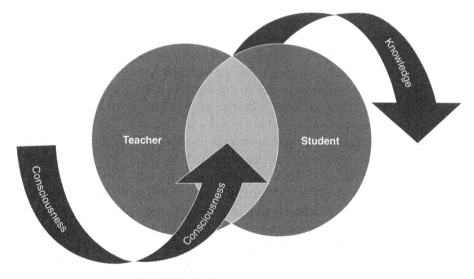

FIGURE 21.3   Emancipatory pedagogy.

the caring moment, and yet another teaching from the heart. We not only openly explore the methodologies and methods that we know, but we also discuss the development of new methods that challenge us to stay fully conscious of our caring human capacities and processes. What an honor it has been to contribute to this creation! This program is in the process of being reinvented as part of WCSI's partnership with University of Colorado (UC). The UC School of Nursing has developed a stream in caring science within its doctoral program and admitted its first students in September 2015.

At the same time that I was deeply immersed in the CNPBC, another opportunity emerged, this time in research. When I was in graduate school, I knew that I wanted to be an academic—I was passionate about teaching. However, I was scared of research, especially orthodox research, and in those days that was the predominant way of doing research. In fact, no one I knew of did any other type of research. I decided that if I was going to be an academic, I would have to overcome my fear. I am thankful to have been guided by some amazing, supportive faculty members and an exceptional supervisor, Dr. Don Knowles. Immediately after completing my beautiful Solomon Four Group Design experimental study examining the personal meaning in knowledge transfer and retention, I was invited to conduct an evaluation for the Ministry of Health of a parenting course I had designed and delivered. Feeling confident now in my newly found research skills, of course, I used a similar design. But I decided on a whim to also interview the parents in this study. When I analyzed the data, I was shocked to find that although the quantitative scales indicated no significant difference in parental behavior or attitude, the data from the interviews indicated a huge impact of the intervention. Parents reported how influential the course had been and how it made a difference in the way they now parented their children. The qualitative data suggested that parents were in more control of their emotions with their children, that they understood their children better, and that they were not as inclined to want to hit their children.

I was left with a dilemma. What was the truth? Had the intervention made an impact? Had it made a difference to these children–parent relationships?

I learned on that day that there are different ways to do research and I began to educate myself in various methodologies, including phenomenological, narrative, and participatory action research. Discovering participatory action research was like coming home for me. The collaborative, emancipatory nature of this approach to research resonated and I discovered that I could now do research based on the same principles as my pedagogy—collaboration and emancipation. I could do research with people, not *on, to,* or *about* them.

Because I had provided leadership in nursing education related to health promotion, when the Tri-Council for Health Promotion Research involving three Canadian provincial universities, was established in 1992, I was appointed as the principal investigator for UVic. That same year, a colleague and I received Research Development Initiative funding to develop a community-based research program. The serendipity of this allocation of funding and other mediating factors prompted us, in 1993, to establish the Community Health Promotion Coalition that brought together researchers, community members, policy makers, and health care practitioners with a shared interest in health promotion community-based research.

About the same time, my colleague and I were awarded a provincial grant to develop and deliver a community-based research program throughout British Columbia. This culminated in our coalition planning and hosting a National Health

Promotion Conference on Community-Based Research (Hills, 2002). Our coalition flourished and was designated a Senate-approved center at UVic in 2004, and I became its founding director. By then, we had been awarded several large federally funded research grants (Hills & Mullett, 1992–2002; Hills et al., 1990–1994; Hills, Green, & Gutman, 1992–1998). There was a national movement at the time to create a Canadian Consortium of Health Promotion Research (CCHPR), and I represented our center at this national organization. I became the codirector and then president of this nonprofit organization, which led me to work closely with Health Canada and the Public Health Agency of Canada. At the same time, I served as a globally elected member of the board of trustees for the International Union for Health Promotion and Education (IUHPE) for 12 years (2001–2013) and, during that tenure, I also served as its vice president of Scientific Affairs for the North American Region. Our research center and the CCHPR worked closely with policy makers on several research projects, including reorienting and increasing access to health services, health promotion effectiveness, effectiveness of community interventions to promote health, and reducing health disparities.

That focus on policy and my working more closely with policy makers, not just with members of the community, led me to question the name "community-based research." We were doing participatory action research, but I felt that the reference to "community-based" did not honor the contributions that the policy makers were making. As a result, we began to refer to our research approach as Collaborative Action Research and Evaluation (CARE). We have recently completed a book chapter on the subject (Hills & Carroll, 2016) and are in the process of writing a CARE textbook, *Collaborative Action and Evaluation (CARE): A Catalyst for Health and Social Change* (Hills & Carroll, in preparation).

Collaborative and emancipatory teaching and research infiltrated everything we did at the center. All of our research grant applications incorporated these concepts, and each summer, we offered an intensive graduate seminar in CARE. We offered this as a both a credit and a noncredit course and collaborated with the local health authority so that practitioners could attend. We applied for and were designated as a World Health Organization (WHO) Collaborating Centre (2008–2013), and my research colleagues and I are in the process of renewing this status. Our current research agenda is multidisciplinary and focuses on health care improvement, health in all policies, intersectoral action for health, social determinants of health, health inequities, and positive youth development. That work continues to this day.

■ MORAL/ETHICAL FOUNDATION

What is most important to me as a nurse is that nursing stay grounded in its disciplinary philosophical and theoretical foundation of caring. If nurses were able to maintain that footing, nursing would be understood to be the discipline of caring, focused on people and their experiences of health and healing. Rather than always following and never leading, we nurses would develop *our own* disciplinary knowledge instead of being attracted to and following the new waves in medicine and education, like evidence-based practice that looks at medical evidence and behavioral education approaches. As the most populous of the health professions, nursing could be the most influential. It is time for nursing to lead health care reform.

I have no doubt that caring is not only the philosophical and theoretical foundation of nursing but also its moral and ethical foundation. When one understands caring as an ethic, as opposed to simply a feeling, one's thinking and actions in practice are guided by caring as the moral imperative to act ethically and justly (Bevis & Watson, 1989). I demonstrate this in *my* nursing practice (education) by teaching students from a caring science perspective and by facilitating their learning to demonstrate this caring foundation in *their* practice.

In addition to having students learn caring in their course work, I also make sure that it is included and evaluated in their clinical performance. Often, evaluation strategies undermine our intended learning outcomes. Having students articulate and analyze their caring assists them to incorporate caring into their daily practice as a moral compass to guide their clinical decision making. For example, when we were developing the CNPBC, we had to develop a clinical appraisal that would not undermine our caring curriculum. The question we struggled with was, "If we are not going to use behavioral objectives, how will we assess students' clinical capacities?"

We recognized that if we did not have a way to evaluate clinical performance other than using behavioral objectives, we would undo all that we had accomplished. We discovered that a group of nurses in Britain had used Benner's (1984) domains of practice to evaluate clinical performance and so we looked into this and massaged Benner's domains to reflect our perspective, as shown in Table 21.1. We created an iterative dialogue process using reflective journals to gather evidence of students' meeting of preestablished

TABLE 21.1   **Benner-CNPBC Domains of Practice With Rationales**

Benner's Domains of Practice	CNPBC Domains of Practice	Rationale for Changes Made
Helping domain	Health/healing domain	To include health
Teaching–coaching function	Teaching/learning domain	To include learning from client
Diagnostic and patient monitoring function	Clinical judgment domain	Combined three domains, as each involved aspects of clinical judgement
Effective management of rapidly changing situations		
Administering and monitoring therapeutic interventions		
Monitoring and ensuring the quality of health care practices	Professional responsibility domain	To capture essence of the domain in language more congruent with curriculum
Organizational and work-role competencies	Collaborative leadership domain	To incorporate language that more accurately reflected a caring science philosophy

CNPBC, Collaborative Nursing Program of British Columbia.

Adapted from Hills (1992, 2001); Hills and Watson (2011).

quality indicators. We used a participatory action research project to develop and change the way we did clinical evaluations (Hills et al., 1990–1994; Hills, 2001). Table 21.1 details the changes that we made and incorporated into our clinical appraisal form.

These five domains of practice still remain constant throughout the program. We developed quality indicators for each semester to level the expectations required (Hills, 1992; Hills, 2001; Hills & Watson, 2011). Students kept journals and presented situations to provide evidence that they had met the quality indicators for each semester. Faculty members read these journals and interacted with students sharing their observations and asking critical reflection questions. This iterative process proved to be very successful in documenting students' clinical competencies and capacities (Hills, 2001; Hills & Watson, 2011).

■ VISION

Although I believe that caring is the ethical foundation of nursing, I fear that, as a discipline, nursing continues to be embedded in a behaviorist, biomedical, positivist paradigm. I believe this to be true in all aspects of nursing—practice, education, administration, and research. As Watson (2012) declares,

> It is critical for nursing . . . to be clear about sustaining a meaningful ethical, philosophical foundation . . ., lest we lose our way in this post-modern era of change. . . . Nurses now are invited to become visionary leaders . . ., [and] shape intentional transformative worldview change, rather than conform to outdated modes that no longer work. (p. 3)

Therefore, the very first task for nursing is to set its roots in that ethical foundation.

I see three other opportunities that nursing should not let pass by. Nursing should integrate health and health promotion into its domain of practice; further develop its understanding of power relations; and, finally, realize emerging opportunities for nurse coaching.

The United Kingdom's Royal College of Nursing (RCN; 1998) has said, "The nursing workforce remains very much a sleeping giant. . . .nurses have enormous potential as agents of social control in promoting health . . . imagine what the impact might be if . . . millions of nurses . . . became empowered, assertive and articulate agents of change for better health promotion" (p. 12). I share this vision with the RCN, but it is even more impressive when viewed in the context of caring science. When nursing focuses on health and health promotion from a caring science perspective, there is an integration of several concepts that work in collaboration with one another. For example, the concepts of wholeness and connection are reinforced by the concepts of caring and health promotion working together in a synergistic alliance.

During the CNPBC described earlier, we had linked caring and health promotion in hopes of strengthening the often-noted misperception of caring as a "feeling" or something "soft." So the question became, "Did students actually practice in a way that demonstrated this health promotion caring perspective?" The results of my research clearly demonstrated that student nurses did practice from this perspective and, furthermore, the centrality of caring became the most predominant theme (Hills, 1998). We concluded that linking health and caring gave students further language to articulate their caring experiences, something needed in nursing education.

Just last week, the importance of this linkage was demonstrated from a student's perspective. I am currently teaching a graduate online course in nursing education on caring science pedagogy. In her weekly discussion notes, while reflecting on her learning in the course, a student wrote the following unsolicited comment. I think she provides a good example of the potential impact of linking health promotion and caring science:

> I felt compelled to discuss ensuring that we, as people, and our patients are not broken down into parts—that we strive to keep wholeness. Beginning this course, I was so challenged by this concept because I prided myself on my understanding of "the parts" and mastering each system, each category of health, and even compartmentalizing social needs of my patients. I was totally broken of this pride when I learned about caring science, and how we need to be inclusive of all areas of the health of our patients, and to also include the personal and loving relationships that nurses embody each day. I had to give myself permission to not be so reliant on science, or the biomedical model of viewing health. Since then, I have become a better nurse, relating better to the mothers and fathers of the infants I care for and have been more conscious of the stages of development of the infants and facilitating bonding. The personal is professional because we are all humans—we . . . all need love and care and we strive for acceptance. It is very easy to fall into the trap of maintaining a boundary with our patients and families, to spare ourselves of the reality of what they are experiencing and how difficult hospitalization is or separation between a mother and her infant. I think it is important to sensitize, rather than desensitize from our patients and families during this time to really care, listen, and strive to see them in their whole state.
>
> This course has helped me see the nursing world differently, in a much more complete, positive, and whole view. I do not know if I will ever truly be able to articulate all I have learned or what caring science means to me, but I am forever changed. (Anonymous, personal communication, N570, 2015)

Health promotion demands that people be empowered to take control of the factors that influence their health. It requires nurses to *share* power with clients, not to hold it over them. Given that nursing is the largest group of health care providers, it seems obvious to me that if nursing could operationalize this one imperative of health promotion, nurses could change existing health care systems throughout the world.

A second area where nursing has yet to realize its full potential is in the area of power relations. Power exists in all relationships; neither health care, health education, nor research is exempt. But there is always a choice about how people use their power (Hills & Watson, 2011) and in almost every situation, power can be negotiated. In caring science, we tend not to pay much attention to this concept, despite the fact that maintaining power *over* relationships is antithetical to the values upon which caring science is built. I believe that, for our future as a caring science discipline, we need to discuss, teach, and research power relations with a view toward more collaboration and emancipation in all endeavors.

Finally, I believe that nurse coaching will become dominant in nursing practice, education, and research (Dossey & Hess, 2013; Dossey, Luck, & Schaub, 2015). Currently, nursing tends to view patient education in all nursing settings as "giving information." Nurses often explain things to patients/clients and send them out the door with a pamphlet; much like the banking concept approach to education shown earlier in Figure 21.2. From a caring science perspective, learning is seen as a relational inquiry process that occurs at the juncture or intersection where the nurse and patient are in a caring relationship and are cocreating knowledge. This transformation of consciousness leads to new knowledge, new insights, new understandings, and new ways of being in the world (Hills & Watson, 2011). For more than 20 years, other professions have explored health and wellness coaching. Surely, given nursing's focus on health and well-being, it is ideally situated to take up the same challenge. In 2013, the American Nursing Association (ANA) supported the publication of *The Art and Science of Nurse Coaching: The Provider's Guide to Coaching Scope and Competencies*, noting that "[t]he professional Nurse Coach and coaching competencies are a fundamental part of nursing practice" (Hess et al., 2013, p. xiii; see Chapters 4, 24, and 27 for more information on nurse coaching).

In the future, I will contribute to advancing the caring science agenda in education and research by completing two books, which I already have under development. My intention with the first textbook, *The Caritas Practitioner as a Health and Healing Coach* (Hills & Watson, in preparation), is to integrate my experiences in caring science, counseling psychology, relationship and family counselling, health promotion, group facilitation, and pedagogy to culminate in a framework for coaching clients from a caring science health promotion perspective. This textbook will be of interest to nurses regardless of their area of practice. My hope is that this will extend the caring science agenda, develop capacity in dealing with power issues, and integrate a health promotion perspective into caring science.

In addition, I will write a second textbook, *Collaborative Action Research and Evaluation (CARE): A Catalyst for Health and Social Change* (Hills & Carroll, in preparation). This book will focus on a new methodology for doing research and evaluation *with* people, not *to, on,* or *about* them.

In closing, I reflect on how, so often in my career, I have been told why something will not work. "We don't have enough money" or "It's not practical" or "No one will follow." But, as I learned to do at my family dinner table all those years ago, I find my voice, push back, and respond: "It *will* work!"

I have a favorite quotation that says it best. It is all about commitment.

Until one is committed, there is hesitancy, the chance to draw back, always ineffectiveness, concerning all acts of initiative (and creation). There is one elementary truth, the ignorance of which kills countless ideas and splendid plans: that the moment that one definitely commits oneself, then Providence moves too. All sorts of things occur in one's favour that would never otherwise have occurred. A whole stream of events issues from the decision, raising in one's favour all manner of unforeseen incidents and meetings and material assistance which no [wo]man could have dreamed would come [her/]his way. I learned a deep respect for one of Goethe's couplets: "Whatever you can do or dream you can, begin it. Boldness has genius, power and magic in it!" (Murray, 1951)

◼ **REFLECTIONS**

1. *What are my experiences with collaboration and emancipation?*
2. *How do I ensure that I am teaching-coaching-leading others from a nursing, as opposed to a biomedical, perspective?*
3. *Upon what foundation have I been basing my practice, research, or education? Is it a nursing or biomedical one? What am I present to now that I was not present to before regarding a nursing-specific disciplinary foundation?*
4. *What experiences have I had leading from beside instead of in front? What have I learned from those experiences?*
5. *How do I see health promotion, power, and nurse coaching affecting my current and future practice?*

◼ **REFERENCES**

Beddome, G., Budgen, C., Hills, M. D., Lindsey, A. E., Duval, P. M., & Szalay, L. (1995). Nursing Faculty, Okanagan University College, Kelowna, British Columbia. *Journal of Nursing Education, 34*(1), 11–15.

Benner, P. (1984). *From novice to expert, excellence and power in clinical nursing practice.* Menlo Park, CA: Addison-Wesley.

Bevis, E. O., & Watson, J. (1989). *Toward a caring curriculum: A new pedagogy for nursing.* Boston, MA: Jones & Bartlett.

Dossey, B. M., & Hess, D. (2013). Professional nurse coaching: Advances in national and global healthcare transformation. *Global Advances in Health and Medicine, 2*(4), 10–16.

Dossey, B. M., Luck, S., & Schaub, B. G. (2015). *Nurse coaching: Integrative approaches for health and wellbeing.* North Miami, FL: International Nurse Coach Association.

Freire, P. (1972). *Pedagogy of the oppressed.* London, UK: Penguin Books.

Gibran, K. (1923/1997). *The prophet.* Ware, Hertfordshire, UK: Wordsworth Editions, Ltd.

Grundy, S. (1987). *Curriculum: Product or praxis.* Lewes, UK: Falmer Press.

Hartrick, G., Lindsey, E., & Hills, M. (1994). Family nursing assessment: Meeting the challenge of health promotion. *Journal of Advanced Nursing, 20*, 85–91.

Hess, D. R., Dossey, B. M., Southard, M. E., Luck, S., Schaub, B. G., & Bark, L. (2013). *The art and science of nurse coaching: A provider's guide to scope and competencies.* Silver Spring, MD: Nursesbooks.org.

Hills, M. (1989). The child and youth care student as an emerging professional practitioner. *Journal of Child and Youth Care, 4*(1), 17–31.

Hills, M. (1992). Collaborative nursing project. *Development of generic integrated nursing curriculum in collaboration with four partner colleges.* Report to Ministry of Advanced Education, Centre for Curriculum and Professional Development.

Hills, M. (1998). Student experiences of nursing health promotion practice in hospital settings. *Nursing Inquiry, 5*, 164–173.

Hills, M. (2001). Using co-operative inquiry to transform evaluation of nursing students' clinical practice. In P. Reason & H. Bradbury (Eds.), *Handbook of action research, participative inquiry and practice* (pp. 340–347). London, UK: Sage.

Hills, M. (2002, April). *Community-based research: A catalyst for transforming primary health care.* 6th National Health Promotion Research Conference. Victoria, BC.

Hills, M., & Carroll, S. (2016). Collaborative action evaluation. In A. Vollman, E. Anderson, & J. McFarlane (Eds.), *Canadian community as partner: Theory & multidisciplinary practice* (pp. 288–301). Philadelphia, PA: Lippincott Williams & Wilkins.

Hills, M., & Carroll, S. (in preparation). *Collaborative action and evaluation (CARE): A catalyst for health and social change.* New York, NY: Springer Publishing Company.

Hills, M., & Lindsey, E. (1994). Health promotion: A viable curriculum framework for nursing education. *Nursing Outlook, 42*(4), 158–162.

Hills, M., Lindsey, E., Chisamore, M., Bassett-Smith, J., Abbott, K., & Fournier-Chalmers, J., (1994). Collaborative Nursing Program, University of Victoria, British Columbia, Canada. *The Journal of Nursing Education, 33*(5), 220–225.

Hills, M., & Watson, J. (2011). *Creating a caring science curriculum: An emancipatory pedagogy for nursing.* New York, NY: Springer Publishing Company.

Hills, M., & Watson, J. (in preparation). *The Caritas practitioner as a health and healing coach.*

Murray, W. H. (1951). Beautiful daily quotes. Retrieved from http://beautifuldailyquotes.com/blog/2015/3/12/whatever-you-can-do-or-dream-you-can-begin-it-boldness-has-genius-power-and-magic-in-it

National League for Nursing. (1988). *Curriculum revolution: Mandate for change* (No. 15). New York, NY: Author.

Rogers, C. R. (1969). *Freedom to learn.* Columbus, OH: Charles E. Merrill.

Royal College of Nursing. (1998). Imagining the future: Nursing in the new millennium. London, United Kingdom: Author.

Shor, I., & Freire, P. (1987). *A pedagogy for liberation: Dialogues on transforming education.* South Hadley, MA: Bergin & Gavey.

Watson, J. (2012). *Human caring science: A theory of nursing* (2nd ed.). Sudbury, MA: Jones & Bartlett.

CHAPTER TWENTY-TWO

Visionary and Reflection Centered: Remaining Open to the Possibilities of Nursing Praxis

Sara Horton-Deutsch

Remaining "open to what is emerging" creates vulnerability and humanity. This persistent, practiced, intentional openness—the quintessence of authentic presence, which is the quintessence of humanity—is also the quintessence of quality nursing. Facilitating the development of authentic presence in nursing requires creating safe spaces for students to explore where they have been, where they are, and where they want to go in their nursing practice.
                    —Horton-Deutsch and Drysdale (2015, p. 152)

■ WHY NURSING?

I was born into a family of health care providers on my maternal side. My grandfather and four of his five brothers were "small-town" doctors, my grandmother managed my grandfather's family practice, and my mother was a nurse administrator in long-term care settings. I never thought of being anything other than a nurse, and in many ways, it seems I always was one. I was the middle of three children and my older sister had been born premature with a number of developmental delays. Looking back, I see it led me to take on many of the roles and responsibilities of the oldest child. Developmentally, I surpassed my older sister within a few years, and this was quite difficult for both of us. We were both too young to understand at the time why my older sister was far from appreciative of my desire to help. However, when my younger sister came along, she was quite receptive to my affection and caregiving, so I directed much of my caring energies toward her.

Both of my sisters and I often spent days off, holidays, and sick days at the nursing home where our mother worked. On weekends, we would stop by and run to the occupational therapy room to dunk our hands in the paraffin while waiting for our mom to resolve a staffing issue. On holidays, we would help the recreational therapists put up decorations, serve the residents snacks, and play games. When sick, my mom would find an empty bed for us to convalesce in. During these visits, it was not infrequent for a staff member to tell us how much they admired or appreciated our mother. She was a single mom and nurse leader known for advocating for her staff and residents. I recall her having the courage to resign from her positions on a number of occasions when the staff or residents were not being treated well and she could not resolve the issues within the system. I loved being with my mom at these nursing homes because it was clear she was in her element; she seemed happy and was making the lives of others better as well. I wanted to be a nurse just like her.

My first recollection of developing a moral/ethical view occurred in high school. I was taking an elective class on society taught by Dr. Jefferies, the only teacher in my high school I recall having a PhD. He was also a lawyer and a bit of a rabble rouser. We studied Kohlberg's stages of moral development (Kohlberg, 1981), and I was struck by how much of our society functioned at the conventional level stages 3 and 4 (conformity and authority/social order). I recall being disappointed that we as society did not do more to understand others and the world around us. I asked myself how we could limit ourselves to such a mediocre level of moral reasoning. Dr. Jeffries taught and challenged students to ask these types of rhetorical and ineffable questions, to imagine what we would do if we were in another's shoes, and to consider what we would believe to be true if we were in their circumstances.

Coincidentally, this same semester, three friends and I wanted to miss one day of school to visit an open house at a college in an adjacent state. The school asked if our parents would be going and we said no. We were informed that our absence would not be excused and we would receive zeros on any tests being given that day. I realized I was being challenged to apply what I was learning in class and I became that much more determined to go. Consequently, all of my teachers gave me zeros that day except Dr. Jeffries. He rescheduled the exam and used my incident as one way to challenge authority. It became something we dialogued about and debated in class. He used this incident to help us develop our own principles to live by—principles that take into account human rights, liberty, and justice. He encouraged us to challenge rules that we determine to be unjust and act because it is right to do so and not merely to avoid punishment. Interestingly, two of the four of us ended up attending that college and ultimately determined it was "the right thing to do."

When I started college, I attended my parents' alma mater, a small liberal arts school with a reputable nursing program in the Midwest. My geriatric nursing professor had been a classmate of my mother's. Another faculty member, Dorothy Stevens, taught my mother and me obstetrics nursing. Dorothy and her partner Thelma (a nursing faculty member who had retired the previous year) led a study-abroad program for 10 nursing students for a semester just before Dorothy's official retirement. I attended and completed my community health and nursing leadership coursework and clinical hours under their guidance. Caring for patients in their homes in Lincolnshire County, near Grantham, England, had a major influence on how I experienced and thought about nursing. I carried firewood into homes, observed home environments, served and drank tea with patients, and learned to genuinely listen to their concerns. There was a palpable sense of mutual respect and unconditional regard between the visiting nurse and patient. The visiting nurse and I would follow up with the patient in a few days and, if needed, reach out to the family. There was no sense of rush or hurry and it seemed everyone was fully present. Looking back, this is where I first noticed the value of reflective practice—a purposeful activity toward realizing one's own vision for practice.

Upon returning to the United States, Dorothy and Thelma made it clear that they had high hopes for me, and I did not want to disappoint. I had one semester of nursing school to complete and returned to my part-time job as a nursing assistant at a nursing home. However, something inside me had changed. I was constantly questioning and challenging the care provided and was now far more concerned with the patient having a voice. I was frustrated and frustrating those around me by constantly challenging the status quo. I changed jobs and went to a different long-term care facility where the residents had more say in their care and day-to-day routine. I was pleased when a newly admitted elderly resident was allowed to continue to have a daily beer just as she had at home. The staff had even put newspaper down around her chair so she could spit on the floor to clear her throat. Yet, it was not enough. Wherever I went, I noticed deeply embedded social norms governed by authority and many of those I worked with were indifferent, resistant, or too afraid to advocate for change. I realized I was never going to make it as a staff nurse in the hospitals where I was completing my clinical hours or the nursing homes where I was employed. Although my mother was able to go far with her baccalaureate degree, I recognized that I needed to go to graduate school in order to have the influence she was having in long-term care facilities.

So, during that last semester of nursing school, I began exploring options for graduate school. Having spent my childhood in long-term care facilities, working as a nursing assistant in a hospital for two years, and nursing homes for three, I figured I was "ready." However, I quickly learned that most universities required formal experience as a staff nurse, so I revised my plan. Knowing I was ready for something bigger, I decided to get a job as a staff nurse in a larger community and applied to graduate school shortly after. I set my sites on either Vanderbilt in Nashville, Tennessee, or Rush Presbyterian St. Luke's Medical Center in Chicago, Illinois. After visiting both and learning about the unification model of nursing at Rush, I decided it was the place for me.

My vision of nursing at the time was largely influenced by both my experiences of going to work with my mother during my childhood and the eye-opening experience of community health nursing in England. In both of these situations, I witnessed nurses with a high degree of autonomy over their practices. Equally important, these nurses demonstrated the value of learning through everyday experiences toward a desirable practice. They were deliberative and intuitive. They worked well with others. When I asked questions, I was greeted with responses to help me more fully understand, to both appreciate and resolve contradictions between what I learned through study and experienced in practice as I dealt with the realities of life.

Although I did not consciously understand it at the time, this vision fit with the Rush unification model and the reason I was drawn to move to Chicago. During my interview, I witnessed the collaboration among nurses, physicians, managers, clinical specialists, social workers, educators, and researchers all on one unit and how this benefited both the patient and unit. There was a sense of freedom and pride among the nurses I had not witnessed since leaving England. I realized it was what I had been missing and sensed it immediately during my interview. At that moment, I knew I wanted to be a "Rush Nurse."

■ EARLY IMPRESSIONS

While in the foreground, my health care experiences had been primarily working with the elderly, in the background, particularly in my personal life, a series of events related to mental illness were weighing heavily on me. First, a very creative, sensitive, and somewhat troubled high-school classmate died unexpectedly with few details of what actually happened. Second, one of my college dormmates made several suicide attempts. And third, my brilliant uncle who worked as a researcher for the National Aeronautics and Space Administration (NASA), who had been diagnosed with bipolar disorder a few years prior, committed suicide while I was taking my state board exams.

The lack of transparency, openness, and dialogue around these events was both troubling and perplexing to me. What these events all had in common were shame, secrecy, and silence. I was angry that nobody in my life wanted to really talk about the intense pain and suffering inflicted on all involved. I turned to my psychiatric nursing faculty and found two people who listened, encouraged me to share what was going on inside of me, and went further by ensuring that my dormmate got the professional help she needed. I developed a deep sense of respect for these faculty mentors who had the courage to have difficult conversations and ask deeply profound questions. I was forever changed by their raw courage forcing the university to address the mental health needs of students. I wanted to be the kind of nurse leader who was not afraid to discuss issues openly. I wanted to be someone who was so grounded in an ethical core that he or she was not afraid to have difficult conversations, ask value-laden questions, and hold others accountable, as needed.

So although my first job at Rush was in the geriatric rehabilitation unit, my college experiences drew me to also want to work in mental health. As a result, I transferred to the psychiatric unit and later the geropsychiatric unit when an opening became available. This provided me the opportunity to combine my interests, a chance for me to focus on both the mind and the body. I spent nearly a decade on the geropsychiatric unit. I began as a staff nurse, eventually becoming a practitioner-teacher. In this role, I guided undergraduate nursing students during their clinical experiences, clinically supervised staff nurses, and became part of the leadership team working with the unit managers to develop continuing education programs and resolve unit and staff issues. I was deeply moved and humbled by my work with patients and their families. I found this same gratification from facilitating growth in students and staff and partnering with colleagues to ensure that patients received quality care. These were phenomenally growth-producing years for me. Along the way, I completed my master's degree in psychiatric mental health nursing, my doctoral degree (which focused on elderly suicide), and postdoctoral studies in psychoneuroimmunology. I had a close-knit group of colleagues whom I dearly loved and who were doing meaningful work. However, once again, something was missing. Looking back, I realize it was the need to address not only the body and mind but also the spirit.

I shared this angst and sense of restlessness with a few colleagues and friends and they suggested that perhaps I was too comfortable at Rush. Reflecting back, I had been there 13 years, completed two graduate degrees, and postdoctoral education. My undergraduate education provided me with a sense of the empathic and caring nature of nursing and my graduate education with the importance of communication and collaboration in providing quality care. However, I was still seeking a way to bring all of these aspects together in a manner that allowed me to have the greatest influence on the patient and the profession. I was ready for a change.

■ PROFESSIONAL EVOLUTION/CONTRIBUTION

Shortly after arriving at Indiana University (IU), I realized how different mental health services were outside of an urban teaching and research medical center; it was like stepping back 10 years in time. My first semester of taking undergraduate nursing students to their clinical experiences at a regional hospital was fraught with moral and ethical dilemmas. There was a lack of mental health education on the part of the staff, and a number of the units lacked nurse leadership. One of the units did have a nurse in a leadership role, but this person was not appropriately educated for the task. This resulted in a unit being run from an authoritative stance and negative reinforcement as the primary tool for behavior management. Furthermore, this carried over to the way the staff were treated and the way they treated the students. My attempt to address concerns regarding the lack of any evidence-based treatments or appreciation for the need for a therapeutic milieu was regarded as an intrusion. I sought guidance from my academic mentors and developed a plan for how to thoughtfully address the nontherapeutic behaviors I observed and at the same time model the way for my students. Since meeting with the leadership team was ineffective, I communicated my concerns to the board of directors and filed incident reports when patients' rights were being violated. I eventually pulled students from their last clinical day and held a retreat at the library. We processed their observations and concerns and went to the literature for answers. Their final clinical papers focused on how to create therapeutic milieus, advocate for patients, and the type of leadership needed to support these efforts. In the meantime, I continued to address my concerns by working through the appropriate channels within the system and began writing about my experiences as a way to learn, grow, and heal. Ultimately, with the support of a senior faculty member, I turned the experience into a publication on the consequences of the absence of nurse leadership within health care (Horton-Deutsch & Mohr, 2001). Professionally, this was when I discovered the dire consequences of avoiding conflict and the value of finding one's moral and ethical voice. I discovered that being an authentic and caring nurse required being deeply rooted in one's moral and ethical values and having the courage to lead. I had also achieved one of my personal and professional goals: to incorporate what I had learned from my psychiatric faculty members in my undergraduate program into my way of being as a nurse.

As a result of this experience, I became curious about how others worked through conflict. Although I had learned a great deal from my personal experiences, I wanted to not only learn more but also to develop confidence and have skillful responses when encountering difficult situations. So I embarked on a grounded theory study of intractable conflict in order to identify ways of responding that promoted growth and/or resolution. This study showed that developing mindfulness was the process that threaded through the phases of working through intractable conflict (Horton-Deutsch & Horton, 2003). This study taught me a tremendous amount about acceptance, focusing attention on what was within my sphere of influence, and letting go of what I could not control.

As a result of this study, I became a student of mindfulness meditation, taking my first introductory course and joining a weekly meditation group. I also attended a conference where Tara Brach spoke and read her work on radical acceptance, aiming to develop what she calls a clear-sightedness and genuine compassion for self and others (Brach, 2003).

Notably, that initial fall semester at IU was the last time I served as a clinical supervisor for undergraduate nursing students completing their psychiatric–mental health nursing practicum. I had inadvertently alienated some psychiatric mental health faculty colleagues who felt I was too direct in my responses to the issues at the hospital. However, in my mind, I could not let apathy or fear keep me from advocating for what I knew to be right. In order to continue to grow (and at the same time not further alienate my colleagues the next semester), I accepted a joint appointment in the school of medicine. I served as the codirector of the psychiatric consultation/liaison program at a university teaching and research hospital. In this position, I had more power, influence, and control over the quality of care and mental health services provided to patients and it expanded my teaching role to include medical students and residents.

Over the next five years, I worked with colleagues from a variety of disciplines to provide quality evidence-based care to patients and modeled this approach to graduate psychiatric nursing students, medical students, and residents. We embraced holistic care and attended three consecutive summer institutes on the use of mindfulness-based stress reduction, integrating this treatment modality into our care of medically ill patients who were suffering from cooccurring mental ailments (Horton-Deutsch, O'Haver Day, & Babin-Nelson, 2005; O'Haver Day & Horton-Deutsch, 2004a; O'Haver Day & Horton-Deutsch, 2004b). Further, we began to appreciate the reciprocal nature of care and integrated self-care practices into our collaborative practice as a way to demonstrate the same compassion for ourselves that we were providing to others.

We eventually had a grant funded to pilot the use of mindfulness-based therapeutic interventions with bone marrow transplant recipients (Horton-Deutsch, O'Haver Day, Haight, & Babin-Nelson, 2007). This study demonstrated that those who engage in mindful practices have a more positive affect, improved concentration, and a greater sense of personal control. This study further taught me the value of presence, acceptance, and letting go, and how embracing these concepts helps to connect the mind to the heart. I was genuinely beginning to integrate my personal and professional life as a nurse and as a person. There was no longer a distinct division between my professional and personal sides. I began to feel more genuinely whole. As a result, I developed more self-confidence; this led to a more authentic way of being with and developing a deeper compassion for myself and others.

After five years of working with this incredible team of colleagues, the budget was cut and our psychiatric consultation/liaison program eliminated. As a result, in 2004, I returned to the school of nursing full-time and was asked to coordinate the advanced practice psychiatric nursing program. Although initially I viewed the termination of the program as a loss, this transition gave me the opportunity to take the work on mindfulness from clinical practice to the educational setting. I readily discovered that reflective practice was a pedagogical approach that offered a conceptual transition. Chris Johns's work strongly influenced my growth in this area through his typology of reflective practices. In his work, one shifts from doing reflection as a technique to being reflective as a way of being within practice or, in other words, mindful practice (Johns, 2004, 2005).

Recognizing my interest in reflective practice, my mentor, Dr. Daniel Pesut (see Chapter 12), who was president of Sigma Theta Tau International (STTI) at the time, knew the value of reflection in education and practice through his own work on metacognition and clinical reasoning. As a part of his presidential call on "creating the future through renewal," he sought to develop a resource paper on reflective practice in nursing. He asked me to join this task force of international colleagues to produce this paper. The task force explored the body of nursing literature to gain a global perspective on reflective practice. The resource paper, titled "The Scholarship of Reflective Practice" (Freshwater, Horton-Deutsch, Sherwood, & Taylor, 2005), solidified my professional and personal commitment to reflection, as it allowed, and continues to allow, me to see my nursing work in new ways. It renews my spirit and connects me at an ontological level to my being as a caring and compassionate nurse. This work was followed by the creation of the *International Textbook of Reflective Practice in Nursing* and a manuscript further illuminating the value of reflective practice in education and leadership development (Freshwater, Esterhuizen, & Horton-Deutsch, 2008; Freshwater, Taylor, & Sherwood, 2008; Horton-Deutsch & Sherwood, 2008).

Having become more broadly informed by these scholarly projects, I felt prepared to transform the nursing curriculum in the advanced practice psychiatric nursing program. Over the next five years, colleagues and I worked to create a reflection-centered framework. At first, our students struggled with the transition. They were accustomed to lectures and, therefore, it took time to appreciate and embrace a more active approach to learning. With time, we moved from lectures to mini-lectures that were followed by reflective exercises and questions, using case studies and vignettes to address the contextual aspects of care. Additionally, we addressed the organizational culture and transformed written assignments to include analyses of students' personal and professional selves, emphasizing the importance of knowing and caring for self as the basis for continued growth in interacting with others (Horton-Deutsch, McNelis, & O'Haver Day, 2012a, 2012b).

After completing this curricular transformation, my only American colleague on the "Scholarship of Reflective Practice" resource paper, Dr. Gwen Sherwood, recommended that we coedit the first American textbook on reflective practice. We both knew of others who were working on or had already developed reflective pedagogies and teaching strategies, so we asked them to collaborate with us by making a contribution to the text. In 2012, Dr. Sherwood and I published the textbook *Reflective Practice: Transforming Education and Improving Outcomes* (Sherwood & Horton-Deutsch, 2012). Interestingly, what gave this work traction were the emerging and eye-opening reports on health care quality and safety (Institute of Medicine [IOM], 2011). These reports outlined that in order to improve quality, we must change how we prepare those who provide care. Further support came from Benner, Sutphen, Leonard, and Day (2010), who described the need for an educational renaissance to transform nursing through innovative approaches to nursing education. Finally, the Quality and Safety Education for Nurses (QSEN) project funded by the Robert Wood Johnson Foundation recommended redesigning pedagogical approaches for students to achieve the knowledge, skills, and attitudes required for quality and safety competencies (Cronenwett, et al., 2007; Cronenwett, Sherwood, & Gelmon, 2009). Our textbook, and the follow-up one published in 2015, provides educators and learners a path to respond to these calls in order to transform nursing education and practice (Sherwood & Horton-Deutsch, 2012, 2015).

The publication of the textbook on reflective practice not only contributed toward the much-needed transformation in nursing education, but it also vicariously transformed my life's work within nursing. In 2013, I received a call from Dean Sarah Thompson at the University of Colorado College of Nursing regarding a position as the Watson Caring Science Endowed Chair. After dialogue with Dr. Jean Watson (see Chapter 16) and thoughtful consideration of the relationship between reflective and mindful practices and caring science, I knew the next phase of my life's work was about to unfold. I recognized that reflective and mindful practices were the bridge and conduit to expanding caring science.

■ MORAL/ETHICAL FOUNDATION

Over the past eight years, while expanding my knowledge and work in reflective and mindful practices, I also engaged in a series of interpretative phenomenological research studies with colleagues from across the country on the lived experience of becoming a nurse faculty leader. Publication of the initial findings occurred in 2011 (Young, Pearsall, Stiles, Nelson, & Horton-Deutsch, 2011), and then two subgroups of the cohort published themes they interpreted in depth (Horton-Deutsch, Young, & Nelson, 2010; Pearsall et al., 2014; Stiles, Pardue, Young, & Morales, 2011; Young, Pardue, & Horton-Deutsch, 2015). During study interviews, we identified that connecting to one's moral/ethical foundation of practice often occurred when nurse faculty were faced with a professional risk and were called to do the right thing.

At one point in this study, we determined we needed to know more about aspects of "taking risks." We reinterviewed six of the original study participants and conducted two focus group discussions among our seven researchers, focusing on taking risks as a nurse faculty leader. In this process, we learned more about taking risks that originated from "doing the right thing." "Doing the right thing" was driven by either a sense of professional responsibility, vision for the future, or being true to both one's values and self. It was during the focus group discussions that I learned a lot about my own moral/ethical foundation. The story I shared in the focus group spoke to my need to be true to both my values and self. Looking back, these values were built through personal and professional experiences, my intuitive nature leading me to seek guidance and help from those who were already doing the right thing, and my desire for lifelong learning and growth. For instance, high school, where I was provided the opportunity to think critically about levels of moral development, and my undergraduate education, where the psychiatric–mental health nursing faculty modeled the way for providing care to those in need, profoundly influenced both my thinking and my growth and development as an ethical nurse.

In addition, during my undergraduate nursing program, students were required to choose a nursing theory that resonated with them and their promising nursing practice. I chose Dr. Jean Watson's Theory of Human Caring (2008) structured around 10 carative factors, now known as the 10 Caritas Processes™ (see Table 16.1). I was drawn to it for both its simplicity—genuinely caring for self and others—and depth—an appreciation for the interconnected evolution of human consciousness and the connectedness of us all. Although my early connection to Dr. Watson's work moved into the background of my mind shortly after undergraduate education, looking back, over the next 25 years, my foreground activities in mindfulness-based stress reduction, reflective practice, and leadership development led me to my own ethical/moral/philosophical foundation for practice, simultaneously bringing me back to the precepts of human caring science (Watson, 2012).

For example, my exploration of mindfulness, the ability to be present in the now, was something I aspired to in order to more fully care for my patients. Using Dr. Watson's language, transpersonal *Caritas Consciousness* requires the same shift in awareness, to the here and now, ensuring that care is more accurate, focused, appropriate, and fulfilling for the nurse and patient (Watson, 2008). Caritas Consciousness also requires that we look for solutions inside ourselves, reflecting on the shadow-and-light side of our humanity, which makes us more deeply human and loving, to ourselves and others. By attending to these aspects of caring and Caritas Consciousness, we grow within ourselves and with the humanity of others. These reconnections, back to caring science, have been a process of coming home for me. It has been and continues to be an amazing journey.

■ VISION

My vision for nursing begins with reconnecting to its core value of caring—a deeper consciousness of caring that responds compassionately and holistically to self and other. This form of caring consciousness provides a deeply rooted foundation for caring and sustains us personally and professionally. It allows us to be open to our own vulner-abilities, share our stories, and connect with humanity. From this place of transparency and unity comes strength. It becomes a way of being-becoming in the world. It helps us to remain connected to our core values, ethics, and philosophy that becomes the keystone of our scholarly foundation. It opens us to the connection between our head and our hearts, where we are able to consciously connect to our internal intuitive know-ing, allowing us to stay calm, self-regulate, and maintain clarity and balance. These enlightened and energy-saving responses, which help us to maintain resiliency, are an important part of caring for self and give us vitality to care for others in a meaningful and balanced way.

By connecting to our own essence and caring nature, we are prepared to more authentically connect with and care for others. Coming from this place of wholeness and feeling grounded in who we are, we are able to bring our fully conscious selves into our relations with others. We become more reflective and able to recognize when our ego or shadow sides of consciousness are surfacing; this recognition allows us to thought-fully choose how to respond. Through the process of learning to notice our ego, and yet respond from a higher level of consciousness, we grow. We grow in a way that not only enables us to recognize the ego and shadow sides of ourselves, but also of others. We can not only have compassion for these human sides of ourselves and others, but can also use our knowledge and understanding to respond in a way that is most helpful for our col-lective learning and growth. This compassionate way of being with self and others allows us to compassionately discern and suspend judgment. We come to appreciate that we are all on our own path to being-becoming more enlightened and fully human.

From this more holistic, balanced, and fully embodied place within each of us and within our profession, nursing reconnects to its shared identity. Having a strong sense of our own identity and the value we bring to health care and healing, we must speak with one voice. Knowing who we are, appreciating what we have to offer, and sharing that with others from a place of humility and strength prepares us to fully partner with other health professionals. Having built a culture of positive energy rooted in a deep sense of knowing, openness, and a reflective stance prepares us for intentional interprofessional partnerships.

Interprofessional partnerships are essential to shifting health care from the sick-care culture to a wellness care paradigm structured upon self-care, healing, and wholeness. Findings from a recent interpretative phenomenological study that interviewed interprofessional nurse leaders revealed that the ability to self-reflect, take deliberate–intentional actions, and have the ability to develop a new mindset were essential to developing common ground with other health care professionals (Stiles, Horton-Deutsch, & Andrews, 2014). Developing a shared common ground serves to build a larger shared culture where health care professionals work together to make this major shift in health care.

Finally, from this place of interprofessional unity, we are prepared to come together around these worldview shifts toward healthy living and life itself. According to Watson (2015), these shifts are "toward inner healing, human caring, mental health, self-caring, self-knowledge, self-control and self-healing approaches, addressing individual and collective human suffering" (Watson, 2015, p. 171). To make these shifts requires an expanded lens toward an energetic view of all life, inner health and healing, healthy communities, and planetary health. Coming together around the idea that health care providers attend to health, healing, and spiritual harmony binds us to a larger shared vision and prepares us for genuine solidarity and collective action toward a more loving and caring world.

The part of my work that has yet to be realized is the creation of an environment of interprofessional unity where all providers deliver competent, caring, compassionate, and respectful health care to those in need. My recent appointment to the Center for Bioethics and Humanities at the University of Colorado–Denver places me in a position to work with colleagues toward this goal as, collectively, we aim to strongly influence health policy, practice, education, research, and community relations. Through an academic leadership council, I will work with six other University of Colorado schools/colleges to integrate bioethics and humanities into existing and new programs across the schools. This appointment provides me the opportunity to integrate caring science into curricula, clinical service, research, scholarship, and community engagement activities. Building a synergy for caring science across schools will positively impact our ability to create an environment for health and healing within health care.

What I did not know early in my career, that I want to share with others here, is the importance of committing equally to both personal and professional development. Although in many ways I did this naturally, it was usually precipitated by an external life event that required further self-examination in order for me to move forward. What I share with students today is the value of adopting reflective, mindful practices that serve to guide them personally and professionally from the beginning. By caring for self (working through shadow sides, having a contemplative practice, developing compassion, and nurturing the soul) while simultaneously pursuing professional goals, one can witness these two aspects of self begin to merge. One no longer feels this separateness between personal and professional life. It becomes a way of being. Through these practices, one develops the foundation for being-becoming a thoughtful, caring, heart-centered, and reflective nurse leader.

■ REFLECTIONS

1. *What connections can I make from my early personal and professional experiences, intuitive nature, and desire for lifelong learning and growth?*
2. *How do these connections reflect my being-becoming?*
3. *How does my personal development influence my professional development?*
4. *What opportunities do I have to open to my own vulnerabilities and share my stories?*
5. *How do I see myself improving my interprofessional partnerships? How might these improved partnerships help move us from a sick-care culture to a wellness care paradigm?*

■ REFERENCES

Benner, P., Sutphen, M., Leonard, V., & Day, L. (2010). *Educating nurses: A call for radical transformation.* Standford, CA: Jossey-Bass.

Brach, T. (2003). *Radical acceptance: Embracing your life with the heart of a buddha.* New York, NY: Bantam.

Cronenwett, L., Sherwood, G., Barnsteiner, J., Disch, J., Johnson, J., Mitchell, P., . . . Warren, J. (2007). Quality and safety education for nurses. *Nursing Outlook, 55*(3), 122–131.

Cronenwett, L., Sherwood, G., & Gelmon, S. B. (2009). Improving quality and safety education: The QSEN learning collaborative. *Nursing Outlook, 57*(6), 304–313.

Freshwater, D., Esterhuizen, P., & Horton-Deutsch, S. (2008). Reflective practice and the therapeutic use of self. In D. Freshwater, B. Taylor, G. Sherwood (Eds.), *The international textbook of reflective practice in nursing* (pp. 157–176). London, UK: Blackwell/STTI.

Freshwater, D., Horton-Deutsch, S., Sherwood, G., & Taylor, B. (2005). *The scholarship of reflective practice.* Indianapolis, IN: Sigma Theta Tau International.

Freshwater, D., Taylor, B., & Sherwood, G. (Eds.) (2008). *The international textbook of reflective practice in nursing.* London, UK: Blackwell/STTI.

Horton-Deutsch, S., & Drysdale, J. (2015). An online teaching framework: Using quality norms and caring science to build presence and engagement in online learning environments. In G. Sherwood & S. Horton-Deutsch (Eds.), *Reflective organizations: On the frontlines of QSEN and reflective practice implementation* (pp. 147–166). Indianapolis, IN: Sigma Theta Tau International.

Horton-Deutsch, S., & Horton, J. (2003). Developing mindfulness: A means to overcoming conflict. *Archives of Psychiatric Nursing, 17*(4), 186–193.

Horton-Deutsch, S., McNelis, A., & O' Haver Day, P. (2012a). Balancing technology with face-to-face interaction: Navigating the path to psychiatric nursing education at a distance. *Journal of the American Psychiatric Nurses Association, 18*(3), 193–196.

Horton-Deutsch, S., McNelis, A., & O' Haver Day, P. (2012b). Developing a reflection-centered curriculum for graduate psychiatric nursing education. *Archives of Psychiatric Nursing, 26*(5), 341–349.

Horton-Deutsch, S., & Mohr, W. K. (2001). The fading of nursing leadership. *Nursing Outlook, 49*(3), 121–126.

Horton-Deutsch, S., O'Haver Day, P., & Babin-Nelson, M. (2005). Integrating insight and understanding with repetitive practices to promote lasting change. *International Journal of Human Caring, 9*(2), 138.

Horton-Deutsch, S., O'Haver Day, P., Haight, R., & Babin-Nelson, M. (2007). Enhancing mental health services to bone marrow transplant recipients through a mindfulness-based therapeutic interventions. *Complementary Therapies in Clinical Practice, 13*(2), 110–115.

Horton-Deutsch, S., & Sherwood, G. (2008). Reflection: An educational strategy to develop emotionally competent nurse leaders. *Journal of Nursing Management, 16*(8), 946–954.

Horton-Deutsch, S., Young, T., & Nelson, K. (2010). Becoming a nurse faculty leader: Facing challenges through reflecting, persevering and learning to relate in new ways. *Journal of Nursing Management, 18*(4), 487–493. doi:10.1111/j.1365-2834.2010.01075.x

Institute of Medicine (IOM). (2011). *The future of nursing. Leading change, advancing health.* Washington, DC: National Academies Press.

Johns, C. (2004). *Becoming a reflective practitioner.* Oxford, UK: Blackwell Science.

Johns, C. (2005). Balancing the winds. *Reflective Practice, 6*(1), 67–84.

Kohlberg, L. (1981). *Essays on moral development: The philosophy of moral development* (Vol. 1). San Francisco, CA: Harper & Row.

O'Haver Day, P., & Horton-Deutsch, S. (2004a). Utilizing mindfulness-based therapeutic interventions in psychiatric nursing practice. Part I: Description and empirical support for mindfulness-based interventions. *Archives of Psychiatric Nursing, 18*(5), 164–169.

O'Haver Day, P., & Horton-Deutsch, S. (2004b). Utilizing mindfulness-based therapeutic interventions in psychiatric nursing practice. Part II: Mindfulness-based approaches for all phases of psychotherapy. *Archives of Psychiatric Nursing, 18*(5), 170–177.

Pearsall, C., Pardue, K. T., Horton-Deustch, S., Young, P. K., Halstead, J., Nelson, K. A., . . . Zungolo, E. (2014). Becoming a nurse faculty leader: Doing your homework to minimize risk-taking. *Journal of Professional Nursing, 30*(1), 26–33.

Sherwood, G., & Horton-Deutsch, S. (Eds.). (2012). *Reflective practice: Transforming education and improving outcomes.* Indianapolis, IN: Sigma Theta Tau International.

Sherwood, G., & Horton-Deutsch, S. (Eds.). (2015). *Reflective organizations: On the frontlines of QSEN and reflective practice implementation.* Indianapolis, IN: Sigma Theta Tau International.

Stiles, K., Horton-Deutsch, S., & Andrews, C. (2014). The nurse's lived experience of becoming an interprofessional leader. *The Journal of Continuing Education in Nursing, 45*(11), 487–493.

Stiles, K., Pardue, K., Young, P., & Morales, M. L. (2011). Becoming a nurse faculty leader: Practices of leading illuminated through advancing reform in nursing education. *Nursing Forum, 46*(2), 94–101.

Watson, J. (2008). *Nursing: The philosophy and science of caring* (Rev. ed.). Boulder, CO: University Press of Colorado.

Watson, J. (2012). *Human caring science* (2nd ed.). Sudbury, MA: Jones & Bartlett.

Watson, J. (2015). Transformational reflective organizations: Front line challenges and changes guided by caring science. In G. Sherwood & S. Horton-Deutsch (Eds.), *Reflective organizations: On the frontlines of QSEN and reflective practice implementation* (pp. 169–188). Indianapolis, IN: Sigma Theta Tau International.

Young, P., Pardue, K., & Horton-Deutsch, S. (2015). Practices of reflective leaders. In G. Sherwood & S. Horton-Deutsch (Eds.), *Reflective organizations: On the frontlines of QSEN and reflective practice implementation* (pp. 49–67). Indianapolis, IN: Sigma Theta Tau International.

Young, P., Pearsall, C., Stiles, K., Nelson, K., & Horton-Deutsch, S. (2011). Becoming a nursing faculty leader. *Nursing Education Perspectives, 32*(4), 150–156.

CHAPTER TWENTY-THREE

Authentic and Creative:
Walking the Caritas Path to Peace

Mary Rockwood Lane

In our lives, . . . we can walk the worn and weary path to war or walk the less traveled path to peace. . . . The Caritas Path to Peace is not the well-worn path, it is a path only angels have treaded. You can't see their footprints—you must make your own.

—Lane, Samuels, and Watson (2012, p. 16)

■ WHY NURSING?

It was my sister who always wanted to be a nurse. She had the medicine bag giving out "happy pills" (gummy bears). She carefully examined my little brother and me whenever we were troubled. My mother was an Air Force Nurse and worked throughout my childhood. The family moved every two years, as my father was a career military officer. As a child, I wanted to be a teacher, artist, or movie star. I clearly had stars in my eyes. My mother was a small Sicilian woman, somewhat progressive, but not quite. I once told her I wanted to be a lawyer and she bluntly told me, "No, Mary, only men become lawyers. Women become nurses, teachers, mothers, and wives. Being a nurse will help you become a better mother and wife, so I would study nursing." In total frustration, I believed her. After a very troubled and rebellious adolescent period, being confused, running away, and getting involved with the wrong boyfriend, my parents decided I needed to be on my own. I needed to figure out a way to survive and get myself through a very painful time in my life.

I always knew I wanted to go to college. That was my goal. I worked part-time, took a full load of classes, and became one of the very first female students in the whole country to be admitted to the Naval Reserve Officers Training Corps (NROTC). Since I was paying my own way, I hoped for a scholarship; every male cadet received a full scholarship. After I marched with these young men for two-and-a-half years in the broiling

Florida heat, training alongside them, learning artillery skills, I was informed that only the male cadets would receive the scholarships. I still remember my gunnery sergeant screaming in my face, nose-to-nose, that I would never make it. Yes, just like in the movies! That is as far as I got to becoming a movie star. That very issue would later be taken to the Supreme Court, but not by me. So I chose to pursue Navy nursing. After my acceptance at nursing school, President Ford suspended the navy nursing scholarships for the next two years. Life has twists, turns, and transformations. Regardless of how I got there, I became a nurse and was committed to serving the profession. I discovered I loved—and still love—everything about it.

How did I, a nurse, get interested in creativity and peace? I was a nurse who became a mother and wife. I discovered that my life as a woman, nurse, artist, activist, and writer was my destiny and spiritual journey. It all seemed to come together on a single day, when I felt a profound inner shift that revealed my true essence; the day that made me realize why I became a nurse in the first place.

It was 9/11 and I watched the World Trade Center come down on television, feeling the fear and paralyzing sensations of shock permeate my bones. It was a turning point in world history. I was unable to comprehend what was happening. It became very evident very quickly that this was a moment in time my country could choose peace or war. I believed in peace, understanding, and forgiveness . . . that was the answer I felt in my heart.

What could I do for peace in this pivotal time? How could I bring in the light? I could combine my nursing knowledge of caring for patients who were very ill or nearing end of life with being an artist, promoting and role modeling the transformative nature of creativity. By this time in my career, I had already delved deeply into the healing dimensions of creativity (Samuels & Lane, 1999, 2000a, 2000b). In a very real sense, war is the ultimate life-threatening illness, and peace the ultimate life-saving treatment and preventive medicine. So, I asked myself, How do nurses call on and apply creativity to take care of patients with cancer who may die? How do we bring back hope in desperate situations, create change for healing, bring the healing power of spirit, and even promote a miracle?

To answer those questions, I looked to my research study at the University of Florida College of Nursing documenting how creativity helped heal patients with life-threatening illnesses. At that time, I had helped to cocreate the UF Health Arts in Medicine program at University of Florida based on Dr. Jean Watson's Theory of Human Caring (see Chapter 16). My research study showed that creativity helped patients find love and compassion. The research revealed themes that creativity helped patients get in touch with their inner wisdom, with their soul or spirit. This access to creative expression gave patients hope, rallied their bodies' own healing forces, and connected patients to something larger then themselves.

Caring and health promotion is simple: It can prevent war. How can nurses make a difference? What do we need to do to stop violence? Nurses are already peace activists. Nurses follow a calling to serve humanity, and they do not do it for money or power. Who better can become the world leaders for peace? Nurses are the global activists for health and caring. Wars kill tens of millions of people. Wars kill innocent women, men, and children. In the 20th century alone, wars killed more than 200 million human beings. Is it not time we stopped? Is it not time we reacted to problems and crises in a new way?

These questions continued to pull at my heart and mind and so I began a book with my coauthor, Michael Samuels, MD, about peace the day after 9/11. First, it was called *The Path to Peace*, and it was about reacting to violence outside us in creative ways, with forgiveness and compassion. We worked on it for several months while continuing to explore and write about other visionary healing tools and practices (Samuels & Lane, 2002). We became committed to the completion of the project as the "war on terror" continued, the Iraq and Afghanistan conflicts persisted, and other militant groups and acts of terrorism threatened the world. This writing became our offering, our prayer, our solace for world peace. It asks simply: Can nurses guide the violence of the world toward a more inner and outer experience of peace?

Dr. Watson invited us to rewrite the book for the Caritas Peace Conference in Hiroshima, Japan, in June 2011. It was in Hiroshima that the International Charter for Human Caring and Peace was shared with the world (Watson Caring Science Institute, n.d.). This experience led us to rename the book *The Caritas Path to Peace*. It is a call to nurses worldwide to stand up as advocates for world peace: a call to stand up and take their place in the global struggle . . . to be empowered . . . to be heard.

In writing the book on peace, we found that we could often substitute the title "Caritas Nurse for Peace" for the words "healer" or "peacemaker." This in itself was a profound teaching. We realized that the Caritas Nurse for Peace is a healer of the self, of relationships with others, and to the world. When you make peace, you heal your own woundedness, you heal others with love, and you prevent more woundedness from being born. Creativity, love, and compassion are powerful tools for both healing and peace.

This is really why I became a nurse.

■ EARLY IMPRESSIONS

After 9/11, I had no doubt who I was. I was not confused. The second it happened, I felt hurt, pain, sadness, and fear. But I also reacted with feelings of peace and forgiveness. I yearned for a creative solution that would not cause war. Every time I heard the cries for violence and revenge, I felt it was a disproportionate reaction; I became filled with sorrow.

I was determined to discover "the caring thing to do" in this situation. What confused me was the sheer power of the image of destruction that was being repeated every day by the media. We were attacked and there was deep pain. I was stunned and kept asking, "Why would anyone do this? What were they trying to accomplish? Did I miss something?" I believe in my heart that we as Americans are a people of greatness. We are a melting pot of the global community, people blessed with prosperity, good fortune, and safety. I had a sense of the strength of who we are. And so I continued to ask, "Why?"

What I eventually realized was that we as Americans had an opportunity to change the world and do something radical that had never been done before. In that moment, there was an invitation to deepen our understanding of ourselves and the impact we could have on the world. We needed to understand what we did not yet know as a nation and, also, to forgive ourselves for what we may have done in the past. We also needed to forgive "them" for their attack. I was aghast, and yet, it was my desire to reach out over the ocean to understand how this could have happened.

How can we do the right thing to heal the world? I searched for what I could do in this moment, after having been assaulted, that could bring world peace. I felt tears in the depth of my soul and a powerful compassion toward the victims. That compassion extended to the people we had inflicted harm on in the years past who felt the need for revenge. I spent the next days dealing with my own feelings. Others around me seemed twisted with hatred. The general consensus was that since the act was violent and hateful, we should react with violence and hatefulness too. It seemed to me that if we were not careful, we would turn into what we were afraid of. I could see that this event had become a crossroads in every person's life that demanded an answer: Will you choose war or peace?

As I looked at my own life, the earliest parts of my life journey, I began to see why I reacted as I did. I believed in caring and forgiveness. I began to understand why caring was actually the choice for peace and war was not. In my personal life I have been raped, physically abused, abandoned, and had my voice repressed, and—finally—I learned to forgive. This was because of my own inner conviction to care and my determination to believe in miracles.

As a little girl of seven years, I lived in Turkey, immersed in the Muslim world. My father was a lieutenant colonel in the Air Force. He was a diplomat, an advocate for the Middle East International Relations. He was in the U.S. military intelligence, representing the Turkish point of view in the conflict between Turkey and Cyprus. As a child of a military officer, I spent most of my life abroad.

During World War II, my father liberated one of the concentration camps in Germany. When I was a little girl, he took us there and showed us the horrific consequences of human ignorance, cynicism, and cruelty. As a child, I felt myself a part of a global world and proud to be an American. I was honored to experience liberty, prosperity, and justice for all. I was just a child with dreams.

But then came the 1960s and another event that formed who I was happened in the American South. The Ku Klux Klan burned a cross in front of the house of a black friend who had been in my fifth-grade class. She told me what it was like to have rocks thrown in the front door and through the windows of her home. She huddled behind furniture in total fear, surrounded by hatred. She asked me, "What do they hate?" I looked at her stunned and confused. I did not understand.

My personal experience of pain and violence continued in high school. During the race riots, I was viciously beaten, kicked, and stuck with pins by eight black girls. I was trapped inside a bathroom in the school being beaten when a tall black boy came in, chasing the girls away, and rescuing me. He picked me up in his arms and carried me to an ambulance. In the chaos, I was feeling both attacked and saved by the same people. The white students came to my house wanting to hunt and beat up the girls who had hurt me. This was not what I wanted to do. I stopped them. No . . . I wanted to forgive them.

As a young teenager, I was in a relationship with a boy who repeatedly abused me. Still, I believed love could heal everything; sadly, this was not the case. Just loving someone does not necessarily change things, but it was a powerful lesson. During the time I was with him, I was beaten, raped, thrown over a balcony, and had my back and arms broken.

I was stalked for months on end. I fell into a spiral of panic, trembling in fear when I was alone. An aggressive prosecutor wanted to put him in jail and wanted me to press charges. I did not want to send another human to jail; that would not help him. I learned from this abuse that love does not necessarily change the other person, but acting out of love does heal your own life. Forgiving someone will allow you to let go and let your life go on. Forgiveness frees you to move on and accept your own pain and suffering and ultimately move beyond. I moved beyond and never looked back.

Many years later, when I was in the midst of a painful divorce process, I was hysterical in despair and fighting. My husband had left me with two young children. I was in total pain, experiencing an uncontrollable anger. The fight raged, my own body was bloodied, and I saw that all my anger did not get me anything. The rage and anger just hurt me more deeply. I saw that in every battle, I came out more wounded than before. I realized that all that happened was I would explode and go nowhere. The essence of life was taken from me by my own doing. Instead of the pain being inflicted on me by others, I was inflicting it on myself. I needed to forgive myself. I finally let go of wanting something I could not have and believed the world would accommodate the dream of what I wanted. One day, in the midst of this letting go and forgiveness, my husband knocked at the door and asked if he could come home. In my heart, I made a decision of total forgiveness and surrender. He came home and the power of forgiveness was born within me deeply.

On that day, I made a commitment to be on a spiritual path, to choose the path of love, compassion, and forgiveness. I did not know what that path was, but each life experience had become a thread, which led me more deeply within. I realized then that my life had become a challenge, a test. This was a commitment to a way of being, not necessarily to a way of understanding. Things can be too complex to understand all the moving pieces. But I could commit to a way of approaching or moving away from the toxicity of emotions that self-inflicted more pain, not necessarily to understanding everything or being able to reach a conclusion. As my life moved forward, forgiveness became embodied. It was my life lesson to learn and it resonated with the core essence of my being. It deepened my understanding of caring.

The crisis of 9/11 changed my life, as it did for countless others. My life lessons had accumulated into something that emerged in that moment. They are not a philosophy or a discourse but a personal experience of what has worked for me. I realized that my own life was the lesson that led me to know forgiveness, caring, and compassion. I turned the experience of abuse into my commitment to being an advocate for world peace.

■ PROFESSIONAL EVOLUTION/CONTRIBUTION

My life's work: I am a Caritas Nurse. I teach others to connect with their inner Caritas Nurse. The Caritas Nurse for Peace is the wise one within. She or he has always been there and spoken to you in your days of despair and pain. She or he was with you during your own birth and the birth of all your children. This wise self holds strong, steady, and still. It has the ability to exhibit compassion, caring, wisdom, and love in every aspect of life. These qualities come forth in relationships with others, in spiritual practice, and in all aspects of clinical work. The Caritas Nurse is an archetypal position in our culture.

The Caritas Nurse stems from ancient times when healers were herbalists, midwives, nurturers, and community activists. The archetypal Caritas Nurse was worshipped as an aspect of the goddess Hygeia. There have been many evolutions of this goddess throughout history, from Hera, Isis, Athena, and Demeter, to the modern founder of nursing, Florence Nightingale, to Dr. Jean Watson. The Caritas Nurse is involved in taking care of others and taps into the ancient traditions and wisdom of the past from the earth. The Caritas Nurse is expanding beyond the traditional nursing roles to include all ways of caring and expressing the ancient peaceful knowledge within. This peace exists as a vibrational energy, which resonates in the body; this energy exhibits in individual ways since every person is different and unique.

Nurses worldwide strive to create health and wholeness for the people they serve. Peace is the cornerstone of wholeness and health and Caritas is an ethical and philosophical foundation for creating peace. Nurses have a covenant with the public to serve and care. The Caritas Nurse is the healer, the teacher, the lover, the giver, the mother, and the father. The spirit of Caritas is deeply connected to the earth, to family, to friends, to animals, to the environment, and to all of nature. We can see the earth deeply; seeing the earth moving through her seasons. We can feel the wind, know when nature stirs, and recognize the beauty inherent in the pulse of life.

■ MORAL/ETHICAL FOUNDATION

Watson's theory (2005, 2008, 2012) and 10 Caritas Processes™ have guided my nursing practice and my life (see Table 16.1). These processes are constantly changing—organic and experiential. They have provided me with the ability to articulate and create a language to shift my way of knowing. They are the essential nature of nursing as proposed by Florence Nightingale more than 150 years ago. They are from the clinical essence of what nurses are actually doing but often do not describe. They make the invisible become visible. The 10 Caritas Processes™ are the foundational steps to living a peaceful life.

The steps do not depend on what political party you vote for or whether you are conservative or liberal. They do not rely on your belief in a specific war or your support of troops; they are based on your hope for peace and come from the spiritual part of you within. The techniques are based on the steps Watson uses to teach nurses loving and caring in hospitals; they come from many of the world's wisdom traditions and from modern practices of psychology and conflict resolution. We believe that the path to peace starts within. From the practice of caring–healing ethic within, we move outward into the world to care and heal for others. First, we change our own understanding and awareness—then we act. First, we change our own consciousness—then we change reality.

You must start by making self-peace. You do this by embracing altruistic values and practicing loving-kindness with yourself. It is the first step toward forgiveness and toward feeling love and compassion for others. In Buddhist meditation, you go to a place where there is total compassion. You go to a place where you re-story your life from a foundation of compassion and love . . . becoming compassionate to yourself by seeing yourself from a distance, from the outside. Stand back and say, "Look at her. She needs . . . ." In a moment of witness, of reflection, see what you need to heal, and complete the sentence on your own. When you see yourself with compassion, you can tend to your body as a sacred vessel and tend to emotions as natural forces that move through you. You can honor intuitions and insights, you can be illuminated to find your place in the world. When you feel the energy of love flowing through you, you will heal yourself and be able to become a Caritas Nurse for Peace. When you feel compassion for yourself, the compassion will flow to others and peace will result. This is an ethical foundation for all nursing practice.

Compassion is a kind of love; it joins your light with another's. If you are ill, it joins you to a healer; if you are a healer, it joins you to the person you are healing; if you are making peace, it joins you to your enemy. When you are in compassion, you flow beyond your boundaries and merge with the person you are with. You see them without judgment, you see them with God's love. You see them as beautiful, as sacred . . . you see their spirit instead of their personality. God's love and compassion are natural, it is a feeling from the heart. It is not God telling you to seek vengeance.

The Caritas Nurse for Peace who sees with compassion sees the enemy in a different way. Yes, you may be angry, but you can teach yourself to see those around you with compassion and invite them to see you in this way too. Your love is felt by everyone and it helps them love you with compassion too.

In compassion, show your light. Compassion breaks the cycle of violence that leads to more violence. There is nothing more ethical than practicing and embracing this way of being and becoming in the world.

■ VISION

The hope is that every nurse, each person, understands the impact of doing his or her own individual peace work on the self and in the world. Integrity, presence, intention, and commitment are states of mind that actualize and inform your way of being and empower your actions. You can greatly increase your ability to live in peace by using these tools. Peace work is inner work projected outward. It is about faith and hope and honoring others. Intention and commitment give us focused ways of increasing our resolve and motivation. They clarify our purpose and make us decisive in our actions.

We can increase our ability to live in peace by using personal integrity. Our ability to live in peace comes from our authenticity as human beings. That is why a Caritas Nurse for Peace has a deep commitment to integrity. The Caritas Nurse for Peace is honest about the presentation of who she or he is. People of peace are sincere in their intention to support the people around them for who they are. They listen to a person and look to see that person clearly. They honor the integrity of a person's actions and respect people for their diversity.

Integrity comes from your core essence. The physical world you experience around you vibrates with the essence of who you are. What you are in the external world vibrates and resonates from your internal world, your essence within. If you stripped yourself down to your essence and built upon that, each step would create integrity. Each feeling, each article of clothing, each authentic act would be an embodiment of Caritas. Integrity is a commitment to yourself and the full expression of that self in the world.

In Caritas, authentic presence is both a way of being and an action. Authentic presence lets you be *Ubuntu*, a term originating from South Africa that relates to humanity and human kindness; it can be translated as, "I am because we are." We are one even with the person we are in conflict with. It is a powerful tool for peace. To be effective is to be present in the here and now. To be totally present, you need to shift away from the ordinary talking in your mind. Pause, slow down, stop your mind chatter. Put aside your daily concerns such as who picks up your child or dealing with your car repair bills. Put aside the things that are distracting your attention. Breathe and deliberately do not focus on distractions. You can deal with them later . . . be present with yourself first.

To use presence as a Caritas Nurse for Peace, face any individual you are working with to make peace. Look at the face . . . look into the eyes . . . look at the person as if this exchange of energy and intention is what your entire life is about in this moment. You are in communion with the person; part of being with the person is seeing him or her. See the color of the hair, the eyes, the skin. Watch the gestures. Allow yourself to be empty, allow the person to fill you up. Use your sense of smell, touch, and sight. See the face unveiling its essence to you. The unveiling of the person's face has to do with the unveiling of your face. You become accessible to yourself at the moment you allow the other to come forward. Presence means the person is inside your own heart. You feel and know him or her deeply as you feel and know yourself.

An important part of becoming an effective Caritas Nurse for Peace is to consciously embody Caritas, intentionally practicing caring in order to make peace real. It means dealing with fears and blockages, with anger and hate, with resistance and personal issues. The Caritas Nurse for Peace way of being is a lived experience, not a theory. It returns us to our earliest impressions, the trajectory of our lives, and professional evolutions. It is the basis of our own moral and ethical foundations.

The Caritas Nurse for Peace is my vision for nursing. It goes up against my most personal issues of ego, anger, faith, evil, confidence, trust, power, and purpose. Being a Caritas Nurse for Peace is about being authentically who you are with intention. That is challenging. This teaching is about healing your own defensiveness and attachments to being right . . . going out in nature . . . meditating . . . learning to hear your own voices of wisdom within. Heal your own life by seeing who you really are and learning to love and accept yourself and others. Trust that this is possible.

Trust is about developing dependable, helping, caring relationships. Let the conviction of your own truth empower you to right action. Let it come from the place of power in your belly. Let it emerge from your center in pure form. Go to the conviction of your own truth and harness that power. The world needs you right now—do not doubt it for one second. Your conviction is like a psychic laser beam of light for the truth. Express it fully in right action. This is how your life manifests your choice for peace. Take your conviction for truth and place it in your gut. Use it to move you forward. Express your pure truth for peace in any form you can—through teaching others, in church, in your business, in conversations with friends, in art, in political action, in civil disobedience. Empower your conviction—you are not alone—you are part of a collective of merging and emerging consciousness. You can change thought and action with this commitment to conviction.

Let us turn the crisis of the moment into the best thing that has ever happened. For the first time in history, people all over the earth are seriously questioning war. For the first time, people are seriously asking themselves if war is an answer, if war can be stopped, if war is a way of being that can continue on earth.

Illness, like war, can be a powerful force for change. A life-threatening illness, such as cancer, can change a person's priorities in a moment. A person can decide to change his or her life, to love family, to change work, to move. Ask yourself what you would do if you had one year or one month or one week to live. This question is not academic. Cancer patients ask themselves this each day. What are your priorities? This introspection is a timely doorway. Let us not turn away from it. Let it bring unity for peace and empowerment to individuals all over the earth.

Forgiveness is a crucial step in creating peace. Forgiveness is about promoting and accepting positive and negative feelings as you authentically listen to another's story. Self-forgiveness is the first step in creating inner peace. First, forgive yourself for not being the person you want to be. Forgive yourself for your apathy, your lack of concern, your turning away from people in need. Forgive yourself for doing business and not making enough time for family and loved ones. Forgive yourself for not feeding the hungry and not working for peace. Forgive yourself for not stopping war. Move on to become a Caritas Nurse for Peace now. Accept and love yourself for your own imperfections. (See Chapters 19 and 26 for more on forgiveness and personal-professional healing.)

Art is the manifestation of our visions for peace. Creativity is about creating solutions and using caring decision making for peace. Use your creative life force to become a source of inspiration and energy that propels you to cocreate Caritas fields of peace with others. The creative process will give you the energy to increase this vibration with passion. Passion helps you tap into the eternal spring of creativity that flows within you. We are the earth and our creativity connects with the earth. Tap into the vortex of your creative energy. When you connect with the power of creativity, it awakens, nurtures, and heals you. As your creativity emerges through you, it heals the earth, as it emerges from the earth. Making art is healing in itself. Making art for peace is the earth making peace.

Prayer, art, and healing come from the same place: the human soul. The creation of art is an act of prayer in which we create harmony and balance within ourselves through extrinsic expressions of the inner world. In the creation of art, we respond to our hopes and problems in a creative way. We create images that emerge from our soul in response to our dreams and visions. We take a vision from our wisdom within and externalize it so everyone can see it. Art was transformative in ancient times; it was the way the shaman helped control the hunt, fertility, and even the weather. Art changes reality by transforming consciousness.

The Caritas Nurse for Peace makes art to learn how to find creative solutions for peace and to heal himself or herself so he or she can do peace work. The process of making art is one of seeing into visionary space; it is the same process the Caritas Nurse for Peace uses as she or he tries to access a heightened plane of problem solving. When a person makes art, the images that come to her or him are creative ideas. They can inform us about what to do next, about decisions and actions. Art can be engaging for an audience; it can rally support and free emotions. A dance for peace can express emotion and move people to action.

Actively reconstruct your own future. Engaging in teaching and learning experiences that honor another's views is a way to peace. Nurses are teachers and they need to be able to meet other persons where they are now. They need to understand where the other is to be able to help; they need to know someone is ready for advice or life change. This is their way of awakening and transforming people's consciousness. The Caritas Nurse for Peace teaches people to move into a new place in the nurse's constructed reality for peace. Move into a place where you construct reality yourself, not where you accept a reality made by another and then blame the other person for it. Move past the old construct of war dominance, hatred, and imprisonment. It is time for humankind to move past this ancient place of territorial hatred. Move to a new place and replace what does not have integrity.

A world based on who is rich and who you know and who has the biggest guns is passé. There is another way. We all know this. The basis of all popular revolutions has been an evanescent glimpse of the new reality over the horizon. Healing environments for peace include basic comfort, removing toxic stimuli, and dealing with cold, hunger, and noise. Healing environments for peace also include therapeutic touch, massage, and love. Dealing with poverty, pollution, ugliness, the destruction of nature . . . these are all crucial to preventing war. Protecting people from war and violence is about basic safety. War is an ultimate destruction of environment, dignity, autonomy, and aesthetic surroundings. War and violence are the opposite of treating the environment as sacred. Indigenous cultures looked at the world, its animals and plants, and the earth as sacred, as our mother.

Creating sacred space is a first step to creating an environment for peace now.

You are sacred.

All of life is sacred.

Let us begin.

■ REFLECTIONS

1. *How do I offer myself? In what ways do I make an offering of my inner wisdom and values?*
2. *What practices of creativity can I cultivate to go into my own inner spiritual and visionary journey, finding my own place of peace within?*
3. *Ubuntu: "I am because we are." What does this mean to me as a person, a nurse, and a peacemaker?*
4. *How do integrity, presence, intention, and commitment inform my nursing practice and healing mission?*
5. *What is peace? What is inner peace? How can I manifest and sustain human caring and peace in my heart, mind, and daily acts?*

■ REFERENCES

Lane, M. R., Samuels, M., & Watson, J. (2012). *The caritas path to peace: A guidebook to creating world peace with caring, love, and compassion.* United States: CreateSpace.

Samuels, M., & Lane, M. R. (1999). *Creative healing.* San Francisco, CA: Harper.

Samuels, M., & Lane, M. R.(2000a). *Spirit body healing.* New York, NY: Wiley.

Samuels, M., & Lane, M. R. (2000b). *Path of the feather.* New York, NY: Putnam.

Samuels, M., & Lane, M. R. (2002). *Shaman wisdom.* New York, NY: Wiley.

Watson Caring Science Institute. (n.d.). *International charter for human caring and peace.* Retrieved from http://watsoncaringscience.org/the-caritas-path-to-peace/

Watson, J. (2005). *Caring science as sacred science.* Philadelphia, PA: F.A. Davis.

Watson, J. (2008). *Nursing: The philosophy and science of caring.* Boulder, CO: University Press of Colorado.

Watson, J. (2012). *Human caring science: A theory of nursing* (2nd ed.). Sudbury, MA: Jones & Bartlett Learning.

CHAPTER TWENTY-FOUR

Informed and Impactful: Stewarding the Environmental Determinants of Health and Well-Being

Susan Luck

At the heart of Florence Nightingale's (1820-1910) legacy is a knowing that our external environment is inextricably interconnected to the health and wellbeing of all species and ecosystems. There is both the urgency and opportunity to address environmental factors that affect the lives of our clients/patients, families, and communities. In its broadest sense, the term "environment" can mean everything, both within and external to each person. When considering the environment, it is imperative to listen and respond to a larger story, not only as practitioners, but also as members of communities, cultures, and humankind.

—Luck (2015b, p. 166)

■ WHY NURSING?

My impulse to become a nurse precedes my earliest memories. My father's recollections give me insight into my life work. When I was young, my mother became ill and I am told that I wanted to offer comfort and help. At age 5, I witnessed her fainting and I ran to get a cool towel to place on her forehead as I held her hand to soothe her and told her she would be okay. Apparently, I knew intuitively what was needed. This was my initiation into the world of nursing and healing.

I can recall as a teenager looking forward to visiting my grandmother in a nursing home and helping the elderly women comb their hair and write letters for them. I can still see their kind yet sad eyes, and remember being deeply touched by their stories and their spirits. In those teenage years, I yearned to see the world and to become independent while finding a direction where I could be of help and make a difference in people's lives. I knew that nursing would allow me the opportunity to learn and know the diversity of people on a global scale.

■ EARLY IMPRESSIONS

I was always interested in the mind beyond the physical being. Early in my nursing career, I was attracted to psychiatric nursing as a way to engage in patients' stories and their uniqueness, their beliefs and rich imaginations. Living in New York City, I was fortunate to be exposed to a diversity of cultures, beliefs, and worldviews and was intrigued and curious to learn more.

These experiences led me to focus my undergraduate study in anthropology. As part of my independent field study, I became part of an emergency field team that worked in the highlands of Guatemala following an earthquake and lived in an isolated Mayan region where my Western beliefs were challenged by shamans/healers calling in ancestral spirits to heal the suffering within the community. I learned and observed the power of beliefs and witnessed the powerful illness of *susto,* derived from the verb *asustar* that means, "to frighten," as the Earth continued to tremble (Luck & Dossey, 2015, p. 340). This disease category was not a Western construct but manifested in symptoms affecting the body, mind, and spirit that would lead to a downward spiral if not treated by local shamans/healers and the community through ritual, prayer, and communication with the ancestors that lived in the mountain caves. It was not until 1975 that the Western medical model recognized these body-mind-spirit connections and it was classified as psychoneuroimmunology.

It was a privilege to be steeped in a culture with an interconnected worldview of how the mind and emotions impact one's health and that of the collective community. As the community healed, I stayed on to work with the women to plant community gardens. I was accepted into their lives in an intimate and personally transformative experience by being invited to be at births, ceremonies, and death rituals.

As I learned more about their way of life in the women's circles of weaving and in the local marketplace, I discovered that their husbands left the highlands to go to the coast to earn money seasonally by working in the sugar and cotton plantations. When they returned, they were often ill with strange skin conditions and various immune, respiratory, and digestive problems. Their offspring often had developmental problems that did not have cultural explanations. Using my community health nursing lens, I began to ask many questions and realized that these men as migrant workers were the victims of pesticide exposures, as spraying the coastal fields was done routinely, and the physiological consequences of these exposures were being passed on to their offspring. As I asked more questions, it became apparent to me that pesticides were poisoning current and future generations. I began to realize that nursing is not only about helping others but also about advocating for creating healthier families and communities through healthier environments.

This began my exploration about the role of the environment and about how the exposure to chemicals affects the health of all people and our planet. I became increasingly aware of the chemicals in the food we eat, the air we breathe, and the water we drink, and the vulnerability of the planet we inhabit. Florence Nightingale's words ring so true for today: The incidence of disease is related to "the want of fresh air, or of light, or of warmth, or of quiet or cleanliness" (Nightingale, 1860, p. 5). As a nurse, I felt it my responsibility to contribute to environmental information and increase awareness toward change so that all people could live healthier lives.

■ PROFESSIONAL EVOLUTION/CONTRIBUTION

Since the 1970s, I have felt an inner tug calling me to examine the many layers of the complexity of living in the modern world. This includes the ecological impact of nature on health and how it involves the health of not only humans but also all species and ecosystems. As I have deepened my knowledge, focusing on healthy environments and nutrition, I clearly see the role of nurses and how they can build upon Nightingale's global legacy of activism, advocacy, and transformation—local to global. With more than 3.4 million nurses in the United States (American Nurses Association [ANA], 2015) and 19.6 million nurses and midwives worldwide (World Health Organization [WHO], 2012). working with individuals, families, communities, and health care workers and their organizations, nurses possess extraordinary possibilities and resources to impact and create a healthy world.

Nightingale was one of the early proponents of the *precautionary principle*. The essence of the precautionary principle is: if there is a suspicion about a harmful environment or exposure, even though all of the evidence is not in, remove the person from the situation or stop the use of suspected harmful exposures (Raffensberger, 1998). It emphasizes that zero tolerance for the contamination of our environment is the acceptable standard, not a minimal or moderate contamination.

Precautionary principle proponents and health policy analysts today advocate that it is incumbent on those introducing a new chemical or technology to demonstrate that it is safe and not the responsibility of the rest of us to prove it is harmful. This is extremely important, since it is theorized that up to 90% of symptoms experienced today have an environmental cofactor (WHO, 2013). This work led to me establishing a nonprofit organization called the EarthRose Institute (ERI).

In 2005, ERI began to bring awareness of the environment's impact on women's and children's health by translating research and information to communities of women and all humanity everywhere (ERI, n.d.). The spirit behind this was my mother, Rose, who died in 1955 while in her 30s of breast cancer. In the 1980s, I began my in-depth research on breast cancer for my own health and well-being and wondered if I had inherited a genetic predisposition. I created a timeline for my mother, as we had no prior family history of cancer. Although epigenetics and the human genome were not yet being discussed and the research was still in its early phase, I began exploring the complexities of lifestyle choices and what triggers could be factors in illness and disease, and how a healthy life and prevention could make a positive impact and difference.

I studied the emerging research on epigenetics and explored how the environment can allow genes to express themselves and unlock our potential predisposition. Two environmental factors in my memories jumped out at me. My mother had been a smoker in the 1950s when smoking was both fashionable and considered safe. Her hair turned prematurely gray and some of my earliest recollections were of accompanying her to the hair salon where she had her hair dyed back to its natural black color. I began to read about black coal-tar hair dyes used in the 1950s and their link to breast cancer (Epstein, 2011). This led me on my own personal environmental healing journey with a passion to share this new body of information with others.

The epidemic of breast cancer continues to grow despite the efforts of the Susan G. Komen for the Cure and its Pink Ribbon Campaign (Susan G. Komen, n.d.). I realize that the public knows little about true prevention and lifestyle habits and factors fueling this public health epidemic, where younger women and more men are being diagnosed with breast cancer at alarming rates. The public is just beginning to get involved in the need to address the chemicals in the environment and in our food chain. Research on chemicals that act as estrogen mimickers, known broadly as endocrine disruptors, is growing. These chemicals, including pesticides and plastics, are taken up at estrogen receptor sites in the breasts, ovaries, prostate, and testes and may be fueling this global health crisis (National Institute of Environmental Health Sciences [NIEHS], 2016). The link between exposure to everyday chemicals and cancer risk in the United States has been grossly underestimated, according to a recent report by the National Cancer Institute (NCI, 2010). The NCI, which advises the president of the United States, has previously focused on better known causes of cancer such as diet and smoking. However, its recent report urges the U.S. administration to identify and eliminate environmental carcinogens from workplaces, schools, and homes. It estimates that there are nearly 80,000 largely unregulated chemicals on the market (NCI, 2010). As nurses work in all sectors of health, we are becoming more aware of the increased risk of exposures in our workplace environments and in our communities.

I have always been concerned with what is recognized today as the social and environmental determinants of health (Luck, 2015a). The *social determinants* of health are the economic and social conditions under which individuals live that affect their health; disease and illness are often a result of detrimental social, economic, and political forces. The *environmental determinants* of health are any external agent (biological, chemical, physical, social, or cultural) that can be linked to a change in health status that is involuntary (e.g., breathing unwanted secondhand smoke), whereas active tobacco smoking is a *behavioral determinant* (Luck, 2015a).

As my passion for health and well-being matured and I continued to synthesize the research and findings of environmentally focused organizations, I conceptualized and created an Integrative Lifestyle Health and Wellbeing (ILHWB) model that is part of the Theory of Integrative Nurse Coaching (TINC; discussed later in this section). The ILHWB model is a personalized approach that deals with primary prevention and underlying causality through a holistic, integrative, and integral perspective. This is a whole-person approach that applies to all people rather than the traditional labels and codes for symptoms and diagnoses of diseases. This means that all interactions are patient centered and the approach honors and emphasizes the individual's unique history, story, antecedents, and triggers rather than medical diagnosis and disease orientation.

There is a deep and powerful interconnectedness where all physiological, mental, emotional, social, spiritual, cultural, and environmental factors impact life and human flourishing. We have an abundance of research now that supports the view that the human body functions as an orchestrated network of interconnected systems rather than compartmentalized systems functioning autonomously and without effect on each other (Luck & Keegan, 2016; Luck, 2015a). Our individuality recognizes the variations in metabolic function that derive from unique genetic and environmental influences among individuals. The ILHWB model considers energy field dynamics, including negative thoughts, persistent stressors, toxic internal and external environments, and a nutrient-deficient diet, any of which may disrupt the human energy field on a cellular level and impair optimal function, contributing to disease processes over time.

The ILHWB model exists on a wellness continuum and can be viewed as a tool to preserve and restore dynamic balance on multiple levels. This approach seeks to regenerate and source our innate reserve as a means to enhance well-being and healing throughout the life cycle. This philosophy and worldview include the promotion of optimizing our internal and external healing environments. It holds that individual human health is the microcosm of the macrocosm in the web of life.

A major component of the ILHWB model has been the exploration of clients'/patients' stories and their cultural beliefs and worldviews, which reveals the multidimensional layers of being human. Exploring my own story and the story of others has also given me many possibilities for growth and change in our shared movement toward wholeness. Beginning in 2010, my ILHWB exploration led me to collaborate with like-minded nurse colleagues, Barbara Dossey and Bonney Gulino Schaub, and to expand this work in the role of integrative nurse coaching. I currently serve with Barbara Dossey as the codirector of the International Nurse Coaching Association (INCA, 2016), a rich journey with many collective successes and more to come (see Chapter 4 for details on our collaborative endeavors and coauthorship of the TINC [Dossey, 2015], the Integrative Nurse Coach Leadership Model [INCLM; Dossey & Luck, 2015], and *Nurse Coaching: Integrative Approaches for Health and Healing* [Dossey, Luck, & Schaub, 2015]; see Chapter 27 for more about Bonney Schaub and Transpersonal Nurse Coaching). This nurse coach collaboration has also inspired the publication of *The Art and Science of Nurse Coaching: The Provider's Guide to Scope and Competencies* (Hess et al., 2013), which led to the national nurse-coach certification process through the American Holistic Nurses Credentialing Corporation (AHNCC, n.d.).

As I continue to explore environmental health and well-being, it is very clear that a nurse coaching lens is needed to assist clients/patients and communities to create new health behaviors and to sustain them over time. A nurse coaching approach opens doors to health and healing as coaching questions assist individuals to reframe their health challenges and/or medical diagnosis. It also helps in exploring the personal meaning of health, illness, dying, and healing, and offers the client the opportunity to develop new insights and a deepening awareness of his or her vulnerability as part of the human condition. By addressing the totality of the individual and interweaving the internal and external environment within the context of community and culture, I have come to learn firsthand the crucial impact of nursing's involvement in community health priorities.

As I have deepened my environmental knowledge and awareness, I also recognized that theory and research must be translated at the grassroots level. I have become involved in my local community as a community health and public health nurse and as a nurse environmentalist. I started an Environmental Impact Committee where neighbors with young children and the elderly along with local politicians have joined together to legislate new environmental codes and ordinances to protect its citizens and build a healthier community. In my Florida coastal community of 5,000 residents, our outcome goals are to assure that our waterways are protected from overdevelopment, the air we breathe is not contaminated by demolition debris, and that the soil being brought in for landfill and for parks is tested and safe. Our local committee work has become a model for neighboring communities and has received national attention.

My role has been to assist citizens to understand environment in its broadest sense. The term *environment* can mean everything, both within and external to each person (Luck, 2010; Luck, 2015a; Luck & Keegan, 2016). When considering the environment, it is imperative to listen and respond to a larger story of all members of communities, cultures, and humankind. I stand proudly as a nurse at our monthly town hall meetings and give voice to my community's environmental concerns. The community listens to my initiating an informed discussion because our nursing profession is not only the most trusted, but it also carries with it an authority of concern, caring, and knowing (Gallup Poll, 2016). These endeavors are built and supported by my moral/ethical compass.

■ MORAL/ETHICAL FOUNDATION

At the heart of our 21st-century nursing legacy is our work and mission to focus on how our internal and external environments are inextricably interconnected with the health and well-being of all species and ecosystems. As previously discussed, Nightingale understood the precautionary principle, and her work can guide nurses' moral/ethical compass so that they take anticipatory actions to prevent harm. Today, nurses must expand on both the urgency and opportunity to address environmental factors that affect the lives of our clients/patients, families, and communities. We are in a new dawn regarding environmental health and activism in the United States and globally. The public awareness and interest in all things "green" is creating a demand for nurses to understand and become more involved in the relationship between human health and the environments in which we live, learn, work, and play. We have moved beyond questioning the science of whether we are in an environmental health peril to almost unanimous consensus that we must act and act now on many of the risks we are all experiencing in our present and for future generations.

As nurses, we are in a position to respond to questions about the environment and its relationship to health with credible, evidence-based information. We provide leadership in making the necessary changes in our policies and practices and can empower our communities to join together to positively impact their health and well-being.

Nurse leadership in environmental coaching, education, and advocacy in health care is rooted in our history (Dossey & Luck, 2015). An expanded role within nursing and nurse coaching is to assist clients and patients to discover and uncover the environmental cofactors contributing to symptoms, conditions, disease patterns, and daily quality of life. Environmental exposures can contribute to one's health challenges, including cognitive impairment, immune dysfunction, hormonal imbalances, impaired digestive processes, weight management, and a host of symptoms often unexplained (Luck & Keegan, 2016).

I believe that each nurse holds a moral/ethical compass and worldview that bring awareness of humanity's place in nature and in society. Part of our role as nurses is to empower individuals and families in creating healthier communities through both individual and collective advocacy and change. Using a nurse coaching approach can explore and promote practices that create healing environments in our homes, workplaces, and communities. It also assists us to recognize that environmental health supports well-being and freedom from illness or injury related to exposure to toxic agents and other environmental conditions that are potentially detrimental to all.

Each of us, as nurses and as global citizens, can act to create safer environments. I envision many nurses becoming involved in environmental stewardship and taking steps toward creating a healthier environment so that we can transform the health of our vulnerable Earth.

Nurses can partner with the clients/patients, communities, and organizations to identify and advocate for the creation of health policies that reduce common exposures in the home or workplace environment. Through a nurse coaching approach, listening to all possible influences in one's life story that might be contributing to current health and life challenges and cocreating new possibilities for changing one's lifestyle behaviors is the keystone of the nurse coach–client relationship. It is about asking questions that increase awareness regarding the connections between the environment and our health and quality of life. Our holistic, integrative, and integral nursing lens offers us new opportunities to use comprehensive assessments and translate these findings, becoming "environmental detectives."

We are challenged to expand our nursing knowledge related to the potential environmental links to many of the issues seen in chronic illness and disease and connect the dots when listening to and uncovering the client's story. To engage successfully, we are challenged to increase our awareness of how our external environment impacts our health and the health of our clients/patients, families, communities, and the planet. As nurses and as frontline health care providers, we have a unique role as advocates within our communities and our health care facilities to create positive environmental change from the inside and to have conversations on how to change health care policies and practices.

The mission of many national and international nursing organizations supports nurses' moral/ethical compass: for example, the ANA, with its *Nursing: Scope and Standards of Practice* (2010), and the ANA *Code of Ethics for Nurses With Interpretive Statements* (2001, 2015b). The ANA has declared 2015 as the Year of Ethics (ANA, 2015a). The ANA has shared its landmark *Principles of Environmental Health for Nursing Practice With Implementation Strategies* (2007) that puts forth a call to action, encouraging nurses to gain a working understanding of the relationships between human health and environmental exposures and to integrate this knowledge into all nursing practice. (The ANA's environmental health principles can be seen in Table 24.1.) It is foundational that human health is linked to the quality of the environment and that air, water, soil, food, and products must be free of potentially harmful chemicals. These principles are applicable in all settings where RNs practice and are intended to protect nurses themselves, patients and their families, other health care workers, and the community, and to recognize their role as environmental health leaders.

The International Council of Nurses (ICN) has a position statement on *Reducing Environmental and Lifestyle Related Health Risks* (2011). It directly addresses the concern of

TABLE 24.1   **ANA's Principles of Environmental Health for Nursing Practice**

1. Knowledge of environmental health concepts is essential to nursing practice.

2. The precautionary principle guides nurses to use products and practices that do not harm human health or the environment and to take preventive action in the face of uncertainty.

3. Nurses have a right to work in an environment that is safe and healthy.

4. Healthy environments are sustained through multidisciplinary collaboration.

5. Choices of materials, products, technology, and practices in the environment that impact nursing practice are based on the best evidence available.

6. Approaches to promoting a healthy environment respect the diverse values, beliefs, cultures, and circumstances of patients and their families.

7. Nurses participate in assessing the quality of the environment in which they practice and live.

8. Nurses, other health care workers, patients, and communities have the right to know relevant and timely information about the potentially harmful products, chemicals, pollutants, and hazards to which they are exposed.

9. Nurses participate in research of best practices that promote a safe and healthy environment.

10. Nurses must be supported in advocating and implementing environmental health principles in nursing practice.

ANA, American Nurses Association.

Adapted from ANA (2007).

the immeasurable human suffering being caused by the growing burden of environmental and lifestyle-related noncommunicable diseases (NCDs), which are largely preventable. The ICN asks that nurses and national nurses associations play a strategic role in helping reduce environmental and lifestyle-health risks related to NCDs. According to the ICN, the concern of nurses is for people's health—its promotion, its maintenance, and its restoration. The healthy lives of people depend ultimately on the health of Planet Earth—its soil, its water, its oceans, its atmosphere, and its biological diversity—all of the elements that constitute people's natural environment (ICN, 2011). The ICN's position statement joins several national and international organizations in their increased focus on and efforts to prevent and control NCDs (WHO & the United Nations [UN] Environmental Programmes, 2013).

To that end, we must prepare all nurses to be a cut above the average citizen with regard to their knowledge of environmental health issues. We must see all nurses as environmentalists and promote steps in educating, advocating, empowering, and coaching for lasting change.

■ VISION

My vision for the future is that nurses increase their copartnerships with clients/patients, interprofessional colleagues, and communities to identify, address, and advocate for change that creates healthier environments in the home and workplace.

I see more nurses engaged in the *Global Green and Healthy Hospitals Agenda* (Green Hospital Alliance, n.d.) in an effort to build on the initiatives happening around the world and engender an approach to sustainability and health that can be replicated by thousands of hospitals and health systems in a variety of countries and health settings. They will explore *Health Care Without Harm* (n.d.) initiatives to promote the health of all people and implement ecologically sound and healthy alternatives to workplace health care practices that pollute the environment and contribute to disease. For example, the incineration of medical waste is a leading source of dangerous air pollutants such as dioxin and mercury, and the use of these hazardous chemicals indoors may contribute to the compromised health of nurses and other health care workers, as well as impede the healing process of our patients.

Our legacy as 21st-century Nightingales is that we bring new health and environmental awareness and health policy initiatives to our workplace and communities in these critical times. I believe the story we want to remember and pass on to future generations of nurses is that we will focus on the following:

- Increase awareness of our place in nature, knowing that we are the microcosm of the macrocosm and understanding that our world is vastly complex and unpredictable.
- Deepen our understanding of how health and the health of our planet are inextricably interwoven.
- Engage in practices that create healing environments in our home, workplace, and community.
- Take risks to challenge the existing structures and maintain values and convictions to create healing environments.

■ REFLECTIONS

1. *What new environmental practices am I willing to bring into my life to support my well-being?*
2. *What environmental lifestyle patterns do I recognize that might influence my health and the health of my family and community?*
3. *What do I see as my challenges in creating a healthy workplace environment?*
4. *How can I become more aware of my environmental choices and behaviors?*
5. *Who are the people in my life who would support me in making healthy changes?*

■ REFERENCES

American Holistic Nurses Credentialing Corporation. (n.d.). Retrieved from http://www.ahncc.org/certification/nursecoachnchwnc.html

American Nurses Association. (2001). *Code of ethics for nurses with interpretive statements.* Washington, DC: Author.

American Nurses Association. (2007). *Principles of environmental health for nursing practice with implementation strategies.* Retrieved from http://www.nursingworld.org/MainMenuCategories/WorkplaceSafety/Healthy-Nurse/ANAsPrinciplesofEnvironmentalHealthforNursingPractice.pdf

American Nurses Association. (2010). *Nursing: Scope and standards of practice* (2nd ed.). Silver Spring, MD: Author.

American Nurses Association. (2015a). *2015: The year of ethics.* Retrieved from http://www.nursing-world.org/MainMenuCategories/EthicsStandards/CodeofEthicsforNurses/Code-of-Ethics-For-Nurses.html

American Nurses Association. (2015b). *Guide to the code of ethics for nurses with interpretive statements: Development, interpretation, and application* (2nd ed.). Silver Spring, MD: Nursesbooks.org.

American Nurses Association. (2015c). *Nurse work force.* Retrieved from http://www.nursingworld.org/FunctionalMenuCategories/FAQs

Dossey, B. M. (2015). Theory of integrative nurse coaching. In B. M. Dossey, S. Luck, & B. G. Schaub (Eds.), *Nurse coaching: Integrative approaches for health and wellbeing* (pp. 29–48). North Miami, FL: International Nurse Coach Association.

Dossey, B. M., & Luck, S. (2015). Nurse coaching and leadership. In B. M. Dossey, S. Luck, & B. G. Schaub (Eds.), *Nurse coaching: Integrative approaches for health and wellbeing* (pp. 387–404). North Miami, FL: International Nurse Coach Association.

Dossey, B. M., Luck, S., & Schaub, B. G (Eds.). (2015). *Nurse coaching: Integrative approaches for health and wellbeing.* North Miami, FL: International Nurse Coach Association.

EarthRose Institute (ERI). (n.d.). Retrieved from http://www.earthrose.org

Epstein, S. S. (2011). *National Cancer Institute and American Cancer Society: Criminal indifference to cancer prevention and conflicts of interest.* Bloomington, IN: Xlibris.

Gallup Poll. (2016). *Ethics in professions.* Retrieved from http://www.gallup.com/poll/1654/honesty-ethics-professions.aspx

Green Hospital Alliance 2020. (n.d.). *Go green.* Retrieved from http://hospital2020.org/Green HospitalVendors.html

Health Care Without Harm. (n.d) Retrieved from https://noharm.org

Hess, D. R., Dossey, B. M., Southard, M. E., Luck, S., Schaub, B. G., & Bark, L. (2013). *The art and science of nurse coaching: The provider's guide to coaching scope of practice and competencies.* Silver Spring, MD: Nursesbooks.org.

International Council of Nurses (ICN). (2011). *Reducing environmental and lifestyle related health risks.* Retrieved from http://www.icn.ch/images/stories/documents/publications/position_statements/E11_Reducing_Environmental_Health_Risks.pdf

International Nurse Coach Association. (2016). Retrieved from http://www.inursecoach.com

Luck, S. (2010). Changing the health of the nation: The role of nurse coaches. *Alternative Therapies in Health and Medicine, 16*(5), 68–70.

Luck, S. (2015a). Integrative lifestyle health and wellbeing (ILHWB). In B. M. Dossey, S. Luck, & B. G. Schaub (Eds.), *Nurse coaching: Integrative approaches for health and wellbeing* (pp. 123–146). North Miami, FL: International Nurse Coach Association.

Luck, S. (2015b). Environmental health. In B. M. Dossey, S. Luck, & B. G. Schaub (Eds.). *Nurse coaching: Integrative approaches for health and wellbeing* (pp. 165–177). North Miami, FL: International Nurse Coach Association.

Luck, S., & Dossey, B. M. (2015). Cultural perspectives and rituals of healing. In B. M. Dossey, S. Luck, & B. G. Schaub (Eds.), *Nurse coaching: Integrative approaches for health and wellbeing* (pp. 335–348). North Miami, FL: International Nurse Coach Association.

Luck, S., & Keegan, L. (2016). Environmental health. In B. M. Dossey & L. Keegan (Eds.), *Holistic nursing: A handbook for practice* (7th ed., pp. 557–587). Burlington, MA: Jones & Bartlett Learning.

National Cancer Institute. (2010). *Reducing environmental cancer risk: What we can do now.* Retrieved from http://www.cancer.gov/cancertopics/understanding-cancer/environment/

National Institute of Environmental Health Sciences. (2016). *Endocrine disruptors.* Retrieved from http://www.niehs.nih.gov/health/topics/agents/endocrine/

Nightingale, F. (1860). *Notes on nursing: What it is and what it is not.* London, UK: Harrison.

Raffensberger, C. (1998). *The precautionary principle, science and environmental health network.* Retrieved form http://www.sehn.org

Susan G. Komen. (n.d.). *Race for the cure.* Retrieved from http://www.komen.org

World Health Organization. (2012). Enhancing nursing and midwifery capacity to contribute to the prevention, treatment and management of noncommunicable disease in practice: Policy and advocacy, research and education. *Human Resources for Health Observer, 12.* Retrieved from http://www.who.int/hrh/resources/observer12/en

World Health Organization. (2013). *Global action plan for the prevention and control of non-communicable diseases, 2013–2020.* Retrieved from http://www.who.int/nmh/events/ncd_action_plan/en

World Health Organization & the United Nations Environmental Programmes. (2013). *State of the science of endocrine disrupting chemicals.* Geneva, Switzerland: WHO Press.

CHAPTER TWENTY-FIVE

Resourceful and Unified: Partnering Across Cultures and Worldviews

Phalakshi Manjrekar

Nurses are the strength of our healthcare system and, today, the need is dire that we learn to care for the caregivers. This will only be accomplished if we keep a small percentage of our time for ourselves—one nurse's wellbeing ultimately helps many.

—Manjrekar (2014)

■ WHY NURSING?

This chapter attempts to reflect the experience of nurses and the dilemmas they go through in developing countries. These countries are vital to the global health care scenario, and nurses are the key health care personnel, the largest sector of direct caregivers, who can move the agenda of health and health promotion to the doorstep of the community. The chapter also emphasizes factors affecting nurses and their various roles and possibilities in decision making, budgeting, planning and conceptualizing, and improvising, to name a few, thus enabling the nurse to call herself or himself a leader to promote these priorities in the absence of systemic support to reach the masses.

Nursing education and its influence on the implementation of idealistic practice, research, and professional development is the second domain emphasized here. In a country like India, basic nursing education is standardized and the only training options available to nurses are limited to what their state of residence has to offer, languages they may or may not speak, and financial support that is not easily available (Chandrachood, 2013). In short, the choices are extremely sparse. Nurse leaders are challenged to meet with and a support a very diverse group of nurse colleagues and collaborate to achieve a wide spectrum of goals in this setting. This, again, may differ by populations, which vary from urban regions to rural placements. Nurse leaders who are unable to meet the linguistic demands of the particular community may not be able to take up an active role as

345

a leader in the absence of fluent communication skills. This further decreases the scope of practice and limits the availability of human resources, increasing a statistic of "failure."

Do nurse leaders have to be female? This may be an outdated question in Western countries where nursing has evolved to the next level. On a more global scale, the world has decided that the gender of the individual is irrelevant to the profession. This is not true in most of the developing countries—nursing is still a female-dominated profession and men do not consider this role as an honorable option (Thomas, 2014). Does this impact nurse leadership? Yes, it does. The dilemma and the preexisting prejudice paralyze many nurses in the leadership role and prevent countless would-be nurses from entering the professions.

Nursing, where I come from in India, is primarily known to be a profession where hard work is expected and appreciated and patients' expressed gratitude is the primary remuneration for nurses. However, society in general still looks upon a doctor's profession to be the superior and more rewarding option. I was fortunate to live in an environment where I saw doctors and nurses working together, but was drawn specifically to nursing because of the compassionate nature of the nursing professionals I observed, which always brought smiles from patients and their families. Unfortunately, in India in 1982, there was scarce literature available for one wanting to know more about this dynamic profession. Using the Internet was not very popular and was inaccessible to many. Very knowledgeable counselors and educators were able to give extensive advice about other professional choices, but knew little about nursing.

Nurses alone were charged with educating the public about nursing. Fortunately, I was able to connect with seasoned and accomplished nursing personnel. I was also able to give factual data about the status of the profession in India and the challenges I would have to face, provided I chose to pursue it. Thinking back, what attracted me to nursing was the opportunity I would have to help "make it work" and show others the myriad opportunities they could have in contributing to the growth and sustainability of nursing. I wanted to be a nurse for the nurses in my society and be an example of how one can be proud to be in this profession.

■ EARLY IMPRESSIONS

The next decision was to choose from the many programs available and take up a curriculum that allowed me to express my vision. In India, the quality of education and credentials attained are based solely on one's financial status (Chandrachood, 2013). Can you imagine how many talents go wasted? How many dedicated caregivers never realize their potential as nurses? At that time, programs that provided very basic nursing and midwifery skills and a nominal stipend, without awarding a degree of any kind, were the best option for young girls who were unable to complete basic school. These girls had little choice but to meet the womanpower deficiencies existing then in most of the hospitals by providing the challenging and exhausting labor needed. The second option was to complete basic school and opt for a diploma in nursing and midwifery, which consisted of a longer duration but the same terms: free of cost, including free housing, a nurse's uniform, and a nominal sum as stipend for all the hard work the nurse student contributed as a part of the coursework (Sharma, 2010).

The third and final option was to enroll in a university program to obtain a BSN from one of the handful of colleges in town and somehow be able to pay the university, accommodation, and library fees (with no scholarship available!). I chose the university option, as I felt I had the financial support to make this decision, and knew the curriculum provided would strengthen the chances of realizing my goals for the future. A distinctive feature of the university curriculum, as per the health care scenario of the nation, was that it provided nurses the real-world experience of visiting homes, door to door, for six months or more in both an urban setting, where the population lived in slum housing or temporary structures made from cloth, tin, or any other available material; and in the rural areas where houses were made of mud or straw. All universities had to contribute to the global strategy of the World Health Organization (WHO) and its international campaign, *Health for All by the Year 2000* (Clement, 2012). This was an eye-opening experience for all young women who planned a future in nursing.

As a graduate nurse, it was an accepted belief that if one wanted to influence thought processes and patterns within the profession, one needed to be an educator (Healey, 2013). A noneducator or clinically based nurse was not in a position to create change easily—clearly a misconception but a strongly rooted popular thought, which tends to dominate all and is often ascribed to blindly. Within a short duration, it was evident that to excel professionally and do justice to my task, basic university education was not adequate. I decided to pursue an MSN, a very difficult decision as scholarship monies for nursing professionals were not easily available, the degree could only be completed as a full-time student, and the fee structure was extremely high.

Thankfully, my family was able to provide me with additional financial aid and I successfully completed the program. Very few nurses at the time had an MSN, and I was able to attain a senior position as an educator in the university. The position in the college was not affiliated with a hospital and in no way was I encouraged to fulfill my vision of promoting nurses to be proud of their profession. I continued to feel there was a gap: The overwhelming majority of nursing needed someone to show them how to be proud of their chosen profession, how to celebrate the work they did, and how to build a strong and inspiring community.

This was when I changed my job to become a part of a hospital-affiliated school of nursing. It was extremely tedious to be a part of a team that maintained the traditional views of nursing as inferior while trying to emphasize nurses' autonomy and create a new view of how essential nursing was to any hospital: difficult, but not impossible. It took me 10 years of hard work to change the lived experience for thousands, who now look back and proudly say that they were and are proud to be nurses. Later, I continued to discover new avenues for my message by being a part of a national nursing organization in India, namely, the Trained Nurses Association of India (TNAI).

I had learned that as an emerging leader, the decisions I made influenced people. I decided that I needed to be a part of a hospital at a senior level and that I had been using nursing education as my crutch without being truly passionate about it. Although I was open and transparent about my goals, I was also surprised to find it was extremely difficult to obtain that position because I was considered overqualified. Traditionally, these senior-level roles could be successfully carried forward by nursing personnel without a university, let alone a postgraduate, education (Healey, 2013). It took multiple meetings and intensive conversations to convince the hospital administration that I would be able to create needed improvements because of, not in spite of, my higher education. One of the hospitals finally agreed and I was able to use my decision-making abilities to create positive and influential changes in the nursing scenario while also allowing a group of hospital administrators the opportunity to reconsider their image of nurses.

As a clinical nurse, the idea of leadership has the tendency to remain a conceptual notion unless one maintains and practices the belief that he or she can lead (Banerjee, 2014). Every nurse makes countless decisions per day, exercising his or her own internal leadership compass. A good decision maker becomes a leader in action, benefiting those at the receiving end and forwarding the goals of nursing. When I started nursing, I met many young people who aspired to be nurses and each had an idea of his or her own individual leadership he or she yearned to implement. This belief had to be applied in varied clinical and practice settings because nursing, itself, is categorically diverse as no other profession can be. In India, a nurse has the option to be a clinician, an educator, or a researcher (Thomas, 2014) and, yet, these young student nurses refused to limit themselves to just one title.

In other parts of the world, young nurses are creating opportunities to use leadership skills and abilities in all settings. But developing countries have their own stories to tell. A country like India, which is dominated by a rural population, requires nurses to provide direct care to 70% of its rural population, where lack of accessibility and inadequate or nonexistent basic resources mean health care may never reach a patient's doorstep (Yalayyaswamy, 2012). Looking back, accessible rural health care would have been possible with an apt nurse leader guiding and redirecting financial and economic decisions to help the situation, unlimited by the restrictions mentioned earlier. Rural nursing continues to be a substantial concern of countries with a poor socioeconomic structure (Clement, 2011). Developed countries that are still attending to the goals set by the WHO are primarily focused on meeting the needs of the overall, more general, population who are more easily accessible due to superior infrastructure and clearer business-minded leadership.

Basic nursing education in developing countries urges students to start asking, "How can nurses help?" A nurse within this system is faced with the dilemma of gathering any adequate resources that are available to him or her and helping all those he or she can physically reach, as I did early on in my career. However, a strong and determined leadership potential informed my sheer inner focus and perseverance that I would get through the masses at the right time to the right person with the right resources.

Out of the hardships of professional restrictions and inadequate financial support arose a nurse who understood that a patient would only receive care if I was able to discover innovative ways of accessing resources and could confidently and readily rely upon independent clinical thinking. This knowledge gave me the liberty to plan and execute what I thought was best, given the situation. I refused to succumb to the circumstances that prevented countless people from receiving care, nor did I relegate my scope to the abilities others thought I should be limited by. Did I need adequate leadership skills to achieve my objectives? Yes. But my instinct to lead had to be trusted in order to fulfill my broader, more humanistic, more global intentions.

Nurse leaders are found at various steps on the ladder—nurses' myriad roles exist on multiple tiers and each level emphasizes a leadership mode. This is one profession where role models are still respected. One who aspires to influence many awakens a broad range of diverse abilities to be shared by all. In many settings, leaders settle for focusing on and limiting nurses to their technical competencies and demonstrated ability to maintain safe standards. But there is so much more to nursing . . . and it requires a transformational leader to create a new environment where all skills and abilities among nurses are nurtured and encouraged to flourish (Blais & Hayes, 2016).

■ PROFESSIONAL EVOLUTION/CONTRIBUTION

Nursing, from the perspective of my early years, needed improvements to standardize basic thought processes and protocols and facilitate better autonomy for nurses. The system as a whole was resistant to substantiate nursing as a profession worthy of such autonomy, as many interdisciplinary partners still believed nursing to be subservient and many nurses did not believe in themselves or know how to articulate their positions. I kept asking, "How to change that?" After asking this question a million times, I somehow realized education was the key. Education needed to be accessible to all! It needed to be affordable with loan and scholarship monies more readily available. Most importantly, university nursing education needed to dominate. This was at a time when hundreds of diploma programs existed in comparison to a mere two university programs. Many provinces did not even have a recognized program (Kaur, 2014).

Aside from school training, there needed to be a system to provide working clinicians with access to continuing education. At that time, there were no opportunities present for necessary and ongoing professional growth. It seemed as if no one believed, as I did, that if nurses received continuing education, they would be capable of providing more efficacious, quality patient care and improve their overall clinical acumen. There was no drive within existing nurse leadership to provide staff with exposure to innovative or cutting-edge practice. This worldview persisted in thousands of nurses practicing age-old processes without any changes, not based on evidence, and becoming maladaptive to advancement of any kind.

Second, I realized it was not just staff nurses who needed to be educated—we needed to educate the world around us about who we were. I quickly started to express and share with health care administration the need to significantly decrease the employment of non-nursing/unregistered personnel who had no formal or recognized training. This allowed only nurses who had received formal education to fill the "nursing" roles in small and moderately large health care systems. With all of the untrained individuals working as "nurses" within countless institutions, no wonder there was confusion about nursing's public image! How could "they" know who we were if "we" presented a broken and inconsistent front?

Trained nurses were better focused to work in the urban areas; rural nursing was not attracting educated staff (Kalita, 2014). Patient and nurse safety in rural areas was a concern; lack of adequate transportation, few collaborating physicians, poor remuneration, and absent resources prevented the delivery of adequate care. It awakened within me a new sense of leadership and responsibility to my profession. I wanted to stop unregistered personnel from presenting themselves as nurses, providing unknowledgeable and even dangerous care to patients, and harming the interdisciplinary and public opinion about nursing. Could legal action be taken against them? Could national nursing bodies stand up for standardizing the profession? Could legislation be put in place to bring a stop to the deregulation that had occurred? Organizational involvement from a national nursing body was overdue.

This was accompanied by several other professional issues and concerns occurring at the time. Should a nurse be a jack of all trades and master of none and be expected to pilot all clinical demands with no significant specialization training? The answer is an obvious "no," but early on this was the expectation and nurses needed an avenue to specialize in clinical arenas of their choice . . . a concept that still appears elusive at times.

Should nurses with higher university education have a forum to demonstrate skills and expertise solely as academicians? Should they be relegated to an academic setting and be forced to sacrifice the rewarding and intimate milieu of clinical practice? This was the question I needed to answer, first for myself, and then for others. Destined to change the trend and provide ample, multidimensional opportunity for all practitioners, I enthusiastically accepted a senior nursing administrative position alongside nursing personnel less qualified and less experienced.

This was my opportunity to prove I was different—to show through my actions what nurses were capable of. I initiated the first step by stating that a need for a separate budget in nursing had to be established. Can you imagine a staff of hundreds bound to other departments by financial mismanagement and a misunderstanding of what the profession provides? This was an example of exclusion through overinclusion; our identity had become erased by being bundled with other disciplines and categorized under their priorities. I procured the separate budget by giving a presentation that delineated nursing's contributory potential to organizational outcome expectations and exhaustive detail regarding how I would accomplish this with an independent, nurse-managed budgetary allotment. I was accepted on a trial. As the temporary period wore on, it was concluded that in addition to a separate nursing budget for staffing purposes, increased needs of student nurses, purchasing of necessary equipment, and various nursing needs should be determined under the auspices of a *nursing* authority/director to better maintain and improve the qualities and outcomes of the nursing department.

This was a mammoth achievement, which was later adopted by many. Today many institutions employ qualified nursing heads who decide nursing budgets. These nursing heads are now recognized at par with other directors in finance, medicine, and general administration to make major budget decisions for the hospitals. I was also recognized for my ability to plan projects; it seemed so obvious to me that just as a nurse in charge of a clinical field is able to implement more effectively if nursing inputs are taken into consideration while planning, a department and institution need a nurse to lead nurses. This was confirmed when the first project was labeled "successful" and that success came because nursing inputs were noted as favorable to the institution as a whole. This allowed for a major impact in the organogram of the hospital and I was considered for appointment to the hospital board of directors. It sparked a major positive impact on the importance and reputation of nursing, and many other hospitals took a similar decision. The presence and relevance of nursing was felt powerfully throughout the interdisciplinary structures of the hospital.

However, successes aside, I am still unable to understand a simple fact: Why is nursing salary consistently below par compared to competitive health care professionals? A common answer to this question, from India's worldview, is that nurses here are from a relatively low socioeconomic strata and will readily agree to work for a minimal salary; they do not demand much, are very disciplined, and work hard without complaining; and they do not insist on comfort, safety, or reasonable working hours with financial remuneration that matches their contributions (Vallee, 2006). My first agenda was to make a difference that required monumental changes. My proposal was very simple: Let us benchmark a standard, map nursing competencies, quantify nursing outcomes, and prove its significance on hospital outcomes. I also wanted to initiate a process that would better nursing salaries from their current status and allow for its sustainability in the annual budgetary plan.

I was the first nursing head among an immediate social circle to have made this statement and it took one-and-a-half years of dedicated planning, multiple presentations, and countless discussions to move it forward. Finally, nursing issues like safety, comfortable working hours, adequate staffing, and, most important, nursing salaries were attended to. I was able to get my workplace to create a salary structure for nurses, which was later classified as the best in nongovernmental institutions. Later, many others cited this example to get salary improvements for their nurses. Maintaining adequate staffing, better safety, and appropriate working hours also followed this in various institutions in the country. To make these changes as a leader is difficult, but as I've mentioned earlier, not impossible. Many others followed or attempted to follow my initiative; it basically depends on one's ability to convince those in decision-making seats. What helps is the potential of the nurse and his or her performance to prove that nurse-driven outcomes are necessary and valuable in the health care sector. This was a considerable achievement, which was attained by a long and healthy debate to let all involved know that nurses are worth it and should not be exploited. Nurses too learned their value and now know their due, which will allow them to see that their worth is appreciated and compensated appropriately. I am now blessed to see that this change is here to stay and though initiated by me, it is not dependent on me . . . it will continue in my absence too.

Nurses are key players in the hospital setting, a fact everyone acknowledges. It is also known that nurses cannot continue to be effective if not developed as professionals in keeping with the ever-developing health sector. Indian nurses are registered to practice; however, the renewal of their registration is through payment of renewal charges only (Umamani, 2011). This does not motivate the nurses to take up self-development activity easily. I took some time to plan an initiative, which included setting up a staff development department with nurse educators who were MSN qualified. They would plan short-term curricula and give on-the-job training programs in continuing education format. These workshops and trainings took place across units. The department would also be responsible to conduct workshops, seminars, and conferences for the nurses and assign nurses to attend other units' trainings as well. They would also be responsible to identify key nursing personnel and recommend them for higher nursing education, which may be a two- or three-year full-time curriculum. The budget for this venture was high and getting it through was a herculean task. My argument was basic: If nurses were better developed educationally in the knowledge and skill sector, they would be better armed to practice and uplift their standards in nursing care. The beneficiaries would be patients and the hospital as a whole.

The nursing time spent for this program was incredibly valuable, as we were hoping and preparing for a result never before envisioned. The entire idea took numerous attempts from my side to be initiated and, finally, I was able to receive the support to put the initiative into practice. The condition: I would be held solely responsible for the outcome. I was confident it would be positive and that there would be wide and varied benefits over a period of time. Competitive nurses started exploring prospects of employment with the hospital because word of mouth had framed the institution to be one that was nurse centered. This was an accomplishment I was able to achieve with active determination and a venture I believed in. Many hospitals followed and were able to duplicate the model successfully. It was later integrated into policy after it was shown to be sustainable; it cannot be changed easily unless it is for the better.

A less publicly visible achievement, but one I keep close to my heart, was 30 years ago when I opted to be a nurse educator for nurses in the villages. It was an opportunity to initiate WHO objectives and I had chosen maternal and child health care. The equation here was simple: In India, 70% of the population was in villages and 70% of the nurses were in cities. Very few nurses opted to take the job—villages were very far; hence, the nurse educators had to reside in the village premises where basic amenities like water and electricity may not be available. Villagers, at times, were resistant to and dismissive of strangers from the city espousing health promotion and often refused to follow basic suggestions like vaccinations for neonates (Joel & Kelly, 1999).

I was able to set an example and achieve multiple targets for four years. My personal achievement here was the smile on the faces of all the villagers—developing a trustworthy relationship that led to the detection and subsequent treatment of many health problems. Developing countries have a long way to go to establish basic health amenities for all. The problems are magnified in a country where the infrastructure remains deplorable and poverty dominates. My contribution here was a drop in the ocean, an effort that requires duplication many times over in order to establish health access as a human right realized for all. I was able to train more than 200 potential nurses, after which students had to choose their potential future job. Unfortunately, many could not take up nursing as a career option due to the absence of job availability or for many of the other limitations mentioned earlier. But I tried . . . and there is satisfaction in that.

With the advent of India's new governmental pay scheme, many job opportunities have surfaced in rural India and bettered nursing services today (Clement, 2012). Over the years, nursing has changed for the better and I strongly believe that each nurse, wherever he or she is, makes an impact and leaves behind achievements, which always benefit someone. I have watched nurses in India evolve from submissive handmaidens to knowledgeably confident professionals. The opportunities for nurses to develop themselves have evolved tremendously; many of these avenues did not exist until a few years ago. A current increase in the number of educational institutions offering nursing education means that students no longer have to travel a long distance to pursue training. University curricula for BSN and MSN are now easily available for a large population in various states (Yalayyaswamy, 2012). More men are adapting to the idea of becoming nurses and the impact is felt positively as the public perception shifts from nursing as a female-dominated profession to a more inclusive one. A change in attitude is always a win for all involved. In most of the developing countries where nursing is considered to be a female-dominated profession in a male-dominated society, a rising ratio of men in the profession has its own way of making a powerful social statement (Newell, 2003).

Another trend that has changed—and was long overdue—is the tilting of the system toward university-recognized education. Remember, nursing in India's earlier years was predominantly a track for those individuals who could not afford education, and a diploma in nursing and midwifery was offered free of cost and included a stipend, free accommodation, and other expenses, such as uniform, library, and so forth. The course was sponsored by hospitals, which were "repaid over time" as nurses were required to work for the hospital for a said duration after program completion on terms decided by the hospital. Many of these nurses, after gaining the necessary experience, would look for opportunities to migrate internationally to the Middle Eastern countries, United States, United Kingdom, or Australia, to name a few. However, once many of these Western countries upgraded their own nursing education standards to baccalaureate-prepared nurses (Black, 2014), the need for BSN-prepared nurses in India skyrocketed. Many nurse aspirants looked for a university-recognized degree program and fewer students opted for diploma programs. Many diploma programs have had to close or restructure accordingly, increasing available programs to hundreds in each state. Education is no longer free and nurse aspirants have to avail themselves of an education loan from banks.

What has also changed due to this trend is the professional, societal, and overall value of nursing; the national status of nurses has bettered as more graduate nurses are able to contribute meaningful work in education, research, development, and practice. Education has also prepared these nurses with rights and empowered them to identify what they are entitled to. This also encourages more nurses to pursue their MSN and attain jobs in ever-expanding colleges of nursing. Those following aspirations of PhD studies are steadily increasing as well. This will ultimately allow nurses to be better armed, to have their say, and to be the ones who matter in their own profession.

All of these progressive changes have allowed me to revise my own opinions and perspectives about nursing for the better. I have new hopes about the potential for myself and for my colleagues. It may be easy for some to say that nursing has changed on a global scale for the better; however, the extent of the progress differs from nation to nation. The development also directly depends upon the economic reforms the country goes through; most of the developing nations maintain poor economic status and the development can be painfully slow.

At times, the language of communication makes a difference in professional unity and evolution. India, for instance, has around 1,721 spoken languages (Chandrachood, 2013) and nursing is predominantly coordinated only in English, a hurdle far too substantial for many to overcome. But over a period of years, many have learned to master or at least get basic knowhow of the language, in order to find a way to enter the nursing education system.

My personal and professional focus on nursing today is on its development, autonomy, recognition, and equality status. No development can be considered as a fixed target that may someday be reached. There is no end to the journey of individual and collective development, especially in the arena of continuous health care advancement. Nurses need to be directed and assisted through an ever-evolving developmental process, be that in a respective clinical field, research, education, or nursing administration. This must be a goal for many nursing heads in order to make it achievable; I have always felt we need to create the beginning we want rather than wait for an opportunistic tide to take us forward.

It is heartwarming to see that nurses have better independence in decision making and now have autonomy in many health care settings. I am personally quite independent in both my organization and my role as head of the Maharashtra state branch of the TNAI. This still has a long way to go, for many hospitals still provide a job description to nurses that undermines their individual and professional skills and limits them to following instructions given by a physician (Black, 2014). Independence to think, to act accordingly, and to be proudly and courageously nurse-centric is what one aims to look forward to one day.

I will continue to work for nurses to get them better recognition as independent professionals. Nursing today is perceived in a much better light than it was many decades ago. It can do still better. It needs to get recognition as a profession at par with any other so-called white-collar profession. A nurse is a vital foundational aspect of health care and has to be recognized for his or her thought processes, contributions, and roles when significant decisions affecting him or her are at stake. Nurses' inputs cannot be overlooked; they hold the answers.

The nursing role is equally important and tantamount in relevance to that of any other health care personnel. Nurses must learn how to be assertive and need to be supported by leaders from across the discipline responsible for taking action to avoid role discrimination.

■ MORAL/ETHICAL FOUNDATION

Ethical considerations are the core of any patient care activity and should always be given preference in clinical decision making. For me, ethical values are the core ideals that all nurses must abide by with every step they take. In a country like India, where ethical practices are often considered optional and reliant on an individual's discretion, the necessity of teaching nurses to adopt morally informed methods of practice as a personal priority and professional responsibility cannot be understated.

Each nurse takes actions related to critical patient decisions on a daily basis and it is the moral responsibility of each nurse to carry out each task ethically. One such responsibility is to be stringent in enforcing a policy decision that would disallow unqualified or nonregistered nurses from practice. Another is to ensure an apt and just nurse:patient ratio; it is unethical to load nurses beyond their capacity and create a situation liable for errors (Blais & Hayes, 2016). It is also important that one does not exploit nurses by giving them substandard salaries. It is important to practice fair wages in nursing, especially in the absence of a legal backup.

Nurses are often torn and apprehensive in decision management after a disaster situation when attending to victims of bomb blasts, earthquakes, and floods (Jamerson, Hornberger, & Sullivan, 2001). It is vital to aid nurses who are at the center of care in making morally grounded and humanely informed decisions. Nurses need to receive such assistance in the form of guidelines and leadership support to avoid enacting poorly rationalized personalized decisions in critical situations. After the 2008 terrorist blasts rocked Mumbai, I stood alongside my clinical nurses who cared for perpetrators and victims alike, helping them to see their role clearly and assisting them in attending to their ethical responsibilities as nurses.

Often I have seen nurses becoming uncertain regarding situations when they have to refrain from sending the patient to the operating room because the patient has not deposited the necessary amount at the cash counter. This is a dilemma found throughout nursing practice in low- and middle-income countries. Nurses hesitate to act and to care for others when they are charged with assessing whether a patient can pay for a service. What is the role we want to remind our nurses of—that of cashier or that of humane provider of care?

Most of the time in India, moral and ethical decisions for the nurse are related to a patient's financial situation (Healey, 2013). Here, the nurse needs clear guidelines when he or she cannot initiate a nursing process or administer a drug that the client cannot afford. We cannot leave our precious clinicians in the dark to fend for themselves on this ethical battlefield. These are times when we assist with processes that allow the nurse to guide the patient's family to seek financial assistance. Here the nurse can be trained to direct the family to various resources that assist with financial aids and loans. This allows the nurse to advocate for the patient in a new way.

Many times, a patient's spiritual beliefs differ from the nurse's. In India, with multiple and still-followed castes, religions, and sects, nurses need to give due importance to the worldview and practices of the patient (Umamani, 2011). Additionally, the gender of the nurse plays an important role, as many female patients will not allow a male nurse to care for them. Similarly, gynecological, obstetrical, or urinary procedures for a female patient may be permissible only to female nurses. The same is applicable when a female nurse has to catheterize a male client. As a nurse leader, I would advocate to have clearly defined policies that benefit the client and also direct the nurse, keeping the sentiments and dignity of all in mind.

Should ethical dilemmas be highlighted in the educational curriculum? The answer here is yes. It allows the nurse to get a clear indication of his or her position, power, and obligation from the very beginning.

■ VISION

What more may be achieved in nursing? On no occasion should we ever say that our goal in nursing is achieved. As an ever-maturing science, nursing is a field where we want to continuously achieve more, primarily because nursing is all about promoting betterment of the human condition, and there is no limit to that possibility.

Nurses need to find their community. I am the nursing director of P.D. Hinduja National Hospital, a charitable hospital in Mumbai, and I oversee more than 750 nurses with the help of only a handful of nursing managers. I know every nurse by name. My goal is that they feel appreciated. I want them to know they matter and that they have a place here . . . as nurses . . . just as they are. This type of community is possible as nurse leaders reassess what is most important to them as people and as professionals.

On a more global scale, community is just as necessary. I sit on the International Board of Directors for the Nightingale Initiative for Global Health (NIGH, 2016; for more information on NIGH, see Chapters 4 and 18). This international forum provides nurses connection and inspiration they may not otherwise have access to. It gives them voices where they are voiceless and opportunities where there are none in sight. We need more of this visionary leadership that helps nurses around the world feel a part of something bigger than themselves.

In the developing countries, many of my colleagues and I envision a period where we can experience a decrease in the international migration of nurses. Nurses of many underdeveloped and developing countries look forward to being in this profession, less for the love of it and more for the economic opportunities they will encounter when they can migrate out of the country to work as travel nurses. Many countries are able to meet their shortfalls by recruiting nurses from these countries, and are able to provide a salary and general infrastructure which are far superior due to better economic conditions. The parent country, however, due to its inabilities to give nurses better status, recognition, esteem, appropriate remuneration, and an honorable lifestyle, continues to lose valuable nurses to international destinations (Thomas, 2014). I look forward to a better reality for nurses within their countries of origin and a future when nurses do not have to emigrate from their homes for want of a feasible lifestyle or much-deserved recognition.

A lot still has to be achieved in India and in the developing countries. The population, in general, still looks upon nurses as dependent on doctors for instructions and directions. I envision a professional status that allows nursing to be fully recognized as having an independent role, dignity within its work force, and its own body of knowledge. A society depends largely upon the cultural scenario at hand and its interpretation of various professions. I hope to continue encouraging nurses who may more positively shift the opinions of the general public by writing in non-nursing newspapers and journals about the profession and its advancements, explaining the roles of specialized nurses and about the impact on society's health when nurses climb the educational ladder. Nurses must learn to use multimedia venues to highlight their achievements and vital role in health care.

Nurses need to feel proud to be nurses. Such a vision is achieved by empowering nurses to stand up for themselves, encouraging them to be assertive, and guiding them to become part of a professional body. To a certain extent, the entire system is responsible. I make this statement based on the existing system of nurse registration in India mentioned earlier, where a nurse registers licensure and renews the registration through payment of designated fees. I recommend a system that promotes and requires professional growth as a necessary component of license renewal. A nurse needs to be motivated to continue self-development through credits achieved via continuing education programs, writing professional articles, attending conferences, presenting papers, and so forth. His or her work with education programs should be recognized by offering him or her credits when renewing. Multiple nurse achievement recognition modalities have yet to be created and honored. This could be one way of enhancing nursing as a fully embodied profession in India.

I think I am very fortunate to say I have been well recognized for the positive changes I have been able and continue to implement in my career. It is what I was *not* able to do that makes me ponder the long road ahead with so much yet to achieve.

I want nurses to know what I never knew when I started my career: Nursing is a career with extremely bright prospects; but do not expect results without working for them. This multidimensional profession has unlimited career pathways to choose from, but you have to take consistent and disciplined efforts and decide on the one that calls your soul.

For prospective Indian nursing students, learn your resources to lessen the strain of taking financial loans. I never knew the support systems available through the TNAI, the Indian Nursing Council, or the Ratan Tata Foundation, all of which offer partial or full tuition fees to help you. Many national nurse leaders support ambitious nurses and if a few lines are penned to them, they will readily help.

I have also learned the hard way that nurses' opinions are respected by all. Nurses need to be encouraged to speak out, whether it be for patients, against the system, or to advocate a positive change. Many stakeholders can be influenced by a solidly informed nursing opinion and will aid in bringing about the necessary change accordingly.

Nursing is a process to which each nurse gets accustomed through the lens of her or his specialty. One must never become so comfortable that one denies the need to mature, evolve, and grow as a nurse. It is a great privilege for me to belong to this great profession and use my best efforts to contribute to it in all ways.

■ REFLECTIONS

1. *Each nurse has a story to tell. Do we, as nurses, have enough people to listen? How can I create an avenue for nurses' voices to be heard?*
2. *Nursing was established by our founder, Florence Nightingale, to care for the ill and vulnerable. Have we, as a profession, lost this foundational platform of caring? How can I help to reintroduce it?*
3. *NIGH is an organization by the nurses and for the nurses. How can I inspire the nurses of my community to partake? What do I envision for the future of NIGH?*
4. *Our patients are our goals. We need to be accountable for our patients' well-being. What needs to be done in order for the system to support nurses in this endeavor?*
5. *In several developing countries, the existence of many languages and many nurses who are not so tech savvy can lead to intraprofessional confusion and disagreement. What is my vision of how nursing can be communicated to all in a way that nurses understand—in a language familiar to them—the language of nurses?*

■ REFERENCES

Banerjee, S. (2014). Transactional analysis. *Asian Journal of Cardiovascular Nursing, 22*(2), 22–24.

Black, B. P. (2014). *Professional nursing: Concepts & challenges* (7th ed.). St. Louis, MO: Saunders.

Blais, K. K., & Hayes, J. S. (2016). *Professional nursing practice: Concepts and perspectives* (7th ed.). Upper Saddle River, NJ: Prentice Hall.

Chandrachood, B. (2013). Concepts and issues—Nurses as policy makers. *Indian Journal of Continuing Nursing Education, 14*(2), 11–15.

Clement, I. (2011). *Management of nursing services and education.* New Delhi, India: Elsevier.

Clement, I. (2012). *Manual of community health nursing.* New Delhi, India: Jaypee Brothers Medical Publishers.

Healey, M. (2013). *Indian sisters: A history of nursing and the state,* 1907-2007. New Delhi, India: Routledge.

Jamerson, P. A., Hornberger, C. A., & Sullivan, E. J. (2001). *Nursing leadership and management in action workbook* (2nd ed.). Upper Saddle River, NJ: Prentice Hall.

Joel, L. A., & Kelly, L. Y. (1999). *Dimensions of professional nursing* (8th ed.). New York, NY: McGraw-Hill.

Kalita, N. (2014). Effectiveness of structured teaching program on the level of practice of communication skill among nurses. *Journal of Nursing Research Society of India, 7*(2), 23–25.

Kaur, N. B. (2014). *Textbook of advanced nursing practice (As per the syllabus of INC for MSc students).* New Delhi, India: Jaypee Brothers Medical Publishers.

Manjrekar, P. (2014, May 12). *Excerpt from International Nurses Day speech* (from author's notes).

Newell, R. (Ed.). (2003). *Developing your career in nursing.* London, UK: Sage.

Nightingale Initiative for Global Health (NIGH). (2016). Home. Retrieved from http://www.nighvision.net

Sharma, M. C. (2010). *Textbook for nursing education for BSc and post basic nursing students: Communication and education technology.* New Delhi, India: Jaypee Brothers Medical Publishers.

Thomas, P. (2014). Indian perspective on migration of health professionals from India. *The Nursing Journal of India, 105*(6), 244–247.

Umamani, K. (2011). *NRHM at crossroads: An appraisal from Karnataka, India.* Germany: Lambert Academic Publishing.

Vallee, G. (Ed.). (2006). *Florence Nightingale on health in India: Collected works of Florence Nightingale* (Vol. 9, No. 9). Waterloo, Ontario, Canada: Wilfrid Laurier University Press.

Yalayyaswamy, N. N. (2012). *Ward management and supervision and professional adjustments and trends for nurses in India.* Bengaluru, Karnataka, India: CBS Publishers & Distributors.

CHAPTER TWENTY-SIX

Awakened and Conscious: Reclaiming Lost Power and Intraprofessional Identity

William Rosa

The core community values that emerge from and define nursing are a matter of consciousness. . . . Such a community implies that nurses [ensure] the integrity of the human experience, serve as advocates of moral/ethical engagement, and are the embodiment of the sacred, if we so choose to honor it.

—Rosa (2014a, p. 246)

■ WHY NURSING?

My mother was an administrative assistant at a local hospital when I was growing up and I often spent my days off from school and weeks of summer vacation with her. I learned how to file, type, answer phones, and how to talk to people. But I also learned a lot about dynamics and power and politics. Coworkers of my mother would constantly approach me with the inevitable "What do you want to be when you grow up?" I would insecurely respond with a childlike ambivalence, "I don't know yet." They would go on to tell me how I could be a physician who managed a hospital, ran a practice, or performed surgery. No one ever suggested to me that I could be, might be, and would end up being a nurse.

I spent years quietly observing the nurse–physician exchange in clinical, administrative, and interpersonal scenarios. I watched as nurses surrendered their seats to physicians, cleared a path for them in the hallways, and stood in silence as they were overlooked in a patient's room. I saw them perch in attention with an obligatory, "Good morning, Dr. Smith," only to receive a fleeting, "Hi, Becky," or, a simple "Becky," accompanied with an inauthentic nod of the head. I sat at lunches and meetings where physicians were lauded for their latest accomplishment or successful money-driving contribution to the institution and led patient rounds in wards where no nurse was welcomed to participate.

There was a definitive power differential established in that young boy's mind; a greater than/less than relationship, painting physicians as wise, worthy, and beyond reproach and nurses as unintelligent, unfit, and incapable. In his mind, nurses were a group of mostly women, considered subservient, and dispensable. There was no notable nursing leadership counterpart to the physician colleague; nursing allowed itself to be defined by Other without any internal compass of pride or intraprofessional sense of Self.

I grew up and became a working actor and dancer for years before experiencing a traumatic hip fracture that rendered me unable to perform. After not walking for several months, I entered massage therapy school for healing, quiet, and reflection. I was honored to have the privilege of therapeutically placing my hands on clients and amazed to see how my applied techniques, care plans, and, oftentimes, just my presence and deep listening, lessened their symptoms. By the end of the education, I was being called to delve deeper into the caring professions and discover a career that would allow me to practice and cultivate healing for my clients, and for myself, in more diverse settings.

My vision of nursing at the time was largely tainted by the experiences of my boyhood. Though I was initially very attracted to the idea of spending extended amounts of time with my patients, the potential flexibility of movement between clinical specialties, and the possibility of advanced education toward becoming a nurse anesthetist or nurse practitioner, I somehow maintained that deep-seated belief that nursing was a profession composed mostly of women, considered subservient and dispensable. At the time, I made the conscious choice to enter a profession that I subconsciously believed was "less than," and there was a part of me that felt like I was settling. I could not quite let go of the impressions left behind by the power differentials witnessed as a young person.

I believed a nurse was someone who dispensed medication, tended primarily to the unpleasant bedside realities of the human digestive system, and worked the hardest with the least amount of appreciation. But for some reason it continued to call me. It called my mind to consider new ways of being. It called my hands toward new ways of doing. And it called my heart to grow in its capacity for human connection and relationship.

Inspired by my newly found call to healing, nursing school created an ongoing quandary for me: How was I to integrate a caring presence and intentionality into the endless to-do list of a staff nurse? I was not sure how the healing moments and person-centered care I shared with clients as a massage therapist would translate into a major urban academic medical center and the organized chaos that often sets the tone for acute patient care settings. In retrospect, I know nothing has opened my heart and mind or clarified my purpose, ethics, and convictions more than the relationships I have fostered with both Self and Other as a nurse.

■ EARLY IMPRESSIONS

My first day on the floor was preceded by two weeks in hospital orientation classes reviewing every bit of anatomy, physiology, and intensive care unit (ICU) intervention that was basic to critical care nursing and would aid me in the day-to-day goings-on of the unit. I was a half an hour early for my shift, as I had heard vivid accounts of staff stampeding toward the elevator bank vying for the rare spot. Safely inside the elevator doors, I closed my eyes and focused on breathing. I tried to think less of how people were knocking into me and stepping on my feet and more on the fact that I was needed here: I was a nurse. I wanted to help people. I just knew I would make a difference. I finally exited the mayhem of elevator world and awkwardly stumbled onto the critical care unit.

People who know me also know it is not characteristic of me to "awkwardly stumble." But I was so caught off guard. I have honestly never seen such seemingly unhappy people in my life. People in white lab coats looking deep in thought as they pondered life-and-death decisions; a rainbow of scrubs running in and out of rooms motivated by something occurring behind closed curtains; visitors looking lost and timidly gesturing to passers-by for help; alarms and bells ringing with nagging consistency; a scary place. This was the place—the scary place, mind you—in which I was to become not only functional but also proficient. It was a place that was recently renovated but had somehow maintained a bare and inhospitable essence.

Upon first experiencing it, there was no human warmth visible to me. That being said, I was a newbie and I am sure my expectations were lofty in comparison to the clinical realities of 12-hour critical care nursing shift. I had no possible way of understanding the emotional exhaustion of caring for patients and families facing health crises, supporting them in making end-of-life decisions, and then being the one to carry those decisions out; the mental drain on the nurse who is balancing the care of two severely ill patients while advocating for early and adequate medical intervention, maintaining practice standards, meeting documentation requirements, responding to emergencies, and managing the multidisciplinary plan of care; the fatigue of one's feet and back after a shift of running up and down the halls, rotating in to do compressions, turning patients, squatting, bending, reaching, and fixing; the spiritual depletion and distress of disagreeing with ethical decisions and seeing human beings be reduced to "objects" and "things" while attempting to ensure the preservation of their dignity; the long-term and multidimensional impacts of witnessing the suffering of Others in a bureaucratically constrained practice environment and the unending Self-interrogation of doubt that ensues, "Did I do *absolutely everything* I could?" How could I have known? It was just my first day.

I remember letting a nurse by the desk know I was here for orientation to see if she could help, and it was made clear to me I was more of an imposition than anything else. During shift report, I heard senior staff discussing other colleagues and defining other nurses' worth by their knowledge deficits. There were open discussions about how "their" skills and, therefore, they as people, were inferior—my first exposure to nurse-to-nurse bullying behavior. I remember a nurse walking by who had only been there a few months, and one more seasoned nurse turned to another while we were standing in the patient's room to say, "That one is an assassin!" He was suggesting that her poor nursing care had been the cause of patient decompensation and injury. How horrible! I could not imagine any environment where that kind of judgment and aggression were warranted. Did he make time to educate her? To mentor her? To help her? No. The pressure was on to pay attention and to be perfect. It was only after being a nurse for some time that I realized perfection does not exist in anything or anyone and we are all accountable for the judgments we hold and express against other people.

All day I remember colleagues being more concerned with my assessment skills than my ability to engage with the human being in the bed. I understand I was a novice and orientation is primarily geared toward building the techniques and the aptitudes required in prioritizing nursing care, but there was a vital component missing from my orientation process, and that was a focus on the very fragile, very humane, and very human work of nursing.

In my first two years as a nurse, I was passionate about learning the science of critical care: ventilators, balloon pumps, continuous renal replacement therapies, pulmonary artery catheters; being effective as a part of the team in patient emergencies; and managing the symptomatic instabilities of multiple pathologies. I had been determined to go to nurse anesthesia school and focused my continuing education on sedation, ventilator weaning, and adequate pain management. As I continued to pursue this goal, I slowly came to realize that my most profound joys came from building meaningful, empathic, and healing relationships with my patients and their families, and not out of a passion for anesthesia. My job became more about spending time with them and knowing them as human beings in need of knowledgeable, expert caring and less centralized around the expertise of any particular clinical skill. Nursing became more about giving people voice, acknowledging their pain, offering them authentic presence amid their vulnerability and suffering, showing gentleness and love in their struggles with fear and uncertainty, and holding a space for them that provided safety, comfort, and an opportunity for hope.

Early in my career, I had an experience that helped me personalize, in a single exchange, the ripple effects of what Watson (2008) calls the *caring moment*, that instance of caring defined by a mutual exchange of shared humanity between nurse and patient that exists in that moment in time, but also transcends that moment, forever becoming a part of the life histories and future life experiences of Self and Other.

> The transpersonal nature of the caring relationship occurs when the nurse is able to connect with the spirit of the other . . . [and] invites full loving-kindness and equanimity of one's presence-in-the-moment, with an understanding that a significant caring moment can be a turning point in one's life. (Watson, 2008, pp. 78–79; see Chapter 16 for more information on caring science)

I was in that crowded elevator I described earlier, gripping my coffee cup for fear of it being knocked and spilled before I had a chance to caffeinate. There were no less than 18 or 20 people in that stifling, suffocating space when from the other side I heard a woman's voice say loudly—with what (to this New Yorker) sounded like a confrontational anger—"You!" And, yes, she was staring right at me. And so everyone else was now staring at me. All I could think to myself as my face reddened and I broke out in a cool sweat was, "I haven't even had my coffee yet!" Like clockwork, all 18 to 20 people exited the elevator on the next floor, and the confrontational, angry woman and I were left alone. I melted as I worked up a weak "Hi."

"You're Billy," she said.

"Yes, I'm sorry, please remind me how I know you."

"You took care of my mother when she was dying in the ICU." I quickly searched the corners and cobwebs of my memory but—nope—nothing. I could not for the life of me remember this woman. I did not recognize her face and I certainly had no clue of her name. I did a quick and detailed ethical inventory. Had I harmed someone? Did I do something wrong? Had I lied or stolen or cheated? Negative. I was completely blank.

As she looked at me, her face softened and she dropped her shoulders. She began to cry and said,

Me and my sister talk about you all the time and how you treated us like we were *your* sisters. We can't talk about my mom without talking about you because you made sure she was treated like a human being when she was dying and you treated us like we were family. You made sure she died well and to see her in peace and not in pain made everything else so much easier. I just can't believe I'm seeing you right now so I can say "thank you."

The elevator stopped at the 15th floor and it was time for me to leave. I looked at her and just said, "It was my honor to be there with you during that important time in your life. Please give my love to your family and thank you for sharing that with me."

And the best part—I left the elevator still not knowing her name or remembering who her mother was. And it did not matter one bit! I had done my job as a human being and as a nurse. I had genuinely cared for another and been open to receiving, embracing, and participating in the journey. I realized I had just experienced the far-reaching mind-body-spirit effects of that transpersonal caring moment.

And I really got it—nursing is so much more than anything we can comprehend at the technical-clinical-medical level. It incorporates expert scientific knowledge and skill and yet transcends it completely. I had affected how this human being saw living and dying, how she thought of her family and related to them, her views on nursing and health care, and how she will forever remember her mother. And now she has forever changed my understanding of my profession, the *real work* of nursing, and the ability of nurses to deeply affect another's life story, at layers and in ways we may never see or understand. She and I are now forever connected through a moment in time that continues to affect how we see and relate to the world around us.

I came to see and understand more and more clearly the depths of unclaimed power that nurses wield unconsciously—the ability we have to guide and direct the wellness and thriving or the stagnation and dehumanization of a fellow human being. I recognized the need for nurses to become more conscious of their gifts and more awakened to their true purpose. I saw the need to reclaim and redefine intraprofessional identity and to educate nurses about how they are integral not just to the circumstantial unfolding of another's illness but also to their lives and to their living.

Being a critical care nurse became increasingly more challenging as I was required to focus exponentially increasing amounts of time on electronic health record documentation, participate in hospital-based initiatives and unit projects, precept new orientees to the unit, and manage the unfolding daily reality of the patient care plan as my many interdisciplinary partners ordered countless consults and procedures. Not only was I witnessing the dehumanization of the nurse–patient environment in action, a setting defined and valued by the tasks accomplished and measurable outcomes determined, but also the degradation of nurse–nurse, nurse–interdisciplinary partner, and nurse–system relationships. Time became of the essence and it became impossible to meet managerial and institutional expectations of work while attending to the continuously emerging needs of the patient's human experience. There was an inner–outer power struggle between my ethical obligation to care for the biological, social, environmental, emotional, mental, and spiritual dimensions of the patient and my ability to ensure the safe, integral, and dignified delivery of such care.

In fact, I had become both detached and angry. In the months after I left the bedside, I pulled nurse colleagues aside and made phone calls to restore my integrity and make amends for my behaviors of the past that were rude or inconsiderate and not reflective of "my best Self." I asked for forgiveness and engaged in self-forgiveness practices. What I had come to realize was that I had become so overwhelmed by the pain I witnessed and the struggles I experienced in trying to advocate for the human being in the bed that I often misdirected it with unrealistic expectations of others, long-standing grudges, and a significant neglect of my own Self-care. Through forgiveness I came to know both my Self and Others again in a new light and learned over time that "by forgiving and reclaiming the power we have lost through harboring feelings of unrest, we create a clearing for the true ethical foundation of personal and professional altruism and loving-kindness to be sparked and nurtured" (Rosa, 2015a, p. 216).

As painful as it was to admit to myself, it was time to move on.

■ PROFESSIONAL EVOLUTION/CONTRIBUTION

Throughout my graduate studies as a nurse practitioner, I became consistently disappointed regarding how the profession was defining itself. It seemed the premise of advanced education in nursing was about validating nurses as useful and necessary health care delivery agents through their mere rote and consistent comparison to other professions. There was little intradisciplinary or intraprofessional celebration of what makes nursing a unique art and science. It is an uncomfortable and somewhat vulnerable thing to admit, but I can legitimately say that by the end of my master's degree, I was unable to articulate what truly made me a *nurse* of advanced practice, and what values, contributions, and discipline-specific skills defined the role, as opposed to that of a technician, physician's assistant, or substandard physician. And I was torn: I did not feel as if the *nursing* part of my education was sufficient (with the exception of one nursing theory class that changed my perspectives on what nursing could be), but I also did not believe the medical–technical skills I was learning were adequate to deliver exemplary *medical* care, and yet the roles I saw advanced practice nurses (nurses in italics please) filling seemed to exist primarily within that *medical* model. It was a personal–professional identity crisis that left me returning to those early insecurities of power differentials and greater than/less than.

I was determined to make sense of it and take a bold stand for my perspectives. Though I was challenged on my choice of graduate thesis because it was not "scientific enough" or "grounded in clinical practice," I felt it was an essential conversation that needed to be had and I did not take "no" for an answer. After proving myself as a writer and showing that this was a topic being discussed at a national level, I was given permission to examine and reexplore Nightingale's first assumption, identified by Fondriest and Osborne: Nursing is separate from medicine (as cited in Dunphy, 2010). The goal of the capstone assignment was to create a publishable paper and I promised that if I was given the green light, I would be determined to see mine in print. As it turned out, I was the first in my class to have my capstone published (Rosa, 2014b), and it was out before the end of my last semester. It meant a lot to me that I had to advocate so hard for my voice to be heard in a way that yielded meaning for me and was overjoyed to see it given space in an international journal. It was a major lesson on holding steadfast to my beliefs and convictions in the face of doubt and disagreement, and the flexibility required to help others see things from my point of view. It was all about saying things in a way that others could receive.

In the capstone paper, "Nursing is Separate from Medicine: Advanced Practice Nursing and a Transpersonal Plan of Care," I highlight the need for further medical and scientific education for advanced practice registered nurses (APRNs) to meet both nursing and physician shortages; discuss society's varying perceptions of the APRN, ranging from "little doctor" to "midlevel practitioner"; and emphasize the importance of a theory-based educational foundation for nursing so that practice is informed from a nursing-specific, humanistic worldview. I suggest that there is a way to inform the administrative, bureaucratic, and medical requirements of bedside nursing and advanced practice alike with the caring, moral/ethical foundations of Nightingalean philosophy, returning the art and heart of nursing to a "spiritual practice of unique and profound character" (p. 81). From my perspective, autonomous APRN practice, prescriptive authority, and expanded scopes of practice are all reflective of needed health care reform and evolution, but there is a necessary and called-for acknowledgment of the core altruistic ideals that do, in fact, provide the cornerstone of our roles as nurses.

Watson (2008) describes the quintessential aspect of nursing as a caring presence, which influences all ways of being, doing, and knowing. If caring is the core of nursing practice, the center from which all skill, technique, and clinical savvy extend, then logic suggests that the absence of such caring perceptions, attitudes, and behaviors is, indeed, the absence of nursing. Understanding the underlying moral and ethical implications of nursing implies that it is irresponsible, disingenuous, and in fact unethical *not* to care (Rosa, 2014c). There is a stark contrast between the doing of no harm and the intentional, impactful doing of good (maleficence vs. beneficence). If nursing fails to do good, to defend, protect, promote, and prioritize the dignified human experience as crucial to ethical praxis, then "we fail to actualize the virtuous possibilities of our own legacy and we become passive" (Rosa, 2014c, p. 265). The passive nurse is that practitioner who may not do outright harm but ceases to cultivate and create environments of good. This is the practitioner detached from the cultural, historical, and foundational roots of nursing.

The absence of this fundamental and idealistic culture of nursing is evidenced throughout the literature in the form of nursing-specific malignancies; pathologies metastasizing throughout the professional community in the form of compassion fatigue, burnout, moral distress, and nurse-to-nurse bullying (Rosa, 2014a). For years, I watched burned-out and fatigued nurses provide subpar care for themselves and their patients, nurse bullies deriving a sense of esteem and power from belittling coworkers, and clinicians being placed in personally divisive circumstances when ordered to deliver care they perceived as unethical. The inability to embody and personalize the aforementioned core values of caring and moral/ethical integrity that give rise to the discipline and delineate nursing's overarching professional scope leads to a depersonalizing, dehumanizing, and degrading of Self, Other, and the collective (Rosa, 2014a). This became clear to me in clinical practice. Nurses required caring and healing environments not only for their patients but also for themselves. A return to the embodiment of ethical praxis honors the universal law that we are each a part of each other's journey, the healing of one supporting and elevating the healing of the whole (Watson, 2005).

Imperative to realizing the unique humane contributions of nursing is an understanding of and relationship with personal/professional healing. Undeniably, Nightingale's primary tenet was healing, a unifying principle for nurses and nursing (Dossey, Selanders, Beck, & Attewell, 2005). While traversing the path of individual healing, one can explore how he or she relates to the values inherent in the 10 Caritas Processes™, as shown in Table 26.1. This personalized inventory guides the nurse to explore Self-care strengths

TABLE 26.1 **Translating the Global to the Personal: In Process With Self**

Global Translations—10 Caritas Processes™	Reflective Caritas Inventory for the Individual Processes of Self-Healing
1. Embrace altruistic values and practice loving kindness with self and others.	*Have I set an intention of self-caring and self-kindness today? Have I centered myself with an act of self-love so that I might be restored?*
2. Instill faith and hope and honor others.	*Am I clear about what I have faith in? Have I reminded myself of the people, places, and spaces that give me hope?*
3. Be sensitive to self and others by nurturing individual beliefs & practices.	*Have I responded to my thoughts and feelings today with gentleness, knowing that my experience is unique and sacred?*
4. Develop helping-trusting-caring relationships.	*Have I empowered myself to release toxic relationships and embrace supportive connections in my life with truth and vulnerability? Just for today, can I trust myself to be there for me?*
5. Promote and accept positive and negative feelings as you authentically listen to another's story.	*Have I authentically accepted my own story? Do I fully embrace all aspects of who I am: the positive and the negative, the light and the dark?*
6. Use creative scientific problem-solving methods for caring decision making.	*Do I recognize how creative I am? Have I celebrated my "me-ness" in how I approach, interact with, and inspire this world around me?*
7. Share teaching and learning that addresses the individual needs and comprehension styles.	*Am I forthcoming about my needs at work and at home? Do I remain flexible and energized or easily tire with my old patterns of rigidity?*
8. Create a healing environment for the physical and spiritual self, which respects human dignity.	*Have I physically or energetically touched my heart today? Have I connected with my own heartbeat, the same heartbeat shared by all of humanity? Have I admitted to myself that my healing starts within?*
9. Assist with basic physical, emotional, and spiritual human needs.	*Have I paused to attend to my own hunger? My anxiety? My worries? My frustrations? Do I recognize my individual needs as valid?*
10. Open to mystery and allow miracles to enter.	*Can I release the need to be certain, to explain, defend, protect, and define? Can I surrender to the moment and allow life to unfold as it will?*

Note: Jean Watson's 10 Caritas Processes™ (Watson Caring Science Institute, 2013) are paired with questions for personalized self-reflection. The Reflective Caritas Inventory, developed by William Rosa, can be used to examine individual processes of self-healing.

and deficits, highlights opportunities to improve Self-reflective practices, and returns Self to a space of inward focus for continued mental-emotional-spiritual well-being (Rosa, 2014d). In essence, the inventory utilizes Self-awareness to encourage and motivate Self-care by relating global and universal principles to the process of Self-actualization. The art of vital, healthy, integrative nursing "requires ongoing inquiry into and cultivation of the true [S]elf, along with a careful tending of that [S]elf, which is the instrument for healing" (Quinn, 2014, p. 20).

Healing of Self remains only one part of recovery of the nursing community's identity loss; there must be concurrent, intentional, and continual focus on healing of the system. The systems we create and sustain are and can be only as healthy as the individuals comprising them; sick nurses lead to sick systems unable to engender healing spaces, healing practices, or healing experiences for patients (Rosa, 2014e). We must strive to illuminate awareness of the systems nurses represent and partake in through the application of systemic inventories, as shown in Table 26.2. This process of relating personal perspectives to the global health of the collective can aid in identifying new mechanisms for how nurses interact with and contribute to their institutional environments, how personal action influences system-wide outcomes, and how health care facilities' treatment of human beings, largely managed and defined by the quality of nursing care, represents to society the moral and ethical intentions of the profession. Table 26.2 pertains more specifically to caring for patients at end of life, but similar system inventories can be utilized to increase the consciousness and awareness surrounding health care delivery across the wellness–illness, living–dying continuum.

It remains vital, in both the midst of current disciplinary circumstances and the anticipation of future professional possibilities, to continually evaluate, question, and correlate Self in relation to system. It is in modifying these reflective inventories to individual needs and work settings for the improvement of Self and system that nurses fulfill their covenant with society to be ethical, sound, dependable, and integral providers of precious human caring (Watson, 2012). It is through applied mindfulness practices, such as inventory work, that nurses will realize that the internal world of thought and the external world of action are one (Sitzman & Watson, 2014); intention is not enough—caring and a commitment to caring practices must become a demonstrated and lived experience.

The story of human caring in the world is the loving result of personal narratives becoming intertwined over time; the merging of individual human paths toward the open road of unitary oneness (Rosa, 2014f). The moment one being engages another, both the carer and the cared-for create an eternal prayer of intimacy, authenticity, and presence essential to the healing of the human race (Watson, 2008; Rosa, 2014f). In fact, in demonstrating compassionate care for another during the cycle of their living-wellness-illness-dying, with the ethical tenets of human caring intact, both the healer and the healed restore their very being, allowing for the potential embodiment of their very becoming (Rosa, 2014g). It is in this transpersonal experience, this evolutionary moment, that nurses and nursing have the humble privilege to personify the humanization of love in action: magnificent, ethical, cosmic praxis. (See Chapter 20 for more on nurse caring as love in action.)

This pinnacle of the nursing experience is the result of aligning thought, behavior, emotion, and intention with a consciousness of caring-healing-loving. In the exchange

TABLE 26.2 **Translating the Personal to the Global: In Process With System**

Conscious Dying Principles©	Reflective Systems Inventory for the Collective Processes of Global Healing
1. Increase beauty, pleasure, contentment.	*Does the system provide space for beauty? Do I see patients having time to value and partake in pleasure?*
2. Provide emotional and spiritual support.	*Have organizations attended to the spiritual needs of the patient today? Has this human being been emotionally seen, heard, and acknowledged today?*
3. Initiate conversations about dying process.	*Are my colleagues and I comfortable talking about the process of death? Is the patient aware that death is a process?*
4. Practice self-care to prevent burnout and emotional fatigue.	*Are the connections clear between my own self-care and the care I provide for my patient? Can I coidentify with the vulnerability of my patient and gently attend to my own self-care needs?*
5. Demystify the stages of the dying process.	*Am I clear about the mental-emotional-spiritual stages of the dying process? Is the patient attended to throughout the spectrum? Is there a dissonance between my knowledge and patient needs?*
6. Acknowledge mysteries, miracles, and unexplained events.	*Am I uncomfortable with the mystical? If yes, am I able to validate and share the patient's subjective experiences within this realm despite my discomfort?*
7. Learn how to be with intense emotions.	*Do systems "lean into" the difficult emotions? Can we guide providers to invest in and engage with the actual, moment-to-moment story of our patients and families?*
8. Honor others' beliefs without them threatening your own.	*Are systems able to release agendas selflessly to support patient beliefs with flexibility? How can we facilitate and empower individualism through compassionate advocacy and empathy?*
9. Be a steward of conscious deaths.	*Do we see systems pave the path for peaceful transitions with integrity? How can we humanize dying by creating an environment of dignity and adequate preparation?*
10. Attend at bedside—no one dies alone.	*Are systems actualizing the needs of human presence and touch? How can we systematically rationalize the unquestionable need to bear witness?*

Note: Tarron Estes's Conscious Dying Principles (Estes, 2011) are paired with questions for the collective processes of global healing. The Reflective Systems Inventory, developed by William Rosa, can be used to reflect on the quality of end-of-life care within health systems.

between a nurse of such consciousness and a patient in need of nursing care, space is created for miraculous realizations of hope, unity, and a deeper understanding of the human–spirit journey. The nurse–patient encounter of such magnitude requires a level of authenticity, presence, and vulnerability in order that such miracles might evolve

(Rosa, 2014h). The possibility of miracles is often overlooked because of a magical, unrealistic connotation. However, this description is essential in discussing the subtle mysteries surrounding our life–death cycles, the fragility of human hope and suffering, and the mental-emotional-spiritual nature of the wellness–illness processes.

These miracles, at their most fundamental level, are truly a repatterning of how one experiences life, a surrender of the Self-defeating habits nurses employ to label and confine the majesty of the bedside experience and a calling on of courage to meet the unforeseeable with vulnerability and compassion. Vulnerability cannot be emphasized enough as a vital component of the transpersonal nursing experience. Brown (2012) assures that the choice to be vulnerable is laden with risk, uncertainty, and even a sense of danger, but nurses know "[t]he gestation of miracles to be birthed in the ordinariness of our everyday lives lies in the womb of vulnerability" (Rosa, 2014h, p. 15). Indeed, the ethical, responsible, and only choice is to nurse from a commitment to embrace vulnerability, a foundation of caring, a core of compassion, and a sense of community-oriented oneness so that the miracle of the transpersonal experience may lead to a personal-professional-universal healing for all.

■ MORAL/ETHICAL FOUNDATION

Ethics is the science of morality. . . . Virtue survives only when it is kept in perpetual practice. . . . Practic[ing] ethics will help you live in harmony. . . . There is no greater comfort than a righteous, virtuous life guided by a clear conscience. Act[ing] [out] of . . . compassion for [others] [is] the path of righteousness (Sivananda, 2013, pp. 157, 162–163).

The *soul work of nursing*—the contributions it makes to humanity at the deepest and most sacred level—is built upon the moral and ethical core of its professional raison d'être. The ethics to which an individual and collective ascribe are not and cannot be limited to scholarly dialogue or written text; they must be lived, witnessed, expressed, and demonstrated in order for them to foster meaning between people and betterment for the global village. Ethics do not flourish in the idealistic terms of intellectual languaging, but in the human-to-human exchanges that permeate our personal and professional lives. Ethics-in-action is what colors our experiences as human beings and defines our professional offerings as nurses. For nursing, a field whose work directly attends to the health, well-being, and healing of the human spirit, ethics becomes the construct for how to be with and do for Self/Other and how to see and know Self/Other.

This exploration has led me to questions such as: What does *nursing* look like? What is that essence of nursing that transcends specialty, educational preparation, and practice setting? What is that thing that makes us "us"? That intentionality and lived virtue that defines nursing in both theory and action? What is the living proof of nursing? What is the ethic-in-action that defines nursing as both art and science?

I believe it is *compassion*.

The Charter for Compassion (Charter for Compassion International, n.d.) acknowledges compassion as the central ethical tenet of all religious traditions, ethical ideologies, and spiritual practices, imploring us to live out the Golden Rule, to treat others as we, ourselves, wish to be treated. Its introduction reads:

> Compassion impels us to work tirelessly to alleviate the suffering of our fellow creatures, to dethrone ourselves from the centre of our world and put another there, and to honour the inviolable sanctity of every single human being, treating everybody, without exception, with absolute justice, equity and respect.

The Charter declares that all human beings, in order to ensure human thriving in a united global community, must commit to the lived demonstration of compassion by refraining from the infliction of pain, learning to appreciate the cultural differences around them, and reconnecting to the shared beauty of humanity beyond boundaries, judgments, and prejudices. It concludes by stating: "Born of our deep interdependence, compassion is essential to human relationships and to a fulfilled humanity. It is the path to enlightenment, and indispensable to the creation of a just economy and a peaceful global community" (Charter for Compassion International, n.d.; you can affirm the Charter for Compassion to promote the principles it espouses at http://www.charterforcompassion.org/index.php/charter/charter-overvew).

Behaving compassionately toward every individual is described in Provision 1 of the American Nurses Association's (ANA, 2015) *Code of Ethics for Nurses With Interpretive Statements* as foundational to nursing practice and is considered central to caring–healing relationships that occur at a spirit-to-spirit level; those nurse–patient partnerships that transcend ego and allow for the realization of a shared humanity (Watson, 2008). In a relationship-centered care model that includes compassion, practitioners are more likely to achieve "the highest level of care" possible (Dossey, 2016, p. 18). The facets and dynamics of compassion and their implications for nursing practice are endless: Research subjects acknowledge that care would not be "care" without the integration of compassion since nursing is a field rooted in emotional engagement (Horsburgh & Ross, 2013); ameliorating the suffering of others through the demonstration of genuine compassion involves embracing vulnerability and refusing to shrink back in the fear of self-protection (Brown, 2010, 2012); there is a noted correlation between self-compassion and emotional intelligence (Şenyuva, Kaya, Işik, & Bodur, 2014); and there is a balance to be found between the satisfaction and fatigue of delivering compassionate care in environments that repeatedly expose nurses to the physical distress and emotional suffering of others (Lombardo & Eyre, 2011; Sacco, Ciurzynksi, Harvey, & Ingersoll, 2015).

Journalist Krista Tippett (2010) suggests that compassion has become misunderstood in the context of modern culture as a soft and sentimental idea that is "potentially depressing" and may even be construed as "pity"; leading society at large to believe it is reserved for the heroic or self-sacrificing and as something that is "too good to be true." She calls us to reconnect with and recalibrate to it as a lived virtue that is visible in its demonstration and "changes the way we think about what is doable, what is possible," significantly different from the overly cerebral and somewhat detached notion of "tolerance." Tippett (2010) suggests that there are component parts that bring compassion to life and magnify its impact in the world around us. Figure 26.1 illustrates these many

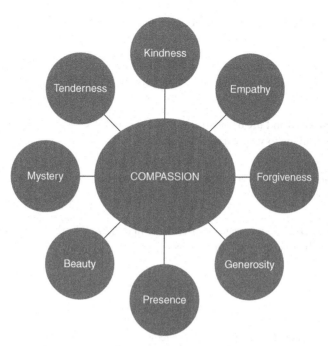

FIGURE 26.1   The component parts of compassion.
Adapted from Tippett (2010).

aspects and virtues that emanate from and contribute toward a compassionate practice both in living and nursing.

To fully understand and embody the far-reaching implications of compassion and a compassionate personal–professional life, it helps to return to the view of nursing as a spiritual practice (Rosa, 2014b). In fact,

> spirituality is inextricable from the sacredness of nursing practice. Both are a search to know God through the continued healing of self and others. Both create a state in which we potentiate and are present to an experience of One-ness. (Rosa, 2015b, p. 24)

Compassion imbues the practices of living and loving and nursing and caring with the breath and wisdom of spiritual clarity. Spirituality does not imply religiosity; it implicates the soul work of nursing, the caring–healing acts of compassion that extend beyond the physical plane and inspire the health and well-being of the mental and emotional, and metaphysical and universal dimensions.

Compassion and its lived experience require practice and patience. Learning to face the humanity of another without turning away or conforming to personal prejudices and judgments is challenging even for the most Self-aware. But as an ethical framework, as a way of life, one cannot help but to recommit to its cultivation again and again. Interpretations of Armstrong's Twelve Steps to a Compassionate Life, which can be utilized and practiced as a starting point for learning the art of compassion and integrating compassionate practices into daily life, appear in Table 26.3.

TABLE 26.3   Interpretations of Twelve Steps to a Compassionate Life

Step 1
Search for the meaning of compassion and its relationship to self in the context of religion, culture, etc.; find compassion's relevance in your personal and professional life.

Step 2
Study your own world and use out-of-the-box thinking to solve today's problems; apply compassionate thinking to your current experience.

Step 3
Have compassion for yourself; accept/own your shadow sides and demonstrate loving-kindness toward self.

Step 4
Demonstrate empathy when engaging with others; find yourself in their story; discover the shared humanity between yourself and others.

Step 5
Be mindful in thought, word, and action; accept the self-limitations inherent in your judgment of others.

Step 6
Commit to action rooted in kindness; acknowledge how your actions, conscious or unconscious, can change a life.

Step 7
Accept that you know very little about the life world of another; seek the truth from their subjective worldview.

Step 8
Be conscious *how* you speak; learn how to listen deeply; question the intention and understand the impact of your speech.

Step 9
Honor all human beings as members of the global village; show concern for all people and advocate for their right to peace.

Step 10
Expand your knowledge of the world at large; humbly seek understanding of cultures and contexts beyond your own.

Step 11
Recognize the universal nature of the human experience; release any self-imposed separation of "us" and "them."

Step 12
Choose to love your enemies by releasing hatred and prejudices; practice forgiveness; role model love; strive for hope.

Adapted from Armstrong (2010).

■ VISION

At the time of this writing, I am living and working in Kigali, Rwanda, as visiting faculty in the country's first master of science in nursing program at the University of Rwanda and as an ICU clinical educator at Rwanda Military Hospital. Nurses here are mandated to the profession based on the results of secondary school testing and provide care within a system that tends to view them as subservient to physicians and inferior in knowledge and skill. As an adult, I know I have the opportunity to confront and reinform the power differentials and the greater than/less than perceptions of childhood on a global, cross-cultural scale. I strive each day to empower nurses to remember who they are as professionals outside of a limiting context and what their potentials are for healing and contributing a unique talent toward the health and well-being of another, and to create a greater sense of collective esteem and collegial support within their ranks. Though Rwanda and the United States, my country of origin, view nursing differently, I see the same themes again and again that prevent nursing from realizing its leadership potentials and fully embodying its role in human healing and caring. (See Chapter 30 for more information on nursing in Rwanda and the practice of cultural humility.)

The vision herein is for the nurse to reenliven its core of ethical praxis and support the profession by reclaiming lost power and rediscovering/recreating/redefining intraprofessional identity. I shared these hopes and aspirations for nurses and nursing during my master's degree valedictory address (Rosa, 2015c) and I share them again here:

> This vision requires that I celebrate what I love most about being a nurse—and that is the time I spend with my patients. As a trained critical care nurse, I momentarily thought my career was all about the IV drips, ventilators, and balloon pumps. I've learned that these modalities aren't enough. They aren't close to enough. They are an extension of my real work. My real work is to use those technologies as tools to be with my patients, to be with their families, to help them heal, to support them through a difficult time in their lives, and to allow them the opportunity to feel seen, heard, and acknowledged. This is the work that they will remember; the work that has changed their lives and mine.
>
> It is our privilege and, in fact, our ethical obligation to breathe humanity into our practice as nurses with each patient, each day, in each moment. It is our right and our gift. It is the foundation upon which we build all other degrees, credentials, titles, and honors. Without it, we cease to be the very embodiment of spiritual practice and human healing that Nightingale envisioned.
>
> So my challenge to all is that whether we are finishing our bachelor's, our master's, or we hold our doctorate, whether we lobby in Washington, manage a business, or educate the next generation of healers—we are nurses first. We attend first to the dignity of the patient and we hold the betterment of society as paramount. All we accomplish and aspire to should move from that starting point; from that foundation of human caring; with the bedside in our hearts and our patients' well-being as our primary professional motivation. Amidst celebrating the possibilities of nursing leadership, I naturally think of my patients; the people in the world who are proof that I have cared.
>
> I think of Percy, a boy with Down syndrome who was in the ICU for eight weeks. He almost died from an internal bleed twice, and a few months ago I received a text message from his dad on a Friday night that read, "Getting ready for the prom tonight. Thinking of you."
>
> I think of Deborah, who had two teenage sons at home who she had adopted from Guatemala to give them better lives in America. Deborah knew

she was dying. Deborah was scared and I had the once-in-a-lifetime opportunity to let her be scared in my arms, to let her feel everything she felt when she wasn't being brave in front of her family, and to let her feel heard before she died.

Lorna, a miracle woman. A woman who decompensated after a C-section and was on the brink of death for several days. The same woman who I was sure had died during my weekend off from work, but instead sat there waiting for me on Monday morning, the most beautiful smile on her face, asking, "What took you so long?"

I think of my Debbie who taught me what love and fun look like, even in the midst of extreme fear and pain. A woman who changed my very perspectives on death and my very values in life.

I think of lying on the floor and praying with parents as they lose their children. Being the hand on someone's back as they remove their wife's life support. I think of celebrating with children while their parents walk again and seeing someone fall asleep because their pain is finally relieved.

I think of the very sacred, human moments that no one else sees or knows about; the moments of human caring between my patients and me that I remember before I fall asleep and in my quiet time. I think of how I have affected the story of another person by my very presence in their life and I think of how my story is forever rewritten because of theirs in mine. I believe it is these small moments, these human caring moments, we share as individuals and as professionals that have the power to change the world.

This is my vision for the fully embodied realization of the nursing profession: Nurses will awaken to the powerful knowing that we are in the unique position to bring human caring to the forefront; to promote, preserve, and protect human dignity, first and foremost and at all costs; to forgive ourselves both personally and professionally in order that we might move forward with clarity and purpose; to use our technologies as tools to more deeply engage our patients; to educate, lead, coordinate, and guide society toward a paradigm of healing and wellness; to humanize ethical values of compassion, kindness, and love; and to become conscious to the humble truth that we continue to light the way because we are, in fact, the light of humanity itself.

■ REFLECTIONS

1. *How do I experience my own moral imperatives in nursing practice? In other words, how do I put my own theoretical aspects of caring into action?*
2. *Is there a collective accountability for the wellness and illness of the profession?*
3. *What is the relationship between my individual mental-emotional-spiritual well-being and the mental-emotional-spiritual well-being of the system in which I work?*
4. *Reflecting upon my practice of compassion in everyday life and using the Component Parts of Compassion and the Twelve Steps to a Compassionate Life, what can I work on to further develop my lived experience of compassion with both Self and Other?*

5. *Who is that patient who has changed how I see the world? How is my life different because of him or her? How is his or her life or how was his or her death different because of me? What miracles occurred that I know to be true in my heart? Take some time to write the story or share it with a colleague and be mindful of how it feels to tell the story.*

■ REFERENCES

American Nurses Association. (2015). *Code of ethics for nurses with interpretive statements.* Washington, DC: Author.

Armstrong, K. (2010). *Twelve steps to a compassionate life.* New York, NY: Anchor Books.

Brown, B. (2010). *The gifts of imperfections: Letting go of who we think we should be and embracing who we are.* Center City, MN: Hazelden.

Brown, B. (2012). *Daring greatly: How the courage to be vulnerable transforms the way we live, love, parent, and lead.* New York, NY: Gotham.

Charter for Compassion International. (n.d.). *Charter for Compassion.* Retrieved from http://www.charterforcompassion.org/index.php/charter

Dossey, B. M. (2016). Nursing: Holistic, integral, and integrative—local to global. In B. M. Dossey & L. Keegan (Eds.), *Holistic nursing: A handbook for practice* (7th ed., pp. 3–52). Burlington, MA: Jones & Bartlett.

Dossey, B. M., Selanders, L. C., Beck, D. M., & Attewell, A. (2005). *Florence Nightingale today: Healing, leadership, global action.* Silver Spring, MD: Nursesbooks.org.

Dunphy, L. (2010). Florence Nightingale's legacy of caring and its applications. In M. E. Parker & M. C. Smith (Eds.), *Nursing theories & nursing practice* (3rd ed., pp. 35–53). Philadelphia, PA: F.A. Davis.

Estes, T. (2011). Teaching careers to access the subtle energies: Breaking into light. *Natural Transitions, 3*(3), 14–16.

Horsburgh, D., & Ross, J. (2013). Care and compassion: The experiences of newly qualified staff nurses. *Journal of Clinical Nursing, 22*(7/8), 1124–1132.

Lombardo, B., & Eyre, C. (2011). Compassion fatigue: A nurse's primer. *Online Journal of Issues in Nursing, 16*(1), 1–1.

Quinn, J. (2014). The integrated nurse: Wholeness, self-discovery, and self-care. In M. J. Kreitzer & M. Koithan (Eds.), *Integrative nursing* (pp. 17–32). New York, NY: Oxford University Press.

Rosa, W. (2014a). Reflections on self in relation to other: Core community values of a moral/ethical foundation. *Creative Nursing, 20*(4), 242–247.

Rosa, W. (2014b). Nursing is separate from medicine: Advanced practice nursing and a transpersonal plan of care. *International Journal for Human Caring, 18*(2), 76–82.

Rosa, W. (2014c). Letter to the editor: It is unethical not to care. *Nursing Science Quarterly, 27*(3), 261–262.

Rosa, W. (2014d). Caring science and compassion fatigue: Reflective inventory for the individual processes of self-healing. *Beginnings, 34*(4), 14–16.

Rosa, W. (2014e). Conscious dying and cultural emergence: Reflective systems inventory for the collective processes of global healing. *Beginnings, 34*(5), 20–22.

Rosa, W. (2014f). Intertwined narratives of the human caring story. *Creative Nursing, 20*(3), 171–173.

Rosa, W. (2014g). Holding heartspace: The unveiling of the self through being and becoming. *International Journal for Human Caring, 18*(4), 59.

Rosa, W. (2014h). Allowing for miracles: The vulnerable choice of intentionality and presence. *Beginnings, 34*(2), 14–15.

Rosa, W. (2015a). Cleaning the slate: Forgiveness as integral to personal and professional self-actualization. *Journal of Nursing and Care, 3*(6), 216. doi:10.4172/2167-1168.1000216

Rosa, W. (2015b). The yamas of nursing: Ethics of yogic philosophy as spiritual practice. *Beginnings, 35*(5), 8–11, 24–25.

Rosa, W. (2015c). Valedictorian address [Author's notes]. Hunter-Bellevue School of Nursing at Hunter College, City University of New York Annual Commencement Ceremony.

Sacco, T. L., Ciurzynski, S. M., Harvey, M. E., & Ingersoll, G. L. (2015). Compassion satisfaction and compassion fatigue among critical care nurses. *Critical Care Nurse, 35*(4), 32–44.

Şenyuva, E., Kaya, H., Işik, B., & Bodur, G. (2014). Relationship between self-compassion and emotional intelligence in nursing students. *International Journal of Nursing Practice, 20*(6), 588–596.

Sitzman, K., & Watson, J. (2014). *Caring science, mindful practice: Implementing Watson's human caring theory.* New York, NY: Springer.

Sivananda, S. S. (2013). *Bliss divine: A book of spiritual essays on the lofty purpose of human life and the means to its achievement* (9th ed.). Tehri-Garhwal, Uttarakhand, India: The Divine Life Society.

Tippett, K. (2010). *Reconnecting with compassion.* Retrieved from https://www.ted.com/talks/krista_tippett_reconnecting_with_compassion?language=en

Watson Caring Science Institute. (2013). Global translations—10 Caritas Processes™. Retrieved from http://watsoncaringscience.org/about-us/caring-science-definitions-processes-theory/global-translations-10-caritas-processes/

Watson, J. (2005). *Caring science as sacred science.* Philadelphia, PA: F.A. Davis.

Watson, J. (2008). *Nursing: The philosophy and science of caring* (Rev. ed.). Boulder, CO: University Press of Colorado.

Watson, J. (2012). *Human caring science* (2nd ed.). Sudbury, MA: Jones & Bartlett.

CHAPTER TWENTY-SEVEN

Vulnerable and Spiritual: Utilizing the Process of Transpersonal Nurse Coaching

Bonney Gulino Schaub

You have within you all the potential for a special relationship that is waiting to be realized right now. It is the relationship between your everyday personality and a deep source of internal wisdom. Sometimes, at night, you might experience this wisdom as knowledge or guidance you receive in your dreams. Sometimes, during the day, a word or phrase or passing mental image might indicate that your internal wisdom is trying to get through to your conscious self. And, on some occasions, in a moment of true grace, a big piece of internal wisdom might break through to your awareness and illuminate reality more fully than you had ever seen it before.

—Schaub and Schaub (2014, p. xiv)

■ WHY NURSING?

I grew up in Manhattan in the 1960s during a time of great social change. I was surrounded by rich cultural diversity and an atmosphere of activism. Feminism and the civil rights movement were vibrant and at the height of expression. The Metropolitan Museum of Art and the Museum of Natural History were a bus ride away and, from an early age, I was able to travel around the city on my own and explore these amazing places.

Attending the public school system in New York City exposed me to students from many cultures. In elementary school, I would talk to friends about why their families had moved to America. Some had left behind the devastation, poverty, and political turmoil of post–World War II Europe. Other families had come for education and work opportunities. I was always curious about what they had left behind and what of their culture they brought with them.

My high school was on the Lower East Side, a place that had been the starting point for waves of immigrants. My own grandparents had arrived there. Two had come from southern Italy and two from Liverpool, England.

My school was one block from Delancey Street, a neighborhood known for its dynamic and diverse Jewish residents, and it was a few blocks from Little Italy and Chinatown. Going out for lunch usually meant buying an egg roll or a small container of fried rice, a slice of pizza, or a knish and a pickle.

Many of the immigrant students in my high school did not speak English. I wondered what it was like to be in a school where you could barely communicate with peers, let alone learn what was being taught. Most of the Jewish students had arrived in America shortly after the war, so they spoke Yiddish as well as English. My friends and classmates shared powerful stories about what had brought them to New York. Some had been born in concentration camps and had suffered the loss of many family members and friends. I listened to stories of the resiliency and courage demonstrated while escaping from this horrific persecution. I witnessed the power of the human spirit to move from utter vulnerability toward new hope and possibilities. Thinking back on this time, I recall that questions like, "Who in your family was killed?" were almost a "normal" topic of conversation for some students.

Later on, in my professional life, when I started working as a mental health clinical nurse specialist, I had many successful adult clients who were the children of death camp survivors. I learned about the process of survivor guilt: the way these children felt the need to be perfect so that they would not cause their parents any more suffering. I also had clients whose fathers were American soldiers who had been traumatized by the unimaginable horrors they witnessed at the end of the war when they arrived at the concentration camps and liberated the camp "survivors."

It is clear that wars never end. The vulnerability and pain continue, often remaining hidden and unexpressed. It is possible, however, to arrive at an attitude of self-compassion and self-forgiveness that allows a person to move forward in his or her life. Clearly this is a psycho-spiritual evolution emerging from a process of transpersonal development.

Recently, my high-school class had its 50-year reunion. It was quite interesting to learn that a very significant majority of my classmates had become health professionals. What role did these early experiences play in their wanting to learn about health and healing? I know that it played a role for me, even though I was not aware of this when I switched my major to nursing.

When I started college at 16 years of age, I was focusing on creative art, art history, and anthropology. I was also practicing yoga, learning meditation, and studying judo. I did not have a clear direction, just a lot of friends and interests.

After two years and three different majors, I reconnected with an aunt who had been living in California for many years. She was a public health nurse. She had moved back to New York City to attend graduate school at Columbia University. She had started her nursing career after graduating from a hospital nursing program, had gone on to obtain her master of science in nursing, and was now enrolled in a doctoral program. She told me about her experience of working in public health and how it influenced her choice to become a nurse educator. Her work had included spending time with families from many different cultures and she thought it might be of interest to me since I was interested in anthropology.

My aunt presented an entirely new possibility for my education. She told me that nursing was coming into its own as an independent profession. She said changes had taken place for RNs in New York State through the establishment of a new definition and scope of practice for the profession. That was why she had moved to New York to pursue her education. This information was surprising to me. It certainly presented a dramatically different image of nursing than that which was depicted in popular culture; for example, the sexy nurse popping out of her uniform and wielding a syringe or stumbling around trying to please the male doctor. This image can still be seen today even though we nurses have made great strides in asserting and owning our importance and what we bring to the health care system.

My aunt's information encouraged me and I decided that nursing would allow me to weave together all my skills and interests and bring them to a field where I would work directly with people. I transferred to Adelphi University where I was taught and mentored by creative and inspiring teachers. I was especially drawn to mental health nursing. My professors were pioneers in opening private practices as nurse therapists and this was an exciting possibility for me to consider.

■ EARLY IMPRESSIONS

I graduated from Adelphi in 1976 and was fortunate to get hired at a hospital that was known for its strong director of nursing (DN). As a student, the word was out that this was the best place to work because the director was very assertive and was implementing the new state mandates in regard to definition and scope of nursing practice. In contrast, we heard of other local hospitals where the doctor was "always right" and needed to be obeyed. There were even places where nurses were expected to stand and offer their seat to the physicians when they entered the nurses' conference room.

This was also a time when the women's movement was impacting our culture. Nurses, practicing in a predominantly women's profession, were demanding respect and acknowledgment of all the knowledge, assessment, and treatment expertise, caring and relationship-building skills, and wisdom that they brought to patient care.

Our DN did not require us to wear white uniforms or caps. We were allowed to wear white or navy blue suits, as long as they were washable, and to have a nametag prominently displayed stating we were RNs. She wanted RNs to be distinctly identifiable as professionals. She did not want every female working on the unit to be referred to as "nurse." It was her passionate determination to discard the image of nurse as physician's handmaiden.

The first clinical setting I worked in was a surgical head and neck unit. It was quite a reality shock experience. I had never seen patients who were being treated for major facial reconstruction because of injuries, deformities, or disfigurement, secondary to head and neck cancer surgery. I had no experience with tracheostomy care. Fortunately, I had an excellent charge nurse who guided me through the process of learning the skills required. I learned to be present in the care of these patients and focus on the task at hand. This also allowed me to recognize and honor the courage of my patients.

One day, I personally experienced the importance of having a strong DN. There was a patient I had been caring for over several days. She had been given two enemas to relieve her constipation. They were not effective but the patient was not in any distress. The attending physician wrote an order for a high colonic to be administered. I did not want to administer this treatment, because the patient was very fragile and fatigued and I was also concerned that she may have had an obstruction. I wanted to wait a little longer, but the doctor insisted I administer it immediately. In expressing my concern to the doctor, I explained that I had been caring for this patient all morning and I would continue to monitor her status closely. The doctor, who had just arrived on the unit for the first time that day, became very angry and ordered me to do it at once. I told him I was the patient's primary nurse and I could not do it because I thought it was contraindicated.

I remembered that during my nursing orientation at the hospital, our DN reassured us all that we could page her if we ever had a problem or question about our role in what was taking place on our unit. I decided I needed to call the DN about this and my charge nurse agreed to support this action. The DN came up to the unit and met with me. After I expressed my reasons for thinking this procedure was not warranted at this moment, she told me she would support me, stating that, as a nurse, I had an ethical commitment to place my patient's needs first. We met with the physician. The DN told him my decision to not do the procedure at the moment was based on my nursing assessment. I did not have to do the procedure and the physician agreed to wait because he did not want to do the procedure himself. My patient did eventually have a bowel movement later in the day.

This incident was a powerful message to all the nurses on the unit. It demonstrated respect for all of us as professionals. It also reinforced the importance of respecting ourselves and taking seriously what we know and what we perceive as we care for our patients. At the same time, it asked us to accept full responsibility for our clinical decisions and actions.

For a period of time, I was working nights on this surgical unit. I was again fortunate to have excellent support from the nursing supervisor on the night shift. The nights were a time when my most vulnerable patients needed lots of attention. The positive part of this shift was that I actually had time to spend speaking with my patients and providing comfort care.

One night I called the supervisor for some advice about my patient, a young nun who was critically ill and close to death. She was frightened and speaking about her spiritual beliefs with confusion and sadness. She was afraid to be alone and was asking many questions about what she could expect. I needed some guidance on how to be with this young woman. The nursing supervisor came to the unit and met with me. She asked me to connect with my breath and give myself permission to just be present in the moment. She told me that the most important answer to all my patient's questions was to reflect back to her, "What are you hoping for?"

I was so surprised by this response. "What will I say if she says 'I want to get better'?" I asked. My supervisor placed her hand on my shoulder and said, "Yes, she might say that, but you may be surprised to know that most people have very specific answers to what they are hoping for."

She went on to say that a person's hope may be to not have too much pain, to see someone one last time, or to know they will not be alone at the end. My supervisor reassured me that my patient would appreciate my asking the question and would then know that I would work with her to help accomplish her request. My mentor went on to write *Using the Power of Hope to Cope with Dying: The Four Stages of Hope* (Fanslow-Brunjes, 2008). In this book, she wrote that

> hope is universally understood to mean something more profound than simply a wish or a goal. But it's not a loaded word, so far, since it has escaped religious or spiritual connotations and therefore people can consider it regardless of their belief system. (p. xii)

That question, "What are you hoping for?" is one I have repeatedly used in my practice and in my teaching. It is truly respectful because it speaks to a person's deepest source of wisdom.

I have gratitude for these two mentors. One taught me to feel empowered and responsible in my work and in my life. The other taught me to be fully present, listen deeply, and trust that people, even in their most vulnerable moments, can be supported in connecting to their wisest source. It was not my job to come up with the answers and I could accept that fact with humility and self-compassion. In reflecting back on these important mentors, I recognize that this was the beginning of my development of Transpersonal Nurse Coaching (TNC).

Eventually, I transferred to working on an inpatient psychiatry unit in the hospital. It was a new learning process for me. I had spent my final nursing school semester interning in an aftercare department in a major psychiatric hospital and so I arrived with some experience. I appreciated being able to spend extended time meeting with patients. I was also reconnecting with my meditation and yoga practice, thinking these practices could be of help to the patients.

Anything associated with "spirituality" was not part of the medical model that existed in the hospital setting at that time. Fortunately, our unit secretary, after hearing me frequently talk about meditation, told me that her brother-in-law, a clinical psychologist, was studying something that included meditation and psychotherapy.

I contacted him and he suggested I read the work of Roberto Assagioli, MD. I obtained Dr. Assagioli's book, *Psychosynthesis: A Manual of Principles and Techniques* (1965). Reading this work was an amazing discovery because it brought together my personal and professional worlds. Assagioli, a neurologist and psychiatrist working and teaching in a hospital in Florence, Italy, created a model of psychological development and psychotherapy that integrated the use of dynamic imagery and meditative practices into a psycho-spiritual approach to working with people. As early as 1909, Assagioli recognized the importance of meditation and spirituality as part of mental health, self-care, and healing.

After reading *Psychosynthesis*, I knew I wanted to immerse myself in the study of this model. I studied psychosynthesis for three years, traveling to the Berkshires in Massachusetts for monthly three-day training sessions. I was especially interested in all the clinical imagery and meditative practices that Assagioli had developed to use with his patients. During this time, I also enrolled in a master's program to become a psychiatric/mental health clinical specialist. I wanted to focus on clinical meditation and imagery and, ultimately, did research on this for my master's thesis.

■ PROFESSIONAL EVOLUTION/CONTRIBUTION

After a number of years working in inpatient settings, I transferred to working in an outpatient substance abuse program in a suburban community. There was a negligible amount of substance abuse treatment available anywhere else in the area, so our patient population was diverse. They were people from middle- and upper-middle-class neighborhoods, from suburban ghettos, from local immigrant communities, Vietnam War veterans, professionals, business owners, high-school and college students, and homemakers.

I did in-depth intakes with physical and psychological assessments on new clients; all being admitted for treatment of substance misuse. The substances of choice included heroin, methadone, hallucinogens, pharmaceuticals such as barbiturates and opioids, marijuana, amphetamines, cocaine, phencyclidine (PCP or angel dust), and alcohol. The typical pattern was use of a preferred drug but other substances as well.

The world of treatment was filled with questions and theories about addiction and dependence. Is there an addictive personality? Is it genetics or a disease? Is it cultural or environmental? Is it family disturbance? Amid all the reading, discussion, and conferences, it was apparent that there was no single answer.

From my perspective, the one common factor I recognized in all the clients was the need to numb their experiences of fear, pain, and loss—their vulnerability. There was a profound need for relief and an end to their emotional suffering. Their vulnerability could be disguised in bravura, anger, or antagonism, but the fact was that they were sitting right there in front of me seeking help.

Through this experience, I developed the Vulnerability Model (VM), which was first described in *Healing Addictions: The Vulnerability Model of Recovery* (Schaub & Schaub, 1997) and can be seen in Table 27.1. This book was part of the *Nurse as Healer* book series, with Lynn Keegan (see Chapter 7) as the series editor. The VM was conceived as a practical and unifying model of addiction and the process of recovery. It recognizes the essential vulnerability that is implicit in the diverse types of addiction. It proposes that there is a need for a holistic and transpersonal component to the healing process, a need for a bio-psycho-social-spiritual model of recovery (Schaub & Schaub, 1997, p. xiv). This is needed to sustain any of the healthful changes that people make as they try to live with more peace and purpose.

Although Table 27.1 lays out an understanding of the VM as it applies to recovery from addiction, it is applicable to other patterns of compulsive behaviors, such as workaholism, gambling, hoarding, and eating disorders, as well as to life challenges, such as illness or disability, retirement, divorce, loss of a significant relationship, grief and bereavement, and unemployment—all requiring a process of recovery. It has also been incorporated into the scope and competencies of nurse coaching (Hess et al., 2013, pp. 2, 63).

Vulnerability is anxiety ultimately rooted in the human condition of being conscious, separate, and mortal. It is a normal emotion based in reality, an elemental aspect of our actual human situation. The theologian Paul Tillich (1952) wrote that the very act of being aware of this reality is to be anxious. He emphasized the importance of having courage and striving toward self-preservation and self-affirmation (Tillich, 1952).

Current brain research provides us with an enlightening map of the interaction between fear and the way in which one's brain, body, and mind react to it. From this

TABLE 27.1 **The Vulnerability Model of Recovery**

- Addiction is a repetitive, maladaptive, avoidant, substitutive process of getting rid of vulnerability.

- This addictive process is triggered by an experience of vulnerability that is believed to be intolerable.

- Vulnerability is anxiety ultimately rooted in the human condition of being conscious, separate, and mortal. As such, this vulnerability is a normal emotion and an elemental aspect of our actual human situation.

- People who have a greater degree of vulnerability (explanations for which include genetic, biochemical, characterological, familial, cultural, and spiritual) have a greater degree of need to get rid of it.

- Getting rid of vulnerability is accomplished by trying to feel powerful or by trying to feel numb. Trying to feel powerful is an act of willfulness. Trying to feel numb is an act of will-lessness. Drugs are selected to help produce these results. Trying to feel powerful and trying to feel numb are both choices. Made repeatedly, they become addictive, producing predictable but brief episodes of relief from vulnerability.

- People in recovery from addiction begin to heal their feelings by recognizing and respecting their vulnerability.

- Continued recovery is based on developing new, nonavoidant responses to vulnerability.

- However, this vulnerability cannot be effectively responded to on a long-term basis by the separate, ego-level, temporary sense of self because it is that sense of self that is at the very root of the vulnerability.

- Advanced recovery therefore requires the development of an expanded sense of self that is communal and spiritual in awareness. Such spiritual development is a normal aspect of adult development, despite the fact that it is ignored by most Western psychology.

- Communal awareness is provided by Alcoholics Anonymous and other 12-step programs through fellowship and service to others in recovery. Spiritual awareness requires development, which has been studied by the world's wisdom traditions and, more recently, by transpersonal psychology.

- Many people in recovery do not experience spiritual awareness, because this aspect of human nature has been neglected and poorly understood in modern culture. Pioneering transpersonal psychiatrist Roberto Assagioli referred to this issue as "repression of the sublime."

- Transpersonal approaches offer insights and practices that can lift repression of the sublime, energize spiritual awareness and increase inner peace, and work at the deepest root of the addictive process.

Source: Schaub and Schaub (1997).

perspective, we again understand that fear/anxiety is normal. It is our natural warning system checking out our world for any signs of danger. It is working hard to keep us alive. Unfortunately, our brain's fear circuitry system is on alert and reacting to all manner of internal and external stimuli. It is not operating from a place of rational thinking. It is vigilant and driven by instinct and survival hardwiring (Shin & Liberzon, 2010; Schaub & Schaub, 2013).

John Welwood, a psychologist and meditation teacher, points out that this shared vulnerability is not all bad. He says it is a state with great potential. Welwood describes "utter vulnerability . . . as the essence of human nature and consciousness" (Welwood, 1982, pp. 132–133). He believes this vulnerability has the potential for being valued as our base emotional experience, as our basic aliveness. It is therefore a common bond among all people and potentially an emotional bridge between ourselves and anyone we meet. Treating our vulnerability with compassion, appreciation, and respect immediately connects us with our world in a loving way. There is untold suffering and pain caused to others by those who put all their energy and will into self-protection, control, and working hard at appearing and feeling invulnerable.

All challenging life events become catalysts for a changed sense of self. How a person understands and negotiates this new self can be immobilizing and defeating—or it can be used as an opportunity to assess what is truly meaningful and of value in life. We all have established patterns of thinking and behaving that allow us to override feelings of vulnerability. We have created this so we can function out there in the world and not be frozen by our fears.

We are making choices that lead to actions all the time. Even "doing nothing," leading to nonaction, is a choice. Making wise choices to behave in ways that will promote growth and well-being is a key recovery technique to whatever challenge is present. It is therefore crucial for a person to become aware of his or her patterns of reactions in response to his or her vulnerability.

Our ability to choose is our free will in action. We may say that we are "willing" to do something. This means we are choosing to use our life energy in taking this action. At other times we may be "unwilling," choosing to withhold our life energy. We may also find ourselves being "willful." This might be thought of as using our willpower to obtain a particular outcome. Alternatively, we may feel we are powerless and have no choice, and so passive inactivity is the result: It is an act of will-lessness.

We can choose to mobilize our life energy in three different ways: willfully, willlessly, or willingly. Addiction psychiatrist Gerald May pointed out that willingness and willfulness are two possibilities when we engage life. The other option is to avoid engagement entirely, a process I refer to as will-lessness (Schaub & Schaub, 1991). *Willfulness* is the forceful use of our energy. *Will-lessness* is the complete withdrawal of our energy. This understanding of the will as our use of life energy empowers the process of making changes and has become an essential cornerstone of TNC.

Willfulness shows itself when we choose to take the following types of behaviors:

- Power over
- Forcefulness
- Exertion
- Strain
- Contraction
- Constriction
- Compression
- Violence
- Manipulation
- Drivenness

If we think of this in terms of "fight or flight" reactions to fear, then willfulness is the "fight" reaction to vulnerability.

Will-lessness shows itself when we make the following choices:

- Numbness
- Collapse
- Powerlessness
- Escape
- Withdrawal
- Surrender
- Immobilization

Will-lessness is the "flight" reaction to vulnerability (Schaub & Schaub, 1997).

We can observe manifestations of willfulness and will-lessness in a person's mental functioning, emotional responses, physical states, and spiritual/transpersonal perspective. This is a bio-psycho-social-spiritual view of the person consistent with holistic nursing philosophy (Dossey & Keegan, 2016).

When reviewing Figures 27.1 and 27.2, it is important to understand that these patterns are universal patterns of response to vulnerable, unsafe feelings. They can be seen in animal behaviors, such as when frightened animals behave in a menacing or violent manner (willfulness) or when they freeze or "play dead" (will-lessness).

From this perspective, there is no judgment about the root of these patterns of reaction. If a person can notice his or her experience of vulnerability without judging it as something bad or feeling shame that it exists, then the possibility of making a wise choice becomes available.

In summary, becoming aware of our habitual choices gives us the option of making new and different choices about how we want to use our life energy. Without awareness, our habits deepen and become set.

The fact that we can observe someone swing back and forth between willfulness and will-lessness in their use of life energy can be recognized as an unconscious attempt to achieve homeostasis. *Homeostasis* is a system of biological hormonal checks and balances that maintains optimal functioning of the system. Achieving a sense of homeostasis contributes to a balanced sense of self, an experience of groundedness, and feeling stable. This is the state of willingness. It is a state of knowing you have your inner resources fully available to you. You can trust yourself and feel that you can be effective in the world.

Willingness is not a static state but rather an active process of balancing between the polarities of willfulness and will-lessness. It is the ideal of dynamic balance spoken of in spiritual and philosophical teachings. It is analogous to:

- The balance of yin and yang energies in Taoism
- The Soto Zen way of effortless effort
- The concept of passive volition in biofeedback training
- The Greek ideal of the golden mean
- The Buddhist path of the middle way
- The advice from Alcoholics Anonymous of finding a place of wisdom from which you know when to change something and when to accept something

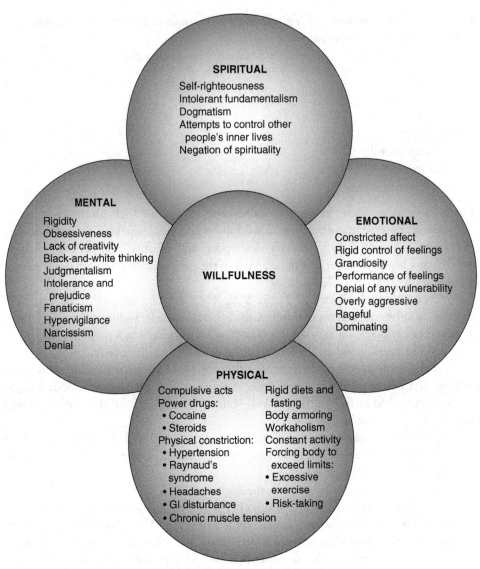

FIGURE 27.1   The spectrum of willfulness.
Source: Schaub and Schaub (1997).

- Assagioli's concept of psychosynthesis—the balance and synthesis of opposing impulses in the personality
- The profound common sense of moderation in all things

Willingness is a balanced, easier, more adaptive response to life. Figure 27.3 presents some of the health-promoting and desirable qualities, behaviors, and emotional, physical, and spiritual experiences of willingness. The model of willingness illustrated in Figure 27.3 is part of the self-care and healing skills promoted in TNC.

The willful and will-less behavioral patterns and responses shown in Figures 27.1 and 27.2 identify the ways people suppress and deny any overt experiences of vulnerability. In accepting that these reactions are coming from the brain's instinctual fear circuitry

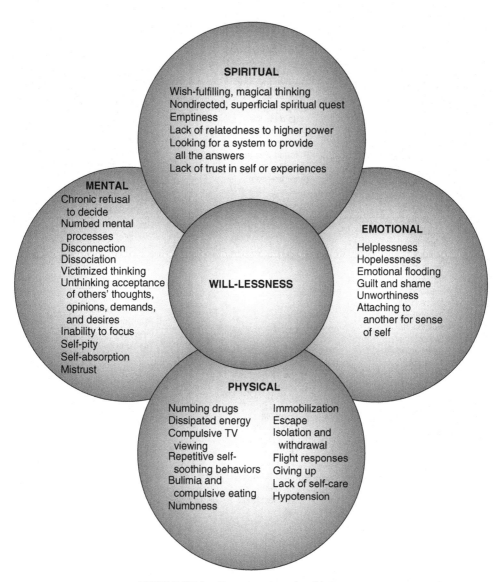

FIGURE 27.2 The spectrum of will-lessness.
Source: Schaub and Schaub (1997).

system, which is on alert, responding to random internal and external stimuli, the next step is to find the antidote to the situation. The cultivation of willingness is the antidote, but how can this be accomplished?

The first answer is *connection*. When we fully recognize that our vulnerability, emanating from the reality of our mortality, is shared with all living beings, we can know that at this basic level we are connected. As conscious beings, we all share in this participation of the cycle of life. Accepting this increases feelings of connection and empathy with everyone and everything around you, including yourself. The experience of connection, empathy, and openheartedness is nourishing and rewarding; it can evoke feelings of love (Schaub & Schaub, 2009).

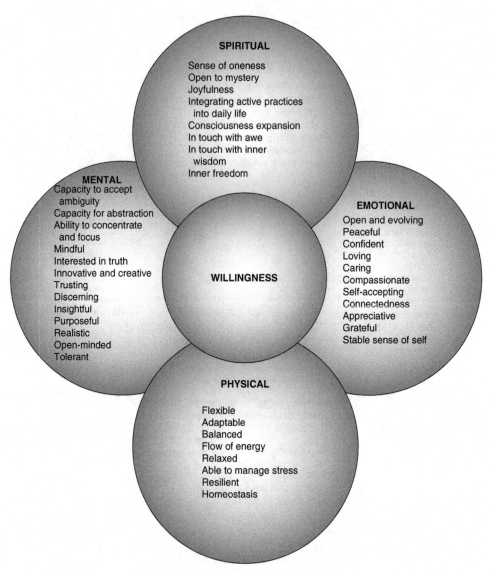

FIGURE 27.3   The spectrum of willingness.
Source: Schaub and Schaub (1997).

I have worked with patients and clients where this perspective has been a relief. This has been particularly evident when working with people in recovery from addictions. Their self-judgment and shame is tempered when they are able to recognize that they were experiencing unmanageable feelings of vulnerability when they began abusing substances. There is an experience of relief in knowing they are not alone.

This perspective is also helpful when dealing with difficult colleagues or coworkers, friends and family members, and in unpleasant interactions with other people. It is helpful to be able to step back and consider that the anger or aggression being directed at you is reflecting how the other person manages his or her own vulnerability. This can tone down your reactivity and allow you to stay centered as you work with the person. These two examples reflect skills that are used in TNC.

As we see in these examples, the first answer to our vulnerability is to recognize and remember that everyone, without exception, is vulnerable. By willingly accepting our own vulnerability, we realize we are connected to everyone's living experience and can let go of any self-centered wish that life should be the way we want it to be. This acceptance starts us on the path to finding a way of harmony with life as life is. We delay this important journey if we persist in willfully using our energy to control life or by trying to will-lessly escape the realities of it.

The second answer is transpersonal development. *Transpersonal development* posits that we already have, in our own deeper nature, the resources to be in harmony with life as life is. The process is one of opening our personality to new discoveries about our deeper resources. The safe, effective, and time-tested way to make new discoveries about our nature is through the clinical uses of meditation and imagery. These skills can be utilized by nurses in any setting, and more will be said in the next section about the uses of these skills in a new vision for nursing, TNC.

The first transpersonal discovery is *inner peace*. This is not a process of relaxation. It is the freedom that comes with experiencing the subtle energy of awareness itself. *Awareness itself* is the natural serenity that becomes available to you when you are freed from the relentless chatter of your fear-based thoughts. Dr. Ching Tse Lee (personal communication, 2015), research psychologist and qigong master, describes this natural serenity as a state of being "at home."

This natural serenity opens you to your inner wisdom. It is a source of inner guidance and an understanding that we each have our own preferred way of perceiving words, images, intuitions, body sensations, and/or energetic experiences. This serenity will allow you to more easily notice your guiding inner wisdom.

As you build your relationship with this transpersonal part of you, you begin to be clear about what is deeply important to you, apart from all the externals that are vying for your attention. This leads to recognizing, understanding, and honoring the meaning and purpose of your life (Schaub & Schaub, 2013).

■ MORAL/ETHICAL FOUNDATION

Before I had any understanding of what transpersonal development meant, I had a strong sense of the qualities and values I respected and wanted to support both personally and professionally. I have always identified with my nurse colleagues, students, and clients who have spoken of their despair that they are not able to fully be the nurse they want to be. They too are very proud of their skills and expertise in patient care, but there is a longing to have the time to make deeper connections with those they are caring for. In their times of deeper connection, some describe an experience beyond the personal (that is transpersonal) that happens between and beyond both the nurse and the patient. They reflect on these times as mysterious moments of oneness. Each nurse expresses the experience from her or his own perspective or belief system, but sometimes it is as simple as "I don't know, but it was amazing." In these moments, their work reconnects them to a deeper sense of meaning and purpose and makes them remember why they went into nursing in the first place.

It is this opening to the transpersonal that forms my own moral ethics and values. I hold that each person has a dormant transpersonal nature, and part of the purpose of any healing exchange is for patients to realize their own healing possibilities. When patients awaken to the transpersonal in themselves, their sense of personal worth and dignity increases and they experience greater courage to face the challenges and suffering in life. As a daily witness to suffering, the nurse is the ideal professional to understand and utilize transpersonal skills to help awaken patients to their healing transpersonal qualities.

Broadly stated, my ethics and values are the honoring of what we brought with us when we came into this world, a potential that waits to be awakened both for the individual and for his or her contribution to the whole. It is the neglect, and even repression, of this potential that causes unnecessary suffering in many people's lives. My advocacy of TNC is based on this commitment to honor each person's innate potential (Schaub & White, 2015). Although I certainly cannot prove it with research-based data, I can speculate that the innate potential in each person is evidence of an evolutionary purpose. Beyond that, the reason for the objective presence of these potentials is a mystery.

◼ VISION

Probably more so than any other helping profession, including medicine, nurses face human suffering every day. As one consequence, nurses need dependable self-care skills to bring their best effort to their work and maintain their own health. An aspect of self-care is the gentle power of feeling that you matter and that what you do has meaning. But a subtler level of self-care is to feel that the work you do is what you are supposed to be doing with your life—that nursing is a form of expression of your life purpose. It is the nagging feeling that you are not doing what you are supposed to be doing with your life that leads to discontent, restlessness, longing for something different, indifference, and burnout.

So, how do we move nursing from being a meaningful job to an expression of life purpose? We do so by realizing that we are partially drawn to nursing because of its arena in human suffering and vulnerability, and our desire to contribute to the alleviation of that suffering. By choosing nursing, you have placed yourself into that arena, but then you are faced with the dilemma of how to actually reduce another's suffering. There are the physical aspects of nursing that reduce physical suffering to the degree possible—but what about the vulnerability that has been heightened in every patient because of his or her health crisis? This is where skills, such as clinical meditation and imagery and an understanding of the transpersonal resources in human nature, become significant to the reduction of suffering.

My vision, based on my own clinical experience and my training of nurses and other health care professionals for 30 years, is that every nurse will:

- Trust and understand that every person, without exception, has a transpersonal nature.
- Possess pragmatic clinical meditation and imagery skills to open patients to their deeper transpersonal resources.

- Realize that the action of awakening the transpersonal resources of peace, wisdom, purpose, and oneness in their patients empowers those persons to get through their crisis with optimal healing possibilities.
- Experience the reduction of suffering through transpersonal work as an expression of their life purpose.

In my own journey, before I had these understandings, I could only address the verbal, rational part of my patients as they spoke of their pain and suffering. I could try to reassure them, and some of them might have believed me, but it was rarely a transformative personal experience for them. With the use of clinical meditation and imagery skills within the framework of TNC, gaining access to the transpersonal part of my patients' natures became possible. I saw patients go from fear to peace and from self-blame and bitterness to honoring their crisis as a point along the journey of their life. These shifts to peace and perspective are possible for both the patients who are suffering and the nurses who are committed to reducing that suffering as part of their purpose in this world.

■ REFLECTIONS

1. *What am I hoping for in my nursing career? And reflecting at an even deeper level, what am I hoping for?*
2. *When do I feel the greatest sense of positive connection with my work and with my colleagues? What can I do to strengthen these experiences?*
3. *What do I recognize as my greatest vulnerabilities? What are my patterns of response to them?*
4. *When am I most in touch with my transpersonal resources? How do I connect with my inner wisdom?*
5. *What is my purpose? How does my work as a nurse help me realize that purpose?*

■ REFERENCES

Assagioli, R. (1965). *Psychosynthesis: A manual of principles and techniques.* New York, NY: Hobbs, Dorman.

Dossey, B. M., & Keegan, L. (Eds.). (2016). *Holistic nursing: A handbook for practice* (7th ed.). Burlington, MA: Jones & Bartlett Learning.

Fanslow-Brunjes, C. (2008). *Using the power of hope to cope with dying: The four stages of hope.* Fresno, CA: Quill Driver Books.

Hess, D. R., Dossey, B. M., Southard, M. E., Luck, S., Schaub, B. G., & Bark, L. (2013). *The art and science of nurse coaching: The provider's guide to coaching scope and competencies.* Silver Springs, MD: Nursesbooks.org.

Schaub, B., & Schaub, R. (1991). Addictive process & the energy of choice. *The International Society for the Study of Subtle Energies & Energy Medicine: Newsletter, 2*(4), 12–15.

Schaub, B., & Schaub, R. (1997). *Healing addictions: The vulnerability model of recovery.* Albany, NY: Delmar.

Schaub, B., & Schaub, R. (2014). *Dante's path: Vulnerability and the spiritual journey.* Huntington, NY: Florence Press.

Schaub, B., & White, M. B. (2015). Transpersonal coaching. *Beginnings, 35*(4), 14–16.

Schaub, R., & Schaub, B. G. (2009). *The end of fear: A spiritual path for realists.* Carlsbad, CA: Hay House.

Schaub, R., & Schaub, B. G. (2013). *Transpersonal development: Cultivating the human resources of peace, wisdom, purpose and oneness.* Huntington, NY: Florence Press.

Shin, L. M., & Liberzon, I. (2010). The neurocircuitry of fear, stress, and anxiety disorders. *Neuropsychopharmacology, 35*(1), 169–191.

Tillich, P. (1952). *The courage to be.* New Haven, CT: Yale University Press.

Welwood, J. (1982). Vulnerability and power in the therapeutic process. *Journal of Transpersonal Psychology, 14*(2), 125–139.

CHAPTER TWENTY-EIGHT

Vocal and Brave: Working Toward No Less Than a Revolution

Tilda Shalof

I no longer differentiate between the person I am and the nurse I've become. Nursing is my profession and my way of life. It is a deep and abiding concern for the human condition.

— Shalof (2007, p. 311).

■ WHY NURSING?

"You're *still* at the bedside? Still just taking care of patients?"

Colleagues and friends are incredulous. Perplexed and disappointed in me.

After all these years, why have I not taken on *greater* responsibilities or *furthered* my education? Why have I not *risen* to leadership, aimed *higher*, or *graduated* to a position of more esteem? My reason is that I have realized these goals doing what I enjoy the most: taking care of patients. Taking care of business—and my business is taking care of patients and being the best nurse I can be at any given moment with each patient entrusted to my care. My other passion is writing about all that I see and do and feel and think as a nurse. I write about the days and nights of nurses and how their professional role affects their personal life and how their personal life affects their professional role and how it all can be political, too. Writing and speaking out publicly about nursing is my way to be a nurse leader. I want to leave a blueprint-manifesto-legacy for younger nurses who are trying to figure out for themselves what this complex and challenging profession—and, I would argue, *way of life*—is all about. For me, it is not about balancing "work" and "life" as if they were separate entities, diametrically opposed. The challenge I have set for myself is bringing the two together as one.

Yes, I am a hands-on, point-of-care, frontline—whatever you want to call it— nurse, and I like it that way. I have never found anything more satisfying or more elusive to master than that. Even after all of these years, it is still fresh, each new shift is different and full of possibilities for me and my patients. Every day or night that I walk into the hospital, I think of the souls that will be in my care and whether I am up to the challenge. Whether their condition improves or deteriorates, if they are to be kept safe or put in harm's way, depends in large part upon me. I continue to learn and be amazed. I cannot believe my good fortune to be a nurse and have a ticket, a passport, a license to this world.

I have been a nurse for 33 years, the past 28 of them in the medical–surgical intensive care unit (ICU) at Toronto General Hospital. I have also been a nurse actor for doctors' practical examinations, an insurance nurse, a flu shot nurse, a traveling nurse, a school nurse, a nurse artist, a nurse writer, and a camp nurse, and now I am a nurse working in a clinic that cares for people living with HIV.

Yes, I have ventured out a little bit . . . an abortive attempt at a master's degree, a short stint in middle management, a brief dalliance with research. Each time, I kept on returning home to what I enjoy most, what to me is the most meaningful and satisfying work I can do as a nurse.

And I have a secret. It heightens my appreciation of this work and of being an "insider." It reminds me that my familiarity with this hidden and restricted world will one day be an advantage to me. I will need my insider information. I never allow it to leave my awareness that one day, someone I love could be a patient, or that I could become one, too. In fact, once I was.

"You stay for the stories," my friends and families tease me. That is true, too. I delight in the connection, intimacy, and implied trust that comes from tending my patients' bodies, witnessing their experience, and receiving and honoring their stories. Being that safe repository for thoughts, secrets, fears, hopes, shames, emotions, failings, triumphs, and dreams is one of the many privileges of being a nurse—even more valuable than my salary, which is pretty decent, too. Oh, and I love the mess, the chaos, the noise, and the full-tilt pace, the urgency of being a hospital nurse. However, I recently discovered that out in the community, beyond the hospital walls, there, too, the stakes are just as high, with just as many life-and-death situations.

I cannot believe how privileged I am to be allowed do the work I do and get to see what I see. I am fortunate to have chosen nursing and to have stayed the course this long, despite ups and downs, challenges and setbacks along the way. These days, a common phrase used to praise a person or a group is to say they "make a difference." That simplistic phrase falls short when applied to nurses. Over the years, I have seen many times where a nurse made *all* the difference. And in every single situation, nurses make not only a difference, but make things better—or have the potential to do so.

Long ago, before I became the dedicated and impassioned nurse I am today, I was a self-absorbed, lazy amateur, de facto caregiver. As a child—an infant, even—I fell into the role of the family "nurse" and my family members were my first "patients." Many days I stayed home from school to take care of my mother, who had Parkinson's disease and mental illness. I monitored my father's blood sugar, gave him insulin for his diabetes, and nitroglycerin for angina. I soothed my brother, who has schizophrenia and suffers hallucinations and paranoia, and back then was always in a rage. Truth be told, I had no real interest in or particular aptitude for caregiving, but that did not stop me from choosing to become a nurse. After all, being around sick people was familiar and surely there would be an unlimited supply of sick people that would make me always in demand, right?

My literary inspiration was Nurse Cherry Ames. Written in the 1950s, this series of books was already hopelessly outdated when I read them in the 1970s. (I dreamed of becoming a dude ranch nurse or ski patrol nurse, like Cherry.) My television role models were the beautiful, brainy Nurse Julia and the spunky, sexy Hot Lips Houlihan on M*A*S*H*. Closer to home, the pink uniform and diver's watch worn by the peppy young nurse who cared for my father when he had a heart attack was also enticing. But my elitist, intellectual family discouraged me. To them, nursing was a low-class, blue-collar job. I think that is what made me want it all the more.

My student years coincided with a rocky time in my life. I was dealing with the end stages of my parents' illnesses, my own depression and anxiety, as well as financial worries. After their deaths, bereft and distraught, I was unable to care for myself. For almost a year, I was homeless, roaming the city where I lived, showing up to a few lectures about nursing theory or microbiology during the day, then riding the city buses and subway alone, late into the night until the last ride. Then I would find a 24 hour diner and eat blueberry pie and drink coffee, and then sleep on a park bench. Yet, somehow I managed to make it to my clinical days and pull it off, despite my distressed state and disheveled appearance. Even at my graduation ceremony, I feared for the safety of the patients soon to be in my care. *Run, run away*, I would telepathically urge my future patients. (I ask you, would *you* have wanted me as your nurse back then? I think not, though now you would.) My goals were simply to not harm anyone (as far as I know, I did not) and to survive, paycheck to paycheck. All the sophisticated concepts of our theoretical frameworks of caring, not to mention "leadership" and "therapeutic communication," that I was learning at nursing school went completely over my head and flew out the window. (Back then, we had windows that actually opened.)

Years passed and my home life and mental state improved. I worked at different hospitals and nursing agencies and was sent to a variety of medical and surgical floors. Initially, like most new graduates, I was ill-equipped to actually take care of patients like my practical and hardworking colleagues, who often reminded me that they were "diploma nurses" and were trained the "right way," by actually working in the hospital. I was scrambling to get the work done and not kill anyone with my bachelor's degree education. Eventually, I caught up with the experienced nurses and the gap narrowed, then vanished. It was due to the fact that I took the word "practice" to heart and worked hard to improve my clinical skills, constantly taking courses, studying in the library, and expanding my scope of abilities. I also wanted to get better at my communication with patients and families and improve my aptitude at handling complex and sensitive situations. I watched in awe the way some nurses could change a dressing, tidy the patient's gown and lines, soothe the patient, explain everything to the patient and the family, and somehow answer all of my questions, too—it was astounding. I tried to emulate that, but for years, I felt overwhelmed and lonely. I yearned to feel competent and I craved the feeling of being part of a team.

After a few years, I stumbled upon an opportunity to take a critical care course and work in the medical–surgical ICU, where I still worked until very recently. Although I was not the least bit technically adept, practical, or emotionally resilient— qualities required of any nurse, but even more so an ICU nurse—the collaboration, the energetic culture, and the fun they seemed to be having pulled me in. Here, the nurses were even more knowledgeable, nimble, and graceful; they could draw arterial blood gases, keep an eye on the cardiac monitor, check the intravenous (IV) flow rate, and assess their patient's breathing pattern while smoothing out the sheets over the patient and answering a distraught family member's question—all at the same time. Best of all, these nurses were empowered. They knew what they knew and they believed in their worth.

Some nurses had *style,* even flair. They knew how to use a combination of their intelligence and common sense, personality, sense of humor, quick wit, their religious beliefs, or even their personal spirituality in their care. Occasionally, when a nurse was requested by name by a family member to be the loved one's nurse, I burned with envy. I wanted to be the nurse requested by family members and patients. I made up my mind that I would become that sought-after, chosen nurse. I would stay in the ICU until I grew into the expert and became the best nurse I could be. I would take care of patients until I mastered it. As I mentioned, I only just left . . . 28 years later.

■ EARLY IMPRESSIONS

In the ICU, patients are unstable, most are unconscious, and all have catastrophic, multisystem, life-threatening illnesses. I have stood by a wife who did not recognize her husband's face, so distorted it was from his illness and our treatments. I have sat with a mother whose son did not wake up after his lung transplant. Months later, when he finally did, he married his sweetheart right there at his side. I have dropped down to the floor to be with children who were drawing with crayons in coloring books under the bed of their mother as she was taken off life support and died. I have plunged into action when a man had a seizure—gave him oxygen, injected 10 mg of Valium into his central line, kept him safe and listened to his daughter praise the doctor who came in afterward. "No," he said with a chuckle, "It was the nurse who saved me." I have cared for a young man who for the first time in his life took an easy, comfortable, breath out of new, transplanted lungs. I laughed with him as he joked that now he would need an alarm clock without the gasping and coughing he had had all his life that woke him up each morning. I have put my arms around family and friends and prayed with them as they gathered around the bed as their loved ones—from ages 18 to 104—were dying. I have tried to stay always mindful and openhearted, and, mostly, I have. The temptation to shut down and turn away from the ever-present sadness, pain, suffering, and death we witness is powerful. I think it must be a means of self-preservation. (I will never forget the patient who took my hand and said, "It's going to be all right," to comfort *me.*) I do not judge nurses or doctors who do keep a distance or cut off their emotions, though this is not the way I choose to handle my feelings. I no longer see my responses as a liability or weakness as I once did. My emotions are the fuel that ignite my passion for this work and sustain me.

Each patient, irrespective of the medical diagnosis, is fascinating to me. Whether it is a patient post-op after a lung transplant for pulmonary hypertension, or a patient encephalopathic from liver failure, or a patient in multisystem organ failure, or one with a metastasized malignancy or a rare autoimmune disease, each is a book to read, a world to discover, a new challenge for me to figure out how to be the nurse for that person, the nurse that person needs. I cannot ever imagine being bored at work. I never tire of wanting to know all there is to know about each one, the challenges he or she faces, and how. Night shifts, day shifts, weekends, Christmas eve, I have shown up, shift after shift, curious and eager.

Because all of these experiences have always been so precious to me, I decided years ago to record as much as I could in a journal. In my paper journal, I give myself complete freedom to express my opinions and impressions without censor or censure. Evidence-based practice is in there, as it organically occurs, but even more is my *practice-based evidence* from all the funny, sad, scary, challenging, and joyful moments, the failures and the triumphs, the patients I will never forget (including a few I'd *like* to forget), and the nurses I admired and a few I did not.

Daily journal writing has always been a part of my life. This form of self-reflection, my method to process my experiences, coupled with regular debriefing sessions in various cafés around town, over coffee (and cake), and sitting and talking and knitting (they knit, I make notes) with my nurse friends has helped me avoid the infamous "burnout" or "compassion fatigue" that the nursing literature states is so prevalent among our ranks. (I wonder if studying and teaching to the extent we do is not almost priming nurses to expect to become burned-out and disillusioned. Same with "lateral violence" and "entrenched hierarchies"—sometimes we look out for what we are taught to expect and inevitably find it to reinforce our preconceptions. What if we focused more on another way, a different vision to shoot for?)

One thing I know for sure: You have to be strong to be a nurse. Physical strength and endurance for the long hours and back-breaking labor. Mental strength for the learning and thinking. Moral courage for advocacy and ethical dilemmas. Emotional hardiness and resilience, for more reasons than I can name. Maturity and spiritual awareness. I was none of these things when I started out, but I am now. Nursing has given me all that—and more.

Every morning, we have team rounds on each patient and, for me, that meeting of the entire team exemplifies all that is healthy and right about a workplace environment. (After all, a hospital will never be healthy for patients if it is not healthy for the people who work there.) In the ICU, morning rounds are like a town hall meeting, just like the ancient Greeks conducted, as described in Plato's *Republic*. A public place where everyone gathers—all members of the team, plus patients if they are able and family if they wish—and all have a chance to listen and to speak. As we move the computer on wheels around the unit from patient to patient, together we review x-rays, CT scans, and lab results. Each nurse presents his or her patients, summarizes the medical history, and then presents a head-to-toe nursing assessment. The guiding motto of our ICU is, "Every voice is valued."

I recall an incident when I was caring for a patient, an elderly man with chronic obstructive pulmonary disease (COPD). After auscultating his lungs and hearing bilateral crackles, I had analyzed his blood and diagnosed a metabolic acidosis. His oxygen saturations had dropped and I suspected a pneumonia was brewing, so I went ahead and ordered a stat chest x-ray. Later that afternoon, our chief physician, Dr. Neil Lazar, stood outside my patient's door and said, "Why was this x-ray ordered? It wasn't needed. Who did this?" Quickly, I realized he was not pulling rank or trying to trip me up and luckily, by then, I did not take anything personally. His questioning was about accountability, clinical judgment, and a rationale for my intervention. For me it was not just about whether that x-ray was needed or not (as it turned out, it was not because of the time lag for certain clinical conditions to appear on an x-ray.). It made me realize how fortunate I am to work in an environment where I can exercise my critical thinking and clinical judgment, even when I am wrong. Unfortunately, not all nurses have this hard-earned privilege, or perhaps they do, but do not believe they do. They blame it on the unfriendly culture or the entrenched medical hierarchies or hostile colleagues, but I think we have to own it. Nurses have to face this fear and find the courage to speak up. Many nurses ask, "Why aren't we listened to?" or "Why don't we get the respect we deserve?" Nurses are not listened to when they do not speak up. Nurses are not respected when they do not exhibit self-respect. Agency, empowerment, and respect are not given; they are earned.

The next phase of my development as a critical care nurse was a period of intense moral distress about end-of-life decision making, specifically situations where I believed we were going "too far," usually at the behest of families requesting that "everything be done." So often we perform invasive and uncomfortable procedures on people during the last few days or weeks of their lives. My angst about this frequently occurring situation was so severe, I thought I would have to leave the ICU for good. But I remember Dr. Lazar saying to a family, "We may choose to withdraw treatment, but we never withdraw care." That was a crystallizing moment when I understood so much, especially what nursing care offers.

■ PROFESSIONAL EVOLUTION/CONTRIBUTION

The years flew by, but I did not just show up shift after shift. I kept myself busy. I started a research committee and journal club. I became editor and contributor to a hospital nursing newsletter and wrote a visitor's guidebook to the ICU. I conducted a small, deeply flawed research study to look at the effect upon nurses of the photographs that families placed at the bedside of their loved ones. At medical conferences, I provided the nursing perspective on end-of-life decisions. I had no position to argue or research findings to present, but I shared my stories and trusted their inherent wisdom. Perhaps what I really wanted to express could only be conveyed in a story or, perhaps, a poem.

It was around that time that I came across a small, red book, a publication of Sigma Theta Tau International (STTI), the Nursing Honor Society. *The Power of Ten, 2011–2013: Nurse Leaders Address the Profession's Ten Most Pressing Issues* (STTI, 2011) is a slight book but hefty in scope and powerful in message. Within it, 10 scholarly, highly credentialed American nurse leaders identify and address the profession's 10 most pressing issues. Topics included were technology, nursing education, and workplace culture. I had ideas and opinions on all of these topics, as most nurses do. Unfortunately, too many nurses believe they do not have the right to contribute to this discussion. Turning the book over, I read the back cover: "Start the Conversation! Nurses tend bodies and minds. They learn; they care . . . [but] nurses are seldom provocateurs. Nursing as a profession has some significant obstacles to overcome. Provocateurs are welcomed and needed." Now, that sounded like something I could do. I liked to start conversations, get discussions going, raise questions, stir things up, and create a ruckus—perhaps I *could* be a nurse leader in some way. I thought of the phrase that Dr. Mary Ferguson-Pare often stated: "Lead from where you stand." She was our nurse CEO and vice president of professional affairs and also a personal mentor to me. Perhaps leadership was possible to work toward, but deep down I did not believe I was leadership material.

As I spent years mulling over that dream, meanwhile, something terrifying happened. It was a worldwide health crisis that hit Toronto especially hard. SARS—sudden acute respiratory syndrome—had erupted and was a lethal pandemic. Toronto, being an international travel and immigration hub, was at the epicenter. The city shut down overnight. Businesses closed. This infectious disease was not like HIV or hepatitis, contracted by intimate contact. It was not transmitted by droplets or, like malaria, through a mosquito vector. No, the SARS virus was airborne—it was in the very air we breathed. Toronto became a ghost town. Many people went into quarantine. Hospitals cleared out—no visitors or management, administration, or maintenance staff were allowed to enter, only frontline workers. It was primarily the nurses who cared for SARS patients. Geared up in big, puffy, astronautlike hazmat suits, plus filters, masks, gloves, and shields to protect ourselves, we still worried about the unknown risks to our lives we were being exposed to.

A side effect to this crisis was that, immediately, nurses were in the news and on the public radar. (We saw a repeat of this scenario during the recent Ebola crisis.) Suddenly, we were seen and heard from, not to mention acknowledged and praised.

It was shortly after this frightening episode that I decided the time had come to take a manuscript of my stories about my life as a nurse to a publisher. I had been writing for years and was used to rejections, so I was completely taken aback when the publisher offered me a book contract on the spot. "This is something new. We never hear this perspective," he said. "Why have we never seen stories in print before?" The funny thing is that all nurses know these stories, but we rarely share them with others, only other nurses. It did feel risky, even dangerous to write so candidly and to expose some secrets and taboos we have always kept within our ranks. "You'll get in trouble," some nurses warned me. "You could lose your job." Naively perhaps, I trusted that telling my reality and being truthful would protect me.

Stories that had haunted me for years made their way into *A Nurse's Story: Life, Death and In-Between in an Intensive Care Unit* (Shalof, 2004): the futile, undignified, and tortuous treatments performed on dying patients; petty nurse-to-nurse bullying; conflicts with family members; abusive and violent patients; incredible recoveries, sometimes against all odds; and sweet, tender moments with patients. Amusing, hilarious moments too. I wrote about errors, nursing and medical ones, and I started with my own—how your heart sinks, your stomach clenches, and your mind races when you realize your careless moment. How you make full disclosure and do everything in your power to remedy the error. How, at the end of it, you go out the door and creep home, mulling it over, and wishing you could just take back those moments "just before." It was important to me to expose the "dirty work" of nursing, specifically about how a nurse moves from feeling demeaned and ashamed into feeling proud of the skill it takes to make a patient feel renewed and clean. Night shift high jinks, popcorn and coffee, and moments of such inexorable exhaustion, you wonder if you are a safe nurse.

Yes, nursing can be an extreme sport. We see human suffering at its most raw and vulnerable and I wanted my stories to reflect that harsh reality and to be real and honest, no sugarcoating, definitely no "angels" or "heroes," and no blaming or complaining either. Just hard-working professionals who are human and—most of them—doing their best. So often nurses lament, "No one knows what we do." I have found that to be true, but it is because we are not telling them. If no one listens to us, it is because we are too quiet, often silent, or completely absent in popular culture, in public forums, and the media. Still, sentimental or sexist images and inaccurate portrayals of what a nurse is persist. Public opinion polls state that nurses are trusted, well-respected professionals, but in my experience, the public does not have any understanding of what we do to keep them safe and help make them better. They praise us for our tender loving-kindness but not for our skills and knowledge.

It is very nice to be modest, but with respect to nursing leadership, here is the problem: Tell a nurse who you believe is an exemplary clinician that he or she has the potential for leadership and, invariably, he or she will demur, deny—even *disdain*—the role. Nursing students and new nurses are told they are leaders. (That's what they told us, too, back in the 1980s.) And yes, with their youthful energy, education, and idealism, they all have the *potential* to be, but will they step up to the challenge? I spoke at a conference once on the topic of nurse leadership and one participant asked, "Do we have to be leaders? Can't we be followers?" Many excellent nurses abdicate leadership, but does not a leader have to claim it, truly own it? Should not a leader want power to make change and take initiative? A true leader does not wait for permission or invitation. Recently I was counseling a young nurse who was thinking of leaving the ICU to work at another hospital closer to her home. "But it might not be like here," she fretted, referring to our lean hierarchy and our healthy work environment. "But you could be the one to lead the way, make change, and empower nurses," I suggested. *Oh yeah, leadership* was the expression on her face. *We studied that at school.* It seemed like it had not occurred to her that she could step up and be a leader herself.

How do you identify a nurse leader or a potential one? A short list of the telltale signs is that a leader sees something missing and steps up to fill the void. A leader inspires others to do better and be better. A leader engages passionately and creatively and invites humor and mirth, even in the bleak atmosphere of hospital. A leader is brave and is vocal when necessary.

A few years ago, something happened that made me realize the courage needed to be a leader. There is nothing like having skin in the game—literally speaking—that makes all of this personal. After 30 years as a nurse, I suddenly became a patient. For almost a year, I had been feeling unwell. Buried in my chest was a secret I had been keeping all my life, even from myself. I had a congenital bicuspid aortic valve and always knew I would need open-heart surgery for a valve replacement, but I was scared like only a nurse can be. We know exactly what to worry about. Sure, "knowledge is power," but also "ignorance is bliss." Which was it? I did not feel power from my knowledge and did not have the luxury of ignorance. What was there to be afraid of? Intubation! Medial sternotomy! Cardioplegia! Adverse events! Medication errors! Nosocomial infections! For starters.

Nurses make the worst patients, do we not? But suddenly I realized my worst fear: nurses. Nurses would keep me comfortable, safe, and prevent complications like a clot, bleeding, or an infection—or not. They would see a problem and do something about it—or not. The surgeon would fix my valve, but it would be up to my nurses to bring me back to life and get me home. I know the power of nursing, but I also know it can be the weakest link, the wild card. There is nothing scarier than a timid nurse. (I know because

I have been that nurse.) A nurse who sees a problem and looks away out of fear of rocking the boat or challenging authority. To survive open-heart surgery, I would need brave and outspoken nurses. Nurses endanger patients when they do not speak up when they see something wrong or when they do not share what they know about their patients.

All went well for me and a few months later, when I returned to work, I realized how being a patient deepened my understanding of fear and trust. I recalled my last shift as a nurse before my surgery. As I cared for my patient and injected 1 mg of morphine for pain relief into the central line close to his heart and as I suctioned his lungs and monitored his cardiac rhythm, I realized the trust required to put yourself in a nurse's hands. I listened to a nearby nurse introduce himself to his patient. "I'm your nurse. I'll take care of you." What a promise of safety that implies! He would steward his patient through the night and do everything in his power to keep him safe. And it is not just expertise and knowledge that create nursing excellence; what about duty, accountability, integrity, honesty, and trustworthiness? We tend to just assume that those qualities are in place—after all, we are *professionals*, are we not? Yes, but we are also flawed human beings, and those noble qualities cannot be taught, measured, evaluated, or legislated. The quality of a nurse's character is also a part of nursing excellence.

These human qualities have a direct impact on patient safety. Safety seems to be on everyone's mind these days, both health care professionals and the public at large, who are all shocked by the reported incidence of errors and adverse events. Once I sat on a panel of experts at a conference on patient safety. The topic was "Heroes on the Frontlines." (Admittedly, a cringeworthy title.) At this conference, held over 3 days and involving more than 100 experts, I was the only frontline nurse to be a conference speaker. Yet, nurses have the most to contribute to this discussion; nursing is about safety. If "Toys R Us," then surely, nurses can claim, "Safety Is Us." Nurses need to own the bailiwick of safety. After all, concern for safety is embedded in everything a nurse does. Of course, every member of the team tries his or her utmost to avoid errors or do harm, but nurses perform certain acts whose express purpose is to keep people safe. It is not that nurses are better at keeping patients safe than others, but they *should* be.

If medicine's credo is "Do no harm," I would say that nursing's credo is "Keep the patient safe." We are the most proximal and spend the greatest amount of time with patients. If patients are to be kept safe, it is in large part due to what we do or do not do. We are the key link in the chain of safety. I hold nurses to a higher standard for patient safety than other professions because patient safety is our job. Nurses are more responsible for safety than is publicly acknowledged.

"Safe" is an essential word in our lexicon. It is embedded in our vernacular. To say a nurse is "safe" is both a minimal expectation and stamp of approval, and a supreme compliment. "Are you safe?" "That's safe," or "That's not safe"—is pure nursespeak. We may be discussing the risks of performing a procedure on a patient with an elevated international normalized ratio (INR) or staffing ratios or workload assignments, but so much of what nurses do—or allow to be done to their patient by others—is determined by attention to safety. Listen to the verbs nurses use: "safeguard," "monitor," "check," (and "double-check"), "watch," "watch over," "watch out for," "look after," "look out for," "listen for," "listen out for," "observe," "care for," "keep an eye on," "trouble-shoot." Any discussion of health care—but especially one about patient safety—that does not include nursing's voice is fundamentally flawed and erroneous.

Here is how you as a nurse start a shift. You enter the room and introduce yourself to your patient and family members. You begin your thorough head-to-toe assessment. You assess your patient's level of consciousness and consider sedation, restlessness, agitation, and look for risks of a fall or ICU delirium. You ensure that the IV fluids and all meds are correct. You study the cardiac monitor and adjust its alarms. You scrutinize the patient's cardiac rhythm, scan for arrhythmias, and check the electrolytes. You examine your patient's skin, especially pressure points, as you assess the risk of skin breakdown. You auscultate your patient's lungs, listening for air entry and any adventitious sounds. You check the position of the nasogastric tube to prevent aspiration. These are actions a nurse does to keep a patient safe. This is not an extraordinary or heroic nurse; it is a picture of doing the job properly. One surefire way to keep patients safe is for nurses to be vocal, brave, smart, and empowered—and for there to be enough of them.

Hospitals are publicly rated on their incidence of nosocomial infections, adverse events, and other parameters, but what about the quality of the nursing care or the nurse-to-patient ratio? We now have an abundance of studies that show a correlation of an increase in the nurse-to-patient ratio with a decrease in mortality, decreased incidence of complications, decreased hospital readmissions, and so forth. But does this data get factored into these hospital performance appraisals? Is the public aware of this metric and its meaning to them, personally?

But first and foremost, in order for safety to be assured for the patient, there must also be safety for the nurse. Hospitals are not "safe" for nurses if nurses do not have a voice or feel that they do not. They are toxic, dangerous places if there is bullying, racism, sexism, or any form of bigotry. Too often, hospitals are inhospitable and punitive—with nurses. Those whose job it is to offer compassion and kindness often do not receive it from the very institution where they work ("Nurses Week" celebrations notwithstanding).

■ MORAL/ETHICAL FOUNDATION

A few years ago, I was offered a golden opportunity that I almost turned down. Dr. Judith Shamian—now president of the International Council of Nurses, but then the CEO of Canada's most revered and influential home care services company—invited me to learn about home care and community nursing. "But I'm a hospital nurse," I reminded her. "I don't know much about home care." That was a lie. I knew absolutely nothing about home care. I had no idea what happened to my patients after they were discharged from the hospital to their homes or the community, or who would be caring for them—or not. Like most hospital nurses, we know little about health care beyond our hospital walls.

As I pondered her offer, Judith told me about "three types of nurses." The first type, she explained, takes care of patients and that is enough for that nurse. The second type of nurse may conduct research, teach, or manage, but separates himself or herself from the real world of nurses and patients. This nurse may even be involved in policy making or political activism, or even volunteerism, but not usually in clinical practice as a nurse. "This nurse has amnesia about being a nurse," Judith said wryly. Then there is a third type of nurse. This is the consummate nurse who can care for individual patients and keep an eye on the bigger picture with a concern for humanity and social justice. This type of nurse swims "downstream" and "upstream." For this nurse, the personal and the political are inseparable.

There was no doubt in my mind that I was the first type of nurse. I worked in a rarified, circumscribed world and rarely, barely, considered the bigger picture. I was a nurse who did not see the forest for the trees. In fact, I was a "leaf" nurse, caring for patients one by one, attending to their "numbers"—oxygen molecules, carbon dioxide levels, and arterial blood gases. My nursing care was down to the cellular level, gas exchange, arteries, and veins.

I decided to accept Judith's invitation and visited nurse practitioners in primary care clinics. I spent time with nurses caring for soldiers with posttraumatic stress disorder (PTSD) and others who care for homeless, pregnant, often drug-addicted young women, and sex workers. I met nurses caring for people in their homes and saw that a home can be a mansion, shack, teepee, or a downtown back alley behind a parking lot. I learned about the toll on family members of around-the-clock caregiving. I realized that all of this, too, was nursing's domain. My eyes were opened to nursing that is every bit as essential, meaningful, and lifesaving as critical care.

For me, all roads lead to nursing. Addressing world problems with a nursing sensibility would go a long way toward their amelioration. A nursing ethos is the antidote for violence, war, and terrorism. Tender, intelligent nursing care will save our endangered planet. The answers are more obvious than we think, but sometimes even the basics elude us. I have to chuckle when I read one of Florence Nightingale's most fundamental tenets about the benefits of fresh air (Nightingale, 1859/1992). Today's hospitals are hermetically sealed vaults filled with recycled air and unpleasant smells. We must move care out from the unhealthy hospital environments to the community and peoples' homes. Sometimes the solutions are cheaper, simpler, and more cost-effective. With the current infatuation with all things "cutting edge" and "high tech," we have obscured the fact that we must first ensure that people's basic needs are met.

■ VISION

The majority of all health care spending, some estimates are as high as 90%, goes to doctors and hospitals, with the remaining 10% going to community and public health. Nursing could lead the way in correcting this unjust imbalance. Kathleen MacMillan (2014), professor of nursing at Dalhousie University, writes,

> Nurses offer community based, low-tech, patient/client-centered . . . and effective [treatments]. . . . The nursing voice is often absent from the system transformation discourse. . . . Of all professions, nursing has the most to gain . . . by shifting care out of institutions to the community, but we are a very meek and quiet voice in the wilderness. (pp. 3–4)

It is hard to disagree with her contention that there is a negligible impact of nurses on system transformation. It starts with voice, presence, and bold leadership. It will take no less than a revolution.

Perhaps the way to light the fire under nurses, to awaken them to lean in and engage deeply with all aspects of the profession, is to start right with nurses themselves. The young generation coming along desperately needs mentors, coaches, and clinical mentors to encourage and guide them, and to pass on the legacy of nursing values. Nursing needs more men in all roles. Men in nursing often tell me how the feminization of nursing, with its emphasis on sentiment, emotion, maternal qualities, and the virtue script, stigmatizes and stereotypes them. It makes them feel disconnected from the profession. Yet nursing desperately needs men for their mental muscle, louder voices, and stronger presence. Balancing the gender demographic of our profession will more powerfully define nursing and help us to rebrand ourselves in accurate ways.

In order for a nurse to do this demanding work and sustain a career, there must be a commitment by institutions, and by nurses themselves, to engage in self-care. Self-care is important for everyone, but *crucial* for nurses and family caregivers. Nursing has the highest rate of work-related illness, injury, and disability of all professions. Forty percent of nurses who are 35 years and older do "double-duty caregiving," caring at work and also at home for relatives (Canadian Institutes for Health Research, 2015, p. 1). These dual responsibilities jeopardize nurses' physical and mental health and put them at an increased risk of committing drug errors or other mistakes in the workplace. Supports—financial, practical, and emotional—must be made widely available for nurses.

My nursing manifesto, my "call to arms," returns always to voice. We are simply too quiet, sometimes inaudible, or even silent. Dr. Shamian poses the question, "Why are so few nurse leaders in management or political power?" Even regarding pure nursing concerns, such as primary care, food security, sanitation, water, vaccinations, and disease prevention, she laments that few nurses are involved at the global, executive level. Yet, if nursing is absent, the discussion will be dominated by other bodies, such as pharmaceutical conglomerates and medical consortia. If nursing is absent, these debates are incomplete, maybe even nullified.

As for me, yes, I am *still* at the bedside, taking care of patients, exactly where I want to be. I do my utmost to stay aware of the bigger issues in our profession and in the world today. Each and every nurse has to decide for himself or herself what the dimensions and scope of the nursing life will be. Will it be microscopic or telescopic? The leaves on the tree, or the trunk and the branches, the whole tree, roots and all, or the vast forest beyond? My nursing career has been about waking up and then waking up again and again. The average person reads the news of the day: wars, poverty, crime, and natural disasters. An ordinary citizen feels helpless and turns to the sports section or the horoscopes. But a nurse knows exactly how these conditions affect the health of people and their communities and society at large. And when you know, it is hard to look away.

There are many nursing theories I know and love. Many of them inform and guide my practice. The works of all of the great nursing theorists are brilliant and have added much to our understanding of our profession, like Benner, Henderson, Parse, Peplau, and Watson (see Chapter 16). However, what guides me now and helps me to understand the core of what nursing is about came from Pope Francis when he spoke about caring for our environment. He stated, "Our purpose on earth is to be a steward of God's creations" (Pope Francis, 2015). *Stewardship*—"the careful and responsible management of something entrusted to one's care" is how the dictionary defines it ("Stewardship,"

2015). That is as good a definition of nursing as any I have heard (see Chapter 24 for more on the role of nurse leaders in stewardship).

Nurses need to wake up to the power and beauty of this profession and become more engaged in their work and expand their territory. We say we are the science of caring, but caring is not just being kind, gentle, and tender; it is also loud, bold, and fierce. Personal and political. Vocal and brave. The subtitle of this book is about evolution, but perhaps what is needed is *revolution*. The world is changing so much and so fast, but is nursing keeping up? If not, we will be left behind, and the beauty, grace, wisdom, witness, safety, and comfort that nurses offer will be lost. This is the challenge that consumes me now.

■ REFLECTIONS

1. *Do I consider myself a nurse leader? Do I aspire to be one? Why or why not?*
2. *Am I a leaf nurse? A tree nurse? A forest nurse? What is the scope and where are the boundaries of my nursing career? Do I try to contract and concentrate them or to broaden and expand them? Basically, is my nurse vision myopic or hyperoptic? Any astigmatism—blurring or distortions?*
3. *What do I consider to be nursing's most pressing issues? What is my "Power of Ten"?*
4. *What is my own "nurse's story"? Have I ever considered writing it or part of it for publication or to share with friends, family, and my community?*
5. *What are the seminal events in my nursing career that made me the nurse leader I am today?*

■ REFERENCES

Canadian Institutes for Health Research. (2015). *Supporting double duty caregivers: A policy brief.* Retrieved from uwo.ca/nursing/cwg/docs/PolicyBrieffinal.pdf

MacMillan, K. (2014). Guest editorial. *Nursing Leadership, 27*(4), 1–4.

Stewardship. (2015). In *Merriam-Webster online dictionary.* Retrieved from http://www.merriam-webster.com/dictionary/stewardship

Nightingale, F. (1859/1992). *Notes on nursing: What it is and what it is not* (Commemorative ed.). Philadelphia, PA: Lippincott Williams & Wilkins.

Pope Francis. (2015). Encyclical letter of the Holy Father on care for our common home. Retrieved from http://www.cruxnow.com/church/2015/06/18/read-pope-francis-encyclical-laudato-si/

Shalof, T. (2004). *A nurse's story: Life, death and in-between in an intensive care unit.* Toronto, ON, Canada: McLelland & Stewart.

Shalof, T. (2007). *The making of a nurse.* Toronto, ON, Canada: McClelland & Stewart.

Sigma Theta Tau International, Honor Society of Nursing. (2011). *The power of ten 2011-2013: Nurse leaders address the profession's ten most pressing issues.* Indianapolis, IN: Author.

CHAPTER TWENTY-NINE

Metaphorical and Passionate: Merging the Personal-Professional for a Unified Self

Leighsa Sharoff

Holistic nursing . . . is a way of being . . . a conscious merger of . . . holism into one's life as well as into one's profession. Self-care, self-responsibility, and self-respect are integrated into . . . one's own life. . . . How can we begin to heal the fragmentation of our profession if we as individuals are fragmented and wounded? (Sharoff, 1997, pp. 11–12). *The reflective practitioner incorporates and integrates his or her vast knowledge base of experience, skills, and attitudes to assist in formulating his or her own practice as a metaphor . . . to create new meaning and provide a deeper awareness into the human spirit* (Sharoff, 2007a) *. . . foster[ing] and promot[ing] self-awareness and enhancement of one's consciousness. Being present in one's life is being able to be reflective. Metaphorical depiction of oneself is an aspect of that reflective process and a powerful expression of self . . . a powerful transformational tool.* (Sharoff, 2009a, p. 271)

I am a phoenix.

■ WHY NURSING?

When I was a little girl, my father was a butcher and he used to come home with bone shards in his hands and fingers. These shards would become infected and my mother had him soak his hands and fingers in hot water and then she would squeeze the pus right out of it. Well, I thought this was the coolest thing I had ever seen! I thought how interesting it was that the body would make this pus and then when it was squeezed out, my father would say that it felt better. I started wondering where this pus came from, why it came out of the wound, and why it felt better when it was not there anymore. How did the body know to do this? I thought that if the body knew how to do this, I wanted to know how it did this also. This was the beginning of my fascination with the human body.

When I was in high school, I was old enough to volunteer as a candy striper (that shows you my age, as we do not call them candy stripers anymore). I volunteered at Coney Island Hospital after school. My friends thought I was crazy since no one they knew ever wanted to go into a hospital. I thought it was captivating. To this day, I still have memories of volunteering there and remember the awe and wonder I felt every time I walked onto the unit. First off, the nurses were in control. They did everything: made all the decisions, took care of the patients and their families, and were always "chatting away" in the nurses' station. The doctors, I noticed, barely spoke to the patients and stayed only a few minutes. It was the nurse who would explain to the patient what the doctor said, would provide the comfort and support to them, and hold their hands when they were scared. I looked at these nurses and thought they were the smartest and most caring people who worked in the hospital. And that is how I began my journey into nursing.

I followed the typical path to become a nurse. I went to a good four-year college and started my training as a labor and delivery (L&D) room nurse. I ventured into the neonatal intensive care unit and enjoyed the hectic pace. I envisioned working as a heli-copter neonatal transport nurse, as I liked the thrill of adrenaline. However, my path took a dramatic detour after an accident that left me on crutches for a year and needing a cane to walk for almost six years. It was during this time that this life-altering experi-ence placed me on a completely different journey than the one I initially had sought out. This transformation of me, not as a nurse but as a person, altered my vision of my life, the very essence of who I was being-becoming. The adrenaline junkie was now looking for meditation, for reflection, for understanding the ways of being that could transform the true core of my life. Who was I to become? For I knew I could no longer be who I thought I was.

This never-ending personal journey was scary, thought-provoking, encouraging, terrifying, and wondrous . . . and transformed every aspect of who I was and why I was. The new path I started on was filled with heavy emotional burdens to unload, rocky per-sonal landscapes to climb over and out of, and honest reflections that tore me apart . . . while healing me to become whole. It was a time of change, of growth, and of awakening to become a new me. And as my new awareness emerged, changes to my professional me developed as well. I no longer felt the need for the adrenaline rush, but instead, the calming serenity of being. I no longer felt the need to run (and was physically unable to run anymore), but learned to breathe and take in the moment.

Thus, who I first was when I became a nurse and who I am now as a nurse are not the same. My initial intention and vision of when I became a nurse was to work in a high-impact, fast-paced, high-stress environment . . . the more adrenaline and intensity, the better. That worked well for me for many years and I loved it. Then, I had to become a different person, a different nurse. So I opened my mind, heart, and spirit and learned initially how to heal myself, how to first engage in self-care and self-reflection, and then I knew I had found the path I was meant to be on. This path led to personal acceptance, professional enhancements, and an intentionality of being who I truly was. So, when I reflect on the memories of those nurses at Coney Island Hospital, remembering how they controlled their unit, how they gave of themselves and cared for their patients, I now ponder, "Did they engage in their own self-care?" Today, I am that mature, giving, and caring nurse, yet I have integrated self-care and self-reflection, for how are we as nurses to engage in the healing–caring processes of another if we cannot first engage in our own self-care?

■ EARLY IMPRESSIONS

When I was a nursing student, I had some incredible nurse educators who, to this day, I still remember. I was not your typical-looking nursing student, it being the 1980s and the emergence of the "punk scene." I was into punk/alternative music and enjoyed the self-expression that it provided. Not all my professors agreed and some took offense at my "individuality." However, the chair of the program in which I was enrolled said that as long as I conducted myself in a professional manner, provided appropriate, efficient, and effective nursing care, and was attentive to my studies, how I wore my hair was of no concern to her or the school (mind you, I graduated nursing school in a mohawk). Another professor of mine, my mental health nurse educator, took me under her wing when I was experiencing some personal issues and needed someone to talk to. Netta was wonderful, teaching me that, as nurses, we need to take care of each other. She showed me that being a nurse was more than just taking care of someone in the hospital; it was caring for people in everyday life.

As a nursing student, I remember going through all the clinical rotations thinking, "This is not what I want to do." I really did not find a connection to any specific area until I had my maternal–child nursing clinical. Once I went to labor and delivery (L&D), I knew this was the area that I wanted to practice in. I did my senior clinical internship in L&D with a wonderful preceptor who shared her knowledge and experience with me. She showed me what it was like to be a nurse and to share your knowledge. She felt that nurses "eating their young" was unacceptable and taught me it does not have to be that way. She even came to my graduation! She was a true role model, and to this day, I share her sentiment that nurses do not have to eat their young. These were some of my first experiences that showed me that nurses are special people, not only to their patients, but as people who care about one another.

As I moved along in my career, going from L&D to the neonatal intensive care unit (NICU), I felt a strong connection to teaching. I would always agree to precept the newly hired nurses on the unit, sharing my knowledge, and telling them that eating the young was a vicious cycle that we could and should stop. I worked in the NICU for many years and I saw a lot of nurses eat the young. As I witnessed some of the new NICU nurses being treated unacceptably by their preceptor, I did ask those preceptors why they acted that way. The response I typically received was, "Well, this was how I was treated." Thankfully, I was given a different vision of how nurses could treat each other and, as such, the pebble I threw into the teaching pool rippled with support and understanding and not maliciousness. I have been fortunate to have wonderful mentors and caring senior nurses who took me under their wing and shared their knowledge, insight, and wisdom with me. And I continue to honor them by instilling the same concept of caring for self and caring for others, be it a patient or a fellow nurse, in those I participate with in the teaching-learning process.

I really loved working in the NICU, caring for the babies and their families. I loved the adrenaline and the rush of stress of working in an ICU. However, my focus changed after my accident. I was not able to work anymore in the NICU; I felt I was not able to work anywhere. What was I to do in nursing if I could not be a *nurse*? I never thought about going into academia as a career, for I was a nurse, and I thought nurses had to work in the hospital. Again, what I thought I would become and who I became are not one and the same. What I needed to change was the perception I had of what a nurse did. What needed to change was my own personal belief of what it meant to me to be a *nurse*. Could I still be a nurse if I did not work in the hospital? Did the saying "once a nurse, always a nurse" mean the same if I was not "nursing" at the bedside? What, really, was *nursing*? This took me on a personal reflective process that I had to embrace if I was ever going to work again.

As I explored what I needed to do to regain my own health, my own way of being, I also began to reflect on what it meant to me to be a nurse. I remembered how much I enjoyed teaching and thought that perhaps it was something I could do. I remembered my psychiatric clinical professor in my bachelor's program. She was so giving, so open and honest about herself and about what it meant to her to be a nurse. So I decided to get my master's in psychiatric-mental health nursing. Once again, the universe provided me with incredible nurse mentors, who gave of themselves so freely. It was due to the power of these nurses, who taught me about nursing, who showed me that nursing is more than just handing someone a pill or inserting a tube into some orifice, that I learned of nursing as the true act of caring. It was through their presence that within me a different perception of what nursing meant to me began to awaken.

Nursing did not have to only mean working in a hospital. Nursing was giving of self to others, of caring for self and others, of honoring self and others, and of doing what felt right for self and others. As I learned to honor this new vision of nursing, I yearned to share my new insights and philosophy. I longed to contribute to the future of nursing by showing, sharing, and caring for the "young nurses" in the ways I was showed. I knew eating the young should not occur and, as a nurse educator, I could begin the continued ripple effect of this concept. I began to explore self-care, reflecting on what it was that I needed to do in order to continue my own personal and professional growth. Simultaneously, while going for my master's degree, I also began my journey into holistic nursing. Knowing that I had to reevaluate my life and how I was to live it, holistic nursing was a path that I chose to nurture and guide my own self-care. I needed to learn how to care for myself, how to be cared for, but, more importantly, I needed to learn it was okay for me to ask for help and accept it. What a precious gift to learn!

My first job as a nurse educator, unfortunately, was in a very un-holistic environment. I could not believe I ended up in such a toxic, unhealthy place. However, the connection I had with my students was beyond anything I could have imagined. My way of being with them was what I had imagined when I thought about a career in nursing education. I also knew I had to leave that toxic environment and find some place that was more holistic and caring. At one time, it had been a caring and giving academic milieu, yet milieus change based on the energy of those individuals in power. It is important to acknowledge this process, accept change, and learn to be aware of how to navigate the fluctuations. My way of being, of honoring myself and my thought processes and of knowing the type of person and nurse I am, has benefited me. I am able to work and continue to be a catalyst of change in self and others. I have an opportunity to share my knowledge, wisdom, and ways of caring with the future of the nursing profession. I only hope their memories of me are as honorable as the ones I have of my teachers.

■ PROFESSIONAL EVOLUTION/CONTRIBUTION

My professional evolution has been one of learning to honor where I am and respect that it might not be where I thought I would be. This has been a tremendous process for me to learn, having learned it by being an observer in my own life, by listening to mentors, but, more importantly, by knowing that I must have some passion for what I am doing. If I do not have passion, a desire to strive to improve myself intellectually by stimulating my mind with personal and professional challenges, then why do what I am doing? Thus, the accomplishment I am most proud of is how I have achieved what I have by being true to who I am, by honoring and respecting my individuality, my singular process in my life. "Learning to trust yourself and appreciate the essence of who you are is the foundation for believing in yourself" (Sharoff, 2008, p. 22).

I have always had a desire to learn, to continue to expand my understanding of life, of how it is affected by all aspects of one's personhood. From the nurses at Coney Island Hospital to the incredible nurse educators I have had the honor to learn from, to realizing what I thought I would do in my career, to what I am actually doing . . . all of these elements helped define who I am as a nurse and person. I used to say that I went into nursing because I needed a job that would provide financial security. Nursing has provided me with that, but now I know that I went into nursing because it is what I am . . . a nurse. When I had to relearn what I thought I would do as a nurse, I really had to relearn who I was as a person. I had to truly delve deep into my own spirit and decide if I was worth the fight. I had to confront my own demons and begin the process of learning to accept myself for who I was, who I lost, and who I was becoming. I had to learn about myself on all different levels. And that is what I try to instill in my students, the ability to honor who they are and learn about themselves while learning about others, thus, growing both personally and professionally.

The evolution of who I am now began when I first decided to become a nurse. Yet life had a different path for me, whereby I had to simply learn to walk again while asking for help should I stumble. What a hard lesson that was for me. The trials of falling and being afraid to go on brought about a fire that fueled my desire to challenge myself and overcome physical, as well as emotional, pain. The need for self-care brought about the ultimate change in my life, for I discovered that there was no separation of my personal and professional lives, as living one's life is an incorporation of the mind-body-spirit connection (Sharoff, 2006a). Being able to integrate the concepts of self-care and honor how I wanted to live an integrated personal–professional life is essential for me. Fostering a way of being that complemented my personal and professional lives resulted in my commitment to the healing process of self and others, the ability to incorporate the concepts and standards of the philosophy of holistic nursing into my life and practice (Sharoff, 2007b). "The need and awareness to work in a nursing paradigm that is congruent with one's own personal and professional beliefs and values are an essential element to the continued development and evolution of one's personhood" (Sharoff, 2008, p. 22). Thus, the continued evolution of who I am is a process of learning to understand and accept who I am, why I behave . . . react . . . respond the way I do, and how I can continually grow to improve the essence of myself. In addition, it is being mindful of how the building blocks of my prior existence, combined with my current being, are all intertwined to create the tapestry of who I am and who I am still becoming.

The journey of my life's work within nursing stemmed from my own need for self-care, self-acceptance, and self-understanding. That was when holistic nursing became a part of my way of being, both personally and professionally. As I ventured further with my own personal and professional development, I maintained a steady course of holism. One major contribution has been my exploration of the connections between holism and metaphors. Metaphorical images of nurses and the art of identifying metaphors can provide nurses with a "better understanding of their skills, knowledge and attitudes, and [serve as a method] to incorporate those characteristics and behaviors into their lives, as well as provide for opportunities to express their thoughts and feelings in a creative way" (Sharoff, 2007a, p. 17). Metaphors "create new meaning and provide deeper insight in the human spirit" (Sharoff, 2007a, p. 14).

Exploring one's metaphor requires being reflective, challenging one's assumptions, and allowing for the continued exploration of one's ways of knowing (Sharoff, 2009b). Metaphors, through narrative inquiry/therapy, can be used for helping individuals during the healing process (Sharoff, 2009b). For me, exploring metaphors helped to solidify my metaphor . . . *I am a phoenix*. I have been able to transform my life, my way of being, and who I thought I was to who I am and am waiting to become. It is a continuous process of awareness and willingness to be open to the process of being and knowing.

> Metaphors provide a unique opportunity to gain a special understanding of self, others, and the universe. . . . [They] can be a form of reflection and transformation, can initiate an honest internal dialogue with the self, can open up a dialogue with others, and can deepen the healing-caring process." (Sharoff, 2009b, p. 316)

I am a phoenix has helped me to accept that my life, both professionally and personally, is always changing, evolving, and transforming; "a reflective practitioner is one who sees with the heart and the spirit and is able to challenge past assumptions and meanings to create, revise, alter and change one's way of knowing" (Sharoff, 2009b, p. 317). It has provided me with the ability to acknowledge that I must not stand still but continually challenge myself to improve my own way of being, my knowledge, and my assumptions. To reflect on one's actions, one's way of being, is to be an auto-researcher in one's practice and life (Sharoff, 2006b). This is certainly no easy task, for it may open up old wounds and cause the scabs with serous drainage to periodically reappear. However, trusting that the healing–caring process will follow, hopefully, leads to enhanced understanding and insight.

As I gain experience in years, I have become more in tune with my ways of being. The old "more comfortable in my skin" adage holds true. I am not that punky 20-something, skipping around with a mohawk haircut or that 30-something with fuchsia wild hair . . . but I am still that same person, the one who likes to express herself outwardly and openly. I am true to who I am, *finally*! What a long and winding road . . . and the journey is far from over. I look to the future now and wonder what it will be. I am a nurse educator/researcher now and I do love it. I really enjoy imparting my knowledge, thinking process, skills, attitude, and ways of being a nurse/person. I enjoy undergraduate students, who are sponges, absorbing all that I have to offer. Sometimes they tell me I am intimidating and have too high expectations of them. I tell them that my expectations are that they will become wonderful nurses and take responsibility for their actions; thus, I hold them to high standards. By the end of the semester, they appreciate me (mostly). I enjoy the advanced-degree students who bring a new vision to the table with new experiences from their careers. I enjoy challenging myself to keep current with new knowledge, from learning about genetics/genomics to simulation to new teaching applications and technologies. If I ever stop learning, then I must stop teaching! Teaching and learning is a two-way process, for I do learn from my students as I hope they learn from me.

For me, as a nurse in academia, I wonder about my students. Did I make an impact on their professional and personal life journeys as I was impacted when I was in school? Will they remember some of the things I have said and reflect on what I have taught them? I can only hope that I have had a positive and meaningful influence on their lives and, as such, helped to mold them into the nurses I would want taking care of me. Reflecting upon my work within nursing, I reflect upon my students and hope that they continue the journey of sharing their knowledge with the next generation of nurses and that the cycle of caring for self/caring for others continues. The ripple effect of teaching nursing students to engage in self-care brings about a new epistemology that will, hopefully, become a normal way of being and evolve into a process of sharing that philosophy with others.

■ MORAL/ETHICAL FOUNDATION

I have a strong moral and ethical foundation of practice, of life. Initially, I knew I had to hold myself to a higher standard of practice in the clinical arena, as I had to prove that I was a good nurse who just happened to have a mohawk haircut. Then, in academia, I knew I had to continue to prove myself, as my dress attire was not the typical Chanel skirt and button blouse. In other words, I walked to my own drummer, valued my individuality, and knew that I had to demonstrate my work ethic and capabilities as my external "look" was not the expected persona of what a "nurse" was. "What a nurse looked like" was something I never truly understood, as we are all people who "look" different. However, the stigma of looking a certain way was/is expected, and as I choose not to follow that path, I knew that I had to prove that I was as good . . . no . . . *better* than expected. So my moral, ethical, and personal values have always been of an extremely high standard.

One of the most important aspects of being a nurse is honoring what a person is going through while, at the same time, honoring what I am going through and then making certain that I can care for them and myself simultaneously. Maintaining and valuing my own individuality while preserving my moral/ethical standards at a high caliber is not an easy task, but one that, at this point in my life, is just another way of being for me. My individuality is the basis of who I am and, as such, I strive to always present myself in the highest regard.

With that said, I do tend to have high expectations of others, and am, very often, truly disappointed when people do not meet my expectations. This is something I have been struggling with as a person and as a professional. What I have learned is that I am holding people to my expectations without telling them what that expectation is; thus, disappointment ensues. When it comes to my students, I am always up-front and clear about my expectations. But with colleagues and in my personal life, I am not always as clear and direct. Why? I honestly do not know, but I do know that I value and respect those who have a high regard for self and others. A strong work ethic, equity, and mutual respect lead to a holistic working milieu that further instills a productive healthy establishment. So, for me, bringing forth a strong holistic and healthy individual self will carry over and assist and support those in need, honoring both myself and the other person at that moment in time.

Being present, being able to provide comfort while caring for someone, and being able to share my knowledge freely and openly while knowing I am making a difference to someone's thinking is what is important to me as a nurse. As a nurse, it is expected that I will be there when someone needs me. However, more importantly, I want to be there! That is significantly different from having it be expected. I do what I do because I want to . . . once I stop loving/enjoying what I am doing, then I know it is time for me to move on. That is why it is important to know who we are and to know what is important to us as individuals, because the personal–professional is always intertwined. Walking around with a big ego, expecting people to treat me a certain way, expecting that I will receive honors and awards, is not who I am. There are those who love to talk about themselves. Then there are those like me who are quiet in the background, but make a large impact when we choose to. Thus, the ethical character that I hold is one of personal attributions . . . personal honor and respect. When I gain the respect of my fellow nurses, I know I have achieved what I hold important.

As nurses are people too, it is hard to pigeonhole what the inherent ethical character is for nursing. However, the overwhelming ability to care for others, to put the needs of others first, is paramount to being-becoming a nurse. And a major corequisite that goes along with that is for nurses to remember to partake in their own self-care. The strong interconnectedness of caring for self while caring for others is what is important for a nurse. Otherwise, burnout, eating the young, negativity, and hostile work environments ensue. And no one benefits from that energy-taking existence.

When I participate in the teaching–learning process of others, I try to instill an understanding of respect, of honoring self and others. Being open to the humane morals of personhood is essential when teaching. Remembering that one's personal and professional lives are always intertwined, that "life happens," and how one reacts and responds to that is what the humane morals of nursing are to me as a nurse educator. For example, I always tell my students to let me know when something is going on in their lives. I am not a mind reader and would not know if they are experiencing personal issues. However, if they let me know, then I will do my best to support them in whatever way I can.

Recently, I had a student taking one of my online classes. Due to a natural disaster in her country, she was unable to participate in the online discussion. She e-mailed me and explained what was occurring in her life. I told her that she should take care of herself and her family and not worry about participating in the online discussion for that week. When she did come back to the class, she was able to be present, fully participate in the discussion, and was not distracted by her personal obligations. That is what I mean by the humane moral character that is nursing: honoring that our lives intersect and realizing the importance of respecting that crossover.

This is the moral/ethical foundation that I hold myself to as a nurse educator—bringing the consciousness and awareness that we are all connected, that we are all persons who care for others while caring for self. Caring for self means that I care for my students as well. How can I not understand when a student is experiencing a difficult time? Was I not cared for by nurse educators when I was a student? We learn by the examples of others, and so the nurse educator should always try to instill a special way of being, for the ripple effect of our actions is continuous.

■ VISION

What will nursing be like in the future? Will it be like it is now, with nurses sitting behind a computer on wheels (COW), dispensing medications, and sitting outside of their patients' rooms? Will it be nurses running around trying to care for more patients than they should be? I certainly hope not. My vision for nursing is about giving more time to be present, to provide support and education that is needed for healing to occur. I believe that nurses will always carry the weight of caring on their shoulders. We will always be looked upon to care for those who need help, for a nurse is always giving.

The profession of nursing needs to bring its wisdom to the table of health care and share the wealth of knowledge of caring. A nurse need to feel empowered by being a nurse. We need to honor that what we do is exceptional work . . . and that we are the backbone of health care. Nursing has always segregated itself by having so many levels of entry into its profession. We have so many layers and divisions that we have fragmented ourselves, leading to a weaker constitution.

I would love to envision nursing as a solid entity, whereby the profession as a whole stands as one. Imagine how strong we can be when we come together globally. Imagine the impact we can make in the world when we stand as one—when we shine our knowledge on what the world as a whole needs! We are only as powerful as we are together. Unfortunately, we have yet to walk or even envision the path of true unity within the profession. Nursing can be such a powerful profession of change. Yet, we are a fragmented form of giving and caring. We, as a profession, are not a unified body for change. We sabotage ourselves by our own fragmented ways, by having numerous levels of entry and degrees. Globally, there are probably more nurses in the world than any other profession. Yet, how connected are we as a core group of like-minded professionals?

So I ask you . . . how can we become as one? How can we learn to share our knowledge, care for others while caring for self, and still remain true to who we are? My mantra is to treat everything with love, honor, and respect, and the Universe will provide. If this were true, if this were taught, if this were practiced . . . that path of professional unity would be clearly delineated and self-maintained by the power and intentionality of such nurses. For me, my little part in the equation is to continually share of myself with my students while being true to who I am.

■ REFLECTIONS

1. *If I had to describe my nursing practice in a metaphor, what would it be? Why?*
2. *Am I who I thought I would be as a nurse? As a person?*
3. *How do I see my personal and professional lives intertwining to bring about the deepest satisfaction for myself?*
4. *Am I honored to be who I am?*
5. *How can we as a profession become more unified?*

■ REFERENCES

Sharoff, L. (1997). Tapestry of the mind-body-spirit: What is holistic nursing? *Pathways: Journal of the American Society of Pain Management Nurses, 6*(3), 11–12.

Sharoff, L. (2006a). The holistic nurse's search for credibility. *Holistic Nursing Practice, 20*(1), 12–19.

Sharoff, L. (2006b). A qualitative study on how experienced certified holistic nurses learn to become competent practitioners. *Journal of Holistic Nursing, 24*(2), 116–124.

Sharoff, L. (2007a). Metaphors: A creative expression of holistic nursing. *Spirituality and Health International, 8,* 9–19.

Sharoff, L. (2007b). Critical incident technique utilization in research on holistic nurses. *Holistic Nursing Practice, 21*(5), 254–262.

Sharoff, L. (2008). Exploring nurses' perceived benefits of utilizing holistic modalities for self and clients. *Holistic Nursing Practice, 22*(1), 15–24.

Sharoff, L. (2009a). The power of metaphors: Images of holistic nurses. *Holistic Nursing Practice, 23*(5), 267–275.

Sharoff, L. (2009b). Expressiveness and creativeness: Metaphorical images of nursing. *Nursing Science Quarterly, 22*(4), 312–317.

CHAPTER THIRTY

Flexible and Responsive: Applying the Wisdom of "It Depends"

Isabelle Soulé

I am uncomfortable with the term cultural competence. . . . I am not dissuaded by the ideals it represents such as receptivity, flexibility, curiosity, inclusivity, understanding context, and humility, but rather that the term inadvertently implies an endpoint. . . . Competence is indeed a worthy goal, but I argue it is not enough.

—Soulé (2014a)

■ WHY NURSING?

The truth is I never wanted to be a nurse. At least not the stereotype of nursing I held in my early years, which consisted of a woman in white stockings, starched white dress and cap, carrying a medication tray, and cleaning up after the infirm. Although I felt nursing might be a noble career for some, it was not my idea of an adventurous life, and I knew I was born for adventure.

I came to nursing inadvertently, or so it seemed at the time. After one year of college, at 19 years of age, I moved to St. Thomas in the U.S. Virgin Islands to teach middle-school math and coach a gymnastics team. It was my first time out of the United States, and I treasured so many things about the experience—the tropical climate, the energy of the seventh and eighth graders, the Volkswagen bug I bought for $60, and, simply, the freedom I felt in an environment much different than the one in which I was raised. At the end of that year abroad, I moved back to the United States with no clear plan other than to finish my college education. My fundamental religious upbringing coupled with that era in U.S. history offered limited career options for women. Honorable professions for a woman included teacher, nurse, or secretary. Artist, poet, and/or dancer, though true to my nature, were not anywhere on my radar, as they were not considered "real jobs" and were therefore unacceptable. Without much conscious awareness at the time I made the decision . . . *I'll become a nurse.*

In retrospect, there was something deeply congruent about my becoming a nurse, as I have come to know the work and the profession over the past three-and-a-half decades. Aspects of my nature, apparent from a very early age, have been consistent threads woven throughout my professional career. My childhood summers were spent on a farm in Wisconsin where we roamed free, played in the barn, and watched the birth of calves and foals, as well as witnessing death when animals were slaughtered for our own consumption.

During those early years, I was also enthralled by the *National Geographic* magazines that came to my family home. I have always been drawn to indigenous cultures, the people, and the rituals, and have resonated most deeply with sub-Saharan Africa. The closest I come to an explanation of this phenomenon is a concept I learned long ago at a conference on the intersection of quantum physics and medicine. The concept, *remembering forward*, refers to moments when we have a powerful response that cannot be understood, at least cognitively, in the context of our history, background, or conscious knowing. It can be thought of as an experience that, instead, relates to our future—thus the term *remembering forward*. For example, once I was wandering in a bookstore and came across an 1886 book entitled *Kaffir (Xhosa) Folk-Lore: A Selection From the Traditional Tales* by George McCall Theal (1886). Immediately, tears began streaming down my face and I stood there stunned for some minutes. Although I felt bewildered by what was happening, at the same time, I recognized that something very powerful had just taken place, and of course, I purchased the book to find out what was there for me. This book is a collection of folktales from the South African Xhosa people, the tribe to which Nelson Mandela belonged. Interestingly, this striking experience happened decades before my first work in sub-Saharan Africa—again the idea of *remembering forward.*

I imagine the roots of my nursing career reaching back into my early years, as the awe of diverse cultures, birthing, and bearing witness to dying and death have been hallmarks of my professional career. Mary Oliver, the renowned American poet, says it best: "You only have to let the soft animal of your body love what it loves" (1986).

■ EARLY IMPRESSIONS

In the spring of 1980, after one term of nursing school, I needed a summer job and interviewed for a certified nursing assistant (CNA) position in a large urban hospital in the northwest. I remember sitting across the desk from the nurse manager who was reviewing my resume. Reluctantly, she said, "I'm sorry, but you've never given an enema." With great urgency, I stopped her and said, "I need someone to give me my first chance. Let me have someone's butt and I will learn." Although it was not my most elegant moment, she did agree to hire me. Wide-eyed, eager, and completely inexperienced, I began my first CNA job.

Do we ever learn more important lessons than in our first nursing work? Yes, I learned to organize myself, do procedures efficiently and effectively, and to document accurately. However, my most profound learning came from hours of talking with clients on evening shift after the tasks were completed and before they went to sleep. Clients on this urology unit were distributed into two main categories: older men with prostate problems and younger men with either paraplegia or quadriplegia. Bearing witness to their varied stories helped shape my early understanding of the meaning clients make of their illness experiences. Over the years, I have remembered that manager with deep gratitude for the exquisite learning she opened to me despite my obvious lack of experience.

After finishing my bachelor's education in nursing, I began working in a level III neonatal intensive care unit (NICU), a field I delighted in for the next 17 years. These were dynamic times in the development of NICUs in the United States and significant discoveries were made that improved the care of premature and critically ill infants such as surfactant, high-frequency ventilation, developmental care, extracorporeal membrane oxygenation (ECMO), and active family participation in the care of their infants. It was a time when I advocated at all levels of the hospital and nursing organizations until fathers and family members could be present with the mother at the time of delivery, a practice largely taken for granted in contemporary U.S. practice.

My role in the NICU shifted throughout those years from bedside nurse, to clinical coordinator, to transport coordinator. With each transition, I was able to broaden and deepen my understanding of the complexity and political and interdisciplinary nature of nursing care and enjoyed working with diverse stakeholders including parent groups, ambulance, fixed wing and rotor wing vendors, the Association of Air Medical Services (AAMS), educators, and hospital administration. I have many wonderful memories of the first half of my career and am grateful for the burgeoning leadership experiences, strong clinical foundation, and the privilege of working closely with the families of critically ill and dying infants, who have been the teachers of some of my most profound life lessons.

In the late 1990s, I had an opportunity to assess how family-centered care was being practiced in a large maternity hospital in Colombo, Sri Lanka. It was a time of civil war in this Asian country and the military tension was palpable. I had never before lived and worked shoulder to shoulder with soldiers carrying large weapons, being stopped anytime to be questioned and frisked, and I felt like an incredible novice and outsider, which of course I was. Returning to the United States from Sri Lanka was a difficult and disorienting experience, one I have come to expect, particularly if I am returning from a low-resource, low-income country. This experience proved to be a pivotal transition in my professional trajectory, as I felt nearly repelled working in such a lavish NICU setting, given the disparity in resources and health I had just experienced between countries. I had been broken open and there was no going back to the comfort of *not knowing*. This profound internal shift led me to leave the much-loved high-tech NICU environment to focus on global health pursuits.

■ PROFESSIONAL EVOLUTION/CONTRIBUTION

My professional and personal evolution cannot be separated, as they flow naturally together, each reciprocally influencing the other. My values, beliefs, and behaviors have been shaped by my being raised White, female, and middle class in the United States, my family of origin and upbringing, experiences with families and their critically ill and dying infants, immigrant and refugee communities, and professional colleagues from around the globe, living and working abroad in diverse countries, my study of Process Work, Deep Democracy, Neuro-Linguistic Programming (NLP), and being a practicing artist. I no longer think of myself primarily as a U.S. citizen, but rather as a global citizen, as I feel I now belong to many parts of the world equally. I have served and been served, held and been held, healed and been healed, and I know that I have made a difference in the lives of families, colleagues, students, and communities over the past 35 years.

Although I feel content with many of my traditional accomplishments in nursing, such as a PhD, publications, and advancement on the academic ladder, those aspects have much less relevance to me today than they did in my early nursing days. As I move toward the end of my professional career, my focus is turning inward and I am becoming more self-aware, reflective, and appreciating the quiet moments of learning where I open myself to a different way of thinking, listen to understand, and bear witness to suffering. I no longer have the need to be the center of attention or to have my ideas approved by others. Instead, I find it a great privilege to be with individuals, families, and communities when they are most vulnerable, and it is those relationships I will be most proud of when I look back on my career.

Although nursing is a rigorous scientific profession, it is also deeply relational. Barbara McClintock, the great genetic scientist, is a fine example of this balanced approach of science and artfulness. She did not objectify her subject but rather entered into relationship with it, assuming that it could best be understood as a communal phenomenon.

> Over and over again she tells us one must have the time to look, the patience to "hear what the material has to say to you," the openness to "let it come to you." Above all, one must have a "feeling for the organism." (Palmer, 1998, p. 55)

Kim and Flaskerud (2007) also addressed the "feeling" of this relational exchange this way:

> This new journey as a patient . . . increased my level of sensitivity . . . especially in encounters with health professionals. Each person contributed to my recovery . . . however there were subtle differences: Some individuals made me feel connected and understood . . . while others were . . . experts in their field yet their efficiency felt strangely insufficient. (p. 931)

I believe that nurses, individually and collectively, are powerful and therefore can either contribute to healing or cause great harm. I have been musing for some years about research designed to evaluate the quality of relationship between nurse and client and/ or family as an intervention toward healing, even when the healing involves the dying process.

One of my most important contributions to the nursing profession has been my research on culture and cultural competence in U.S. health care, which, of course, is directly related to my desire to work skillfully with diverse groups around the world (Soulé, 2014b). In this chapter, I highlight portions of that work, including the impetus for the burgeoning literature on culture and cultural competence, conceptualizations of culture, underpinnings of cultural competence, and moving beyond cultural competence toward cultural humility.

Increasingly, culture and cultural competence are being discussed in health care literature, as recent political and economic crises have resulted in a major surge of people migrating across international borders, expanding contact among groups of people with widely varying backgrounds and worldviews. Because different cultural groups prioritize values differently, mismatches in understanding may result from not appreciating basic cultural differences such as gender roles and positions of authority, sense of self and space, communication, relationship to time, relationship to others, learning styles, and spiritual practice. Within the health care system, these differences exhibit themselves in how health and illness are perceived and manifested; what is thought of as cause; how, when, and where communication occurs; the roles of health professional, client, family, and community; and how treatment is negotiated, implemented, and evaluated. Inevitably, individuals and communities brought up in widely varying contexts and backgrounds live in widely different realities or "truths." As a result, health professionals are now being called upon to alter traditional ways of working with clients, families, and communities and to begin thinking differently and "being" differently as they encounter new relationships across cultures both domestically and internationally.

The concept of culture is complex, and each individual, family, and community represents a unique blend of dynamic, overlapping, and nested cultures that influence their perceptions, attitudes, and behaviors. A *constructivist* view recognizes culture as a dynamic process, evolving and changing over time as individuals and communities move in and out of various and multiple cultures. For example, from a constructivist perspective, health care providers not only address issues related to physical and mental health, but also examine experiences related to migration, dislocation, and adaptation to unfamiliar circumstances and settings. A constructivist view of culture consistently directs attention to social and political factors, in addition to individual ones, acknowledging the multidimensional nature of human experience. A constructivist view of culture can also include recognizing the limits of our knowledge before the mystical nature of health and illness and the expertise of the accumulated wisdom and resilience of clients and their communities.

Regrettably, common notions of culture in U.S. health care literature often reflect an *essentialist* view, wherein culture is portrayed as a static set of traits generally associated with an ethnic minority group. The intention of this literature is to give information to health professionals about health beliefs and practices of diverse groups entering, or already in, the health care system. However, the paradoxical result of this superficial understanding and approach to culture is that instead of engendering respect as originally intended, it promotes stereotyping of the client, family, and community. Finally, when health care focuses narrowly on an essentialist view of culture by limiting its focus to the beliefs, customs, and traditions of immigrant, refugee, or ethnic minority groups, it can obscure the interlocking systems and oppressive relations that establish and maintain systems of imbalanced power in which certain groups are systematically privileged and certain groups are systematically devalued. Health care professionals individually and collectively must become centrally concerned with the underlying systems that maintain power imbalances and that keep structural disparities in place around the globe (Gray & Thomas, 2006; Soulé, 2014b). Table 30.1 summarizes the key elements in these two conceptualizations of culture.

TABLE 30.1   **Conceptualizations of Culture in Health Care Literature**

Constructivist	Essentialist
Complex	Simplistic
Dynamic	Static
Unknowable	Known
Multiple cultural identities	Single cultural (ethnic) identity
Influences all individuals	Resides in client, family, community
Unique responses to health and illness	Predictable responses to health and illness
Mindfulness (conscious)	Mindlessness (unconscious)

As a field of study, cultural competence has evolved from and, therefore, been deeply influenced by U.S. values. For example, in the United States, there is a shared understanding of individualism that is so pervasive, revered, and deeply ingrained that it is seldom recognized, let alone questioned. *Individualism*, rooted in a belief in the separation and autonomy of individuals, recognizes the individual, and not the group, as the basic unit of survival.

In contrast, many clients residing in the United States and around the world come from cultures that value a collectivist viewpoint. Collectivists perceive themselves as intrinsically part of a group and emphasize interdependence over independence, affiliation over confrontation, and cooperation over competition. *Collectivism* recognizes the group, and not the individual, as the basic unit of survival. Both individualism and collectivism have equal, albeit different, merits. However, of salient importance here is the understanding that each standpoint relies on different mechanisms and values in decision making.

The exploration of individualism and collectivism has been described using myriad lenses. The German philosopher Martin Buber (1958) made an important distinction in his classic work *I and Thou* as he explored the relationship of subject and object that is also relevant in the conceptualization of cultural competence. He wrote about two primary worlds, the "I-It" and "I-Thou." Buber differentiated between these worlds, claiming that the "I-It" world interacts on the basis of subject-object, representing separation and disconnection between the two, similar to an individualist's view of the world. Buber believed that thinking and behaving from this standpoint fragments both the self and the surrounding world. In contrast, the "I-Thou" world interacts on the basis of being interconnected with others and the surrounding world, comparable to a collectivist view of the world.

Being sensitive to the cultural context, beliefs, and values and behaviors of clients, families, and communities is considered a cornerstone of culturally competent practice. Although this call for sensitivity may seem intuitively correct, it implicitly denotes culture as residing outside of the health care professional and health care system. Embedded in this view is a dichotomizing of *us* and *them*, where what is labeled *them* is considered diverse although *us* is considered the norm or culturally neutral. Consequently, when the focus of cultural knowledge is outward, toward the client, the implied corollary belief is that biomedicine and the U.S. culture in general, where most of the cultural competence literature has emerged, are culture-neutral. This failure to concomitantly identify the beliefs, behaviors, and customs in the culture of biomedicine and the United States is a major flaw in the cultural competence literature, since each of these cultures warrants careful examination, as they are not neutral backgrounds against which other cultures can be measured.

Biomedicine, the belief system that drives U.S. health care, is a relative newcomer to the healing professions. This system, based on a belief in the power of science and technology, of personal autonomy, and of the capacity to overcome disease, has been effective in generating public health measures that have resulted in improvements in health and life expectancy for many and eradicated a number of major worldwide diseases. In the world of biomedicine, the more ancient healing traditions are collectively referred to as complementary and/or alternative medicine (CAM). In the past, these more traditional modalities have been thought of as nonrational and superstitious, thus reducing them to appendages of the main body of "real" or biomedicine.

For much of the world, however, biomedicine is the alternative model, as it stands alone in conceptualizing health as belonging to the individual separated from the social fabric in which she or he is interwoven. This separation dissects the physical, mental, and spiritual aspects of a person, and the person from the family and community in which he or she is embedded. In addition, the values that underlie biomedicine may conflict with more traditional models by distrusting any *real* value in the mystical and metaphorical aspects that are highly revered in many cultures of the world. For example, clients' choices to use complementary and alternative healing practices, spiritual healers, and community-based support mechanisms as primary sources for health maintenance or healing can be at odds with the beliefs and practices of many U.S. providers whose explanations and approaches to health and illness differ markedly.

As discussed earlier, when culture is perceived as residing in the client, family, and community, what emerges is biomedicine imagining itself not as a culture but rather as fact, reality, or truth. Taylor (2003) identified this conceptualization of biomedicine as perceiving itself to be a "culture of no culture" (p. 557). This lack of understanding of biomedicine as a culture unto itself is thought to maintain power imbalances that may be endemic to client–health care provider interactions.

Until recently, most cultural competence education focused on ethnic group affiliation as the predominant cultural variation. This view is superficial and inadequate; instead, experiences should be designed to help health care providers perceive themselves as situated in a specific social and economic location in order to appreciate the influence that this positionality has on interactions with clients. However, this level of accurate and reflective self-scrutiny flies in the face of the objectivity that many providers believe they possess, no matter what the client looks like, how she or he acts, what she or he believes in, or what she or he wants.

The term *competence* is a familiar one; in fact, it is one of the most common terms in U.S. health professions today. *Competence* refers to proficiency, ability, skill, and mastery. It is based on a model of active volition, moving forward, and becoming competent or skillful. This model often places the health care professional in the position of expert and "knower" and conceptualizes cultural competence in a unidirectional flow from provider to client, family, and/or community. It is generally thought that all individuals are influenced by culture, yet Yan and Wong (2005) noted a dichotomy in the cultural competence literature where health professionals are able to transcend the limits of cultural influence in order to help clients in culturally appropriate and specific ways. In this subject–object framework, health professionals are represented as *active* human subjects learning from clients' culture and experience as they are helping *passive* clients who can be understood and helped. This biased underlying assumption, most often outside conscious awareness, can reinforce the power differential nearly always present in a client–health professional encounter.

Cultural competence, a subset of competence, most frequently addresses the knowledge, attitudes, and skills of the health professional. This predominant focus on knowledge, attitudes, and skills suggests that cultural competence is a performance-centered (vs. person-centered) approach and conceived as a cognitively based technical solution to cross-cultural challenges. Western professional culture, embedded in individualism, competition, and cognitive knowing, is often unreachable by alternate ways of knowing or traditional wisdom. Today, because the United States values cognitive knowing over other types of knowing, cultural competence may be thought of primarily as an intellectual activity centered on the pursuit of knowledge and skills. However, health care education and professional systems that primarily emphasize competence vis-à-vis empiric and cognitive understanding can generate a climate of arrogance and exclusivity, with the unintended consequences of a false security in *knowing*, which can inherently be a state of closure. Consequently, new inquiry and discovery can be blocked, as can the capacity to understand and accept the worldview of another.

Importantly, when one of the primary foci in the cultural competence literature is cognitive knowing, implicitly the body, including sensations and visceral responses, is excluded as another important way of knowing (Soulé, 2014b). Cultural knowledge alone is insufficient for successful engagement with others. It is also necessary to become sensitive to the individual lifeworld of others in order to build interpersonal relatedness. This ability to physically experience one's own and another's experience is termed *embodiment*. Lakoff and Johnson (1999) addressed the physical aspects of culture in *Philosophy in the Flesh: The Embodied Mind and Its Challenge to Western Thought*:

> There exists no . . . person . . . for whom . . . embodiment plays no role in meaning, whose meaning is purely objective . . . and whose language can fit the external world with no significant role played by mind, brain, or body. Because our conceptual systems grow out of our bodies, meaning is grounded in and through our bodies. (p. 6)

Rather than primarily cognitively based, cultural competence is best thought of as embodied and relational, fostering high-quality relationships that require awareness, intellectual, attitudinal, and behavioral flexibility and humility. This includes being open to learning, conceiving of alternate sets of values, appreciating how mindsets develop, and understanding that all behaviors make sense in context. Humility includes respecting difference and recognizing that all perspectives have value. Difference is legitimate and different ways of expressing oneself and enacting health and illness are just as valuable as our own. Respecting different viewpoints as equally valid can serve health care providers in revealing where their own viewpoints may be incomplete or limited. In addition, interacting in a nonjudgmental way with people who have different ways of looking at things requires asking more questions than simply giving answers—a crucial skill in the development of trust and empathy.

Humility, not often addressed in professional circles, can be thought of as an accurate assessment of oneself, an ability to recognize and acknowledge limitations, and a willingness to be influenced by alternate values and worldviews. Humility may not be simply overlooked in U.S. health care, but may actually be perceived as antithetical to competence, professionalism, and professional practice. Because many health professionals are educated to think in these terms, they may be quick to misunderstand or reject teachings that offer an unrecognized worldview or alternate set of truths. Moreover, building partnerships where health professionals respect the expertise of the client, family, and community in their own health care decisions runs contrary to how professionalism is taught and role modeled in U.S. schools and professions today.

Understanding the role of arrogance can also help illuminate the concept of humility. *Arrogance* can be thought of as exaggerating our own importance, feeling that our own ideas, thoughts, and unique ways of viewing or understanding the world are superior to others. This "arrogance of absolutism" (Palmer, 2004, p. 126) is not only a human tendency but is also reinforced through U.S. health care education and practice. Interacting from this place of limited vision or one-sidedness can narrow our understanding, limit creative alternatives, and generate distance between us and others, making it difficult, if not impossible, to negotiate a collaborative plan of care or work effectively on multidimensional international health and research projects.

Interacting from a starting point of humility rather than professional expertise (competence) can generate a very different type of health care encounter that, in the end, can be more satisfying to client/family/community as well as health care providers. Humility is rooted in passive volition, receptivity, and being open to learn from another. *Passive volition* is not "passive" in the traditional sense of being inert or docile, but rather of using conscious engagement in the experience of another without inserting oneself or one's own experience or knowledge to dominate the dyad. Passive volition is the context of unknowing or creating space in our knowing that allows for the ability to move into the perceptual perspective of another and to know differently. *Unknowing* requires that we know that we do not know and that the individual, family, or community that stands before us does not fit neatly into some preconceived idea or package. This deep and profound knowing of another emerges when the nurse remains in a place of curiosity and willingness to understand and experience another differently. With this understanding, every encounter can be fresh and unique.

The Spanish language elegantly captures this difference in separate words for knowing. The first, *saber*, refers to the intellectual or cognitive knowing of a concept, person, or place. It is a knowing *about* something or someone, a *head*-knowing, such as, "I know the capitals of the 50 United States." In contrast, *conocer* refers to an *embodied* knowing or *experiential* knowing, as in the way a parent knows the scent of his or her own child or someone knows a beloved friend. It is a *heart*-knowing. Such intimate knowing requires a desire on the part of the health care professional to experience the lifeworld of another and feel humble in their presence, to be in the place of learner, and to know and understand differently in order to create a context where client, family, and community feel understood and healing can occur in a way that makes sense to them.

To embody cultural humility is to have an understanding that every encounter is a cultural encounter. Each individual brings to the encounter the unique life experiences that have shaped his or her current values, perceptions, attitudes, and beliefs. These a priori understandings may be in the conscious awareness of the individual, or (more likely) they remain predominantly in the unconscious awareness. Cultural humility requires an accurate self-appraisal, not overestimating or underestimating our unique gifts, abilities, and achievements. Honesty, integrity, and authenticity require that we recognize our failures, but there is no reason to construct our life stories around our less-than-elegant moments. Cultural humility is a characteristic of persons who are connected to their roots, know who they are, are content to be who and what they are, and accept their inherent nature gracefully. Because of this genuine comfort in a sense of self, lies, exaggerations, and evasions are not needed in order to inflate their importance in the eyes of colleagues or to prop up self-esteem. Being the center of attention is unnecessary and contentment is found in remaining in the background and supporting the success of others. This background position is not one of passivity but rather of being fully present with astute perception and wisdom. The tendency to regard others as competitors or rivals has been overcome, and there is no time wasted envying those who possess different qualities. Individuals who manifest cultural humility are not at war with themselves but are gracious, accepting, and forgiving of both self and others. There is a lack of self-absorption and an ability to transcend the self in an outward focus toward others. The experience is often one of wonderment, appreciation, and deep gratitude. Self-awareness is a dynamic process and requires a lifelong commitment to engagement in deep, honest, and ongoing self-reflection.

A necessary component of cultural humility is the ability to experience, in our own body, the lifeworld of another. It requires a movement from a mere cognitive understanding to a visceral understanding and an interconnectedness to the other's experience. This transcendence of one's own experience is uncomfortable and unfamiliar to the Western mind, which often separates cognitive function from bodily experience. In formal academic programs, there is often even a trained incapacity to see that heart and mind work as one and that they cannot be treated separately. The phrase "walking in someone else's shoes" is used to represent an embodied experience, yet an important distinction is required here. If I "walk in someone else's shoes" and imagine how I might experience the situation, looking through my own eyes, values, and beliefs; my own spiritual understandings; my own life experiences; my perceptual position remains centrally about me and I have not been moved to a place of embodied cultural humility. This perspective is referred to as *sympathy*. If, however, I can cognitively, emotionally, and viscerally move into the lived experience of another, seeing as if through his or her eyes, experiencing the situation through his or her values and beliefs, life experiences, and spiritual understandings, I have been able to make a transformational shift in my understanding of his or her experience. This perspective is referred to as *empathy*.

Experiencing another in this profound and physical way inevitably alters us at our deepest reaches, and knowing in this way is always communal. However, to elevate the position of humility in U.S. health care education and systems, radical transformation will be required. A beginning point can include creating safe places for colleagues to discuss and learn from their less-than-elegant cultural moments (incompetence) without judgment and with emphasis on openness (humility) and deep learning. Remen (2000) echoed this theme in her work with the terminally ill as medical director of the Commonweal Cancer Help Program.

> The medical model I was taught focused on what I as a physician thought. . . . I no longer . . . diagnose. I simply . . . listen. Something will emerge . . . that is a part of a larger coherent pattern that neither of us can fully see in this moment. So I sit with them and wait. (p. 90)

■ MORAL/ETHICAL FOUNDATION

As I have grown as a professional, what is most important to me has shifted significantly and I am much less "certain" than I was as a young woman, my certainty being based on a specific positionality uninformed by diverse points of view or diverse experiences. In short, my edges have softened as I have learned more about myself, my colleagues, and the communities I work with. My highest priority now is to lead an undivided life and practice exquisite self-care. Those priorities will enable me to continue to be in service to others throughout the remainder of my career.

The primary fuel for my work is a desire to contribute to reducing health and health care disparities around the world, specifically as they relate to women's and children's health. I have a deep and ongoing commitment to social justice, gender equality, and reducing violence against women and children in the global context.

Now, a very common response for me is "it depends," which reflects my embracing varied values, beliefs, and behaviors. I have come to understand that there are many right ways to be a nurse and that each of us must enact nursing through our most authentic selves, because if we are not "real" with clients (or with ourselves), it creates an energetic dissonance that can disrupt the relationship and, therefore, the healing process. My experience is that this resonance or dissonance with others can transcend language and customs and that living and working abroad provides unending opportunities for self-reflection.

I am currently in my second year living and working in Rwanda, East Africa, coordinating the first master of science in nursing program at the University of Rwanda. (See Chapter 26 for more about nursing and the cross-cultural exchange in Rwanda.) Each day brings a blend of bewilderment, excitement, frustration, and deep joy in varying proportions. I still feel the visceral welling up of "being right" until I consciously put that aside in order to open myself to alternate ways of thinking, perceiving, and behaving from this particular cultural context. I notice when I am trying to inform, fix, or enlighten Rwandans and remind myself that I am the invited guest here and that my primary work is to open myself up, learn new ways of being in the world, and add new ways of thinking and skills to my personal and professional repertoire. So again . . . it depends.

For example, my many years of working in NICUs in the United States embedded in me the impulse to actively resuscitate critically ill infants. It remains almost a primal or automatic response. Underpinning these actions is a belief in U.S. health care that goes something like "living is winning" and "dying is losing" or a slight variation on that theme. Given the disparity in physical and human resources between the United States and sub-Saharan Africa, it is essential for me to get off of "automatic" in order to respond mindfully from this cultural context and these cultural values. If a critically ill infant is born in a rural health center, he or she needs to be transported, by a variety of means, to a higher level of care. The chances of surviving the trip are marginal at best, as there is no oxygen available during transport, and certainly, there are no ventilators, intravenous (IV) fluids, medications, and so forth. The infants are bundled and held by the transporting nurse who, upon arrival at the hospital, sometimes discovers that the infants have died along the way. Furthermore, family members provide food and clothing to mothers and infants in the hospital, so if mother and infant are transported, there is no food available when they arrive at the district hospital unless another family voluntarily shares. Finally, if the infant dies, the mother cannot take the body home on the public bus, and she is unlikely able to pay for a taxi to return her to her community depending on the distance. These circumstances are very real in sub-Saharan Africa, requiring a different set of norms in making important moral and ethical decisions about clinical care. In this context, I frequently consider the distinction between "doing the thing right," which might mean a competent resuscitation, and "doing the right thing," which may require stepping back and supporting the family as their child dies in the embrace of loved ones and community surrounding them. Again, there is no single right way to do things.

Early in my career, altruism was a common motive for individuals, predominantly female, to join the nursing profession in the United States. However, after the financial crisis of 2008, I began seeing a shift in the incoming nursing students where I taught in an accelerated baccalaureate program. Many students had lost their jobs as engineers, journalists, marketing specialists, lawyers, business people, and so forth, and they turned to nursing as a viable career to support themselves and their families. Their moral and ethical reasons for joining the profession likely varied significantly. However, this infusion of diversity in gender and background disciplines added a depth and breadth to the complex and dynamic discussions that occurred both inside and outside of the classroom.

The idea of being individually passionate about nursing may be a Western cultural construct, where individuals likely have more choices available to them. Here in Rwanda, the government assigns students to nursing and midwifery based on their marks in secondary school, and the impetus to practice high-quality care is often more aligned with being in service to one's community and country (collectivism) than to individual passion (individualism).

■ VISION

My vision for the future of nurses and nursing education around the world includes:

1. Embedding global competencies into health care education and continuing education in order to prepare nurses to work successfully in a globalized world. Competencies should include but not be limited to global health disparities, health care disparities, donor/recipient nations, migration and diaspora, conflict negotiation, and the role of power and privilege in the provision and receipt of health care.
2. Raising the perceived value of what has historically been referred to as "soft science" in health care education, including relationship building, self-awareness, positionality, cultural competence, and cultural humility. This is because unless we as health care providers are able to skillfully work across differences,

clients, families, and communities will seek alternatives where they feel understood and respected.

3. Inviting and incorporating interdisciplinary viewpoints into health care education and practicing with inclusive consideration of anthropology, sociology, political science, the arts, and so forth.

4. Exploring the role of the body and techniques grounded in the body for their usefulness in supporting the development of cultural competence and cultural humility in health care education (Soulé, 2014b).

These significant shifts will require letting go of familiar ways in order to embrace new thinking and encourage collaborative innovation across disciplines and nations. Academic centers can play a major role in enhancing creative partnerships that will be crucial to eliminating the enormous health disparities that are present locally and worldwide.

I have learned two important pieces of wisdom over the years that I would like to share with both novice and seasoned nurses. First, "It's not about you," referring to the tendency for some health care professionals to take up too much space in the room, dominate individuals and families toward their way of thinking, and somehow become the center of attention (the helper, the rescuer, the expert, etc.). I believe our highest work as nurses is to support and care in leading individuals and families to solutions that work for them even when they are not decisions we might make for ourselves in similar circumstances. *It is not about you.*

Second, "It depends." There are many right ways to be a nurse and to enact nursing depending on your own background; the desires of the client, family, and community; the resources available; and the values, beliefs, and priorities of the culture. Quick solutions to complex questions regarding health and illness are often both premature and superficial and can create distance between provider and client, and in the end, actually cause harm. A mindful pause is needed to consider alternatives, listen to understand, and develop culturally appropriate solutions in partnership with client, family, and/or community. *It depends.*

I have always valued being a nurse and feel that it has afforded me an intimacy with clients, families, and communities that few professions can equal. At this point in time, I have come nearly full circle, a fitting next-to-the-last chapter in my professional career. Living and working in East Africa blends the two major halves of my career, NICU and African immigrant and refugee health, as I prepare the first cohort of master of science in nursing students with a neonatal specialty focus in Rwanda. I believe my highest contribution to the nursing profession is yet to come and I expect to have one more culturally enlightening destination of professional work before retirement. I do not know exactly what that work will be; however, I have some clues . . . "Another world is not only possible, she is on her way. On a quiet day, I can hear her breathing" (Roy, 2003).

■ REFLECTIONS

1. *What assumptions am I making? What are the roots of these assumptions?*
2. *How else can I think about this? Who do I know who can help me think about this differently?*

3. *Which assumptions get in my way of connecting with this person, family, and/or community?*
4. *How might the other person/family/community be thinking about this? What meaning does it have for them?*
5. *What am I pretending not to know?*

■ REFERENCES

Buber, M. (1958). *I and thou*. New York, NY: Simon & Schuster.

Gray, D. P., & Thomas, D. (2006). Critical reflections on culture in nursing. *Journal of Cultural Diversity, 13*(2), 76–82.

Kim, S., & Flaskerud, J. H. (2007). Cultivating compassion across cultures. *Issues in Mental Health Nursing, 28,* 931–934.

Lakoff, G., & Johnson, M. (1999). *Philosophy in the flesh: The embodied mind and its challenge to Western thought*. New York, NY: Basic Books.

McCall Theal, G. (1886). *Kaffir (Xhosa) folk-lore: A selection from the traditional tales*. London: S. Sonnenschein, Le Bas & Lowrey.

Oliver, M. (1986). Mary Oliver. Retrieved from http://www.mrbauld.com/oliverpms.html

Palmer, P. (1998). *The courage to teach*. San Francisco, CA: Jossey-Bass.

Palmer, P. (2004). *A hidden wholeness*. San Francisco, CA: Jossey-Bass.

Remen, R. (2000). *My grandfather's blessings*. New York, NY: Riverhead.

Roy, A. (2003). Confronting empire. Retrieved from http://www.ratical.org/ratville/CAH/AR012703.html

Soulé, I. (2014a). Exploring the meaning of cultural competence. *Advances in Nursing Science Blog*. Retrieved from http://ansjournalblog.com/2014/03/20/exploring-the-meaning-of-cultural-competence

Soulé, I. (2014b). Cultural competence in health care: An emerging theory. *Advances in Nursing Science, 37*(1), 48–60.

Taylor, J. S. (2003). The story catches you and you fall down: Tragedy, ethnography, and "cultural competence." *Medical Anthropology Quarterly, 17*(2), 159–181.

Yan, M. C., & Wong, Y. L. R. (2005). Rethinking self-awareness in cultural competence: Toward a dialogic self in cross-cultural social work. *Families in Society: The Journal of Contemporary Social Services, 86*(2), 181–188.

CHAPTER THIRTY-ONE

Engaged and Expressed: Storytelling as a Way to Know and Be Known

A. Lynne Wagner

*Reflective process guides one to a stillness of inner space where the mind [and heart] can contemplate the essence and wholeness of an experience. Stories (narratives) are a form of reflection on life experiences. How stories are told affects what they can teach about life. . . . Aesthetic [interpretation of story] . . . expands the power of reflection to explore self in story more deeply. The uncovering of hitherto unknown essential meaning in everyday relationships between self, others, and world occurs. An experience re-lived through an aesthetic sense of the narrative is freed of trappings and cognitive constraints and is turned to its essence, a unity of core beliefs, values, actions, and spirit. . . . A new sense of being **in the world** rather than **of the world** emerges.*

—Wagner (2008a, p. 24)

■ WHY NURSING?

I knew as a young child that I wanted to be a nurse and help others. Although I preferred outside activities, a favorite inside activity was making paper dolls, creating healing environments for them, and feeling responsible for their well-being. I was a curious child, always asking, "Why?" At a young age, I was intrigued with everything alive, especially with the amazing human body. This interest morphed into my love of biology, microbiology, and zoology. I built models of human anatomy and conducted experiments on growing plants under different conditions and the effect of different foods and household remedies on microscopic amoebas and euglenas. Loving nature, having pet dogs, growing up across from a dairy farm, and raising rabbits, sheep, and chickens for the 4-H club, I experienced early in life the cycles of birthing, dying, and all the living that evolves in between as a natural part of life and the interconnected universe. On summer nights, my mother invited us to lie on a blanket and study the sky. I developed a deep sense of caring, appreciation for nature's beauty, and a reverence for life.

With loving-kindness, my childhood heroes taught me about well-being, the human spirit, and the mysteries and miracles of life. Being loved and cared for set the stage for my caring for others. My role models provided a moral compass. Some touched my life constantly—my parents, grandmother, aunts and uncles, special teachers, and mentors. Others I knew only from my reading, such as nurse Cherry Ames, Dr. Tom Dooley, Albert Schweitzer, Gandhi, Mother Theresa, Florence Nightingale, and Heidi. So many other real and fictional characters followed over the decades to help me understand the coherence of love's healing, the energetic power of presence and cultural sensitivity, of human relationship, and the sacredness of caring.

I grew up in the 1950s and 1960s, a time when career choices for women were expanding. Although nursing was still portrayed as a subservient job, in the 1960s, baccalaureate nursing programs and the notion of nursing as a professional career were just emerging. My mother, a college graduate, created an innovative career in dental hygiene and research and encouraged me to also be creative in my career, which, she warned, often leads to challenging the status quo. Parallel to my nursing and science interests was a talent for writing, creatively and poetically. As a little girl, I would sit under a tree and write poems about caterpillars. Literature and music were part of our home life. Thus, I knew I wanted to learn in an expansive college environment to fulfill both my right- and left-brain needs. Knowing that the liberal arts would enrich my sense of nursing science, against the advice of my guidance teacher, who believed the traditional hospital–school diploma nursing programs made the "best nurse," I applied to two BSN programs, choosing one in a rural area, knowing the setting would feed my spirit. And there I flourished, attending to my aesthetic sense with English courses and a semester at Oxford University in England, studying poetry and drama, while learning the science and art of nursing in a holistic and forward-thinking baccalaureate program.

Along this early path, I experienced two personal events that strengthened my resolve to be both a competent and compassionate nurse. After my freshman year, I stepped out of school for a year for surgery and a long hospitalization to correct a congenital back condition. Although not a welcomed detour, being a patient and feeling the impact of both caring and noncaring practices became invaluable experiences in my coming of age as a nurse. In my third year of nursing school, my father had a heart attack while I was home on semester break and died later that day. This event had a deep influence on my resolve to practice a more humanized kind of nursing than what I experienced that day in the mechanized task-oriented world of medical care, watching as my dying father was separated from his loved ones who filled the waiting room. We were allowed five-minute visits, one at a time, once an hour. Many of us never got to say goodbye and my father died among strangers, swallowed up by the institution.

I had always envisioned nurses needing an expansive knowledge of body and disease, of clinical skills and machinery, and perhaps team skills of working together in a crisis. I witnessed nurses following doctors' orders, doing treatments, passing medications, cleaning utility rooms, feeding and washing patients, attending to all bodily functions, and being part of patients' most vulnerable and intimate lives. Most nurses who cared for me over my three-month hospitalization, during which I was bedbound and totally dependent, were a mainstay and demonstrated constancy in my physical and emotional well-being. The time and ways they spent caring for my needs, listening to my stories, and sharing their stories anchored me and provided healing beyond what the doctors' skills offered. But life was not perfect in this microworld. Although many nurses appeared to love their job, some appeared tired and short-tempered and unable or unwilling to respond to my call light. When I asked if they were having a bad day, some shared that they were disheartened, feeling they were no longer making a difference in people's lives as more of their time and touch disintegrated into hurried tasks. The days they cared for me were difficult. These two personal experiences with health care during my "nurse-becoming" demonstrated deficiencies in caring for the well-being and human spirit of both caregivers and the patients and families they served. Even as a young student, I knew it could be a different experience for the *carer* and the *cared-for*, but I did not know how or what to change or how I would survive in such a career.

■ EARLY IMPRESSIONS

Fortunately, my education and role models empowered me to have the courage to challenge the status quo of subservient medicalized nursing practice and the overlooked and accepted burnout of nurses. As a budding, competent, caring professional practitioner, I was able to step into the health care arena with confidence in my nurse identity and skills to holistically care for others. Initially, my journey was rocky, as my ingrained professional model of nursing clashed with the lingering traditional diploma nursing model. In my first job on a medical–surgical unit in a small community hospital, which offered no orientation or in-service education, I was challenged by a system that assigned nurses to clean the utility room, although I had been taught and believed that my time should be with patients, supporting them before surgery, hearing their stories, teaching, and advocating. I was disciplined by a physician for teaching basic diabetic home care to his very anxious patient, newly diagnosed with diabetes and about to be discharged on a Friday without any preparation. The doctor asserted that I had overstepped my responsibilities in patient teaching that he had planned to do on Monday in his office. However, through my patients' and their families' response to my caring, advocacy, and teaching-learning, I began to define my *nursing role* as encompassing empirical knowing and skilled tasks, along with compassionate presence, trusting relationships, and human dignity. Experienced nurses I worked with told me not to rock the boat. The dissonance between what I knew nursing practice *could be* and how others appeared to define it *for me* drove me to be reflective and brave enough to search for an environment in which I could flourish in both the science and art of nursing.

Although I was drawn to maternal–child health, I decided to accept another job in medical–surgical nursing that would foster a strong foundation of my basic nursing skills and knowledge. The attractive bonus was that this large teaching hospital offered a year's internship for BSN graduates, which included mentoring and opportunities to rotate to different units every three months. I experienced caring for patients with orthopedic, neurological, medical, and surgical challenges. At the end of my year's internship, I chose to work on a large men's medical unit that featured an open ward with curtains separating the beds and a smaller observation room across from the nursing station for critically ill patients, as well as isolation rooms for those with infections. This nursing experience of intense eight-hour shifts, rotating between day, evening, and nights, challenged me to grow into my multidimensional nursing roles, uncomfortably stretching me to expand and blossom as a leader and patient advocate, a skilled confident practitioner, a learner, and teacher.

But more important, the spirit of the unit, shared stories, the closeness of the patients who often supported each other, the daily acuteness of life and death struggles, and the necessary collaborative interdisciplinary team effort—despite the hierarchical medical world—taught me about nurses' essential role and voice in patients' healing and in the quality of their living or dying experiences. In the days before advance directives, one poignant experience was my ability to help interns humanely listen to the plea of a very ill patient who wished not to be resuscitated again after his many repeated experiences, which then opened opportunity for the interns to make new decisions *with* the patient. In essence, I excitedly came to know the art of nursing and the shared face of humanity and interconnectedness of carers and the cared-for at this large teaching hospital.

My first two jobs, one negative and one positive, helped me fall in love with nursing and cemented a humanistic foundation and philosophy for my nursing career. Two events followed these jobs that would shape the rest of my career. The first was spurred by my marriage and move to the suburbs. The commute to Boston and the changing shift work challenged daily life. Looking for balance, I found myself drawn to my growing love of and strength in teaching and mentoring, feeding my continued desire to make a difference. Calling upon my courage and my creative artistry once again, I drafted a plan and curriculum for a nursing in-service program, featuring orientation and educational support, based on what I had experienced as essential at the large teaching hospital. I made an appointment to meet with the director of nursing at the hospital where I first worked, which still offered no in-service education. She hired me with my proposal, creating a new position, which eventually became a department of nursing education that would change the landscape of nursing in this small hospital.

The second event arose from my decision to stay home for 12 years with our children, inventing a new way of sustaining my nursing career, meshing my love of teaching and maternal–child health nursing. After taking prepared childbirth classes, my husband and I had an amazing birthing experience together at a time when most women were inhumanely heavily medicated, given general anesthesia, strapped to the delivery table, and separated from husband and baby. Again, wanting to make a difference for other women and their families to know and witness the beauty and humanity of birthing, to be empowered and educated to shape their own birthing experience with their medical team, I apprenticed with the nurse-midwife who taught our childbirth classes and who became a lifelong mentor. As I gained experience, I earned my certification as a Lamaze Childbirth Educator, teaching childbirth and parenting classes in our home. This work was so important to me and to the families I touched in my community that I continued to teach these classes in the evenings for 30 years, even amid my returning to graduate school, working, and family life with three growing sons. I also became a teacher-trainer for Lamaze International to prepare new Lamaze instructors. In my day-to-day work, I realized I was fostering changes in my nursing practice, small but steady, that increased the quality of life for both nurses and patients/clients.

■ PROFESSIONAL EVOLUTION/CONTRIBUTION

My professional evolution began in nursing school, fired by visionary professors who believed in and lived nursing as a growing discipline founded in caring science. My nursing was evolving into a fabric of many colors and textures of personal and nursing experiences, adventures and opportunities, failures and successes, but always bound together by the threads of caring. An important step was learning to honor my wholeness, realizing I cannot separate myself by roles or interests, but that I must bring all of who I am to every situation, like the fragments in a kaleidoscope that enrich the wholeness of the viewed image. For instance, when I let the poet in me meet the nurse in me, I was able to see beyond the empirical, discovering multiple ways of knowing myself and my shared humanity with others.

When our third child was of school age, I completed a master of science, family nurse practitioner (FNP) program and my first venture into research. Again, I felt like a pioneer, forging into new territory on two fronts. First, in the early 1980s, the concept of nurse practitioners was in its infancy. Second, one professor, who impacted nursing progress at the university and my personal evolution, encouraged master's nursing students to participate for the first time in a formal research thesis process, rather than the expected shorter route of "research project." Accepting the challenge, along with several others, our small group was then encouraged to individually apply for a competitive university research grant. I was one of the first graduate nursing students to receive the grant. My master's thesis, *Socioeconomic Status, Career Satisfaction and Anxiety in Primiparous, Postpartal Women Planning to Return to Work* (Wagner, 1984), emerged from my many conversations with pregnant women about their struggles to decide whether to return to work after their first baby. The nursing program valued quantitative research and, thus, I was required to use this research methodology. I learned important aspects of research and contributed to understanding that job satisfaction, more significantly than socioeconomic status, inversely affected the mother's anxiety about leaving her baby to work. However, I sensed that the statistical findings did not represent or honor the wholeness of the mothers' complicated dilemma around their decisions to return to work that their stories reflected. A qualitative study would have captured a richer understanding of the phenomenon. This experience impacted my future research.

As an FNP, I worked in a large obstetric–gynecological practice. Again, at the cutting edge of redefining nursing roles, I was challenged by a system that wanted a "mini-doctor," not appreciating the "nurse" part of "practitioner"; a system that appeared to value the "bottom line" of closely timed visits more than the flexibility needed to hear the story behind visible bruises or invisible pain after the loss of a baby. I was caught in the rational medical model. I was asked once, with all my years of education and hard work, why did I not just become a doctor? This one question brought me back to my nursing soul and commitment.

After two years, disillusioned, I left my FNP position to teach community health and maternal–child health nursing in a BSN program for 20 years. In the education setting of combined teaching and clinical practice, I found my niche to grow and discover a deeper sense of self and nursing through caring science, making a difference now for students and future nurses. I was launched into an evolving journey through my discovery of caring theory and literature, meeting the revolutionary pioneers of the caring movement, including Dr. Jean Watson (see Chapter 16). The journey would bring me back to my roots and heart, giving me language to name what I had been doing and being for so many years. This helped me to be present to my students, learning from them about nurturing the spirit and soul of becoming a nurse by creating a healing environment of transpersonal teaching and learning that sustains human dignity. I explored multiple ways of knowing myself and viewed students, patients, and colleagues as cocreators in discovering nursing's potential to change lives and the world. I began to reclaim the holistic primacy of knowing caring as the essence of nursing (Benner & Wrubel, 1989; Carper, 1978; Leininger, 1976; Tanner, 1988; Watson, 2012). My practice and worldview philosophically shifted from epistemology to ontology, expanding the question of "How do I come to know?" (e.g., my nursing science, myself, the patient) to "How do I find meaning in what I know?" (Wagner, 2000a, p. 7). Such reflection also honors the mystery and unknowns of human suffering and healing and leads to further exploration of the shared meaning of profound human experiences (Silva, Sorrell, & Sorrell, 1995; Watson, 1999, 2005).

One way to explore experiences is through story (Sandelowski, 1993). In the early 1990s, I was diagnosed with my second bout of breast cancer. Unlike the first time, I decided that part of my healing through decision making, treatment, and life changes required me to engage in reflective journaling and conversations with myself (Watson, 1985), which helped me sort out decisions to be made, honestly explore feelings and reactions, and find hope. I wrote day after day "of illness and fear, choices and confusion, despair and pain, newfound strengths and resources, and the healing celebration of life. . . . Through my writings, which flowed with inexplicable ease and artful poetry, I touched my core of humanness" (Wagner, 1994, p. 178).

I always felt better releasing my thoughts. My journal stories were private and safe and never meant for public scrutiny. I rediscovered my journals two years after the crisis. Reading my own raw, detailed personal story and poetry of pain and joy was a surreal out-of-body experience, as though it came from another's soul. But I intuitively knew there was something important here to share. On one level, here was a story from beginning to end of a woman experiencing breast cancer, a story that moved beyond textbook descriptions, a profound narrative that captured the depth of the human spirit in turmoil and triumph. Nurses usually see patients at disjointed periods of diagnosis, treatment, or after treatment, seldom hearing their full story. On a second level, I had rediscovered my poetry-writing gift and the power of poetry to capture the essence of human experiences. Insights gained were carried into practice.

With another leap of faith and a colleague's encouragement, I presented my story, "The Color of Hope: A Woman's Journey with Breast Cancer" (Wagner, 1993), crafted from my journal writings, poetry, and photography at the International Association for Human Caring (IAHC) conference in Portland, Oregon. The audience's standing ovation and the personal comments from nursing leaders and caring theorists who were present—Dr. Jean Watson, Dr. Madeleine Leininger, Dr. Delores Gaut, Sister Simone Roach, Dr. Ann Boykin, and others—affirmed my belief that story and poetry are powerful ways to learn about shared human lived experiences. "A good story is like hugging each [listener], for it individually touches the person's intimate sense of self and leaves an afterglow of connectedness" (Wagner, 1994, p. 180).

This experience of finding both an organization and people leading a revolutionary caring movement was a momentous turning point in my personal and professional life. My nursing contributions blossomed in new ways as I dived into studying caring as a concept and practice model, qualitative research methodologies, and reflective practice. I began my journey in exploring the power of reflective inquiry via story and aesthetic expression to inform self and others through three avenues that fostered deeper meaning of nursing: (a) *Nurse-Self as Artist*: developing a personal reflective practice and aesthetic worldview to explore my own experiences of life and nursing from a more intimate inside-out perspective; (b) *Practicing Nurse as Artist*: teaching student nurses and nurses to use story, poetry, and art making to reflect on practice; and (c) *Nurse-Researcher as Artist*: collecting narrative data and developing an aesthetic interpretive heuristic methodology—use of poetry/art to interpret and share data findings—to get "inside the story." Poetry serves as a vehicle to make visible the unknown and to expand the consciousness of self in relationship with others, which, in turn, captures the essence of meaning in the human experience that can then be shared with others.

First, as *Nurse-Self as Artist*, I continued to reflect through a poetic lens on my life experiences, which included caring for patients. These poetic images are powerful testimony to what nurses encounter daily, but seldom share, touching the heart of the story that the objective facts do not reveal. Caring for a mother who held her dying newborn infant, I wrote a poem about that sacred, boundless moment of love I witnessed. Art has the capacity to heal (Picard, 1997). When I gave the mother the poem, she described the poetic image as a "treasured photograph":

Saying Goodbye With All Machines Turned Off
Mother rocks with baby, still wet,
gazing, stroking with deep love,
melding dreams with body heat.
Child is one with mother,
encased in arms and breast,
and cordless connection of kiss.
Mother tears baptize infant with grace
before death steals him away.
Breath is labored for both,
as mother sings a lullaby
for baby's long sleep to come.
"Goodnight" became "goodbye,"
as child leaves home,
twenty years too soon.

(Wagner, 2000a, p. 10)

Another example comes from my early nursing days when I was occasionally floated to the emergency room where my nursing skills were challenged by inexperience. One encounter haunted me as profound, but not until I reflected on it years later did I realize what it taught me about being a nurse. Through poetic reflection on this past experience (Johns, 2013; Schon, 1983, 1987), I captured what Watson (2008) calls the *caring moment*, an experience that connects two human beings as cohealers, both in the moment and beyond:

The Lady Who Sings
She arrived in that crack between night and day,
When all the world yawns,
some yearning for sleep,
some stretching to consciousness,
but somehow connected in the dawn's shadows.
Sirens heralded her thrashing entrance
and swirling red lights magnified her mania.
She laid on an ER stretcher,
but resided somewhere we did not know.
Raging, nameless, ageless,
we simply called her "the lady who sings."
She smelled like day-old garlic;
her body was as tattered as her clothes,
harboring unwelcomed life that jumped at us
as we removed the faded cloth to treat her wounds.
All the time she sang a tune unknown
with words that made no sense,
except to give a rhythm to her writhing soul.

As I placed a pillow beneath her head,
just once her eyes met mine,
a small window that invited me in.
I went and saw her fear, understood.
I listened and heard her words in jumbled song,
then gently said, "You must love to sing."
She quieted for an instant
as I waved away the doctor
who had come to sedate her.
"I will stay and listen to your song,
until another nurse moves to your rhythm."
Her cautious smile, framed by blackened teeth,
ridiculed our presumption that white sheets alone
could heal her wounds so deep.
Yet a sliver of her pain slipped away
as she reached for my hand.

I never saw her again, but this her gift:
In three hours when two worlds overlapped,
bonded in mysterious human ways,
when light and darkness fuse through touch,
I was pulled outside my shell,
and knew God's face beyond what shadows tell.

(Wagner, 2000a, p. 11; 2002b, p. 83; 2005, p. 143)

In another example, documenting my caring for my mother during her last six years of life, as she struggled with dementia, evolved into sharing multiple times with large audiences of nurses and community groups an aesthetic presentation of story, poetry, and photography, *The Mother-Daughter Dance to Unspoken Caring Needs: A Lesson in Caritas* (Wagner, 2008b, 2008c, 2009, 2011a, 2011b, 2012, 2013a, 2013b), framed by Watson's (2008) 10 Caritas Processes™ (see Table 16.1). A large rehabilitation medical center contracted me to present the work repeatedly over a couple of months during the three nursing shifts. The center required all hospital employees to attend one of the sessions during their transition period in adopting Watson's caring science as their practice care model. What attracted so many to the presentation is that the story explored a common experience of caring for a loved one or patient with dementia in everyday language and in ways that touched the heart and soul of long-term care through a caring lens.

Similarly, I documented a year's journey with grief and healing after my mother's death through journaling, poetic story, and a metaphorical relationship with a tree outside my skylight window. Photographing and witnessing the tree, I found a kinship between my grief journey and the tree's changing seasons. Healing was viewed through the four tasks of human healing (Watson, 2005) that I experienced as winter surrendering, spring forgiveness, summer gratitude, and autumn giving and receiving of compassionate service. Originally crafted into a presentation, *Healing Conversations With a Tree During a Journey With Grief: Framed by Watson's Theory of Human Caring,* and presented nationally and internationally, I was encouraged by conference attendees to write a book. Thus, *Four Seasons of Grieving: A Nurse's Healing Journey With Nature* (Wagner, 2015) was published, "capturing the essence of my healing spirit on a grief journey" (p. xviii). The book invites nurses and other readers to reflect on their own stories, and also offers suggestions for healing self and helping others to heal from loss through a caring science framework.

A second way I implemented aesthetic ways of knowing was to encourage nursing students I taught and nurses who attended workshops to be *Practicing Nurse-Artists,* to write about their caring moments or noncaring moments with patients or others and then to translate their story into a poem, drawing, or drama skit. In 1994, I entered a doctoral program in educational leadership, already knowing I wanted to study how nursing students develop their caring-self. My new adventure encouraged the opportunity to more deeply study philosophers, educators, and nursing scholars who added new dimensions to my understanding of caring science. My dissertation, *A Study of Baccalaureate Nursing Students' Reflection on Their Caring Practice Through Creating and Sharing Story, Poetry, and Art* (Wagner, 1998), explored how students learn about themselves and their caring experiences through reflective journaling, translation of their stories into poetry and art, and sharing their stories and aesthetic representations in class. A typology of three modes of reflection—cognitive, affective, and collective— used to explore caring-self in nursing practice emerged from the data, describing different activities, processes, and outcomes of reflective storytelling that lead to a fuller understanding of experiences can be seen in Table 31.1 (Wagner, 2002a).

Knowing does not necessarily come directly from experiencing a situation. We need to intentionally reencounter the experience through reflective processes of exploring the many aspects embedded in any human experience—the facts, emotions, relationships, and differentiation between self and others in the event, ripple effects, and outcomes.

TABLE 31.1   **Typology of Reflective Levels Used to Explore and Grow Caring-Self**

Levels of Reflection	Reflective Activity	Process	Outcome
Cognitive	Descriptive story writing and telling of nursing experiences	Rational process; recall of experiences; asks, "What happened?" remembering details; relives experience	Organization of details; identifies self and others; experience available for deeper reflection
Affective	Creative expression of experiences through poetry and art	Nonrational analytic process; forced to go inside the story; confronts feelings and relationships; asks, "What is going on here?" "What is important?" Sifts through the detail of story to find "essence" of experience	Deeper relational meaning becomes known to self; connecting to patient; healing emotions; therapeutic
Collective	Sharing stories; dialogue	Allows self to be heard; listens to others' stories; forms collective story; asks, "Why did you do it that way?" Discovery of alternative ways of doing and revelation of shared humanity	Therapeutic; support; revealing to others; circular; reaffirming; connects us to others through our shared humanity

Adapted from Wagner (2002a).

In essence, we need to come to know the mind-body-spirit meaning of what happened and what more was possible. Encouraging students and practicing nurses to engage in such exploration of their experiences, personally and collectively, allows experiences to teach them through critical reflective practice (Johns, 2013). Additionally, the human lived experience can also be known through other poets' and artists' work (Fox, 1997; McNiff, 1992; Styles & Moccia, 1993; Wagner, 2008a; Watson, 1994; Young-Mason, 1995). Thus, I began to use poetry reading and art museum assignments in my teaching as aesthetic sources of knowing human suffering and healing, despair, and joy.

Third, I grew into *Nurse-Researcher as Artist* through my dissertation work. The differences between quantitative and qualitative research are obvious. However, from my research and practice, I started to see a pattern of knowing a phenomenon through different pathways within qualitative research, as depicted in Figure 31.1. My work had brought me to the nonrational approach of heuristic inquiry, using self as a way of knowing. My method of "poetic dialogue" and interpretive aesthetic inquiry emerged in new research projects.

In one study (Wagner, 1995), I interviewed 11 women experiencing breast cancer, exploring through narrative their perception of how the medical system was caring for them. I created a cyclic "poetic dialogue" with the women via a process of inviting women's storytelling; recording, listening, and reflecting on each story; using poetry writing to interpret the "data," along with emerging themes; and then inviting the

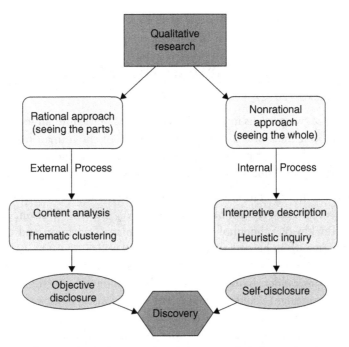

FIGURE 31.1   Qualitative research rational and nonrational pathways leading to discovery.

storyteller to reflect on the transcribed data and poem for accuracy. The continued dialogue created space and openness for a deeper understanding of the story as told and the story's meaning as it evolved in the telling and listening, creating a shared interpretation. One woman, who felt that she received good "medical care," but was degraded by poor communication and insensitivity to her family's problems and fears, told me with tears after reading the poem I had written to her story, "Your poem shows you really listened to me."

Where Is the Caring?
I called the doctor and was put on hold,
left listening to the echo of my breath.
Where is the caring?

I sat in his waiting room for an hour,
background music and *Ladies Home Journal* padded empty time.
Where is the caring?

He listened to my heart, palpated my scars,
but never asked about my family's fears.
Where is the caring?

Exam complete, "You're fine." said he,
not a chance to tell him how I hurt inside.
Where is the caring?

Breast gone. Hair gone. Tired. How can I look fine?
Through what special glasses is he looking at me?
Where is the caring?

(Wagner, 1995, p. 75)

According to Watson (2012),

The union of two persons in which the conditions of the human soul and feelings have been transmitted allows for liberation of the human mind, spirit,
and soul that leads to a greater sense of strength, power, and human capacity
for finding . . . meanings in existence and illness. (p. 84)

My aesthetic interpretation of the woman's story was able to capture the essence
of her feelings and create for both of us a shared *caring moment* (Watson, 2008) or *nursing situation* (Boykin & Schoenhofer, 2001) of human connection and discovery. This
woman found strength in being heard.

The same method of inquiry was used to explore elders' experiences of growing
older in three settings: elders living in their own homes, those in assisted living, and those
in long-term care settings (Wagner, 2000b). The study consisted of two visits to each participant. During the first interview, I listened to their stories, which I then translated into
a poem, distilling out the essence of their story. At the second visit, I presented the poem
to them, with each one affirming that the poem meant I had really heard their story. The
poem also engendered expanded story, deeper details, and feelings that spoke of growing
trust fostered by authentic presence. "Shared storytelling often softens the boundaries
between different realities, allowing each to know the other more wholly within the context of mutual humanness" (Wagner, 2005, p. 37). An 85-year-old woman in a long-term
care setting told me in factlike manner about her stroke and loneliness without family.
My poem transcends the factual story and captures a deeper intricacy of *being with* this
woman and *knowing* more humanly her lived experience.

Mrs. O'Malley: Pain
You sit, lap covered with frayed blanket,
framed by two wheels,
one leg firmly against metal plate,
the other shortened by disease
not knowing where it belongs;
face twisting at bright light
that streams through your window
filtered by cobwebs on the glass
and cloudy cataract vision.
You sit enjoying a moment of warmth
that brings late afternoon memories.
But then the pain,
that pain whose source is deeper
than ulcers on your leg,
merges past and future with present space.
Your swear word breaks the sacred mood of brief escape;
reality beckons you to pay attention,

nudging you back to prison
that you describe as shrunken world
of chair with wheels that go nowhere.
                              (Wagner, 2005, p. 37)

Being immersed in caring theory, practice, and research, I was able to apply my expertise in developing and facilitating a unique Caring Mentoring Model for Nurses (Wagner & Seymour, 2007) that sustains human dignity, respect, and mutual growth for both mentor and mentee. For more than 10 years, I have developed mentoring programs for schools of nursing, hospitals, and a statewide nursing organization, each time founding the programs on the tenets of caring science (Watson, 2008): loving-kindness, authentic presence, building of trusting relationships and healing environments in which to grow, transpersonal teaching and learning, and being open to unknowns along a relationship path that is cocreated by both mentee and mentor. My model has been used by others to frame their mentoring programs. It serves as a foundation for my teaching/mentoring new Caritas Coaches in the Caritas Coach Education Program (CCEP) at the Watson Caring Science Institute (WCSI) since 2008, which is now centered at University of Colorado's Watson Caring Science Center. My caring work further extends to locally mentoring individual nurses in applying caring science in their doctoral work and practice. In 2013, a natural outgrowth of my expertise in caring science and mentoring practices was my founding with a colleague of the Massachusetts Regional Caring Science Consortium, a grassroots initiative that invites nurses and other health care providers to gather periodically for dialogic sharing and exploration of caring practices.

■ MORAL/ETHICAL FOUNDATION

I came to nursing with a strong moral, ethical foundation of caring for others, with a sense of respect and compassion that was fostered by my caregivers, role models, mentors, and growing spirituality throughout my life. However, my deeper understanding of moral responsibility and ethical guidelines matured as I grew into nursing, tested caring in a wide variety of nursing situations, and embodied caring for myself and others. The American Nurses Association (ANA, 2015) defines values and explicitly addresses RN behaviors of caring for self and others through professional nursing standards and a code of ethics. Many state licensing boards of nursing, such as in Massachusetts, also legally mandate an ethical foundation that guides moral nursing behaviors. Considered important guides for the nursing profession, it was the wise caring leaders mentioned in the following text who have helped me to translate the seemingly task-oriented moral duties into heart-centered intentional caring ways of being and practicing loving-kindness and compassion, and of connecting with patients and students, families, and colleagues through a shared humanity of valued wholeness and sustained human dignity—essential ingredients of a healing practitioner. This worldview of caring science also calls forth a moral responsibility to be open to the mysteries encountered in living and dying, suffering, and healing.

Boykin and Schoenhofer (2001), whose Theory of Nursing as Caring emphasizes that "all persons are caring by virtue of their humanness" (p. 1), posit, "This belief . . . entails a commitment . . . to know self and other as caring person. . . . Moral obligations arise from our commitments; therefore, when I make a commitment to caring as a way of being, I have become morally obligated" (p. 2).

Similarly, Roach (1997, p. 16) declares, "Caring, as the human mode of being, is caring from the heart; caring from the core of one's being; caring as a response to one's experience of connectedness." Likewise, Watson (2008) describes nursing as the "intersection of technical competencies and emotional/intellectual literacy of human caring skills of *Being-caring*" (p. 27), which embodies "relational caring as ethical-moral-philosophical values-guided foundation" (p. 29). Further expanding the universality of caring, Watson (2005, 2008) describes caring as promoting meaningful transformative relationships with expanding consciousness of the inseparable bond between caring and love and the resulting spiritual, energetic field of healing presence and connectedness that each nurse is capable of influencing in daily care *for* and *with* others. This commitment to care shapes all actions and prevents me from reducing any human being to an object—a diagnosis, a bed number, a failure.

Roach (1992, 2002) describes six attributes of caring to be compassion, competence, confidence, conscience, commitment, and comportment. All six attributes are a constellation to inform morally based caring responsibilities that humanize the otherwise objective scientific–technological experience of being cared for. Watson (2005, 2008) advances Roach's attributes, emphasizing caring for self and others through her 10 Caritas Processes™ that both name and guide specific caring–moral actions. Compassion emerges from practicing heartfelt loving-kindness and equanimity that promotes human flourishing of mind-body-spirit. Competence requires knowledge, judgment, and skills in both nursing and caring sciences that foster transpersonal and collaborative teaching-learning and creative finding of solutions to challenges. Confidence embraces developing trusting–healing relationships with sensitivity to self and others. Conscience is a continually growing moral Caritas Consciousness that each human being is worthy of loving care. This, in turn, fosters a commitment to be authentically present to each person and to *become* the healing environment, in which all ways of knowing and all voices are honored. According to Watson (2008), the love for humanity that we carry in our hearts matters and shapes our caring moments. Finally, comportment speaks to the necessity of attending to our own well-being, setting caring intentions throughout the day, recentering for each new situation, and consciously using Caritas language and communication processes that respectively honor each person's wholeness.

Guided by this philosophy of caring, I am morally bound to honor my patients' and students' life paths and frames of reference, to help myself and others grow (Mayeroff, 1971) toward self-actualization, competency, connectedness, and discovery. As a nurse educator, this stance helps me to dialogue with students about the dissonance of what they are learning and what they may see in practice. It guides me to empower students to value honesty, beliefs, caring values, and the importance of their knowledge of nursing skills that safeguard patients' well-being and to be advocates and change agents for themselves and their patients by living their values.

One such example is my caring for a senior nursing student who was close to failing the semester and came to me for advice. I consciously put away the rules and regulations, closed my office door for privacy, sat next to her instead of behind my desk, and invited her to tell me her story, to tell me why she thought her grades were falling and what she thought the solution might be. I was present to her story without interruption as she expressed both positive and negative feelings about becoming a nurse. Her feelings were highlighted with meaningful experiences as a nursing student but were overshadowed by the fact that she never wanted to be a nurse. It was her parent's dream she was living, not her own, and failing was her solution to "getting out and doing her own thing." She was angry. Acknowledging her dilemma and honoring her feelings and perceptions, I asked her to reflect on the meaning of her decision; on the meaning of her nursing experiences, not as a career, but as a human experience; and what alternatives she saw for herself. Led by her reflections, we explored together her journey, her strengths and successes, and her choices and possible outcomes. In the end, she decided to stay, to catch up, and study so she could graduate. She was not sure if she would ever practice as a nurse, but she had discovered for the first time some personal meaning in caring for others. She felt she was making her own decision now and knew her degree, almost within her grasp, would give her more options. Tearfully, she thanked me for listening to her story, never told before, and for making it safe for her to release it. I thanked her for having the courage to explore her story. I witnessed her slowly let go of her anger and move toward forgiving her parents as she realized their decision for her was out of love and desire for a good career. I witnessed the student expressing appreciation for what she had learned in nursing. I witnessed the beginning of healing and discovery of what more was possible.

Likewise, my work with narrative and poetic inquiry has fostered Caritas practices. Storytelling is a sacred trusting act of revealing spirit and soul of self, facing our shared humanity, which honors the "Ethics of Face" (Levinas, 1969), and creates healing environments of belonging. One powerful testimony of the healing power of face-to-face shared humanity is embodied in a story I heard. A nurse from New England was working in a Midwest hospital, caring for a man who was dying. He was restless, noncommunicative, alone, and angry. The nurse sat with him one day and asked about his life. He told of many regrets, one being that he would never see the ocean now. Using her moral self and artistry of caring–healing practice, the next day the nurse brought in a seascape painting and hung it on the patient's wall. At her lunchtime, she sat with the patient, playing a recording of ocean sounds and described her walks along the beach in great detail—the sights, sounds, sensations, smell, beauty, and sailboats catching the wind. He smiled, cried, hugged the nurse, and fell asleep for the first time in days.

> The nursing model of transpersonal caring-healing more fully accommodates the human-nature-life processes of the mindbodyspirit unity, the art and science which returns a sense of sacred, harmonious, beautiful, ritual, archetypal unity as the ground of our being as healers . . . (Watson, 1999, p. xxvi)

■ VISION

Florence Nightingale gave structure to nursing as a valued profession of specific knowledge and training. She provided evidence that nursing care and nurse caring—based on assessment, principles of health, knowledge of the patient and human suffering, and healing environments—were critical in "putting the patient in the best condition for nature to act upon him . . . [for] nature alone cures" (Nightingale, 1969, p. 133). This suggests that healing is a complex phenomenon of interconnections between medical diagnosis and treatment, nursing care and caring, and the often mysterious dimensions of nature and the human spirit that aid in the healing of body-mind-spirit unity. Over time, nursing has advanced in knowledge, and required technical skills, new roles of practice, communication, and interdisciplinary collaboration. However, nursing still struggles today to separate itself from objective medical–technical practices and define its discipline of competent care within a caring-ethical-moral philosophy. And importantly, the public still struggles to know what nursing is and what nurses do, at least until they become patients. Much of the public's image of nursing comes from TV characters and nurses in the news when disciplined for a wrongdoing. I think nursing as a profession is one of the best-kept secrets, and it is up to nurses to become their own advocates in claiming their unique healing place in health care.

The challenge is that nursing has always been about caring, about being with the patient, but questions still linger around what constitutes nursing care: what theory guides practice; how nurses are prepared to care for others in complex health care systems; how evidence is gathered; what distinguishes nursing from other health professions; and how we honor the very essence of nursing-caring for the wholeness of each person and sustaining human dignity through transpersonal relationships. Without an informed discipline, a fully developed science, and nonconflicting paradigms that guide nursing education, practice, and research, the nursing profession suffers an identity crisis (Watson, 1999, 2008, 2012). My vision includes nurses coming to terms with these questions and educating each other and the public, defining who we are and what we do through our stories, public presentations, and publications, and serving in our communities to spearhead changes. Change takes courage to join the conversation and action.

I have been privileged to witness, to know revolutionary voices and visionaries who started to emerge in the 1970s to challenge the status quo of nursing image, practice, education, and research, to start provocative dialogues about reclaiming the essence of caring as central to the nursing discipline, and to provide blueprints for action. Voices from other disciplines also echoed similar challenges. A small seminal book, *On Caring,* by philosopher Milton Mayeroff (1971), which outlined the major ingredients, meaning, and characteristics of a caring life, became a talking point for nurses. Nursing leader and theorist on Culture Care Diversity and Universality, Madeleine Leininger (1976) named care as the essence of nursing and Watson (1979, 1985) began to develop her Theory of Human Caring founded on a philosophy of caring science. In the 1970s, educators Nel Noddings (1984, 1992) and Paulo Freire (1997) challenged all schools to cultivate caring environments, nurturing pedagogy and dialogic opportunities of building on individual strengths through caring for self, others, and the larger world of life and ideas. Likewise, nurse leaders were also challenging nursing education to adopt curricula based on humanistic theories and models to prepare nurses to reclaim caring as essence, to reawaken the humanism of Nightingale's vision (Bevis, 1989). At this same time, nursing organizations that still exist today were forming, such as the IAHC in 1978 and the American Holistic Nursing Association in 1981 to support and promote caring practice and research.

Over the past 40 years, I have participated in the conversation and contribution to understanding caring as the essence of nursing. I am heartened that practice is changing, demonstrated by the growing number of Magnet®-designated hospitals that have adopted caring practice models; the WCSI Affiliate Hospitals; the increased number of nursing schools, including those at University of Colorado and Florida Atlantic University, adopting caring curricula; nurse educators attending caring conferences; the growth of holistic nursing; and the more than 300 graduate Caritas Coaches from the Watson CCEP, who are practicing, teaching, and role modeling in health care institutions.

Hope is found in Watson's (2012, p. 17) observation,

> Even though nursing is still evolving and has yet to actualize the ideas and ideals of the early nursing leaders . . . most contemporary theories of nursing generally promote converging ideas about nursing . . . expanding unitary, ethical, philosophical views of person-nature-environment-universe; expanding, evolving human consciousness, and life-sustaining caring–healing knowledge, patterns, and processes.

We are moving forward, but more work has to be done in anchoring caring curricula in all schools of nursing to nurture caring and help our new nurses develop their heart-centered caring-self, in changing practice arenas to caring–healing environments for staff and patient flourishing, and in honoring the role of qualitative methodologies to gather evidence about the wholeness of the lived experience. My vision is that nurses will fully come to know and practice caring as a way of being and unify to reclaim their focus on transformative well-being and healing, nurturing trusting relationships as they care for humanity with loving-kindness. This includes educating the public about nursing and increasing nursing's presence as the voice of patient-centered care at health care decision-making tables and on legislative committees (Chinn, 2001).

On a personal level, my work will continue in mentoring and teaching, evolving my Caring Mentoring Model, and sharing my gift of storytelling and aesthetic ways of knowing to gain deeper insights into the human lived experience. With new vision, the grassroots Regional Caring Science Consortium that I cofounded in 2013 is maturing this year from small, short bimonthly gatherings to two half-day conferences annually to offer more interactive sharing and participation to wider audiences. Many have responded, a testimony of the hunger out there for nurses to return to their caring roots and to work in healing environments. My vision comes from what I have experienced and what is still possible. The vision is inspired and guided by the lives I have touched and the lives that have touched mine:

- The more than 3,000 couples who attended my childbirth classes, many of whom I continue to meet in my community decades later and who tell me how their empowerment changed their lives. Little do they know how their shared birthing experiences of joys and losses changed mine.
- The 20 years of teaching nursing students beyond the textbook, beyond the task; empowering them to be competent and present doing their first injections at flu clinics and their first home visits, and introducing them to the mystery and wonder, the humanness and love that transcended their fear and inexperience of their first-time caring for a woman birthing or a patient dying.

- The uncounted patients, in little and big caring moments, who taught me about courage, about suffering, about healing and dying, about miracles, and about myself and how to care and who touched my heart and gave me confidence that my caring makes a difference. I particularly remember as a new nurse the first dying patient I cared for during his repeated admissions, a man courageously living with scleroderma who taught me how to be present in healing ways.

> **Touch Transformed**
> He lay so still, stiffened by disease,
> mask-like face unable to respond
> to passing time beneath white sheet,
> filling bed, deformed, alone,
> frequent guest to the ward.
> A friend for whom I cared
> as disease claimed space under skin,
> reaching inward to vital spots,
> pulling, tensing, molding, rigid.
> He labored in his last hour
> to capture healing peace.
> I held his hand, stroked his face
> that once had laughed with me.
> He sighed with effort,
> as though to drive my touch to soul,
> smiled, I think, relaxed,
> let go of pain, closed his eyes,
> to hold the present in his heart.
> Breathing stopped.
> Love held the space.
> Wagner (2011c)

In summary, change takes time and change begets change. It takes one nurse, one unit, one system, one nursing organization to create the spark; to fire up the conversation; to share caring wisdom and to bring that wisdom to practice; and to stand up, speak out to other nurses, health care professionals, and the public through dialogue, publications, and actions to say, "I have had enough of being defined by others. I am a healer whose expertise is nursing and caring science founded on a healing-loving-humanistic-relational caring philosophy that sustains human dignity. I am a nurse who makes a difference in people's lives like no other profession."

My rich and varied career continues to be a journey of learning, giving, and receiving; a journey of reflection, love, caring, and being cared for; of misalignment with others' expectations and a coming into my gifts of teaching and an aesthetic way of knowing; of advocacy and courage to be in "right relationship" with myself and others; and of creativity and discovery. I know why I am a nurse, why I came, what I do, and why I stay. The challenge is always sustaining the connectedness of who I am, the meaning in what I do, and the wholeness of my being, all of which will shape my relationship with myself and others, and thus open new possibilities for human healing. In the end, that is the essence of nursing.

■ REFLECTIONS

1. *What in my journey created a career discomfort or disillusion that made me move on to another opportunity? What ethical–moral guidelines helped me make my decisions? How did this experience help me grow?*
2. *Everyone has a creative part in him or her, an aesthetic/right-brain way of viewing the world. What is my creative side? How have I aligned my creative aesthetic part of me with my nursing practice? How has my creativity enriched my nursing practice?*
3. *In what way are the stories of nurses, patients, students, nursing leaders, educators, and people in the community important in understanding nursing's past and nursing's vision, nursing's unique contribution to humanity?*
4. *Who have been the mentors in my life? How have they helped me grow? Who have I mentored in nursing? If I have not mentored, who could I mentor toward developing a heart-centered caring nursing practice?*
5. *What is a situation during which I experienced a caring moment with a patient or a person in my life, a moment that touched my heart and soul and increased my consciousness of shared humanity? Write a story about this caring moment and translate the story into a poem or drawing. How does the poem or artwork further my awareness of the moment and what I have learned?*

■ REFERENCES

American Nurses Association. (2015). *Code of ethics for nurses with interpretive statements.* Silver Springs, MD: Author.

Benner, P., & Wrubel, J. (1989). *The primacy of caring.* Menlo Park, CA: Addison-Wesley.

Bevis, E. (Ed.). (1989). *Curriculum revolution: Reconceptualizing nursing education.* New York, NY: National League for Nursing.

Boykin, A., & Schoenhofer, S. O. (2001). *Nursing as caring: A model for transforming practice.* Sudbury, MA: Jones & Bartlett.

Carper, B. A. (1978). Fundamental patterns of knowing in nursing. *Advances in Nursing Science, 1*(1), 13–23.

Chinn, P. L. (2001). *Peace and power* (5th ed.). Boston, MA: Jones & Bartlett/National League for Nursing.

Fox, J. (1997). *Poetic medicine: The healing art of poem-making.* New York, NY: Jeremy P. Tarcher/ Putnam.

Freire, P. (1997). *Pedagogy of the oppressed* (Rev. ed.). New York, NY: Continuum.

Johns, C. (2013). *Becoming a reflective practitioner* (4th ed.). Oxford, UK: Wiley-Blackwell.

Leininger, M. (1976). Caring: The essence and central focus of nursing. *American Nurses Foundation: Nursing Research Report, 12*(1), 2, 14.

Levinas, E. (1969/2000). *Totality and infinity* (14th printing). Pittsburgh, PA: Duquesne University.

Mayeroff, M. (1971). *On caring.* New York, NY: HarperCollins.

McNiff, S. (1992). *Art as medicine.* Boston, MA: Shambhala.

Nightingale, F. (1969). *Notes on nursing: What it is and what it is not.* New York, NY: Dover.

Noddings, N. (1984). *Caring: A feminine approach to ethics and moral education.* Berkeley, CA: University of California Press.

Noddings, N. (1992). *The challenge to care in schools.* New York, NY: Teachers College Press.

Picard, C. (1997). Walk in beauty: Aesthetics, caring and spirituality. In M. S. Roach (Ed.), *Caring from the heart: The convergence of caring and spirituality* (pp. 149–162). New York, NY: Paulist Press.

Roach, M. S. (1992). *The human act of caring: A blueprint for the health professions.* Ottawa, ON, Canada: Canadian Hospital Association Press.

Roach, M. S. (1997). Reflections on the theme. In M. S. Roach (Ed.), *Caring from the heart: The convergence of caring and spirituality* (pp. 7–20). New York, NY: Paulist Press.

Roach, M. S. (2002). *Caring, the human mode of being: A blueprint for the health professions* (2nd rev. ed.). Ottawa, ON, Canada: Canadian Hospital Association Press.

Sandelowski, M. (1993, March). We are the stories we tell. *Journal of Holistic Nursing, 12*(1), 23–33.

Schon, D. A. (1983). *The reflective practitioner.* New York, NY: Basic Books.

Schon, D. A. (1987). *Educating the reflective practitioner.* San Francisco, CA: Jossey-Bass.

Silva, M. C., Sorrell, J. M., & Sorrell, C. D. (1995). From Carper's patterns of knowing to ways of being: An ontological philosophical shift in nursing. *Advances in Nursing Science, 18*(1), 1–13.

Styles, M. M., & Moccia, P. (Eds.). (1993). *On nursing: A literary celebration.* New York, NY: National League for Nursing.

Tanner, C. (1988, October). Curriculum revolution: The practice mandate. *Nursing & Health Care, 9*(8), 427–430.

Wagner, A. L. (1984). *Socioeconomic status, career satisfaction and anxiety in primiparous, postpartal women planning to return to work* (Unpublished master's thesis). University of Massachusetts, Lowell.

Wagner, A. L. (1993, May 16–18). *The color of hope: A woman's journey with breast cancer.* Podium presentation at International Association for Human Caring 15th Research Conference, Portland, OR.

Wagner, A. L. (1994). A journey with breast cancer: Telling my story. In D. Gaut & A. Boykin (Eds.), *Caring as healing: Renewal through hope* (pp. 178–182). New York, NY: National League for Nursing Press.

Wagner, A. L. (1995). Unleashing the giant: The politics of women's health care. In A. Boykin (Ed.), *Power, politics, & public policy: A matter of caring* (pp. 63–81). New York, NY: National League for Nursing Press.

Wagner, A. L. (1998). A study of baccalaureate nursing students' reflection on their caring practice through creating and sharing story, poetry, and art. (Doctoral dissertation, University of Massachusetts, Lowell). *Dissertation Abstracts International, 99*(05), 334. (University Microfilms Inc. No DAO 72699)

Wagner, A. L. (2000a). Connecting to nurse-self through reflective poetic story. *International Journal of Human Caring, 4*(2), 7–12.

Wagner, A. L. (2000b, July 2–4). *The elder storyteller and the nurse-poet: A collaborate understanding of growing older.* Poster presentation at the International Association for Human Caring Research Conference, Boca Raton, FL.

Wagner, A. L. (2002a). Nursing students' development of caring self through creative reflective practice. In D. Freshwater (Ed.), *Therapeutic nursing: Improving patient care through self awareness and reflection* (pp. 121–144). Newbury Park, CA: Sage.

Wagner, A. L. (2002b). Two poems: "The Faces of Oklahoma City" and "The Lady Who Sang." In M. C. Wendler (Ed.), *The heART of nursing: Expressions of creative art in nursing* (p. 83). Indianapolis, IN: The Center Nursing Publishing.

Wagner, A. L. (2005). Three poems: "The Faces of Oklahoma City," "The Lady Who Sang," and "Mrs. O'Malley: Pain." In M. C. Wendler (Ed.), *The heART of nursing: Expressions of creative art in nursing* (2nd ed., pp. 37, 146–147). Indianapolis, IN: The Center Nursing Publishing.

Wagner, A. L. (2008a). A caring scholar response to "uncovering meaning through the aesthetic turn": A pedagogy of caring. *International Journal for Human Caring, 12*(2), 24–28.

Wagner, A. L. (2008b, April 6–9). *Mother-daughter's dance to unspoken caring needs: A lesson in caritas.* Podium presentation at 30th Conference of the International Association for Human Caring, Chapel Hill, NC.

Wagner, A. L. (2008c, April 10–11). *Mother-daughter's dance to unspoken caring needs: A lesson in caritas.* Podium presentation at International Caritas Consortium, Scottsdale, AZ.

Wagner, A. L. (2009, March 19). *Mother-daughter's dance to unspoken caring needs: A lesson in caritas.* Keynote presentation, Goldfarb School of Nursing/Barnes-Jewish College/Washington University, St. Louis, MO.

Wagner, A. L. (2011a, June 4). *Healing conversations with a tree during a journey with grief: Framed by Watson's theory of human caring.* Plenary Presentation at the International Association for Human Caring 32nd Annual Conference, San Antonio, TX.

Wagner, A. L. (2011b, October 14). *Healing conversations with a tree during a journey with grief: Framed by Watson's theory of human caring.* Plenary Presentation at the International Caritas Consortium, Woodlands, TX.

Wagner, A.L. (2011c). Touch transformed. Unpublished poem.

Wagner, A. L. (2012, November 10). *Healing conversations with a tree during a journey with grief: Framed by Watson's theory of human caring.* Keynote presentation at Winter Haven Hospital, Winter Haven, FL.

Wagner, A. L. (2013a, July 18). *Healing conversations with a tree: A year's journey with grief framed by Watson's caring science theory.* Presentation at Nursing Grand Rounds, Massachusetts General Hospital, MA.

Wagner, A. L. (2013b, September 10). *Healing conversations with a tree during a journey with grief: Framed by Watson's theory of human caring.* Podium presentation at the Reflective Practice Conference, Swansea University, Wales, UK.

Wagner, A. L. (2015). *Four seasons of grieving: A nurse's healing journey with nature.* Indianapolis, IN: Sigma Theta Tau International.

Wagner, A. L., & Seymour, M. E. (2007, September/October). A model of caring mentorship for nursing. *Journal for Nurses in Staff Development, 23*(5), 201–211.

Watson, J. (1979). *Nursing: The philosophy and science of caring.* Boulder, CO: University of Colorado Press.

Watson, J. (1985). *Nursing: Human science and human care: A theory of nursing.* New York, NY: National League for Nursing.

Watson, J. (1994). Poeticizing as truth through language. In P. L. Chinn & J. Watson (Eds.), *Art & aesthetics in nursing* (pp. 3–18). New York, NY: National League for Nursing.

Watson, J. (1999). *Postmodern nursing and beyond.* New York, NY: Churchill Livingstone.

Watson, J. (2005). *Caring science as sacred science.* Philadelphia, PA: F.A. Davis.

Watson, J. (2008). *Nursing: The philosophy and science of caring* (Rev. ed.). Boulder, CO: University Press of Colorado.

Watson, J. (2012). *Human caring science: A theory of nursing* (2nd ed.). Sudbury, MA: Jones & Bartlett Learning.

Young-Mason, J. (1995). *States of exile: Correspondences between art, literature, and nursing.* New York, NY: National League for Nursing Press.

Endnote: What Are We Leading?

Diana J. Mason

I am writing this endnote after reading a November 8, 2015, *New York Times* report by Marc Santora on the almost 30 million children throughout the world who have been displaced from their homes because of war and conflict. The story of 9-year-old Chuol in South Sudan left me close to tears. Here is a boy who fled to the swamps with his grandmother after witnessing his father and grandfather being burned alive, girls being raped, and warring soldiers killing with abandon. He still wants to find his mother, who was lost in the chaotic flight of his fellow villagers. He has moments of respite at a United Nations Children's Emergency Fund (UNICEF) camp that has established a "safe space" for children to study and play.

While the United States is not South Sudan, our nation has a growing income disparity that is leaving 22% of children living in poverty, according to the National Center for Children in Poverty (NCCP, 2016). Their lives are often filled with trauma and stress. Indeed, we now know that "toxic stress" in childhood results from chronic stressors, not necessarily one major traumatic event. The Harvard University Center on the Developing Child (2016) reports that chronic elevated stress hormones can actually change the structure and processes of the brain, leaving a child disadvantaged cognitively and in other ways. And imagine the effect on the child's spirit when parents are stressed and depressed from life's daily struggles. These children are at risk for failure in school and, in the long term, for adult onset of conditions such as diabetes, chronic obstructive pulmonary, and heart disease.

So when I think of the children of the world—including the children of the United States—I have to reflect on nursing's mandate for leadership. What are we leading? What is our mission? And if you argue that our mission is to advance the nursing profession, I will ask you, to what end?

Throughout the pages of this book, you have examples of nurses who have been visionary leaders in advocating for the health of individuals, families, and communities. Indeed, these and other nurses are continuing a legacy and mandate that nursing has established to put the public's interests before our own. Consider Florence Nightingale, who transformed the British military and civilian health systems in her lifetime. She knew that good nutrition and a clean environment were essential to health and that medical statistics could help one understand where improvements are possible.

Or think about Lillian Wald, who founded the Henry Street Settlement House on Manhattan's Lower East Side at the turn of the 20th century. She and her nurse colleagues served a poor immigrant population that had no access to health care. She was also a leader in the development of the first federal Children's Bureau, at a time when forced child labor was a growing problem. In addition, Harriet Tubman was born a slave and was a nurse during the Civil War; she became an ardent orator on the importance of freedom and human rights. She knew that you cannot have health without freedom.

Contemporary nurses have followed in their footsteps. Ruth Watson Lubic and Kitty Ernst are two nurse midwives who have been outspoken advocates for community-based childbirthing centers that are run and staffed by midwives and provide women with an alternative to more expensive hospital-based perinatal care. These hospital-based options for women have resulted in excessively high rates of Cesarean sections, infants with low birth weight, and prematurity, as well as lower rates of breastfeeding.

Or consider Lauran Hardin, a clinical nurse leader who has been designated an "Edge Runner" by the American Academy of Nursing (AAN; 2014) for designing a model of complex care that reduces emergency department visits and the rate of hospitalizations, producing significant cost reductions for patients, hospitals, and insurers. Lauran will tell you that addressing social determinants of health outside of the hospital is crucial for helping people to live healthier lives.

The Robert Wood Johnson Foundation (RWJF; 2001–2015) has launched a major initiative focused on building a "Culture of Health" and focusing our attention on working with individuals, families, and communities to create the conditions that will allow health and well-being to flourish. This is an aim that Nightingale, Wald, and Tubman would have embraced. Although I see the work as foundational to nursing, others outside of the profession do not see us as leaders in promoting health. Indeed, a 2010 Gallup Survey of key leaders in health care found that most do not see nurses as influential in reforming health care. We are still fighting to get to the table, whether boardrooms, policy advisory groups, commissions, conference headliners, or health system leadership positions.

Fortunately, 2011 was also the year that the Institute of Medicine (IOM, 2011; now the National Academy of Medicine) issued its now landmark report *The Future of Nursing: Leading Change, Advancing Health* that challenged our profession and society to make sure that nurses were prepared to be leaders in redesigning health care and improving the health of the nation—and had the opportunity to serve as such leaders.

As the implementation of the report's recommendations continues at the state and national levels under the umbrella of the Campaign for Action (n.d.), it now behooves us to be clear about why we are advancing nursing. It is not for our own sakes. It is for promoting the health of children and families, of struggling communities, of a nation and of a world that is rife with conflict. We can expect nothing less of ourselves than to continue down the paths of leadership that the contributors to this book have described. I urge you to contemplate where and how health is created and then to examine the leadership knowledge, skills, experiences, and opportunities that you need as a 21st-century leader in promoting health.

■ REFERENCES

American Academy of Nursing. (2014). *Raise the voice: Edge runners*. Retrieved from http://www .aannet.org/edgerunners

Future of Nursing: Campaign for Action. (n.d.). *Building a healthier America through nursing*. Retrieved from http://campaignforaction.org

Gallup. (2010). *Nursing leadership from bedside to boardroom: Opinion leaders' perceptions*. Retrieved from http://newcareersinnursing.org/sites/default/files/file-attachments/Top%20Line%20Report.pdf

Harvard University Center on the Developing Child. (2016). *Key concepts: Toxic stress*. Retrieved from http://developingchild.harvard.edu/science/key-concepts/toxic-stress

Institute of Medicine (IOM). (2011). *The future of nursing: Leading change, advancing health*. Washington, DC: National Academies Press.

National Center for Children in Poverty. (2016). *Child poverty*. Retrieved from http://www.nccp.org/topics/childpoverty.html

Robert Wood Johnson Foundation. (2001–2015). *Building a culture of health*. Retrieved from http://www.rwjf.org/en/how-we-work/building-a-culture-of-health.html

Santora, M. (2008, November 8). The displaced: Chuol. *The New York Times*. Retrieved from http://www.nytimes.com/2015/11/08/magazine/the-displaced-chuol.html?_r=0

Index

Printed in the United States
By Bookmasters